THE DISLOCATED BRAIN:

A NEW PERSPECTIVE

THE DISLOCATED BRAIN:

A NEW PERSPECTIVE

Innovation in Traumatic Brain Injury and Irrigation

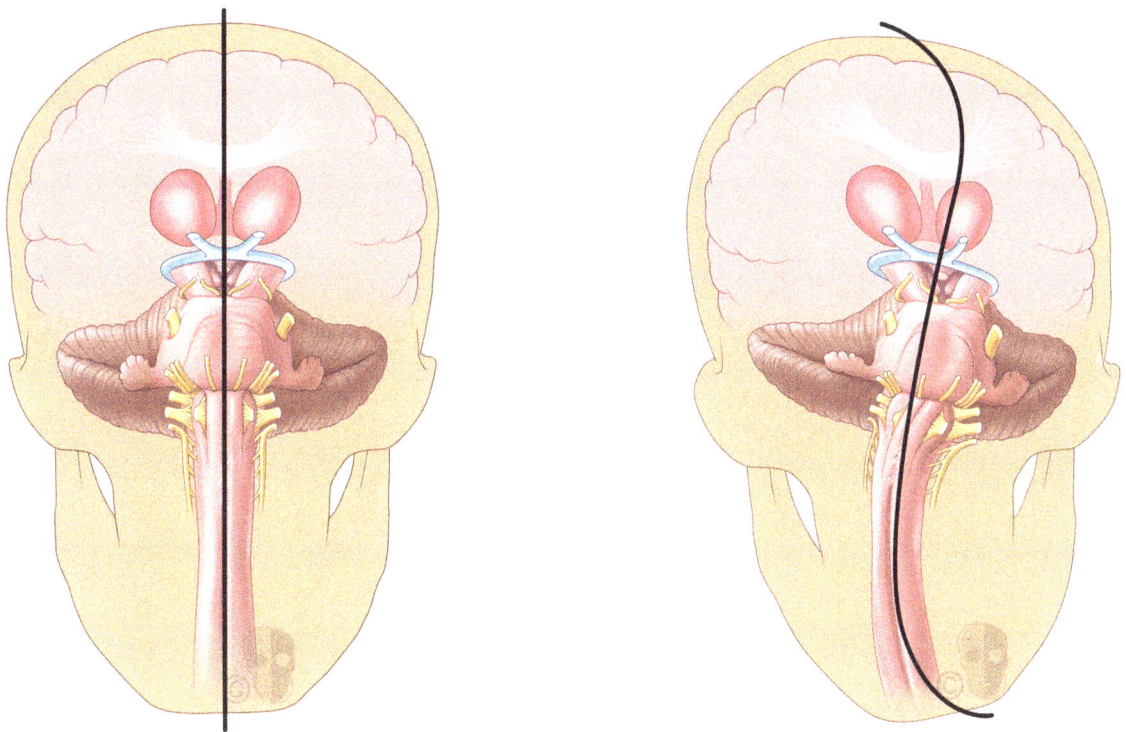

JONATHAN M. P. HOWAT

DC, DICS, FICS, FCC (PAEDS), FCC (CRANIO),
FEAC (CRANIOPATHY), FBCA

First published in Oxford, UK, by Jonathan M. P. Howat 2021

www.craniofascialdynamics.com

ISBNs hbk 978-1-9993295-4-9
    pbk 978-1-9993295-5-6
    ebk 978-1-9993295-6-3

Illustrations © Jonathan M. P. Howat. Original artwork by Mandy Miller (www.mandymiller.co.uk) and Paul Banville (www.paulbanville.co.uk); annotation and manipulation by Jonathan Howat.

Typeset and designed by www.ShakspeareEditorial.org

DEDICATION

To my family for their enthusiasm, patience and support all the way through this project.

Arline, my rock, providing me with the most valuable human resources a man could wish for in a marriage – her amazing care and dedication throughout our lives together.

Josh, whose numerous discussions, ideas and encouragements have contributed to our collective passion for cranio fascial dynamics.

Kate, whose invaluable contributions have been instrumental in the formation of this lecture programme, dedicating tireless hours of her time, scrutiny, expertise, teaching and leadership to this journey.

Juliet, who spent hours filming, directing and producing and then editing the on-line course to produce a very professional and user-friendly credit to the world of cranio fascial dynamics.

All these contributions will, I hope, add to the dialogue and narrative between the various professions that treat traumatic brain injury, in the anticipation that humanity will be better placed to resolve the terrible effects of this worldwide problem on so many family units.

CONTENTS

LIST OF ABBREVIATIONS

A to P	anterior to posterior	**LH**	luteinizing hormone
ACA	anterior cerebral artery	**MCA**	middle cerebral artery
ACTH	adrenocorticotropic hormones	**MSH**	melanocyte-stimulating hormone
ADD	attention deficit disorde	**mTBI**	mild traumatic brain injury
ADH	antidiuretic hormone	**NOT**	neural organisational technique
ADHD	attention deficit hyperactivity disorder	**NPH**	normal pressure hydrocephalus
ANS	autonomic nervous system	**OCD**	obsessive compulsive disorder
ASIS	anterior superior iliac spine	**OPG**	orthopantomagraph
BBB	blood–brain barrier	**PCA**	posterior cerebral arteries
BP	blood pressure	**PNS**	peripheral nervous system
CN	cranial nerve	**PRL**	prolactin
CBF	cerebral blood flow	**PSIS**	posterior superior iliac spine
CFD	cranio fascial dynamics	**PSNS**	parasympathetic nervous system
CMRT	chiropractic manipulative reflex technique	**PTH**	post-traumatic hydrocephalus
CNS	central nervous system	**R plus C**	resistance plus contraction
CO	centric occlusion	**RH**	releasing hormones
CPP	cerebral perfusion pressure	**RTM**	reciprocal tension membranes
CR	centric relation	**SCM**	sternocleidomastoid
CRH	corticotropin-releasing hormones	**SNS**	sympathetic nervous system
CRI	cranial rhythmic impulse	**TBI**	traumatic brain injury
CSF	cerebrospinal fluid	**TFL**	tensor fasciae latae
CTE	chronic traumatic encephalopathy	**TL**	therapy localises
DJD	degenerative joint disease	**TMA**	transcortical motor aphasia
EX	external	**TMJ**	temporomandibular joint
FSH	follicle-stimulating hormone	**TMJD**	temporomandibular joint dysfunction
HGH	human growth hormones	**TRH**	thyrotropin-releasing hormone
HPCFD	Howat Protocols of Cranio Fascial Dynamics	**TS**	temporo-sphenoidal (line)
		TSA	transcortical sensory aphasia
HR	heart rate	**TSH**	thyroid stimulating hormones
HRV	heart rate variability	**VE**	vacuum extraction
ICP	intracranial pressure	**VEN**	von Economo neuron
IN	internal	**VVP**	vertebral venous plexus
LOA	left occipital anterior		

THANKS AND ACKNOWLEDGEMENTS

Mandy Miller – this book would be incomplete, if it were not for the beautiful, accurate and lifelike graphics that have been created and captured by the medical artist Mandy Miller – my thanks to her is without reservation.

Lesley Wyldbore, thank you for your early contribution to the book.

Erika Gadsden, thank you for taking the manuscript and working so tirelessly on editing and proofreading it from beginning to end to make it readable and understandable.

Fiona Evans, thank you for continuously updating and revising the HPCFD website as an ongoing exercise.

Alison Shakspeare, thank you for the task it has been to publish this work and make it aesthetic in its appearance and tying up the numerous graphics with the relevant narrative and discourse.

Thank you to Igor Grgic, Joe Porter and Chris Vickers for their invaluable contribution and time proofreading this enormous manuscript.

To my PA, Geraldine Blackburn, who integrated, collated and managed the project with the help of the aforementioned, I want to thank you for your personal commitment and dedication.

Finally, to my students over the last three years, whose passion and understanding on this subject have added to its clinical application and efficacy for the dislocated brains we come across daily in our practices.

PREFACE

I have been in clinical practice for over 50 years and personally involved with the treatment of hundreds of patients. I have become critical of conventional treatment regimens prescribed for countless people who have suffered, possibly many times in their lives, with traumatic brain injury. The causes and manifestations of this type of injury are many and varied and, in my opinion, the vast majority never receive any form of treatment that leads to some form of positive resolution.

Some of that number are surgical patients in life or death scenarios, ultimately reliant on the amazing skills of the surgical teams who determine their survival. Apart from this small group of severely brain-damaged patients, the majority of traumatic brain injury patients have sustained their injuries through physical trauma. Severely damaged patients who end up in Accident and Emergency rooms around the world, often return home simply with a word of caution from medical professionals; often they are treated with pharmaceutical agents in the form of analgesics, anti-inflammatories and steroids, then later with psychotics, antidepressants and opiates. All are chemicals and produce iatrogenic changes to an already depleted system – akin to pouring WD40 over a smashed-up car after an accident and expecting it to work again!

Head and neck injuries from whatever physical aetiology (during birth and throughout life) damage and involve all the central brain-core components – hence saying the 'brain dislocates'.

The following list gives an idea as to what the 'dislocated brain' may manifest as long-term changes to the core brain components. These changes can involve a combination of neurological, structural and vascular deviations that alter the normal physiology of the brain core, possibly with devastating consequences:

- The cervical spine – the trigeminal spinal nucleus
- The cervico-cranial junction; the atlanto-occipital membrane – brain drainage
- The spinal cord, medulla oblongata, the pons and the midbrain – fourth ventricle
- The ventricular system and its boundaries; the hypothalamus and the thalamus – third ventricle
- The hippocampus and the amygdala – memory and emotion
- The caudate nucleus – executive control of movement
- The fornix – the limbic system
- The corpus callosum – interhemispheric communication
- The cingulate gyrus – processing emotion and behaviour
- The frontal, temporal, parietal and occipital lobes – the vast storage houses of necessary information and processing
- Critically, brain perfusion – blood and oxygen absorption
- The neurological pathways – the nerve conduits and neurological communications between cortex and spinal cord and vice versa.

These are all physically displaced and their function disrupted, and yet prevailing treatment does nothing to reinstate this physical damage, nor does it recognise the necessity of doing so. As a result, these injuries progressively deteriorate and alter nervous system activity. The neurological syndromes that plague the elderly, and the not so elderly, along with cardiac failure and stroke (the world's biggest killers), have their origin in these long-overlooked physical injuries.

This book discusses these anomalies and presents the innovative protocols of cranio fascial dynamics (CFD). CFD addresses traumatic brain injury and physically attempts to reverse traumatic distortion and the subsequent failure of brain drainage, thereby reinstating normal physiological function.

CFD deals with the 'central brain core components' that make up the intricate neurological pathways that service all aspects of brain function. It includes: the understanding of early (from day 16 to day

23) embryological development of the 'primitive streak' (brain and spinal cord); the development of 'mesenchyme', which is the future fascial covering that encapsulates every part and component of the body; the ventricular system (producing cerebrospinal fluid), supported by the retrieving and processing components as listed above. CFD shows the hierarchical importance of these structures in human development. These areas are fundamental to normal brain function, namely, the retrieval, processing and dissemination of neurological information.

Traumatic brain injury torques the spinal cord and the brainstem (the 'central brain core component'), and therefore disturbs the homeostasis of normal retrieval, processing and distribution of neurological information through the now distorted and corrupt neurological pathway system. This is the first primary deficit to neurological imbalance, which I call 'the dislocated brain'.

The effect of torque on the neurological pathways is not unlike the build-up of scale in water pipes, gradually depositing 'fur' and reducing the flow of water. Similarly, in the brain this torque will inhibit the normal retrieval, processing and dissemination of neurological information.

The purpose of this book is to give the reader the physiology and the understanding of the reinstatement of the 'central brain core component' by the removal of the central brain core component torque, which is the deep-seated ultimate 'subluxation'. The body and brain are now in a position to accept the numerous techniques that aid in the recovery of the neurological deficits, visceral changes and extremity distortions with far more effective outcomes.

Without reinstatement and removal of that vital torque, the efficacy of all applied techniques cannot achieve their optimum results and the true efficacy is not reached or appreciated. This 'reinstatement' allows improved neurological pathways to be re-established, it permits the evidence of true indicators and a more accurate account of what is happening in the body, and therefore achieves a better end result. In other words, the neurological 'blur' created by the central brain core torque is no longer an issue.

'The Howat Protocols of Cranio Fascial Dynamics' (HPCFD) have been designed to facilitate brain drainage – removing cytotoxic waste and allowing restoration of the central brain core components – the definitive and crucial changes to brain core function.

THE DISLOCATED BRAIN

PART I

CRANIO FASCIAL

DYNAMICS

'BRAIN BALANCING'

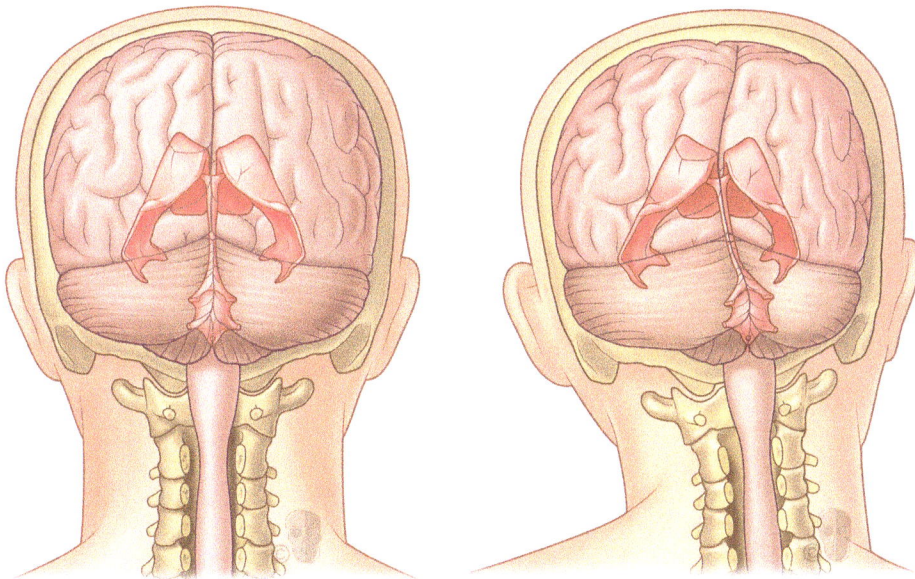

CONTENTS PART I

ILLUSTRATIONS PART I

CHAPTER 1

CEREBROSPINAL FLUID CIRCULATION

OVERVIEW OF CSF CIRCULATION

Homeostasis

The most important aspect of our biological system is to ensure that homeostasis is maintained at all levels. Homoeostasis is defined as that state of physiologic equilibrium in the living body – including temperature, chemical content, respiration, pH and so on – under variations in the environment.

The Dural Meningeal System

The dural meningeal system consists of three layers:

- Dural mater – the outer/external layer
- Arachnoid mater – the middle layer
- Pia mater – the inner layer

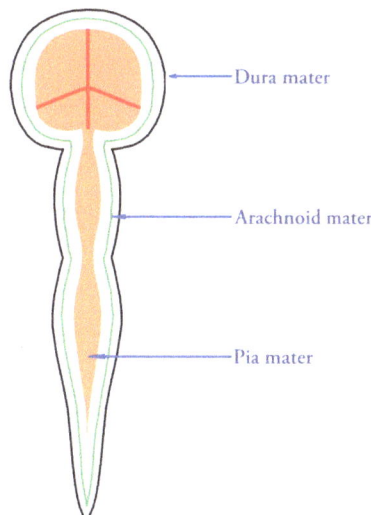

Figure 1.1. Dural Meningeal System: Meninges of the brain and spinal cord

The dura mater, the external layer is a thick, tough durable membrane. In the brain it consists of two layers: the internal layer, which covers the inner surface of the skull; and the endosteal layer, which exits through the sutures of the skull and becomes the periosteal dura on the outside of the skull. The inner layer of the dura mater covers the brain surface and is called the meningeal layer.

The arachnoid mater, the second layer, is a thin transparent membrane composed of fibrous tissue and is impermeable to fluid. It has the appearance of a spider's web.

The pia mater, the third layer, is a very delicate membrane, adhering to the surface of the brain and spinal cord, and covered on its outer surface by flat cells impermeable to fluid.

Inter-meningeal spaces

Between the arachnoid mater and the pia mater is the subarachnoid space, which is filled with CSF. The space between the arachnoid mater and the dura mater is called the subdural space, filled with small veins that connect the two membranes. After trauma to this area these vessels tear and blood will collect, causing a subdural haematoma. The epidural space between the dural sheath on the spinal cord and the bony surroundings is filled with fat and small blood vessels.

Ventricular Function

CSF is generated in the tela choroidea, of the choroid plexuses of the two lateral ventricles – the third and fourth. CSF is moved from the two lateral ventricles into the third ventricle through the interventricular foramen of Munro. CSF is then moved from the third ventricle to the fourth ventricle through the aqueduct of Sylvius.

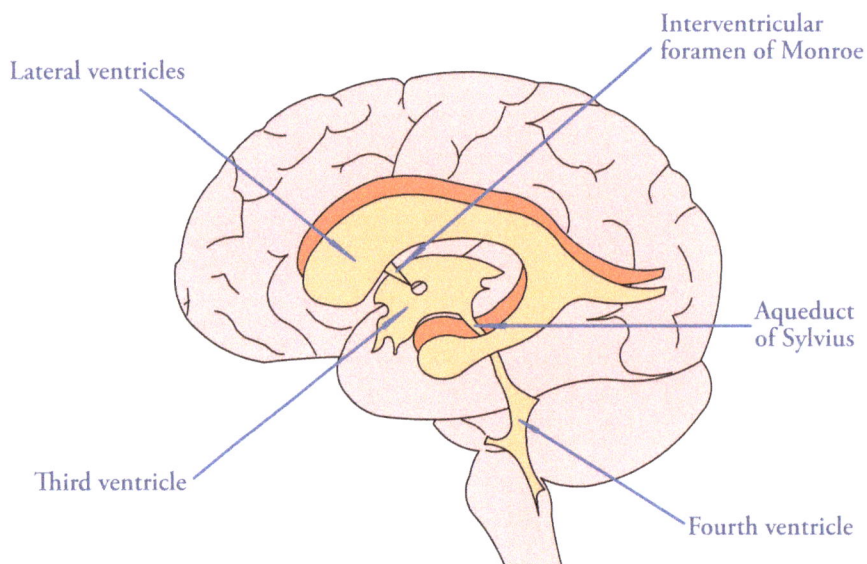

Figure 1.2 Ventricular Function

CSF Circulation

From the fourth ventricle CSF is moved into the cisterns through the aqueducts of Luschka and Magendie and the central canal. From the central canal, CSF moves down towards the sacrum into the subarachnoid space. In the aqueducts of Luschka and Magendie, the CSF moves into the cisterns and down in a helical motion towards the second sacral tubercle, then up in a cephalad direction in the subarachnoid space.

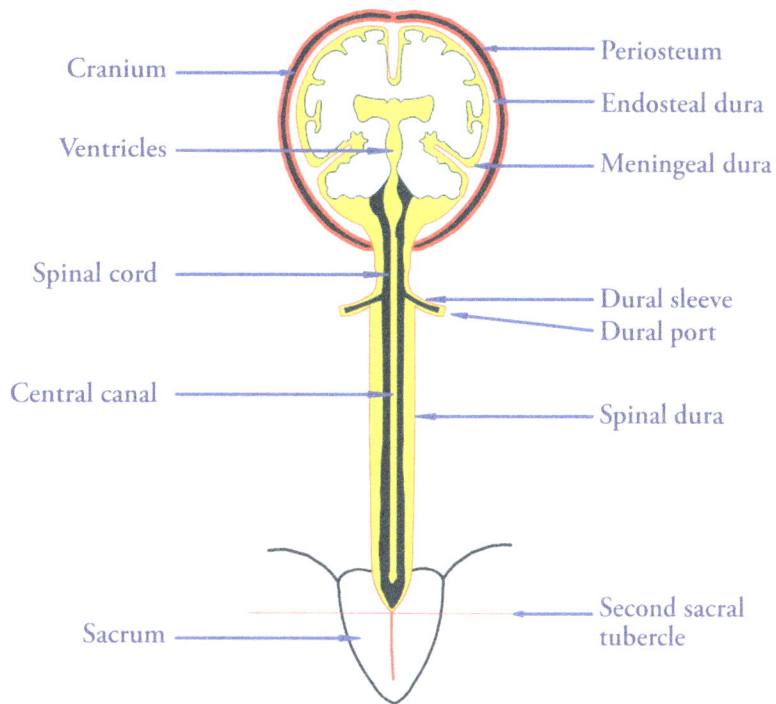

Figure 1.3 Cerebrospinal Fluid Circulation: Dural meningeal system

Superior Sagittal Sinus

Venous blood and CSF are absorbed through the arachnoid granulation of the subarachnoid space into the superior sagittal sinus. This is the collection point for all the superior anterior venous blood.

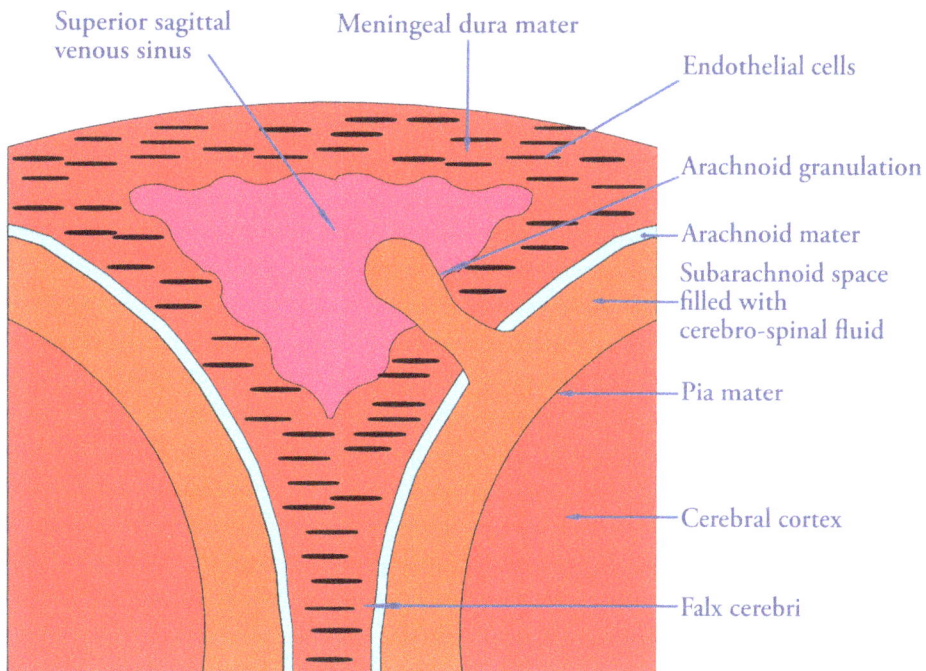

Figure 1.4 Superior Sagittal Sinus

Venous Sinus System

From the superior sagittal sinus, CSF drains down the posterior area part of the brain to the confluence of the sinuses. Venous blood also flows from the inferior sagittal sinus, through the great vein of Galen, into the confluence of the sinuses. From here blood travels bilaterally through the transverse sinuses into the sigmoid sinuses and finally into the internal jugular veins where the blood leaves the brain. The whole membrane system – the venous sinus system – is covered and supported by the dural membrane. As there are no valves or locks in this entire drainage system, a pressure gradient dictates where volumes of blood and CSF are required.

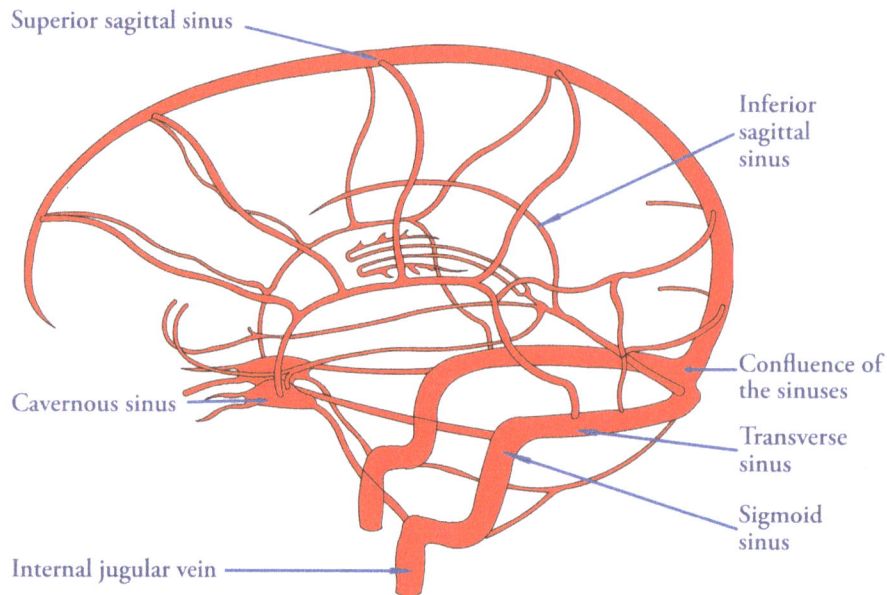

Figure 1.5 Venous Sinus System: Encapsulated in dural membrane

EMBRYOGENESIS

Embryogenesis 0–7 Days

On the day of conception, day 1, the egg and the sperm cell come together, with the sperm cell penetrating the cell membrane, and fertilization takes place.

On day 2 the two-cell stage develops with the formation of the zygote. Cell division now takes place at a rapid pace, with the zygote going from 2 cells to 4 cells to 8, then to 16, to 32, to 64, to 128, to 256, to 512, to 1,024 and so on, which gives rise to the morula on day 3.

By day 4, the early blastomere has formed, and the multicell body has entered the uterine cavity. The cell division and multiplication has reached a stage where there are many more cells, always decreasing in size, and now arranged in an outer cell mass and an inner cell mass.

By day 6 the embryo is going through the early stage of implantation, and the uterine endometrium is depicted in the progestational stage. The embryo is a blastocyst.

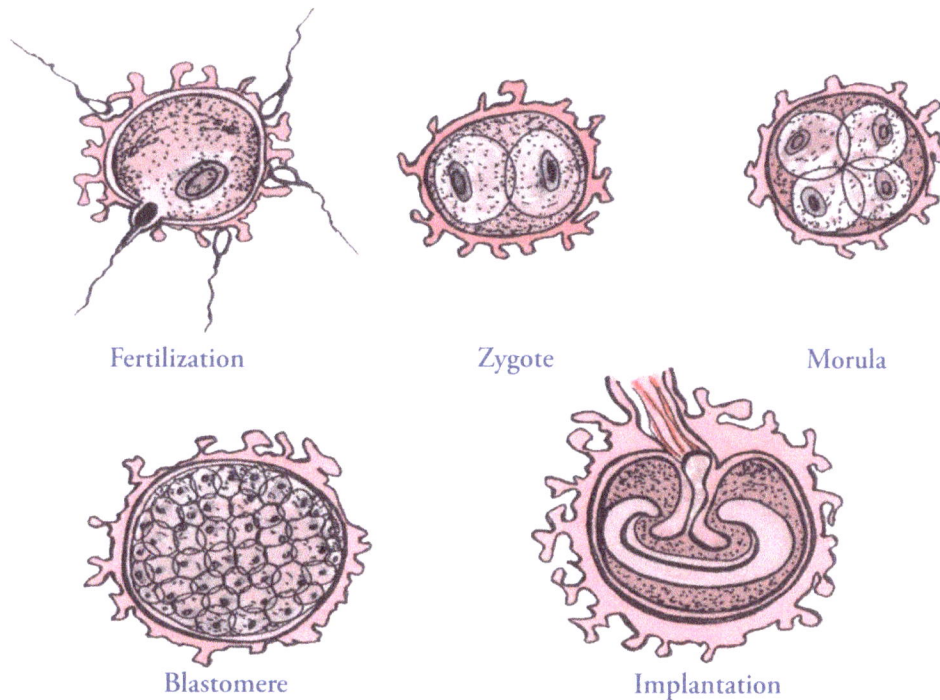

Figure 1.6 Embryogenesis 0–7 Days

Embryogenesis 0–3 Weeks

This is the embryological developmental process that occurs in the first three weeks, and includes:

- Fertilization of the egg
- Zygote forms in 24 hours
- Morula – the multicellular structure – develops in 48 hours
- Blastomere – further multiplication and cell division – 72 hours later
- Implantation into the endometrium starts at the end of week 1
- Full implantation is complete by the end of week 2
- Primitive node, pit and streak by day 16.

Embryogenesis 3–8 Weeks

Primitive streak – end of week 3 gives rise to:

- Mesenchyme – embryonic connective tissue – cling film – day 18
- Gastrulation – end of week 3 – three germ layers; endoderm, mesoderm and ectoderm
- Neurulation – end of week 3; neuroectoderm, neural groove, neural plate, neural tube.

Brain vesicles – week 4:

- Prosencephalon
- Mesencephalon
- Rhombencephalon.

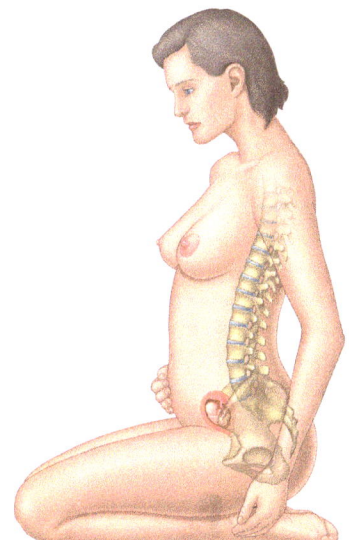

Figure 1.7 Embryogenesis 3–8 Weeks

Pharyngeal arches – week 4, day 23. All mixed cranial nerves:

- Trigeminal nerve
- Facial nerve
- Glossopharyngeal nerve
- Vagus nerve.

All the mixed cranial nerves are generated on day 23 of embryological development. The remaining cranial nerves are not developed until week 6.

MESENCHYMAL DEVELOPMENT

Fascia is a single and continuous laminated sheet of connective tissue that extends without interruption from the top of the head to the tips of the toes. It contains pockets that allow for the presence of the viscera, muscles and skeletal structures.

Facts about the fascia lamina:

- The fascia lamina is continuous; each viscera has its own fascia. The fascia is generated during embryological development and precedes all other tissue, as it evolves before other tissue is developed
- It is a slightly mobile connective tissue organ
- Dysfunctional injury reduces localised fascial mobility
- Loss of fascial mobility produces a drag upon the fascial system; this loss of mobility thus alters the craniosacral mechanism.

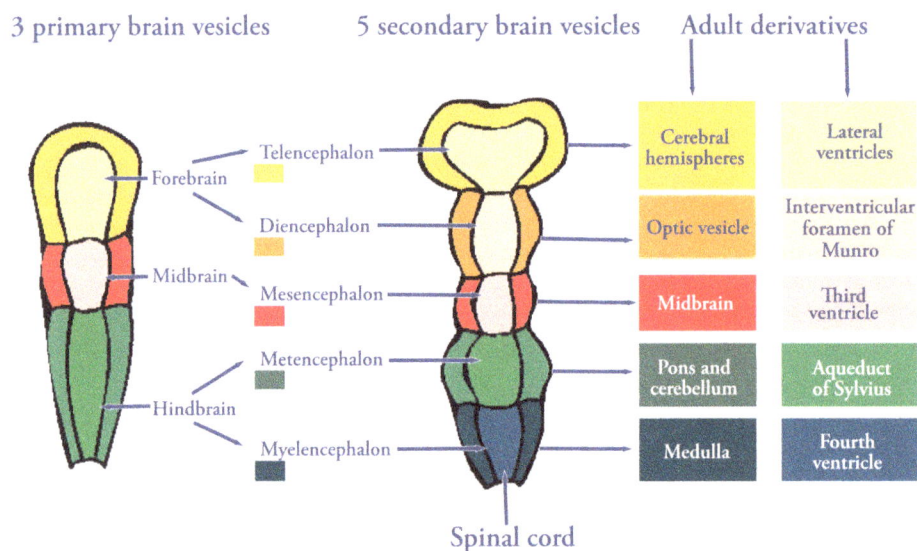

Figure 1.8 Central Canal at 5 Weeks: The ventricular system becomes the central core support of the brain

Extracellular matrix

In biology the extracellular matrix is the extracellular part of the tissue that usually provides structural support to the cells and includes the interstitial matrix and the basement membrane.

Interstitial matrix

The interstitial matrix is present between the intercellular spaces and is filled with gels of polysaccharides and fibrous proteins. These act as a compression buffer against the stress placed on the extracellular matrix.

Basement membrane

The basement membrane consists of a thin sheet of fibres that underlies the epithelium, which lines the cavities and surfaces of organs, including the skin and the endothelium, covering the interior surfaces of blood vessels.

Embryonic mesenchyme

By the end of week 3 somitomeres appear at the cephalic region of the embryo. From the occipital region, caudally, these change into somites and continue to develop in a cranio caudal sequence (approximately three per day) until at the end of week 5, when 42–44 pairs are present. By the beginning of week 4, cells differentiate and become known collectively as the sclerotome, and form a loosely woven tissue known as mesenchyme.

Mesenchyme

The primitive streak gives rise to mesenchymal cells, which form loose embryonic connective tissue called mesenchyme or mesoblast at the end of week 3, usually on day 18. Gastrulation follows this process.

Gastrulation

The mesenchyme spreads and develops laterally and cranially, forming the trilaminar germ layers:

• Embryonic endoderm
• Embryonic mesoderm
• Embryonic ectoderm.

Note that this differentiation takes place three weeks after mesenchyme is generated.

Properties of mesenchyme

• Initiates the gastrulation process
• Supports the gelatinous extracellular matrix
• Forms other types of tissue – connective, bone and cartilage
• Develops other types of structure – blood cells, endothelial cells, smooth muscle cells, circulatory and lymphatic system.

All organs in the body contain mesenchyme and mesenchyme contains:

• Collagen – abundant protein in the extracellular matrix
• Fibronectins – proteins that connect cells with collagen fibres in the extracellular matrix
• Elastins – give elasticity to tissues that are required to stretch as part of their function
• Laminin – these are sheets of protein that form the substrate of all internal organs and assist in cell adhesion and bind other extracellular components; it is the glue that holds tissues together.

ECTOMESENCHYME

• Has similar properties to mesenchyme;
• Is derived from neural crest cells;
• Formed in the cranial region between weeks 4 and 5 of embryological development.

The primary and fundamental structure of the pharyngeal arches in preparation for the mixed cranial nerves (see Figure 1.9).

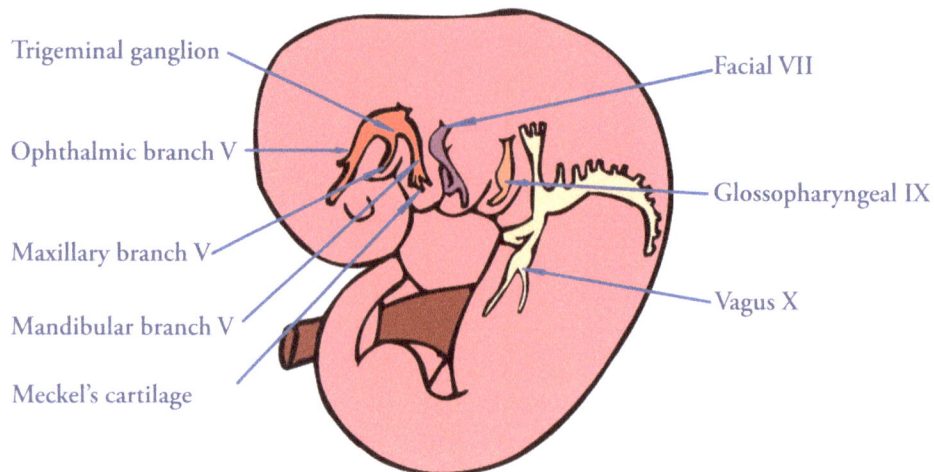

Figure 1.9 Week 4 of Cranial Nerve Development in the Pharyngeal Arches: All the mixed cranial nerves

On the twenty-third day of embryological development, the formal mixed pairs of cranial nerves evolve from the pharyngeal arches; these are the four mixed cranial nerves with both motor and sensory function:

- First pharyngeal arch produces the trigeminal ganglion which comprises the ophthalmic, maxillae and mandibular branches. Meckel's cartilage also arises from the first pharyngeal arch and is the cartilage that developes into the mandible
- Second pharyngeal arch produces the facial nerve
- Third pharyngeal arch produces the glossopharyngeal nerve
- Fourth pharyngeal arch produces the vagus nerve.

The balance of the cranial nerves are only found in week 6.

The hierarchical development

The hierarchical development is embryologically very important, as it indicates the priority of each of the components in a chronological order of importance.

Day 1: fertilisation occurs with the egg and sperm cell coming together and this marks the conception of the embryo – egg and sperm cell unite.

Day 16: the primitive streak emerges as an indentation in the blastocyst and is the beginning of the brain and spinal cord.

Day 18: mesenchyme appears and represents the initial stage of cranial dural fascia.

Day 23: as above.

FOETOGENESIS

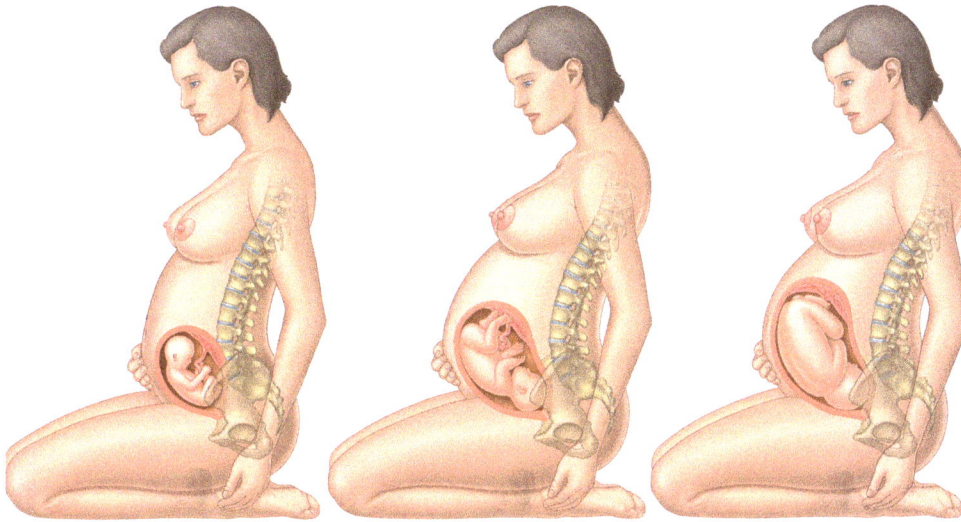

Figure 1.10 Foetogenesis (left to right) 9–20 Weeks, 20–30 Weeks, 30–40 Weeks

Foetogenesis 9–20 Weeks

Embryogenesis is considered as the embryonic growth phase from conception to the completion of embryonic development at week 8. This phase presents the highest risk of teratogenesis – malformations and other deformities which result from alcohol, drugs and nicotine.

Foetogenesis is considered as the foetal development phase beginning at week 9 and concluding at birth:

- Weeks 9–12 – the foetus grows in length
- In week 9 erythropoiesis occurs in the liver, and by the twelfth week it is taken over by the spleen
- By week 11 the intestines are formed in the abdomen
- Weeks 13–16 – there is rapid growth of the trunk, lower limbs and head
- Weeks 17–20 – there is foetal movement known as 'quickening', and vernix caseosa and downy hair known as 'lanugo' are in place.

Foetogenesis 20–30 Weeks

There is substantial weight gain, the foetus becomes better proportioned, and the lungs start producing 'surfactant', which gives the lungs patency and starts to sustain breathing.

- Week 25 – life is sustainable
- Weeks 26–29 – lungs are capable of supporting respiration, the nervous system regulates body temperature and breathing, and erythropoiesis can be found in the bone marrow.

Foetogenesis 30–40 Weeks

Between weeks 30–34 the foetal head becomes heavier than the rest of the body, so it inverts and engages in the mother's pelvic ring. The pelvic ring acts as a template for the baby's head and, as such, from here until birth all the dynamic pressures applied to the foetus through the diaphragm and abdomen cause the inverted foetus to continue to engage in the pelvic ring. Over the next twelve weeks the head will become moulded to the shape of the pelvis. If the pelvis has an external flare on the right side and an internal flare on the left side this will create an external and internal rotation of the cranial bones respectively, possibly on the occiput and/or temporal bones.

- Week 32 – the foetus will survive on its own as all the systems function
- Weeks 35–38 – the foetus is orientated towards light, has a firm grasp and the pupillary reflex of the eyes is present.

BIRTH PROCESS

Labour

The process of labour involves the adaptation of the foetal head to the various segments of the pelvis. As the foetal skull engages into the pelvis at 32 weeks its shape is controlled by the pressure dynamics of the often asymmetric pelvic ring of the mother. The first changes to cranio fascial dynamics may occur during a traumatic, artificial and unnaturally induced birth.

Induced Birth

The most common method of inducing labour is surgical rupturing of the foetal membranes:

- Forewater Rupture – bulging membranes in front of the head
- Hindwater Rupture – membranes behind the presenting part are ruptured.

Another method of induction is by using pharmaceutical agents to artificially stimulate uterine activity:

- Oxytocin infusion (synotocin) induces uterine contractions
- Prostoglandins (prostoglandin E2) ripen the cervix.

These procedures are usually followed by a sweep of the cervix.

Maternal Pelvis

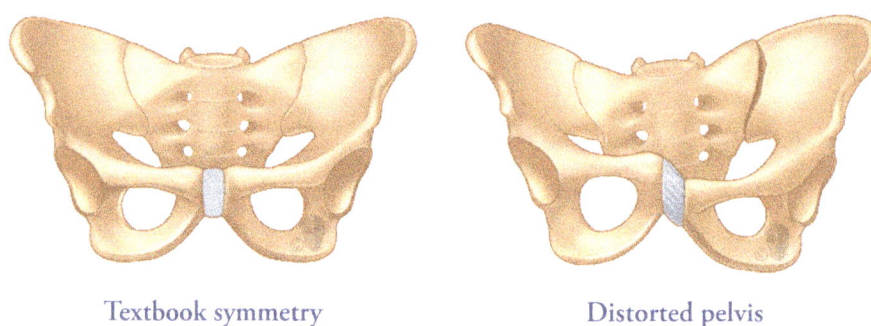

Textbook symmetry   Distorted pelvis

Figure 1.11 Maternal Pelvis

In Figure 1.11 on the left, the normal maternal pelvis, shows symmetry of both the ilia, and a level horizontal sacrum. Both sacroiliac joints are even and appear compactly joined to their iliac components. The obturator foramen are both even and equal in appearance, the symphysis pubis is central in its placement with the sacrum, and both crests of the anterior part of the ilia are horizontal. Both acetabular notches are even and symmetric.

The graphic on the right of Figure 1.11 depicts the usual distorted pelvic arrangement. The ilia on the right has gone posterior and external, while the ilia on the left has gone anterior and internal. The sacrum has moved into an oblique/diagonal position and is no longer level or horizontal. Both sacroiliac joints are disarticulated, separated and what one would classify as being a lesion. Both obturator foramen appear uneven and distorted, while the symphysis pubis is patently distorted and the acetabular notches are asymmetric.

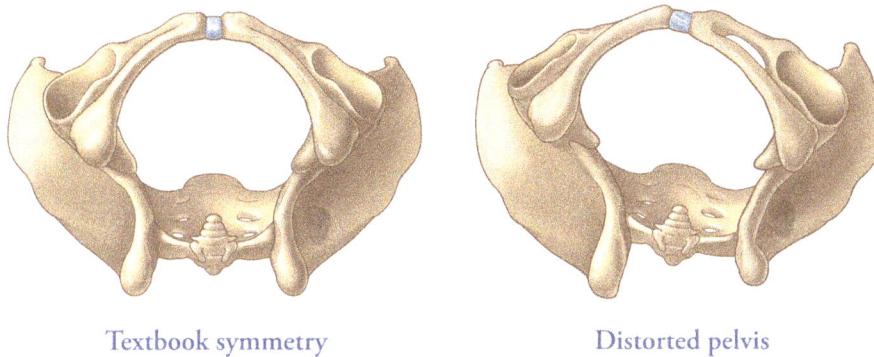

Textbook symmetry   Distorted pelvis

Figure 1.12 Inferior View of the Maternal Pelvis

In Figure 1.12 the normal pelvic ring on the left appears normal, even and symmetric, while the pelvic ring on the right is distorted and asymmetric. Notice the horizontal line of the sacrum on the left where it appears to be horizontal and evenly distributed between the two ilia. The sacrum on the right lies at an acute angle and is asymmetrically arranged with the two ilia on either side. This view clearly illustrates the distortion of the symphysis pubis on the right, and how it does not coincide with the sacral base on the opposing side of the pelvis.

Foetal Head Engaged

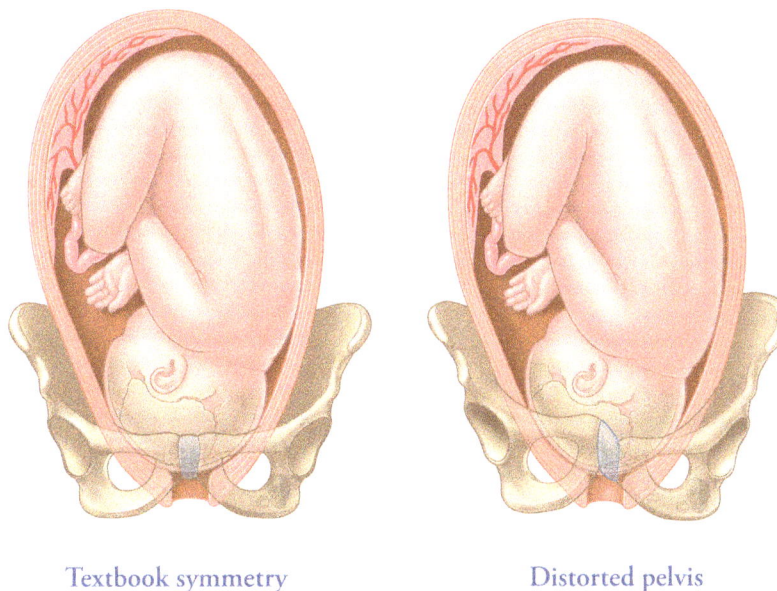

Textbook symmetry   Distorted pelvis

Figure 1.13 Foetal Head Engaged at 32 Weeks

As mentioned earlier, between 32 and 34 weeks the head of the foetus becomes heavier than the rest of the body and the foetus inverts. The head then becomes engaged into the pelvic ring. Figure 1.13 on the left shows a uniform engagement of the head within the pelvic ring, and the foetal body is maintained in a vertical position. In contrast, the foetus on the right shows a collapse of the neck and shoulders into the left pelvis and the body of the foetus lies in a curved posterior position. The position of the foetus will be maintained in this position for the next 8–10 weeks. Dynamics in the form of abdominal pressure, as well as a mother's breathing, coughing and sneezing, will continue to press the foetal head into the pelvic ring, ultimately producing a distorted cranium.

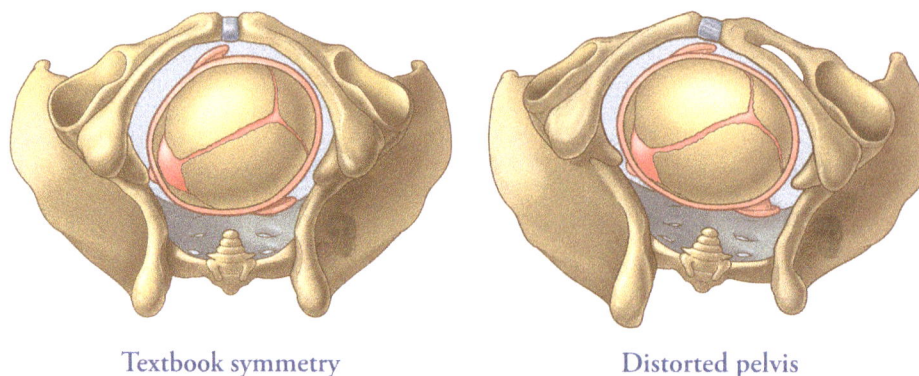

Textbook symmetry   Distorted pelvis

Figure 1.14 Inferior View of Engagment

The inferior view of the pelvis in Figure 1.14 shows the cranial head engaged in a normal pelvis and in a distorted pelvis. On the left, the head in the normal pelvis is lying in an oblique position, where the sutures and fontanelles are symmetric. The view of the pelvic distortion on the right also shows the cranial head, but the fontanelle and sutures are distorting and twisted. Underneath the cranial skull bones/ cranial plates lies the endosteal dura, and within that endosteal dura lies the superior sagittal sinus. The uniformity of the diagram on the left would indicate a superior sagittal sinus with unrestricted drainage, while the graphic on the right shows a superior sagittal sinus which is torqued and the diameter of the lumen is diminished, resulting in restricted drainage.

Crowning Presentation

The crowning presentation (Figure 1.15) shows the infant skull as it makes its appearance through the cervix and into the vagina. Again the normal pelvis on the left shows a uniform presentation, while the diagram on the right shows the distorted cranial skull preparing to pass through the similarly distorted pelvic ring.

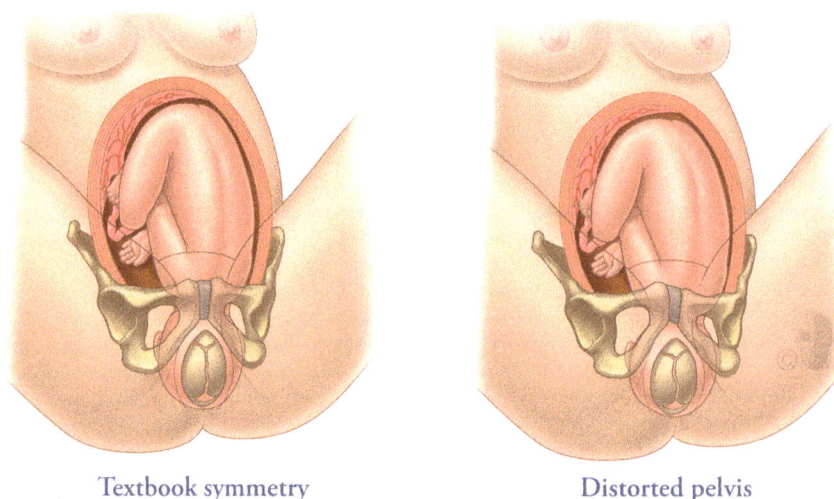

Textbook symmetry   Distorted pelvis

Figure 1.15 Crowning Presentation

First Phase Rotation

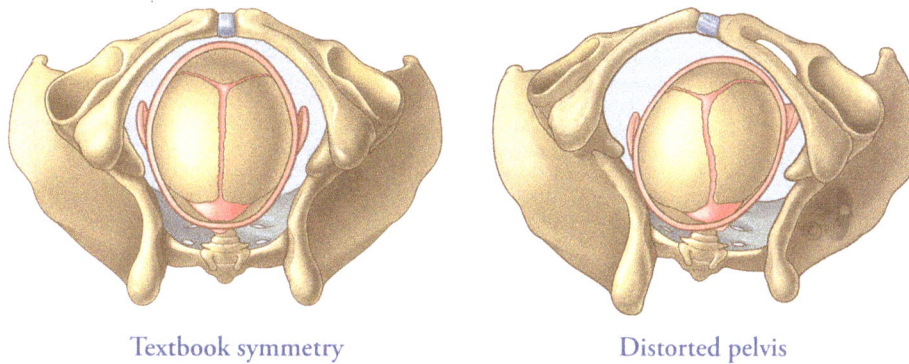

Textbook symmetry   Distorted pelvis

Figure 1.16 First Phase Rotation

First phase rotation shows the infant cranium going through a 45° turn, preparing for a left occiput anterior delivery. It can be appreciated looking at this angle that the skull on the left side moves in an uninhibited fashion, while the skull on the right comes into conflict with two parts of the pelvic ring. In terms of birth trauma, the distortion of the membranes, the uterus, the distorted cervix and the vagina, will involve a torsional dynamic during delivery that could result in the head becoming stuck at worst, or cranial abrasions at the least. Subsequent restriction of the skull's passage may necessitate the invasive use of forceps or ventouse.

The birth process involves the following dynamics as a cranium is delivered from the cervix and prepares to move through the pelvic ring. The descent of the head is followed by the flexion on the skull as it attempts to rotate through the pelvic ring. This is followed by the internal rotation of the head, extension of the head and its eventual delivery. Once the head is clear it rotates to allow for the delivery of the shoulders.

Head and Shoulder Presentation

Once the head is clear of the pelvic ring, it rotates to allow the shoulders to follow and will remain in that rotational position until the pelvis is expelled. As was mentioned earlier, the membrane distortion in the uterus, the position of the head early on in the pelvic ring, and the inability of a distorted pelvis to facilitate a normal birth, are all factors that can lead to a traumatic birth.

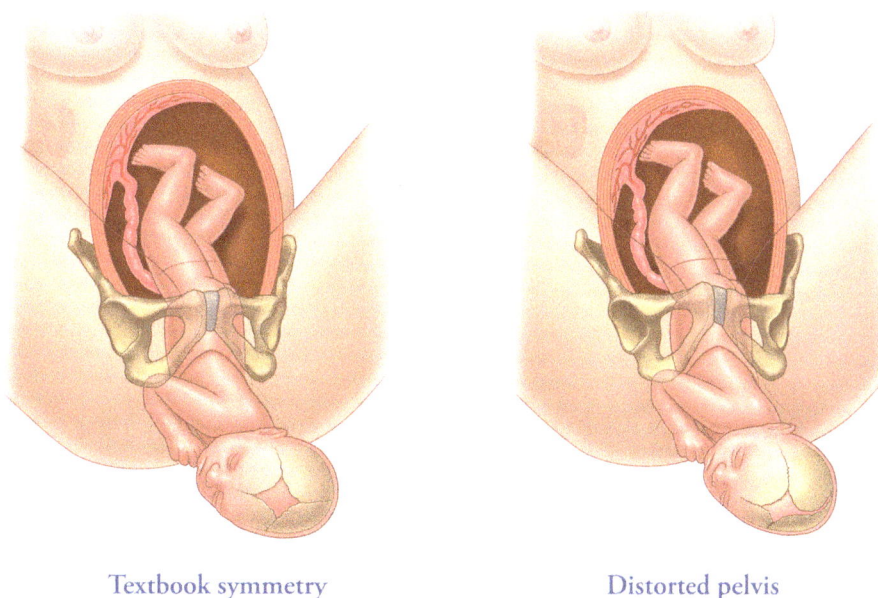

Textbook symmetry   Distorted pelvis

Figure 1.17 Head and Shoulder Presentation

The invasive use of instruments in birth trauma depends on several factors and the choice of instrument will be guided by the distress of the baby, the baby's head position and the mother's status and resilience.

Forceps

In a forceps delivery, the forceps (shaped like a large pair of salad spoons) are applied to the baby's head to help guide it through the birth canal. A forceps delivery poses a risk of injury to both mother and baby. If a forceps delivery fails a caesarean delivery might be necessary.

Ventouse

Ventouse, also known as vacuum-assisted vaginal delivery or vacuum extraction (VE), is a method to assist birth using a vacuum device. The ventouse is used in the second stage of labour if the labour has not progressed adequately. The vacuum cup is applied to the baby's skull and a vacuum is induced by use of a pump to help force baby's head through the birth canal. If the ventouse fails a caesarean delivery might be necessary.

Caesarean Section

A caesarean section is a surgical procedure where an incision is made through the mother's abdomen and uterus to deliver the baby. Caesarean section is utilised if vaginal delivery might pose a risk to the mother and the baby. If the mother's pelvis is considered to be too small for a vaginal delivery, then an elective caesarean can be scheduled at about 40 weeks. However, if there are complications during the birth process, then an emergency caesarean may be carried out.

Complications during the birth process could include: position of the foetus in the birth canal; prolonged labour or failure to progress; foetal or maternal distress; cord prolapse; problems with the placenta; uterine rupture; umbilical cord abnormalities; hypertension and tachycardia.

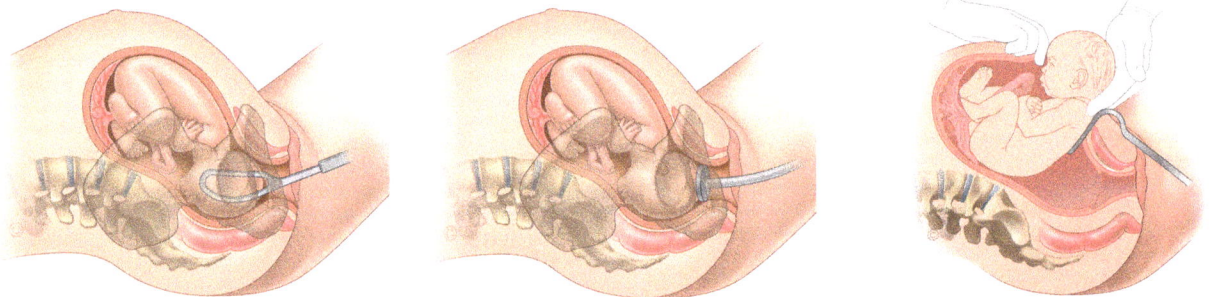

Figure 1.18 (left) Forceps Trauma: Compressing the parietal, temporal and sphenoid bones; (centre) Ventouse Trauma: Pressure on the superior sagittal sinus, bregma and lambda; (right) Caesarean Trauma: Vaginal delivery not possible; emergency or elective

CHAPTER 2

INFANT CRANIUM

INFANT CRANIAL PLATES

Almost all anatomy textbooks will illustrate an infant's cranial plates as shown by the normal cranium in Figure 2.1. It defines the anterior and posterior fontanelles, the superior surgical suture, the bregma, the lambda, the two frontal bones, the two parietal bones and the occipital bone. Most anatomists will assume that the symmetric presentation of the cranium, as depicted in this view, is normal. The illustration on the right however, shows distortion of all the cranial plates, the fontanelles and the sutures – the coronal, the lambdoid and the sagittal.

After twenty years of research the author has concluded that the left occipital anterior (LOA) birth presentation indicates a consistent left counterclockwise torque, consistent in all the abnormal/distorted appearances of the cranial plates, sutures and fontanelles. This follows the consistency of the pelvic rotation depicted above, as having an external right ilium and an internal left ilium.

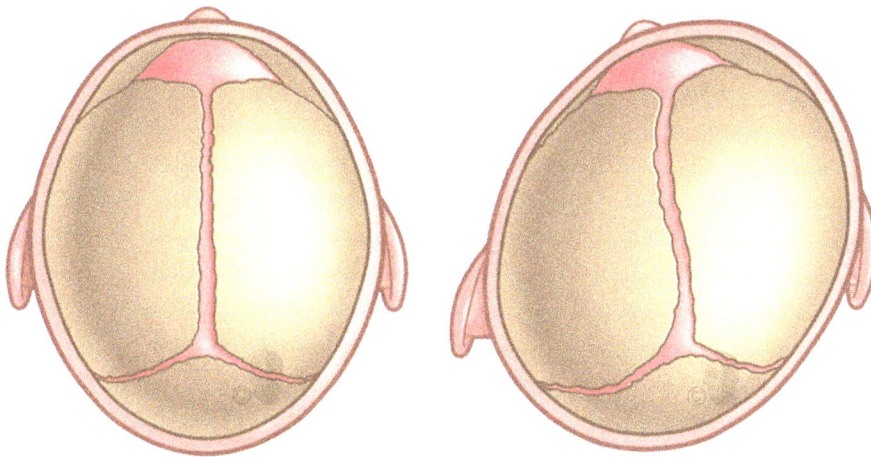

Textbook symmetry   Distorted cranium

Figure 2.1 Infant Cranial Plates

INFANT SKULL

The LOA presentation produces the skull as a left external occiput and a right internal occiput. This results in a right frontal external rotation and left frontal internal rotation, a right maxillary external rotation (flexion) and a left maxillary internal rotation (extension).

This produces a normal right eye/ocular orbit and a left compressed ocular orbit with the appearance of the left frontal bone dropping into the orbit. Compare the right and left superior orbital fissure, where some of the major cranial vessels traverse. The left superior orbital fissure virtually collapses and the lesser wing of the left sphenoid pulls the orbit inferiorly and pulls the eye posteriorly, in the direction of the anticlockwise torque. As the greater wing of the sphenoid becomes depressed and moves inferior and posterior, the temporal bone moves into external rotation, taking the mandibular fossa posteriorly and pulling the mandibular condyle posteriorly, and deviating the mandible from right to left, compressing the left temporomandibular joint (TMJ).

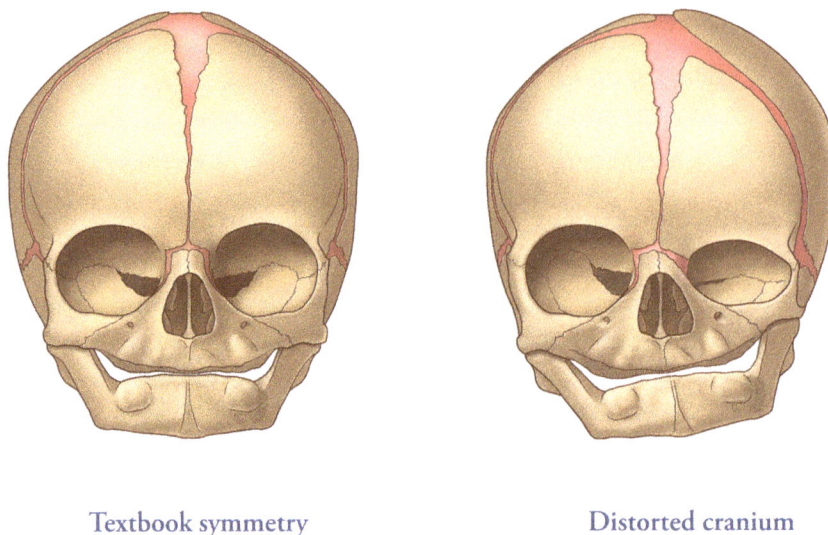

Textbook symmetry   Distorted cranium

Figure 2.2 Infant Skull

CRANIO FASCIAL DISTORTION

The facial distortion in Figure 2.3 is the result of the cranial distortion seen in Figure 2.2. Most notable in this picture is the large externally rotated ear on the left, in comparison to the right internally rotated ear which follows the right internal temporal bone. The right eye appears anterior and larger, while the left eye appears posterior and smaller. The right eye is more engaging and alive, while the left eye is definitely the accompanying eye, and not taking much part in proceedings. Notice also the evidence of the left mandibular deviation.

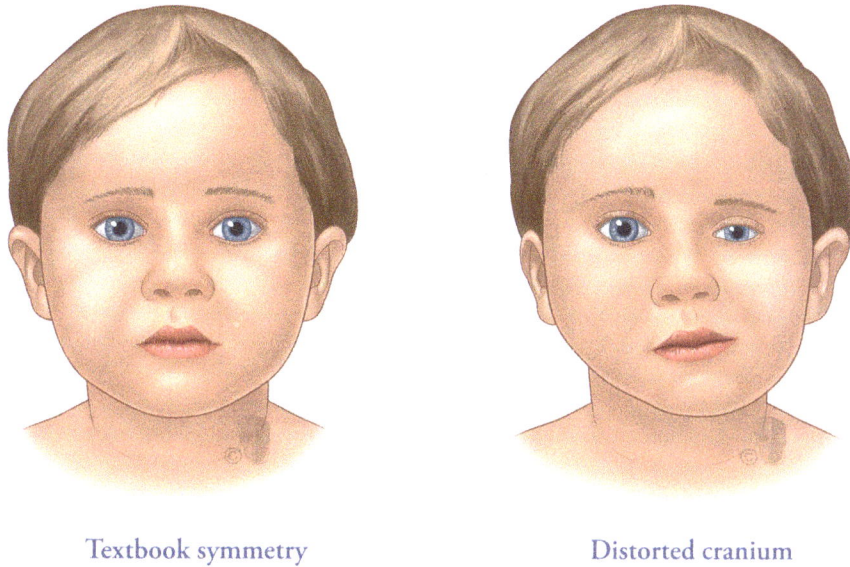

Textbook symmetry   Distorted cranium

Figure 2.3 Cranio Fascial Distortion

The superior view of the cranium in Figure 2.4 shows symmetric frontal, temporal and occipital bones, with the central position of the sphenoid body and the greater wings anterior of a symmetric foramen magnum.

Once again, the graphic on the right shows a very asymmetric superior view of the skull. One notices a right external frontal bone, complemented by a left internal front bone. The left greater wing of the sphenoid is depressed, while the right greater wing of the sphenoid is elevated. The left temporal bone is externally rotated, along with the left half of the occiput, while the right temporal bone is internally rotated, along with the right occipital bone. The crista galli of the ethmoid bone, the anchor point for the falx cerebri, is markedly distorted, as are the two petrous portions of the temporal bone – left and right. The final distortion in this view is the internal occipital protuberance – the junction point for the confluence of the sinuses – the horizontal anchor point for the tentorium cerebellum, and the reciprocal tension membranes (RTM), supporting the brain within the cranial vault.

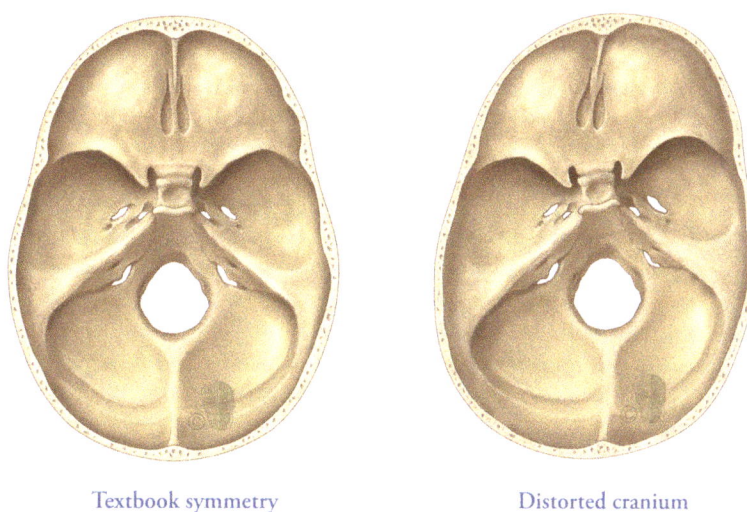

Textbook symmetry   Distorted cranium

Figure 2.4 Superior View of the Cranium

TENTORIUM CEREBELLUM AND FALX CEREBRI

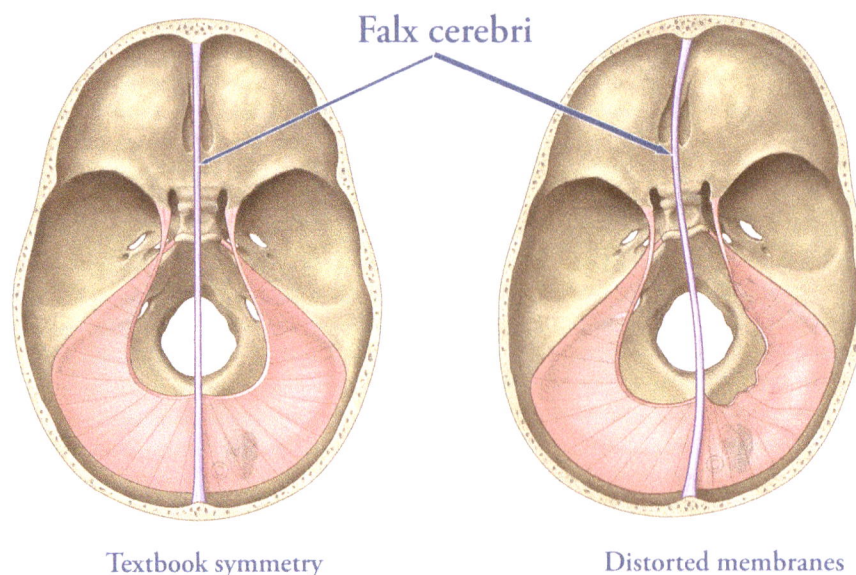

Figure 2.5 Tentorium Cerebelli and Falx Cerebri

The tentorium cerebellum is the horizontal membrane that is attached at the anterior and posterior clinoid processes of the sphenoid bone anteriorly, and at the transverse sinus bilaterally of the occipital bone, and bilaterally at the sigmoid sinuses of the temporal bone on the petrous portion. The sinuses, the transverse, sigmoid and the internal jugular vein are housed within the peripheral margins of the tentorium cerebellum. On the right graphic in Figure 2.5 one can see how taut the membrane is on the left external temporal/occipital bone, while on the right temporal/occipital internal bone the membrane is quite loose and concertinaed, which means the transverse and sigmoid sinuses and the internal jugular vein lose their functional diameter, which then reduces their ability to drain efficiently. The falx cerebri, represented here as a straight line between the crista galli of the ethmoid bone and the internal occipital protuberance, is the vertical membrane. This membrane separates the left and right cerebral hemispheres. The graphic on the right shows the distortion of this membrane which now has an 'S' shaped appearance. This vertical membrane carries the superior and inferior sagittal sinuses and its drainage efficiency becomes more compromised when the membrane becomes distorted and flaccid.

Superior View of the Brain

This view of the brain in Figure 2.6 shows the left and right hemispheres being separated by the falx cerebri, the vertical membrane that supports the superior and inferior sagittal sinuses. Cranial tissues that are part of the central brain are placed in a midline position so that they have access to both left and right cerebral hemispheres.

Input from both the left and right cerebral hemispheres, allows the brain to retrieve information from all sensory areas of the body. This information is collected from the various cranial organs, processed and retained/discharged to other components within the brain or other parts of the body. Where the falx cerebri is symmetric, the communication between left and right hemispheres is exact and accurate, and the transfer of information is completed with efficiency. However, when the falx cerebri is distorted, or the cross-membrane communications become inefficient and inaccurate, the transfer of information from hemisphere to hemisphere becomes compromised and affects the physiology of that organ.

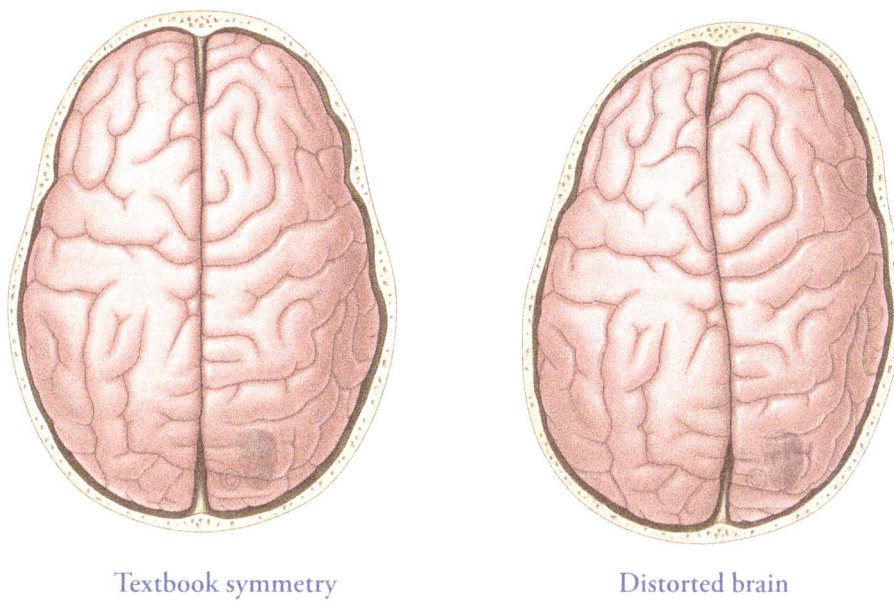

Textbook symmetry   Distorted brain

Figure 2.6 Superior View of the Brain

Optic Chiasma and Optic Tracts

Cranial nerve two, the optic nerve, takes information from both retinae and transfers that information through the optic chiasma to the occipital lobe where the visual centres are maintained. The optic chiasma takes information from each eye, both central and peripheral, medially and laterally, combining one half of each nerve's axons as it enters the opposite tract, making it a partial decussation at the chiasma. This system allows for parts of both eyes that attend to both visual fields, left and right, to be processed in the brain. The resulting information is exchanged across both brain hemispheres.

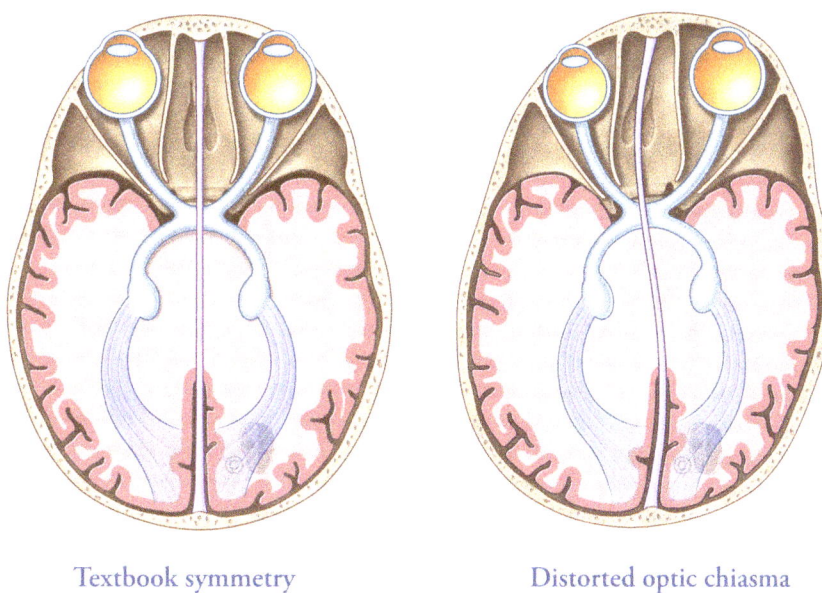

Textbook symmetry   Distorted optic chiasma

Figure 2.7 Optic Chiasma and Optic Tracts

PITUITARY

The pituitary is a small endocrine gland that is an extension of the hypothalamus at the base of the brain and is found in the sella turcica of the sphenoid bone body. The diaphragma sellae is a horizontal layer of dura that is an extension of the tentorium cerebellum and secures the hypophyseal stalk of the pituitary in the sella turcica, between the anterior and posterior clinoid processes of the sphenoid bone.

The pituitary is made up of two lobes – the anterior and the posterior. When cranio fascial distortion occurs, the tentorium cerebellum and diaphragms sellae become distorted, twisting the hypophyseal stalk – the infundibulum – reducing the blood flow and affecting the parvocellular neurosecretory system.

The anterior pituitary is derived from ectoderm, while the posterior pituitary is derived from neuroectoderm. The anterior pituitary synthesises and secretes hormones – releasing hormones (RH) under the influence of the hypothalamus:

- Somatotropins: human growth hormones (HGH)
- Thyrotropin: thyroid-stimulating hormones (TSH) are released under influence of hypothalamic thyrotropin-releasing hormone (TRH), and inhibited by somatostatins
- Corticotrophins: adrenocorticotropic hormones (ACTH) and beta-endorphins are released under the influence of hypothalamic corticotropin-releasing hormones (CRH)
- Lactotrophins: prolactin (PRL)
- Gonadotropins: uteinizing hormone (LH) and follicle-stimulating hormone (FSH)
- The intermediate lobe synthesizes and secretes melanocyte-stimulating hormone (MSH).
- The posterior lobe secretes magnocellular hormones
- Antidiuretic hormone (ADH) is secreted from the supraoptic nucleus of the hypothalamus
- Oxytocin is released from the paraventricular nucleus in the hypothalamus.

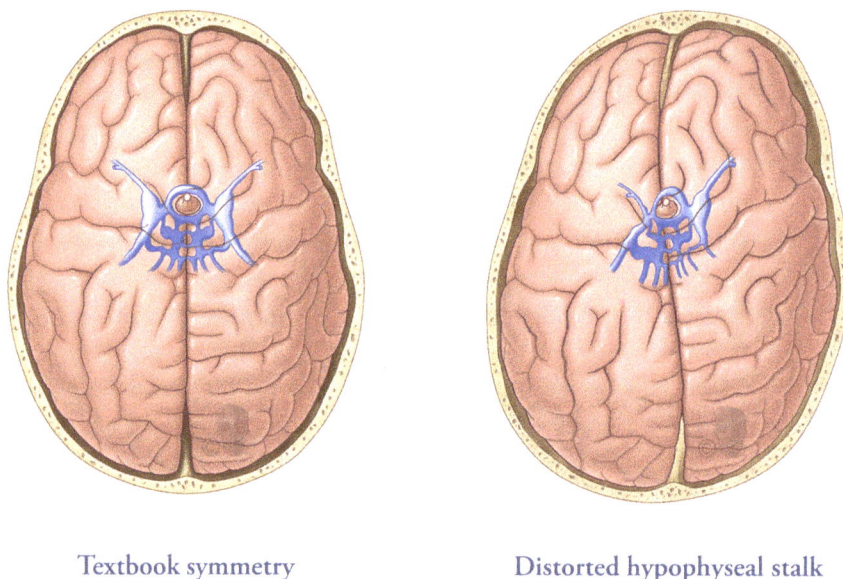

| Textbook symmetry | Distorted hypophyseal stalk |

Figure 2.8 Pituitary and Hypophyseal Stalk

Hypophyseal Stalk

The hypophyseal stalk (infundibulum), is a system of blood vessels that carry regulatory hormones from the hypothalamus to the anterior pituitary lobe, and blood directly from the heart to the posterior pituitary. The hypophyseal stalk is kept in place by the diaphragma sellae attached to the anterior and posterior clinoid processes of the sella turcica – the body of the sphenoid.

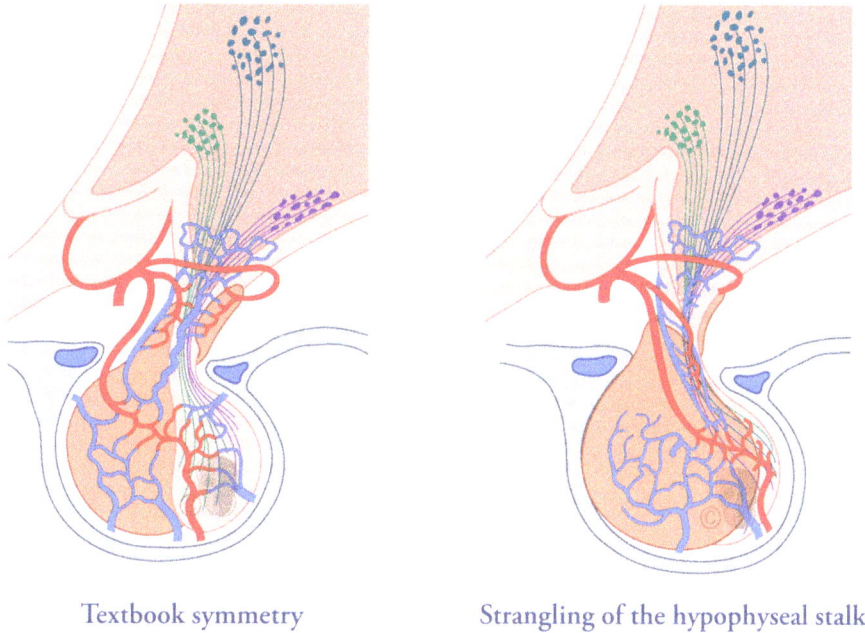

Textbook symmetry   Strangling of the hypophyseal stalk

Figure 2.9 Pituitary and Strangled Hypophyseal Stalk

CORPUS CALLOSUM

The corpus callosum is a wide flat bundle of neural fibres beneath the cortex. It connects left and right cerebral hemispheres and facilitates interhemispheric communication. It is the largest white matter structure in the brain. The posterior part of the corpus callosum is called the splenium, the anterior part the genu, and the part in between the body. The part between the body and the splenium is the lamina terminalis, which represents the cephalic end of the early neural tube and extends from the roof plate of the diencephalon to the optic chiasma. There are three different types of fibres.

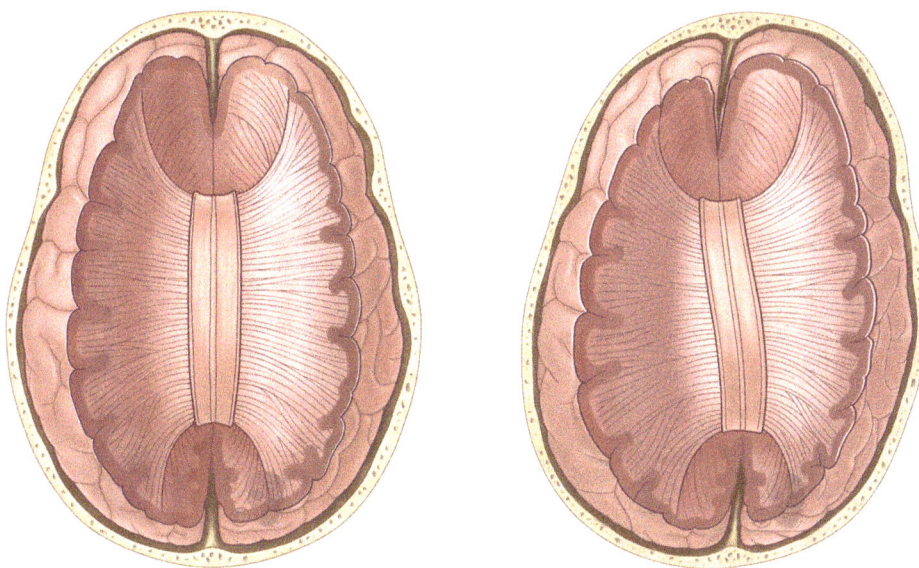

Textbook symmetry   Communication fibre distortion

Figure 2.10 Corpus Callosum

CEREBRAL FIBRES

Commissural Fibres

The commissural fibres pass from one hemisphere to the other. The largest group of these fibres integrates and facilitates the information being passed from one cerebral hemisphere to the other and provides the most important integrative pathways to the brain. It appears in week 10 of development and connects the non-olfactory areas of the left and right cerebral hemispheres.

- Anterior commissure – connect right and left anterior temporal lobes and subconscious brain nuclei (amygdala), unifying and integrating the emotional responses from each side of the brain. The amygdala serves important functions in motion autonomic and neuroendocrine circuits of the limbic system
- Hippocampal/fornix commissure – connects the left and right hippocampi to the laminar terminalis closest to the roof plate of the diencephalon. The hippocampus appears to be critical to memory formation, consolidation and retrieval
- Posterior commissures – interhemispheric fibres connecting the superior parietal lobes involved in the integration of physical sensations to the legs, the arms and the stomatognathics
- Habenular commissures – connect right and left nuclei of the other midbrain areas, providing integration of subconscious processing
- Collicular commissures – fibres that synchronise eye, head and neck movement, providing a stable foundation for visual focus.

All these commissural fibres occur across the midline and are connected to both left and right cerebral hemispheres. Cranial fascial torque has a huge influence on the neurophysiological outcome when the commissures become distorted and misrepresented. Learning and memory lapses can be attributable to corpus callosum dysfunction, while emotional behaviours and changes in neuroendocrine function can be the result of hippocampus, amygdala and anterior commissural changes.

Association Fibres

These fibres connect areas of the cerebral cortex within the same hemisphere. They are white matter fibres that run between the front and the back of the brain.

- Long fibres – connecting the front and back of the same hemisphere
- Short fibres – U-shaped fibres linking adjacent cortical areas in the same hemisphere (i.e. arcuate fibres)
- Occipitofrontal tracts – integrating association between the visual centres at the occipital lobe with the pre-motor areas controlling the eye muscles.

Projection Fibres

Fibres that connect the cerebrum and other parts of the brain and/or spinal cord. These are white fibres deep within the subconscious core that project up into the conscious cortical areas – where our subconscious emotions enter our consciousness. Similarly, cortical fibres transmit conscious desires deep into the subconscious limbic system to parts of the brain, which perform these desires.

Projection fibres lead from the motor cortex into the spinal cord through corticospinal tracts, providing voluntary control of movement. The reverse is also true when sensory projection fibres from the extremities relay impulses through the spinal cord sensory areas of the cortex, identifying these sensations. Cranio fascial torque will create distortion of these fibre activities and affect the neurological outcome.

BASAL GANGLIA

These are the neuronal cell bodies deep within the white matter. Basal ganglia are groups of paired brain nuclei that play a crucial role in the integration and organisation of coordinated motor activity. When integrated with the cerebellum, the basal ganglia turn the derived conscious activity into reality.

Included in this group of brain nuclei is the corpus striatum which is made up of:

- Caudate nucleus – which has both cognitive and motor functions, controlling eye movement with corresponding motor movement (e.g. a tennis player hitting the ball)
- Tailed nucleus
- Lentiform nucleus – runs predetermined motor programmes
- Outer part – the putamen-motoric
- Inner part – globus pallidus, the output structure of the basal ganglia.

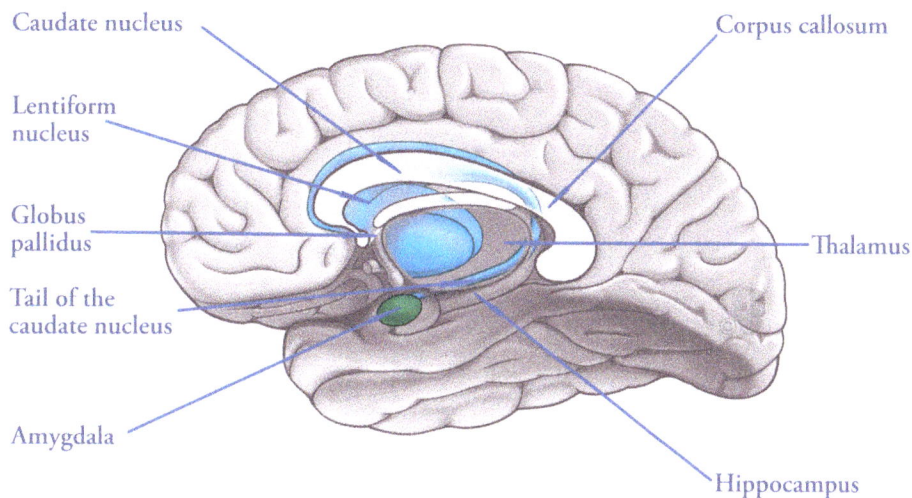

Caudate nucleus

Corpus callosum

Lentiform nucleus

Globus pallidus

Thalamus

Tail of the caudate nucleus

Amygdala

Hippocampus

Figure 2.11 Basal Ganglia

These areas govern the subconscious functions carried out by the basal ganglia controlling automatic movement. All motor patterns rely upon subconscious input from the cerebellum to smooth out and coordinate muscle activity. The cerebellum reacts to impulses from the subconscious senses in the muscles, joints and fascia, which tell it what the body is doing so that, along with the cerebellum, the basal ganglia acts as an interface between sensory and motor systems, permitting the brain to perform complex movements almost subconsciously.

Cranio fascial distortion will affect the delicate balance and transmission of these processes and render them incomplete and dysfunctional.

HYPOTHALAMUS

The hypothalamus is that section of the brain responsible for the production of many of the body's essential hormones and chemical substances that help control different cells and organs. Physiological functions (such as temperature regulation, thirst, hunger, sleep, sex drive, mood, blood pressure, respiration, intestinal peristalsis and the release of other hormones within the body) are controlled by the hormones from the hypothalamus. It has master control of body metabolism because it is in charge not only of the autonomic nervous system but also of the nearby pituitary gland. The hypothalamus has central control over visceral autonomic functions.

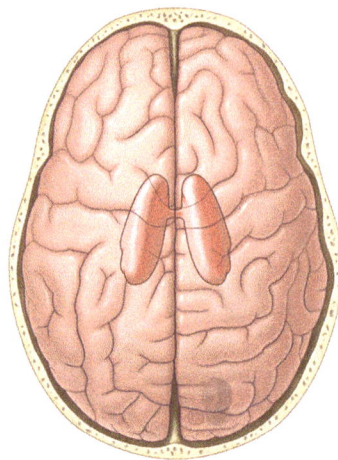

Textbook symmetry

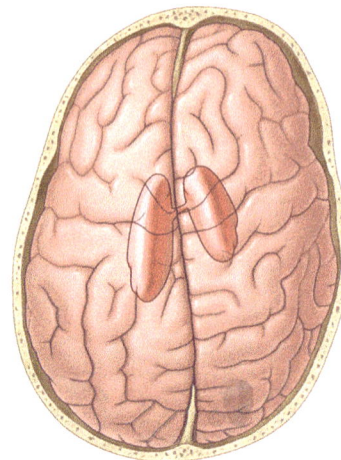

Distortion of hypothalamus
'junction box'

Figure 2.12 Hypothalamus

a. Parasympathetic control from the anterior hypothalamus:
- Increases digestive motility
- Decreases heart rate
- Constriction of the pupils

b. Sympathetic control from the posterior hypothalamus:
- Increases heart rate
- Increases vasoconstriction
- Decreases digestive motility
- Dilation of the pupils
- Piloerection and sweat gland activity

c. Endocrine control:
- Directly – via neuron axon extensions from the posterior pituitary
- Indirectly – via neuro hormones to control the release of anterior pituitary hormones.

Subdivision of the Hypothalamus

The hypothalamus nuclei are found in the region of the hypothalamus, superior and posterior of the optic chiasma and an intermediate area above the infundibular stalk.

a. Anterior area:

- Supraoptic nuclei
- Paraventricular nuclei
- Preoptic nucleus
- Intermediate area
- Dorsomedial nuclei
- Ventromedial nuclei
- Arcuate nuclei
- Tuber Cinereum

b. Posterior area:

- Mamillary bodies
- Posterior nuclei.

Subthalamus

Found under the lateral interior aspect of the thalamus and includes the following nuclei:

- Parvocellular region of the red nucleus
- Superior portion of the substantia nigra.

The subthalamic nucleus (corpus Luysi) sends and receives fibres to and from the globus pallidus of the telencephalon (part of the extrapyramidal system).

The reason for outlining all these nuclei is that the medial borders of this area (the thalamus, the hypothalamus and the subthalamus) are bordered by the lateral margins of the third ventricle and the interventricular foramen of Monro. Fluctuations in intracranial pressure within the third ventricle by CSF congestion will have a detrimental effect on the optimum performance of all these nuclei.

LIMBIC SYSTEM

The limbic system is the centre of our subconscious emotional processing and comprises the cingulate gyrus, lying just above the corpus callosum, the orbitofrontal and subcallosal gyri of the basal frontal lobes, the dentate and hippocampal gyri and the para hippocampal, entorhinal and perirhinal cortices of the medial temporal lobes.

In addition to the cortical limbic lobe, the limbic system also includes subcortical areas: the mammillary bodies of the hypothalamus; the amygdaloid bodies of the basal ganglia; and the anterior thalamus nuclei of the thalamus septal nuclei of the basal forebrain. Many of the messages coming from the subcortical limbic nuclei are then relayed through the cingulate gyri on the way to the cortex. Likewise, cortical messages to the subconscious limbic system are delivered via the cingulate gyrus.

The cingulate gyrus acts as a major interface between the conscious and the subconscious. Also located within the anterior cingulate gyrus is the centre that suppresses feelings of anger and rage, which when destroyed renders us incapable of suppressing rage.

The hippocampus formation is the central processing unit for memory and this same information can be processed by the amygdala – the seat of our subconscious emotions. Subconscious emotions, often triggered by memory, thus initiate a physiologic cascade from the hypothalamus of both the autonomic nervous system signals and hormonal flows that creates our physical sensations. It is also due to the widespread connections of the limbic system to the hypothalamus, basal ganglia, thalamus and cerebral cortex that our emotions have such profound effects on our visceral and gut functions, such as ulcers, muscle tone and neck posture, sounds, taste and smells that define our moods.

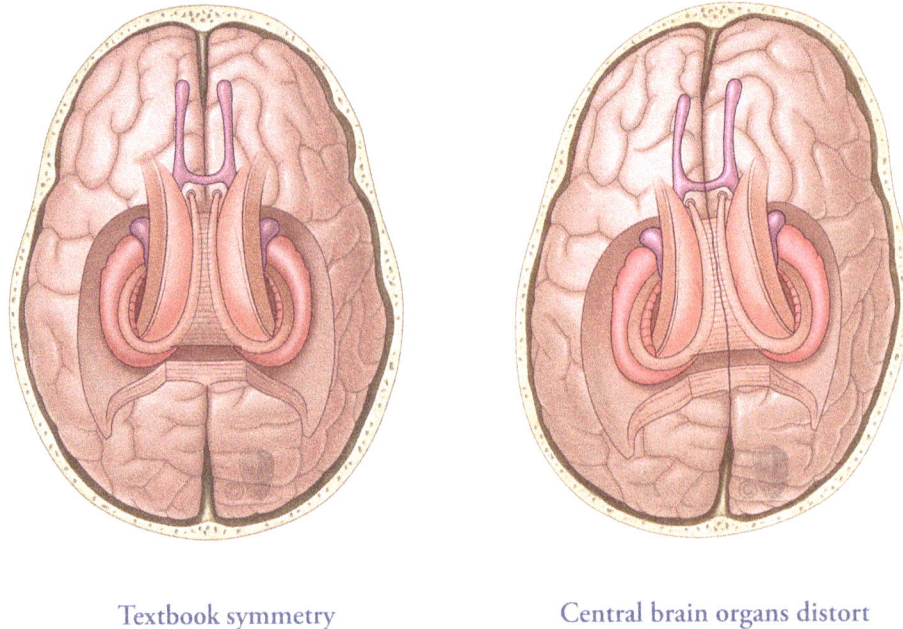

Textbook symmetry   Central brain organs distort

Figure 2.13 Limbic System

THALAMUS–MIDBRAIN–PONS

The thalamus consists of two nut-shaped collections of nuclei that lie immediately on either side of the centre of the brain, surrounding the ventricular system. The thalami play a major role as the relay station for all information transmitted to and from the body. The thalamus on each side is the final processing station where all sensory input, except olfactory, is relayed or filtered before transmitting to the cortex where it may become conscious. Because the thalamus acts as a junction box it can, if necessary, filter information that is still below conscious awareness. The subconscious therefore has the ability to filter what is being sent to the cortex.

Research has shown that not only is the thalamus the major relay centre for information, but that conscious awareness of crude sensations (such as pain, touch and temperature) begin in specific thalamic nuclei and are then relayed to specific areas of the cortex, where more detailed subconscious perception is formed.

As well as receiving sensory input, motor sequences from the basal ganglia and cerebellum are forwarded to two specific nuclei of the thalamus. These thalamic nuclei relay this motor information to the pre-motor cortex and/or the primary motor cortex, which sends signals to activate the individual muscles via the corticospinal tracts running down the spine.

The thalamus lies just above the brainstem, which is made up of the midbrain, the pons and the medulla oblongata.

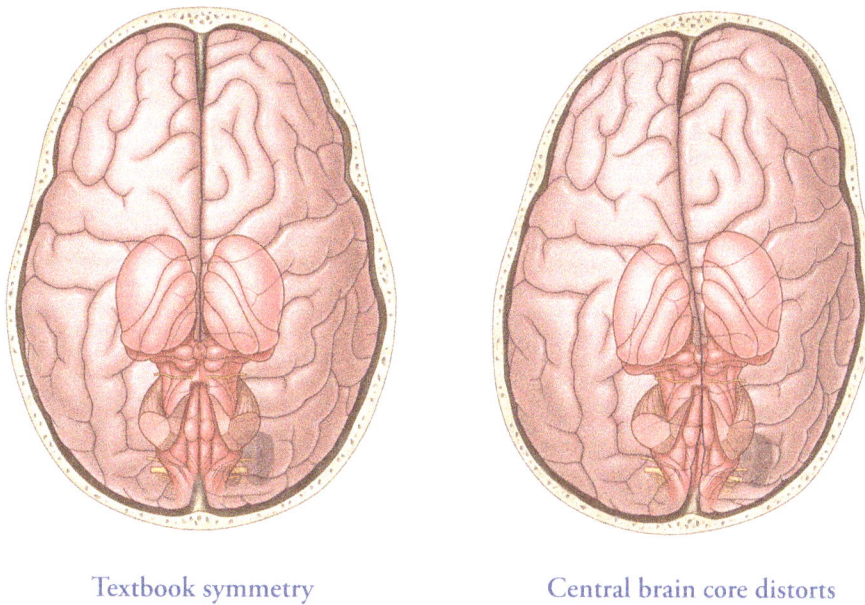

Textbook symmetry   Central brain core distorts

Figure 2.14 Thalamus-Midbrain-Pons

The hypothalamus is a region of many small nuclei with diverse functions located above the midbrain and below the thalamus. The hypothalamus makes up the ventral diencephalon and is composed of numerous fibre tracts and nuclei situated around the third ventricle. The diencephalon is an embryonic region of the vertebrate neural tube that gives rise to posterior forebrain structures. By synthesising and secreting neurohormones, the nuclei of the hypothalamus act as a conduit between the nervous system and the pituitary gland, regulating homeostatic functions such as hunger, thirst, body temperature and circadian rhythms.

VENTRICLES (CENTRAL CANAL AT 5 WEEKS)

The brain vesicles (the prosencephalon, the mesencephalon and the rhombencephalon) basically form the forebrain, the midbrain and the hindbrain. Within those structures are formed the dominant system, the two laterals, the third and the fourth ventricles.

The ventricles produce CSF. The two lateral ventricles feed into the third ventricle through the interventricular foramen of Monro, and from the third to the fourth ventricle by the aqueduct of Sylvius. From the fourth ventricle, CSF flows laterally through the two apertures of Luschka and medially through the aperture of Magendie.

Within the lining of each of the ventricles are areas known as choroid plexuses, which are derived as double layers of pia mater richly invested into tuft-like processes called the tela choroidea, which emerge from the linings of each of the four ventricles.

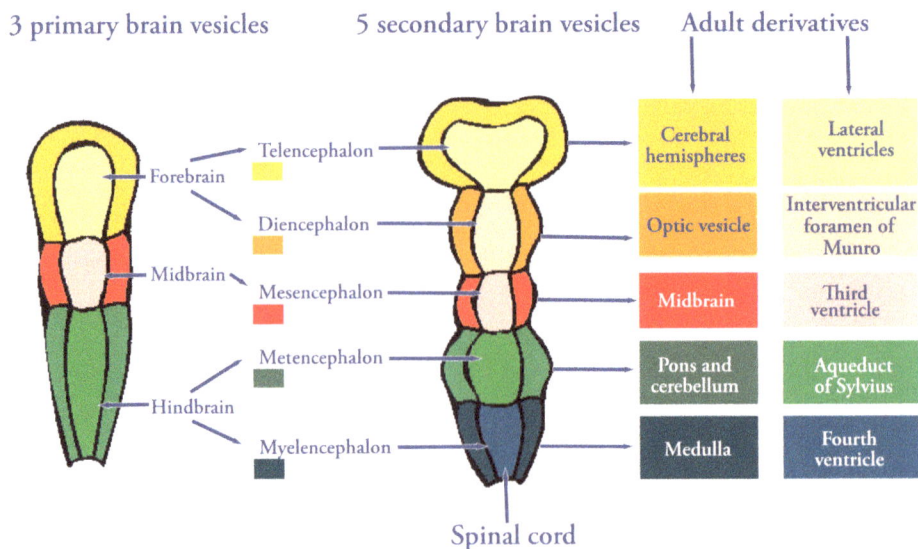

Figure 2.15 Vesicles of the Brain at 5 Weeks

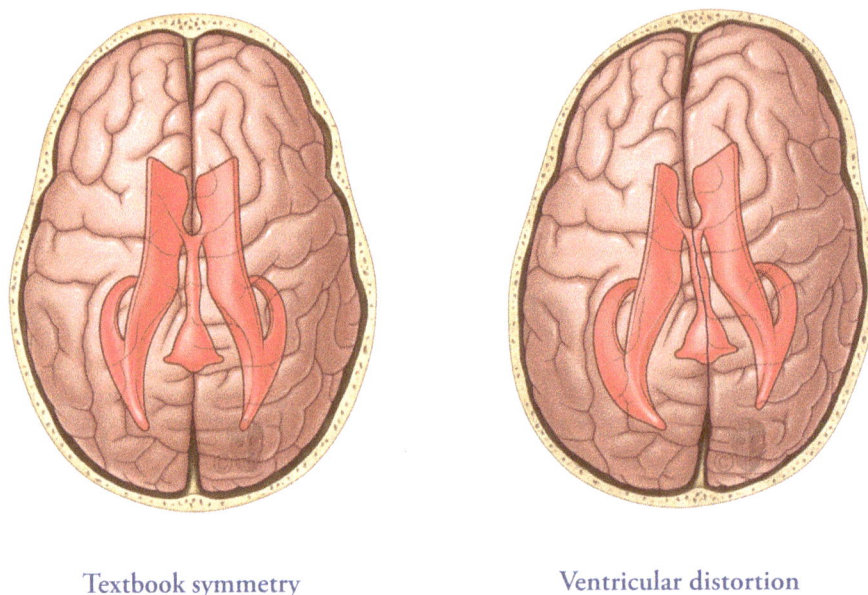

Textbook symmetry   **Ventricular distortion**

Figure 2.16 Ventricular System

The ventricles receive their vascular supply via the circle of Willis. The two lateral ventricles are fed by the two internal carotid arteries, the third ventricle is fed by the basilar artery, and the fourth ventricle by the posterior inferior cerebellar arteries. These arteries are developed from embryonic mesenchyme of the third and fourth pharyngeal/branchial arches during weeks 4 and 5 of embryogenesis.

While the two lateral ventricles lie in the left and right cerebral hemispheres, the interventricular foramen of Monro lies in the midline of the brain and joins the third ventricle. The third ventricle and its drainage into the fourth ventricle, the aqueduct of Sylvius, are all affected by cranio fascial distortion compromising the ability of the dominant system to drain efficiently and effectively.

CEREBELLUM DISTORTION

The cerebellum lies in the occipital fossae, under the tentorium cerebellum, and is separated down the midline of the cerebellum by the falx cerebellum. The tentorium cerebellum is the crescent shaped sceptre of the meningeal dura that separates, horizontally, the occipital lobes superiorly and the cerebellum inferiorly. Its interior concave border is free and between it and the dorsum sellae of the sphenoid there is a large oval opening called the tentorial incisura, which is occupied by the midbrain and the anterior part of the superior vermis of the cerebellum.

At the petrosphenoid articulation and beneath the cavernous sinuses is a recess that is created by an anterolateral evagination of the lower section of the tentorial membrane called the trigeminal cave. It forms a dural pocket that enfolds with the roots and sensory ganglion of the trigeminal nerve.

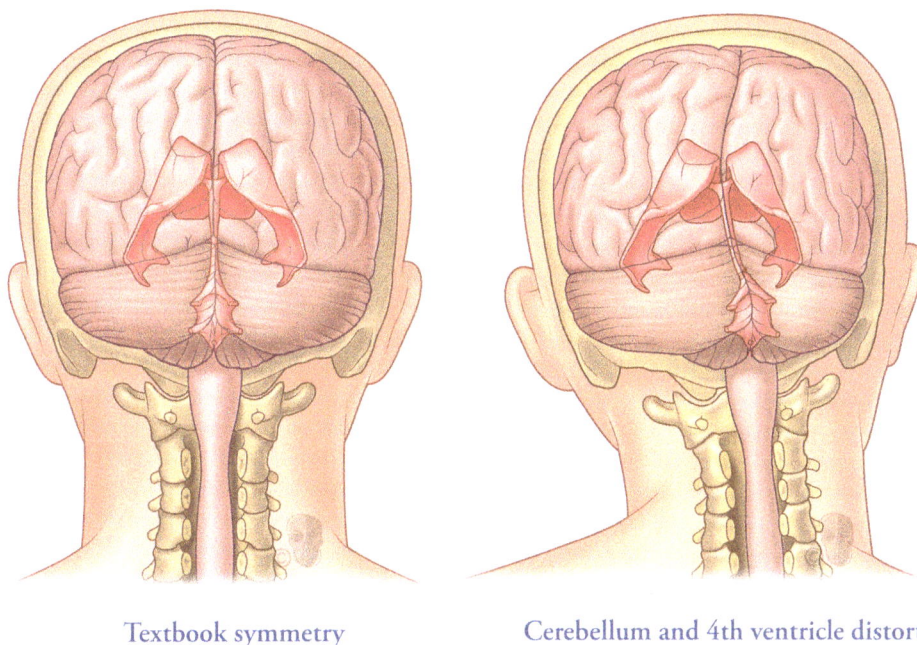

Textbook symmetry   Cerebellum and 4th ventricle distort

Figure 2.17 Cerebellum Distortion

The vertical torsion displayed by the falx cerebelli affects the cerebellar hemispheres, and cerebellar dysfunction is characterised by awkwardness in intentional movements:

- Ataxia – awkwardness in gait and posture
- Asthenia – muscles tire more easily
- Tremors – emphasised jerky movement
- Nystagmus – oscillating movement of the eye (tremors)
- Basal ganglion disorders – Parkinson's chorea (rigid tremor)
- Athetosis –a succession of slow writhing movements
- Hemiballismus – jumping about (flailing) on one side of the body.

Changes at the pons and the brainstem are brought about by a restriction of the dural membrane at the foramen magnum and the endosteal dural membranes and, of course, CSF changes at the cisterna basalis, magnus and pontis that provide the brainstem with a waterbed.

CRANIAL FLOOR VENOUS SINUSES

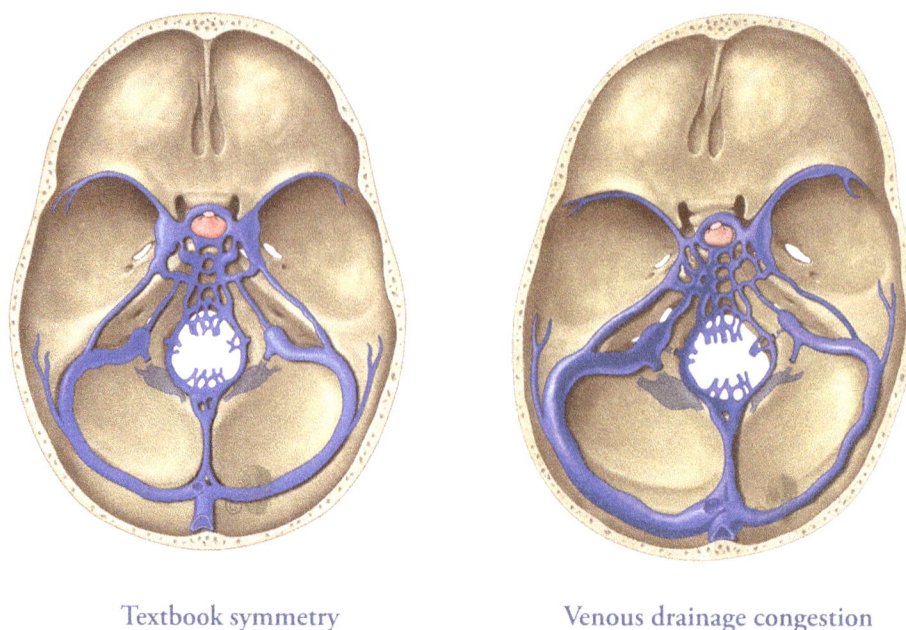

Textbook symmetry   Venous drainage congestion

Figure 2.18 Cranial Floor Venous Drainage

The anterior inferior drainage of the brain occurs at the cavernous and intercavernous sinuses that drain through the basilar plexus and the superior and inferior petrosal sinuses into the transverse sinus and the sigmoid sinus respectively.

The anterior superior drainage of the brain occurs through the superior and inferior sagittal sinuses that drain into the confluence of the sinuses and then through the transverse sinus, the sigmoid sinus and into the internal jugular vein.

Around the foramen magnum the vertebral venous sinuses collect blood from the basilar plexus, the occipital vein and the sub-occipital cavernous sinus.

With cranio fascial distortion the left external temporal gives a far greater drainage potential than the right internal temporal, so the left transverse sinus and the sigmoid sinus leading into the internal jugular vein carry a greater volume of ischaemic blood than its counterpart on the right. This potential is created by the open jugular foramen on the right following the external temporal and occipital bones, while the jugular foramen on the left is more constricted, following the internal temporal and internal occiput.

The depression of the greater wing of the sphenoid also allows more drainage potential than the elevated greater wing on the right, which affects the left cavernous sinus removing more ischaemic blood from that area than on the right side.

TENTORIAL VENOUS DRAINAGE

The tentorium cerebellum encapsulates both the transverse and sigmoid sinuses along the internal occipital boundaries and the petrous portion of the temporal bone, which is where the tentorium is anchored.

As cranio fascial distortion comes into effect, the left temporal and occipital bones move into external rotation and the bilateral taut tentorium is subjected to a torsional twist giving a far greater surface area on the left, opening the transverse and sigmoid sinuses. This allows for a greater volume of blood than its counterpart on the right that now becomes more flaccid and crimped distorting the transverse and sigmoid sinuses as the right temporal and occipital bones go into internal rotation, thus reducing venous flow.

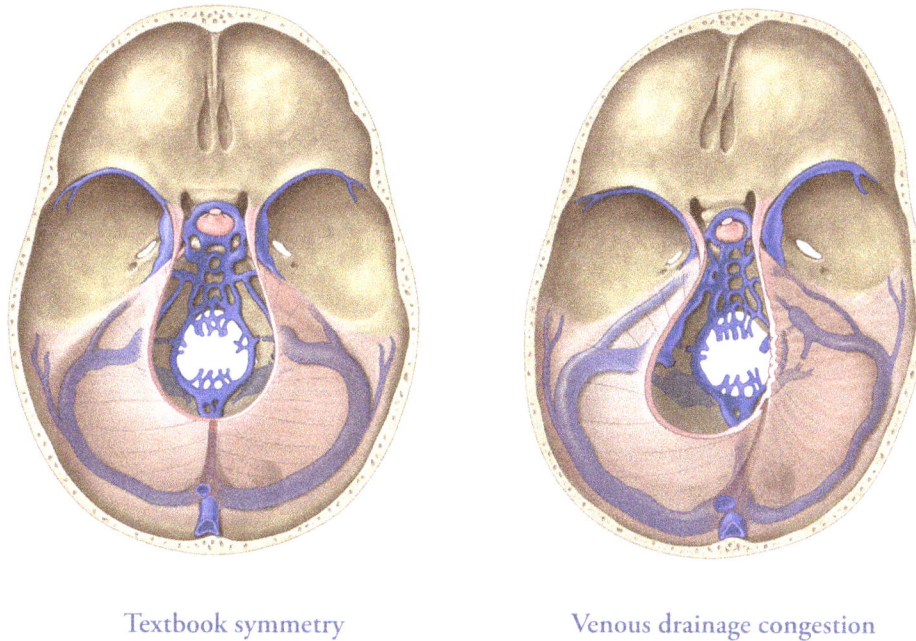

Textbook symmetry   Venous drainage congestion

Figure 2.19 Tentorial Venous Drainage

HAEMODYNAMIC EFFECT OF VENOUS SINUS DRAINAGE

According to *Gray's Anatomy*, the confluence of the sinuses has two separate and distinct passages of drainage flow. While there may be a couple of anastomotic connections between the two pathways at the confluence of the sinuses, they are in fact two separate pathways. The superior sagittal sinus drains into the right transverse sinus, then into the right sigmoid sinus and into the right internal jugular vein – this is the anterior superior drainage. The inferior sagittal sinus drains into the straight sinus, then the left transverse sinus, left sigmoid sinus and into the left internal jugular vein – this is the anterior inferior drainage.

Gray's Anatomy also states that the superior sagittal sinus is a larger vessel than the inferior sagittal sinus and, furthermore, the right transverse and sigmoid sinuses are larger vessels than their left counterpart. Scientific studies also confirm that there is a greater volume of venous blood draining through the right side of the brain at the right internal jugular vein than on the left side of the brain at the left internal jugular vein.

This differential in blood volumes suggests that there is a propensity for the right drainage to drive the brain into a counterclockwise direction, giving rise to a benign counterclockwise asymmetric torque, which is supported by the fact that cranial plates in infancy are islands of osseous bone, encapsulated by periosteal dura and through the influence of brain's counterclockwise activity means these islands of cranial osseous bone are also driven in a counterclockwise direction, giving rise to the larger ocular orbit on the right and a smaller ocular orbit on the left. The sphenoid bone torques in a counterclockwise direction meaning the greater wing on the right moves anterior and superior, while the greater wing on the left moves posterior and inferior, changing the balance of the tentorium cerebelli.

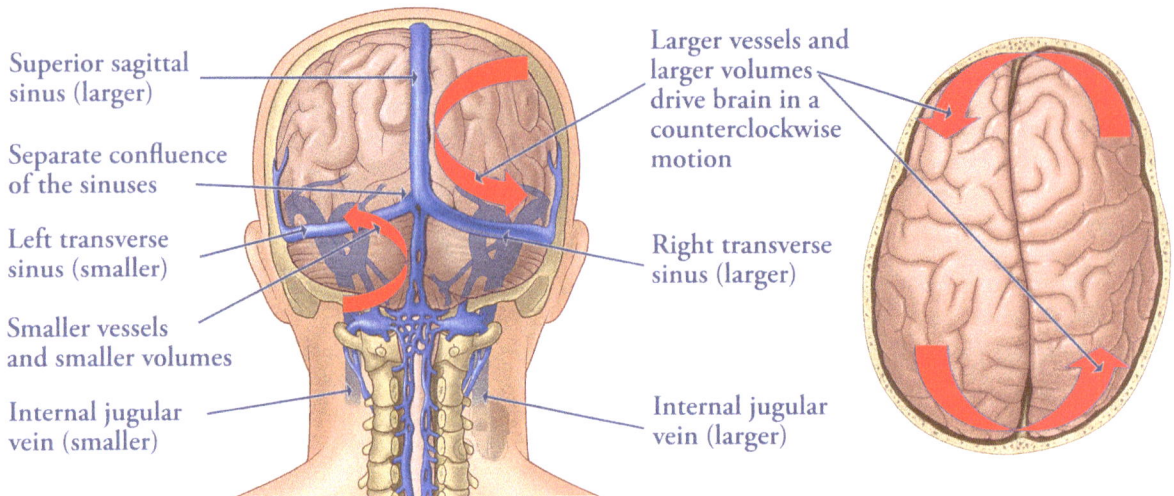

Figure 2.20 Propensity for the Haemodynamic Drainage to Drive the Brain Counterclockwise

This drainage process occurs between weeks 32 and 34 of foetal development and so becomes an integral part of the counterclockwise motion seen in the neonate and throughout life. The outcome is a benign asymmetric counterclockwise torque of the cranial vault.

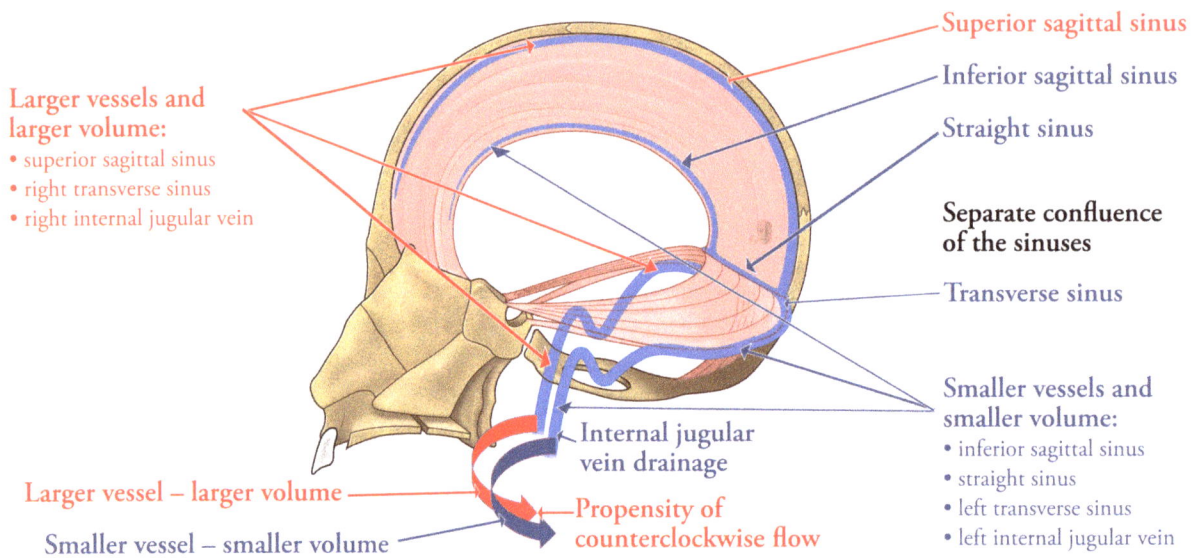

Figure 2.21 Haemodynamic Forces Influence Counterclockwise Motion of the Brain

The right eye is in a bigger orbit and has all the cranial nerves passing through a larger superior orbital fissure. The posterior wall of the socket is made up of the greater and lesser wings of the sphenoid, propelling the eye anterior, superior and more prominent. By comparison, the left eye is compressed posterior and inferior by the smaller (closed) superior orbital fissure on the left. The mandible deviates to the left, as the left glenoid fossa is relatively posterior to the right glenoid fossa.

CONCLUSION

The infant cranium consists of the anterior and posterior fontanelles, the superior sagittal suture, the bregma, the lambda, the two frontal bones, the two parietal bones and the occipital bone. The temporal bones with the frontal and parietal bones form the anterior lateral fontanelle, while the parietal, temporal and occiput form the posterior lateral fontanelles. The fascial distortion in Figure 2.3 is the result of the cranial distortion seen in Figure 2.2.

Tentorium Cerebellum and Falx Cerebri

The tentorium cerebellum is the horizontal membrane that is attached at the anterior and posterior clinoid processes of the sphenoid bone, anteriorly, and at the transverse sinus bilaterally of the occipital bone, and bilaterally at the sigmoid sinuses of the temporal bone on the petrous portion. The falx cerebri, represented in Figure 2.6 as a straight line between the crista galli of the ethmoid bone and the internal occipital protuberance, is the vertical membrane that supports the superior and inferior sagittal sinuses.

Cranial nerve two, the optic nerve, takes information from both retinae, and transfers that information through the optic chiasma to the occipital lobe where the visual centres are maintained.

Pituitary

The pituitary is a small endocrine gland that is an extension of the hypothalamus at the base of the brain and is found in the sella turcica of the body of the sphenoid bone.

Corpus Callosum

The corpus callosum is a wide flat bundle of neural fibres beneath the cortex. It connects left and right cerebral hemispheres and facilitates interhemispheric communication.

Cerebral Fibres

All the commissural fibres are across the midline and are connected to both left and right cerebral hemispheres.

Basal Ganglia

These are the neuronal cell bodies deep within the white matter. They are groups of paired brain nuclei that play a crucial role in the integration and organisation of coordinated motor activity.

Hypothalamus

The hypothalamus is that section of the brain responsible for the production of many of the body's essential hormones and chemical substances that help control different cells and organs.

Limbic System

The limbic system is the centre of our subconscious emotional processing and comprises the cingulate gyrus lying just the above the corpus callosum, and the orbitofrontal and subcallosal gyri of the basal frontal lobes, the dentate and hippocampal gyri and the para hippocampal, and the entorhinal and perirhinal cortices of the medial temporal lobes.

Thalamus

The thalamus consists of two nut-shaped collections of nuclei that lie immediately on either side of the centre of the brain. The thalami play a major role as the relay station for all information transmitted to and from the body. The hypothalamus is a region of many small nuclei with diverse functions located above the midbrain and below the thalamus.

Ventricles (Central Canal at 5 Weeks)

The brain vesicles, the prosencephalon, the mesencephalon and the rhombencephalon basically form the forebrain, the midbrain and the hindbrain. Within those structures are formed the ventricular system, the two laterals, the third and the fourth ventricles.

Cranial Floor Venous Sinuses

The anterior inferior drainage of the brain occurs at the cavernous and intercavernous sinuses that drain through the basilar plexus and the superior and inferior petrosal sinuses into the transverse sinus and the sigmoid sinus respectively.

Tentorial Venous Drainage

The tentorium cerebellum encapsulates both the transverse and sigmoid sinuses along the internal occipital boundaries and the petrous portion of the temporal bone, which is where the tentorium is anchored.

Haemodynamic Effect of Venous Sinus Drainage

The venous sinus drainage, due to the propensity of the force from the right side of the brain, drives the brain into a benign asymmetric counterclockwise torque.

CHAPTER 3

SKELETAL CHANGES

SKELETAL CHANGES

As cranio fascial dynamics (CFD) ensue and become more settled over time, the entire fascial system becomes compromised by the torsional effects of fascial distortion. Being aware of this problem, one has to challenge all the systems that are covered and protected by what was once mesenchyme, as every component, every organ, every vessel, muscle, ligament and tendon, as well as the entire skeletal system will, and does, become influenced by the torsion. Every trauma, whether chemical, emotional or structural will have a compound effect on the efficiency of the entire human body. The partial correction of only some discrepancies will simply render the body less capable of changing the dynamics and the system will continue to deteriorate. One needs to address primary issues, not those which are secondary or tertiary. Primary issues are normally only fascial in nature and these need to be unwound if any headway is to be maintained in the healing process. Dealing in secondary and tertiary issues only produces more compensations and adaptations and confuses body functionality even further. One of the major problems in dealing with the human body is that the early intervention of fascial torsion is not understood and is therefore not taken into account.

NEUROCRANIUM

The neurocranium is divided into two components. These components are devised to maintain the dynamics from the internal structures of the body and the external pressures that are applied to it through its normal everyday function.

The skull is made up of cartilage at the base of the skull in which all the apertures for all the vessels and nerves need access. The cartilage in the early days of growth and development allow for enough rigidity to support and protect all the components that pass through these apertures. As the skull ages and matures the cartilage becomes bone and remains bone throughout its life.

The superstructure of the cranium lies above the cartilaginous element, and this is made up of membrane. The membrane component has a certain amount of agility, which allows the membrane to flex and vary according to the dynamics applied to it during its lifetime. In the early days, while the skull is growing and developing, the sutures and fontanelles that lie mainly in the membranous areas, adapt and compensate, expand and contract, and absorb much of the physical traumas that are applied to them. The membranous part of the skull will always remain as memory and although the fontanelles close there will still be sufficient movement within the sutures to allow the membranes to respire.

RECIPROCATION

When one looks at the spine in front of a plumb line, one is looking to see where the midline plumb is going. Ideally, one would like to see the plumb line bisect the sacrum, the thoracic spine and through the external occipital protuberance, with a level head, shoulders and pelvis. In an ideal world this would represent a physiological norm, as the lines define the vertical line of the pelvis and spine, and the horizontal lines of the base of the cranium, the shoulder girdle, the diaphragm and the pelvic girdle.

The author believes that this model may be misunderstood by anatomists and physiologists, and that for too long the human body has been expected to maintain itself vertically against gravity and the other dynamics that are applied to it.

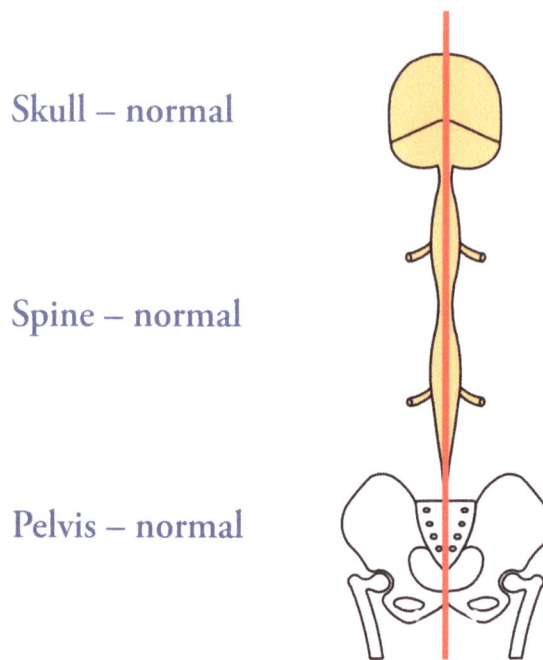

Skull – normal

Spine – normal

Pelvis – normal

Figure 3.1 Reciprocation

SKULL–PELVIS TORQUE

On consideration of the vertical plane assumed by the musculoskeletal system, there are also horizontal planes within that model. One needs to look at the torsional twisting dynamics of the spinal cord, the RTM supporting the brain and the venous sinus system (its drainage), and then the cavitation dynamics of the heart, as one of the hydrostatic systems, and then the liver and its irrigation dynamics as the second cavitation system. When the body is synchronised and structurally balanced, the cavitation of these two systems can work in a homeostatic environment and balance each other in a reciprocal manner.

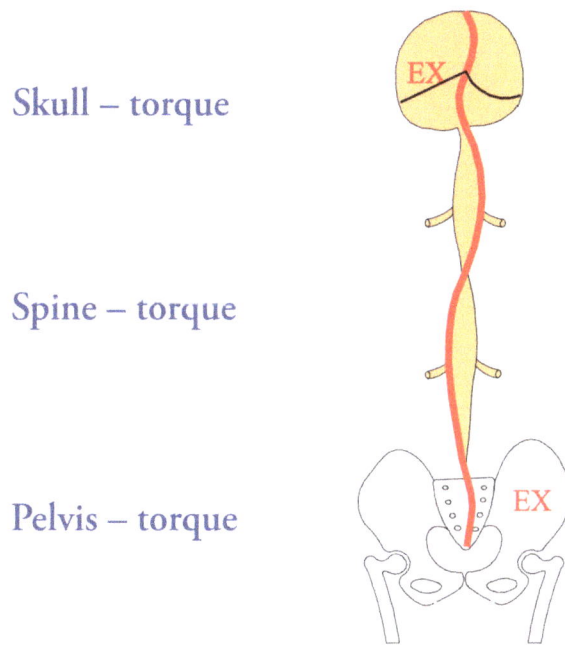

Skull – torque

Spine – torque

Pelvis – torque

Figure 3.2 Skull–Pelvis Torque

INFANT SKULL

Normal Infant Skull

The anterior view of the normal infant skull shows the anterior fontanelle, the coronal suture, the frontal bones, and the two ocular orbits, surrounding the superior orbital fissures between the body and the lesser wing of the sphenoid bone. The face shows the two maxillae bones, the two lacrimal bones and the nasal septum, while the lateral aspect shows the two zygomatic (malar) bones, which act as the lock bone of the skull. The sutures of the frontal bone are the frontozygomatic, the temporozygomatic and the maxillo-frontal. And in this format, the frontal bone keeps the other facial bones in place, acting as a shock absorber when there is activity of the maxillary and mandibular bones, such as chewing, bruxing or grinding. Notice that the mandibular bone is in symmetry with the rest of the face, meaning that the condyles of the mandible are set in their juxtaposition within the mandibular fossae.

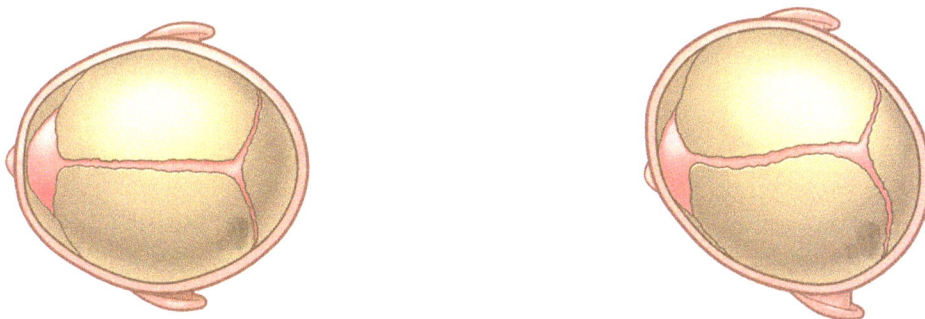

Figure 3.3 Infant Skull: (left) Textbook symmetric; (right) Cranial distortion

Infant Cranial Distortion

The distorted anterior view of the skull shows the right frontal bone in external rotation while the left frontal bone is in internal rotation. Notice too, that the anterior fontanelle has slipped and has moved inferior on the left side. The greater wing of the spheroid has gone superior on the right side and inferior on the left side, meaning the sphenoid bone has slipped. The temporal bone on the left has gone into external rotation taking the mandibular fossa posterior and the mandibular condyle posterior, which is why the mandible deviates to the left in this example. Notice too, the superior orbital fissure on the right is open and that the superior orbital fissure has closed on the left side, compressing all the vessels that pass through that fissure. The left maxillary bone has, as a result, moved posterior and is in internal rotation, while its counterpart on the right side has moved into external rotation.

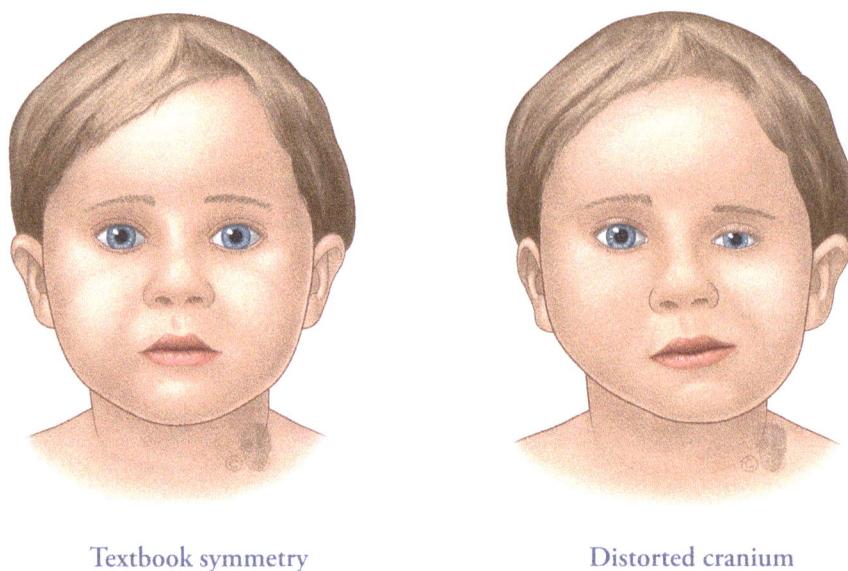

| Textbook symmetry | Distorted cranium |

Figure 3.4 Cranio facial distortion

The facial appearance of the normal skull shows both popular orbits being even and as a result both eyes are attentive and focused. Both ears are externally rotated following the external rotation of the temporal bones bilaterally. There is no deviation of the nasal septum or the nose and the mandible sits evenly and in a balanced position.

The facial distortion of the infant on the right shows the left eye in a posterior position, sunken, inattentive and out of focus. The mandible has deviated to the left, taking with it the labial crease and pulling the mouth over to the left. The left ear is in external rotation following the external temporal bone, while the right ear has gone into internal rotation and has the appearance of being flattened. The right eye is still attentive, focused and appears to be anterior of the left eye.

CAVERNOUS SINUS

Sphenoid

The sphenoid sinus is one pair of four paired paranasal sinuses found in the body of the sphenoid bone under the sella turcica. The cavernous sinus surrounds the sphenoid sinus and is traversed by a number of vessels, including the internal carotid artery. It is bordered laterally by the temporal lobes and the sphenoid bone and is lateral to the sella turcica. The cavernous sinus is filled with venous blood collected from the superior and inferior ophthalmic veins from the eyes and the orbits, discharging through the basilar plexus posteriorly, into the superior and inferior petrosal sinuses then the internal jugular vein. The internal carotid, on leaving the cavernous sinus, turns superiorward to form the anterior communicating artery, then the anterior cerebral artery and the middle cerebral artery of the circle of Willis.

The circle of Willis lies just above the sella turcica and encircles the pituitary stalk, and so lies above the sphenoid body. Torsion to the sphenoid bone with its fascial connectors to the circle of Willis, potentially results in a torque of the circle of Willis, which may explain the high incidence of aneurysms in the anterior and middle cerebral arteries.

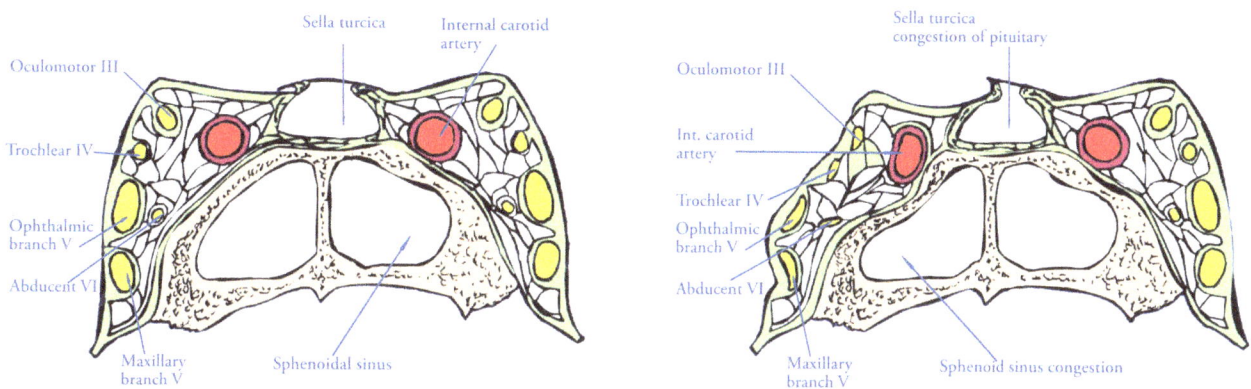

Figure 3.5 Cavernous Sinus – Sphenoid Bone: Distorted sphenoid on right, showing congestion of all nerve and vessel apertures

Figure 3.8 shows a coronal view of the body of the sphenoid bone surrounded laterally by the superior orbital fissures. The superior orbital fissures contain the oculomotor nerve (CN III), the trochlear nerve (CN IV), the ophthalmic division of the trigeminal nerve (CN V 1), the abducens nerve (CN VI) and the maxillary division of the trigeminal nerve (CN V 2). The internal carotid artery lies in the superior position of the superior orbital fissure. The sella turcica lies in the sphenoid body and houses the pituitary gland, suspended by the infundibulum/hypophyseal stalk, while the two sphenoidal sinuses lie just below.

Movement between the greater and lesser wings of the sphenoid would change the dynamics of the superior orbital fissure and cause compression and distortion of the various apertures.

Distorted Sphenoid

The collapse of the right sphenoid body shows congestion of all the apertures through which the aforementioned cranial nerves and internal jugular artery traverse; the collapse of the right sphenoid sinus causes congestion and pressure, while the sella turcica pulls on the infundibulum, distorting and congesting the pituitary. The anterior and posterior clinoid processes surrounding the sella turcica will become distorted and change the position of the tentorium cerebellum, the horizontal dural membrane. This sphenoid distortion can be brought about by direct trauma to the face, changes in the occlusion and the jaw-to-jaw relationship, or trauma to the cranium changing the dynamics of the RTM.

RIGHT SUPERIOR ORBITAL FISSURE AND OPTIC FORAMEN

The superior orbital fissure lies between the greater and lesser wings of the sphenoid bone. This fissure provides the apertures for the following cranial nerves and the ophthalmic artery:

- Trochlear nerve (CN IV)
- Frontal nerve

- Lacrimal nerve
- Ophthalmic nerve (CN V 1) – branch of the trigeminal
- Superior division of the oculomotor nerve (CN III)
- Nasociliary nerve
- Abducens nerve (CN VI)

Then through the optic foramen in the lesser wing of the sphenoid go:

- Optic nerve (CN II)
- Ophthalmic artery

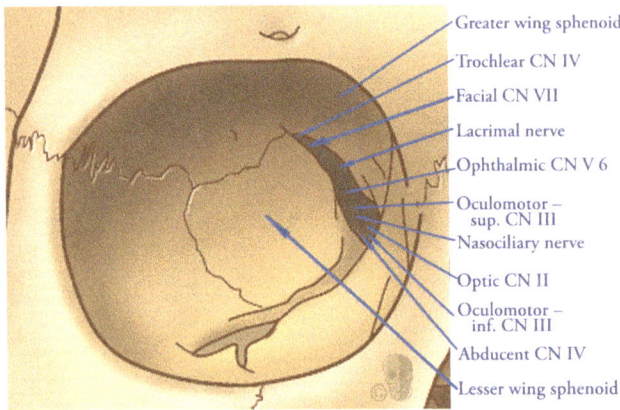

Figure 3.6 Textbok Right Superior Orbital Fissure

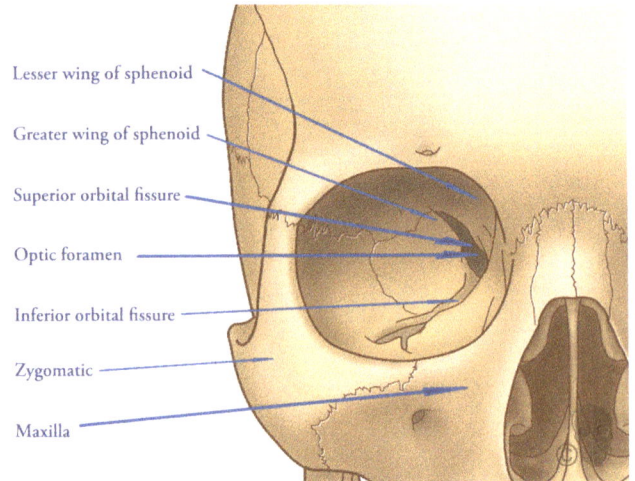

Figure 3.7 Textbook Anterior View of Right Orbital Cavity

The anterior view of the right orbital cavity shows the superior orbital fissure in its relationship with the greater and lesser wings of the sphenoid bone. The superior orbital fissure with all its contents was discussed previously. The greater wing of the sphenoid frames the eyeball and as such directly influences its position. When the greater wing of the sphenoid becomes distorted and rotated then the eye is pushed into a pronounced position (exophthalmic) or compressed. This will obviously cause tautness in the optic nerve and in the other three cranial nerves responsible for positioning the eye within the socket. The inferior orbital fissure acts as a housing for the lateral pterygoid muscle.

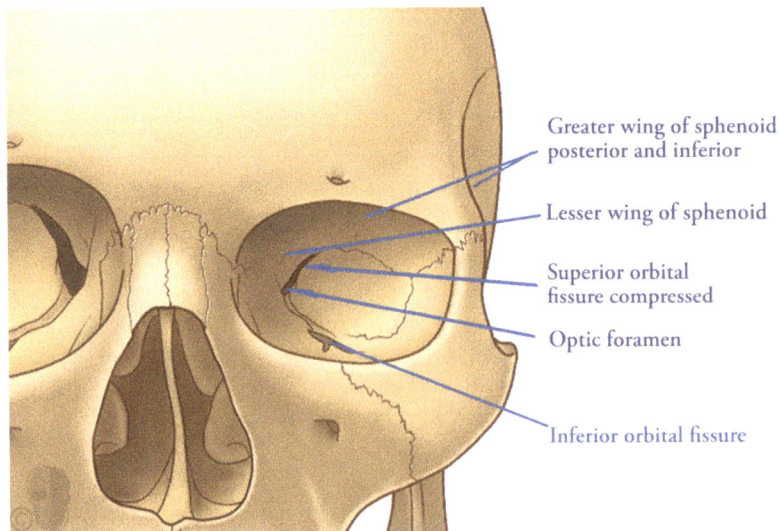

Figure 3.8 Distortion of Left Ocular Orbit

Distortion of the left orbital fissure

Distortion of the left orbital fissure usually occurs when the sphenoid bone collapses on that side and follows the external temporal and the posterior mandibular fossa. This usually suggest that the condyle of the mandible has been jammed posterior against the retrodiscal tissue and creates temporomandibular joint dysfunction (TMJD), ultimately affecting the vestibular mechanism, changing hearing and balance. The superior orbital fissure that contains several cranial nerves and the ophthalmic artery, will ultimately be compressed and compromise the optimal function of those nerves. As the greater and lesser wings of the sphenoid become torqued, one twists left with the other twisting right, shifting the anterior surface of the greater wing of the sphenoid anterior on one side and posterior on the other, affecting the orientaion of the eye in the socket.

INFANT SPHENOID

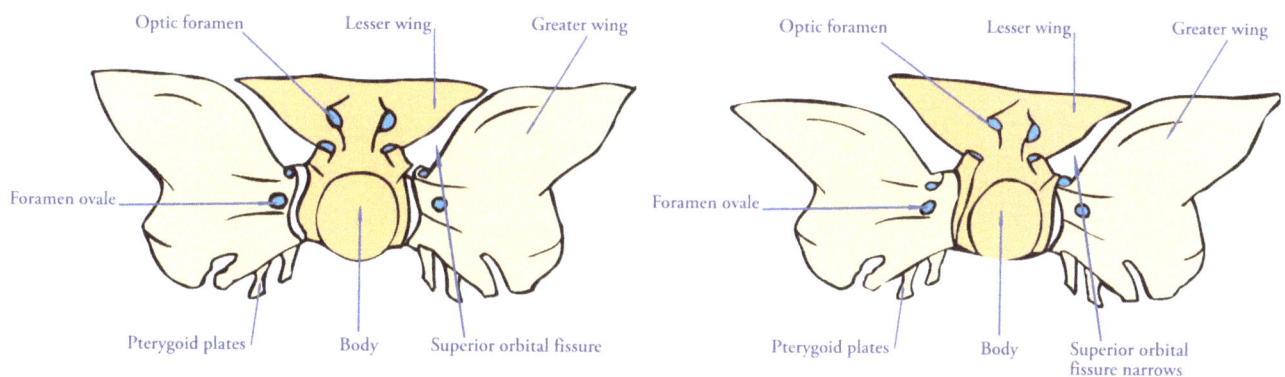

Figure 3.9 (left) Textbook Symmetric Infant Sphenoid
Figure 3.10 (right) Distorted Infant Sphenoid: Foramen occlude, congesting cranial nerves; pterygoid plates distort affecting pterygoid muscle tonus

Normal Infant Sphenoid

The normal infant sphenoid is made up of three components: the body, which is generated in cartilage and will become bone; the lesser wing of the sphenoid (also generated in cartilage); and the greater wing of the sphenoid, generated in membrane (which remains as membrane throughout life). Attached to the greater wings of the sphenoid are the lateral and medial pterygoid plates. These are the origins for the medial and lateral pterygoid muscles. Both these muscles are attached to the condyles of the mandible and have the effect of pulling the mandible either laterally or medially, depending on the occlusion. Malocclusions will change the dynamics of the pterygoid muscles, which then change the position of the greater wing of the sphenoid, changing the position and spacing of the superior orbital fissure and affecting all the nerves and arteries traversing that aperture. The body of the sphenoid contains the sella turcica that houses the pituitary gland, and around the perimeter are the anterior and posterior clinoid processes, the attachments for the tentorium cerebellum. The optic chiasma lies over the body of the sphenoid.

Distorted Infant Sphenoid

The fact that the sphenoid bone is the central bone of the skull, means that it comes under many influences from many different directions. The tentorium cerebellum, with its posterior anchor at the occiput and attachments at the temporal bone (along the petrous portion), is a significant force which, when one considers its anterior anchor, points at the anterior and posterior clinoids of the sphenoid. Changes in the sacrum distorting the occiput change the tentorium and torque the sphenoid. Similarly, changes with the ilia have a torsional effect on their reciprocal temporal bones, particularly with the petrous portion and its interlinkage at the sphenobasilar junction. The temporal torque will also affect the tentorium and again the sphenoid.

Anteriorly any change to the ethmoid/sphenoid junction will affect the stability of the sphenoid. From the maxillary/mandibular junction, tooth to tooth contact at the occlusion can change the bite, altering the smooth movement of the mandible, and affect the lateral and medial pterygoid muscles, which attach from the mandibular condyles onto the lateral and medial pterygoid plates of the sphenoid, again changing its juxtaposition. Fluctuations in components of the sphenoid may change the body, the lesser wings and the greater wings, altering the optimum function of several cranial nerves, the cavernous and intercavernous sinuses, the carotid artery, the optic chiasma and the pituitary.

TEMPORAL BONE AT BIRTH

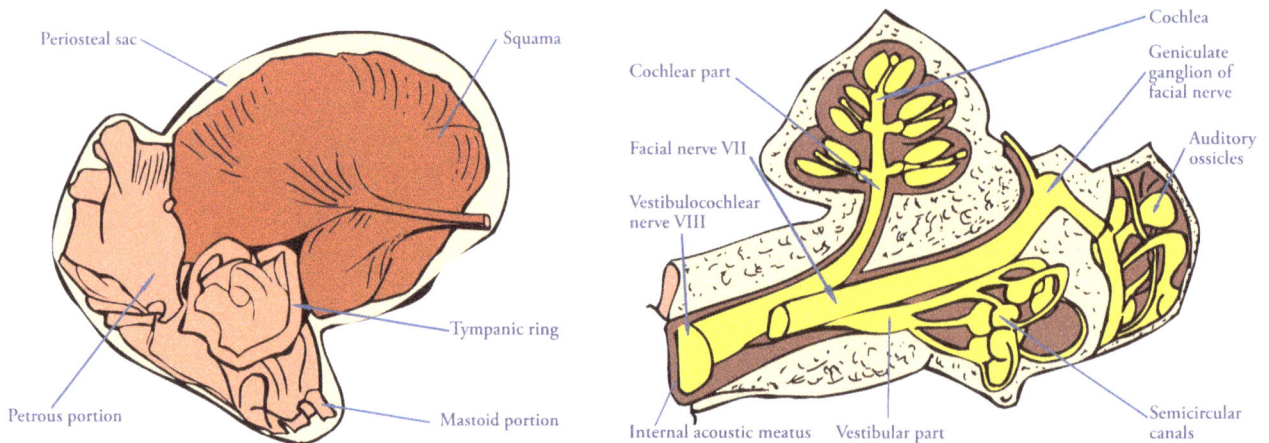

Figure 3.11 (left) Textbook Temporal Bone at Birth: Outer aspect
Figure 3.12 (right) Textbook Internal Acoustic Meatus of the Temporal Bone

At birth, the temporal bone comprises three different embryological components. The mastoid portion, including the petrous portion, are made from cartilage (later to become bone), and the temporal squama and the tympanic ring are made from membrane and remain as membrane throughout life. These three components are generated embryologically and retained in a periosteal sac, through birth until ossification of the skull at about three years old. Probably 90% of the cranium will ossify around this age and the remaining 10% will take place over several years to allow the brain to grow and adapt normally. Until the age of three there is a stiffening of the sutures when a more protective covering ensues, as the brain enlarges and needs further protection. The petrous portion of the temporal bone acts as a conduit, and is called the internal acoustic meatus, and contains the facial (CN VII) and acoustic (CN VIII) nerves. The peripheral vestibular system is an integral part of the labyrinth that lies in the otic capsule in the petrous portion and consists of five distinct end organs: three semicircular canals sensitive to head rotation and position; and two otolith organs sensitive to linear (straight) movement. The mastoid functions as an origin for the sternocleidomastoid (SCM) muscle.

Distortion of Infant Temporal Bone

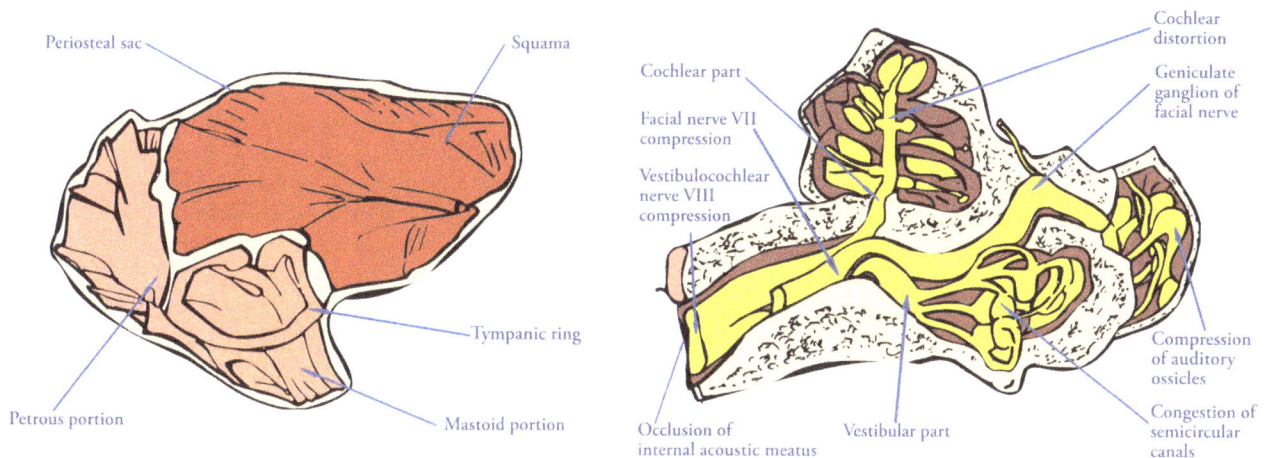

Figure 3.13 (left) Distortion of Infant Temporal Bone: Distortion of internal acoustic meatus, affecting hearing components and cochlea vestibular mechanism
Figure 3.14 (right) Distortion of Internal Acoustic Meatus of the Temporal Bone

Birth trauma can disturb the periosteal sac containing the three components of the temporal bone. Disturbing their individual balanced relationships can change the internal acoustic meatus and affect both the facial and the acoustic (vestibulocochlear) nerves, the cochlea (auditory portion of the inner ear), auditory ossicles (incus, stapes and malleus, which transmit sounds from the air to the cochlea), and the semicircular canals (balance and head position). When this happens early on in life, the child could be handicapped by poor hearing (thus affecting speech), learning disabilities, hyperacusis and balance problems (learning how to walk). Behavioural issues and social exclusion are also part of this syndrome. Later on in life these problems can arise as a result of cranial distortion, TMJD and physical trauma. Tinnitus, as a result of mandibular condyle congestion in the mandibular fossa could possibly cause excessive wax to build up resulting in poor hearing. Invariably, this is resolved by syringing out the ear and reducing the wax (i.e. treating the effects not the cause), resulting in a loss of hearing at the top and lower ends of the range, ultimately deafness, loss of balance and that person, not wishing to become a social pariah, becomes a recluse. Tic douloureux, Bell's palsy and trigeminal neuralgia are also by-products of temporal bone distortion and vestibular changes.

NORMAL INFANT OCCIPUT

The normal infant occiput is made up of four components. The basilar and two condylar components are made up of cartilage – which becomes bone later on in life – and the occipital squama is made up of membrane – which stays as membrane throughout life. These four components surround the foramen magnum through which the brainstem exits the skull. On either lateral side of the condylar components, where the occiput joins the temporal bone, lies the jugular foramen through which the glossopharyngeal (CN IX), the vagus (CN X) and the spinal accessory (CN XI) cranial nerves exit. A very important drainage vessel, the internal jugular vein, also exits through this aperture. The hypoglossal (CN XII) cranial nerve exits through the hypoglossal canal that lies adjacent to the condyles. The condyles of the occiput articulate with the condyles of the atlas, while the vertebral venous plexus and the vertebral arteries are contained by the atlanto-occipital membrane. The basal portion of the occiput buttresses against the body of the sphenoid bone, and early in life the sphenobasilar junction acts as an expansion joint for the base of the skull and allows full flexion and extension of the cranium.

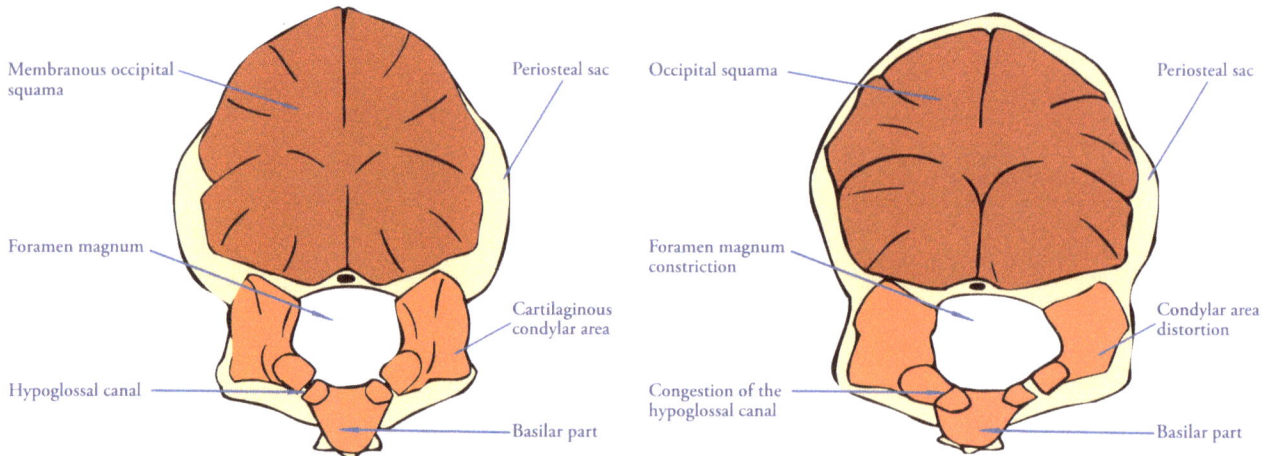

Figure 3.15 (left) Textbook Infant Occiput
Figure 3.16 (right) Distorted Infant Occiput: Misaligned relationship between occiput and atlas; constricted brainstem and medulla oblongata

By the age of 18 the sphenobasilar junction ossifies and consolidates the strength of the cranial base. The internal occipital protuberance attaches the conference of the sinuses, joining the straight vein of Galen to the transverse sinuses – the major drainage vessels of the brain. At the same point on the external surface of the occiput lies the external occipital protuberance – a heavy outcrop of bone – which extends bilaterally to form the nuchal line, where all the paravertebral muscles attach. These two junction points on either side of the occiput allow the head to be kept vertical and straight by the paravertebral muscles externally and counterbalance the internal dynamics of the tentorium cerebellum.

Distorted Infant Occiput

Early trauma to the occiput will change and distort the four components of the occipital bone. When the squama distorts, the internal and external occipital protuberances shift and change the equilibrium of the tentorium internally, and the nuchal line externally, changing head posture and cranial drainage, as well as twisting the atlanto-occipital membrane, crimping the two vertebral arteries and the vertebral venous plexus, congesting the sub-occipital drainage potential. The condylar components, when distorted, change the alignment of the condyles with the condyles of the atlas, creating a subluxation at the atlanto-occipital junction. The effect of this subluxation impinges on the spinal nucleus of the trigeminal nerve and will always have a negative effect on trigeminal function. The hypoglossal canal distortion will also compress the hypoglossal nerve. The jugular foramen will also distort bilaterally, compressing the three pairs of cranial nerves that exit through this foramen and the internal jugular vein, affecting brain drainage. The sphenobasilar junction will also distort the cranial base at the sphenoid junction, changing the juxtaposition of the sphenoid and affecting all its neurology.

CONCLUSION

Skeletal Changes

As CFD develop and become more established, the entire fascial system becomes involved in the torsional effects of fascial distortion.

Basement Membrane

As in any building construction, engineers working on site construct scaffolding to establish a template as a basis for the future building. This template will include levels (horizontal and vertical), weight-bearing structures to maintain the load, moments to clarify structural support for the roof, windows and doors.

Concrete Pour

Once the template has been built and checked, concrete can be poured into the channels that will eventually replicate the walls, the arches and the superstructure of the building.

Concrete Cure

Once the concrete has been cured, the engineered structure will be rigid and resilient, and at this stage the reinforced scaffolding can be removed. This concrete structure now resembles the architectural design given to the engineers for building on site.

Neurocranium

The neurocranium is divided into two components. These components are devised to maintain the dynamics from the internal structures of the body and the external pressures that are applied to it through its normal everyday functions. The skull is made up of cartilage at its base through which all the apertures for all the vessels and nerves need access.

Reciprocation

When one looks at the spine in front of a plumb line, one is looking to see where the midline plumb is going. Ideally, one would like to see the plumb line bisect the sacrum, the thoracic spine and through the external occipital protuberance, with a level head, shoulders and pelvis.

Skull – Pelvic Torque

When one considers the vertical plane assumed by the muscular-skeletal system, there are also horizontal planes within that model, from cranium to pelvis.

Infant Skull

- Normal skull
- Distorted infant skull

Cavernous Sinus – Sphenoid

The relationship between the cavernous and intercavernous sinuses around the anterior body of the sphenoid.

Superior Orbital Fissure

The aperture created by the greater and lesser wings of the sphenoid to carry vessels to the eyes, palate and forebrain.

Infant Sphenoid Bone

Showing the embryological formation of the sphenoid, with the body, pterygoid plates, and the lesser wings and greater wings. The early sphenobasilar junction, where flexion and extension of the infant skull occurs during growth and development, before the adult skull appears, forming an ossification of the sphenobasilar joint at about 18 years old, where this junction becomes fixed.

Infant Temporal Bone

The tympanic ring shows the cartilaginous component of the temporal bone, including the petrous portion, where the temporomandibular joint is formed, and the external auditory meatus and the specialised and delicate tympanic membrane reside. The membranous components are the mastoid and squamosal portions of the temporal bone, which allow for flexibility of the dural membrane system, after the strong anchor point areas along the petrous portion of the temporal bone.

Infant Occipital Bone

The occiput is in four segments.

The two condylar areas are made of cartilage that articulates with the condyles of the atlas – strong weight-bearing components for supporting the weight of the skull around the foramen magnum – and carry the main arteries and blood into the brain, and the various veins and venous plexuses that drain the brain.

The basilar portion of the occiput is also generated in cartilage to provide a strong link to the sphenoid body – the sphenobasilar junction – which in the early infant skull allows for compensatory movement and adaptation before puberty. Between these two bones lies the petrous portion of the temporal bone, also generated in cartilage to obtain maximum movement at the jugular foramen and the carotid canal.

The occipital squama lies to the posterior part of the foramen magnum, up to the internal occipital protuberance and along the insertion for the tentorium cerebellum. This consists of cartilage and provides strong attachments both inside the skull for the tentorium cerebellum, and outside the skull to form the nuchal line supporting the strong erector spinae muscles holding the body upright. Above that line the rest of the squama is made of membrane, again allowing flexibility and compensation for the pubescent years.

CHAPTER 4

RECIPROCAL TENSION MEMBRANES

The RTM comprise the vertical membranes – the falx cerebri, the falx cerebelli, and the horizontal membranes – the tentorium cerebellum and the diaphragma sellae. These membranes support and maintain the brain in a normal homeostatic position within the cranium, as well as supporting the venous sinus system, the important irrigation system of the brain. The RTM also place the brain in a position to facilitate all the cranial apertures and allow full access for all the arteries, veins and nerves to work at their optimum. These RTM are also part of the dural meningeal fascial system that supports the spinal cord within the spinal canal of the vertebral column, allowing the twenty-four pairs of spinal nerve roots to exit the intervertebral foramena at each vertebral level for normal neurological transmission from the brain to targeted organs. CSF bathes the entire brain, spinal cord and all the spinal nerve roots, from the ventricles to the cisterns to the subarachnoid space and finally into the superior sagittal sinus, completing the CSF circulation and drainage.

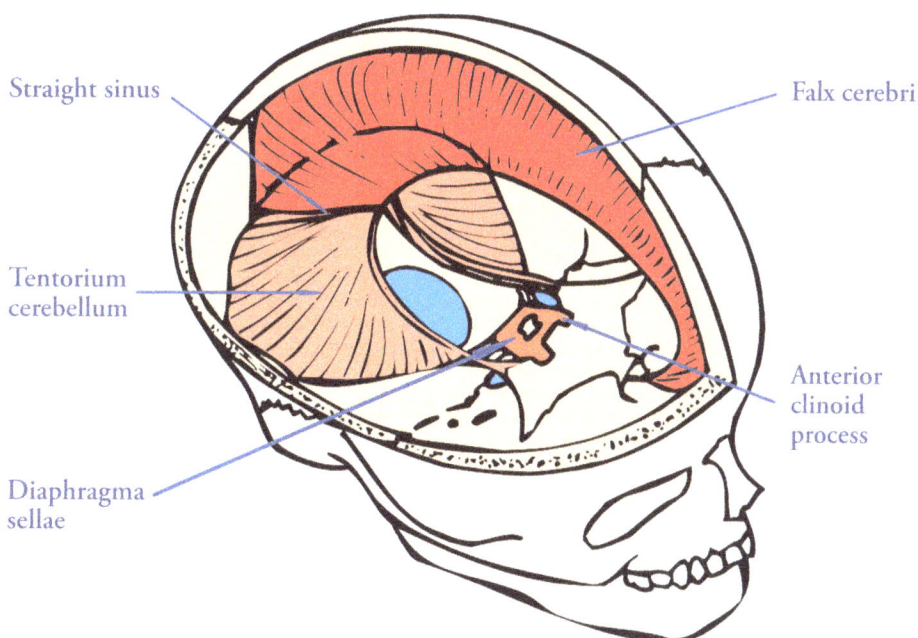

Figure 4.1 Reciprocal Tension Membranes

The RTM attach to all the cranial bones within the cranial vault. The vertical sickle-shaped falx cerebri and falx cerebelli separate the left and right lobes of the brain and cerebellum and support the superior and inferior sagittal sinuses. The anterior attachment is at the crista galli of the ethmoid bone while the posterior attachment is at the internal occipital protuberance. The superior sagittal sinus lies directly beneath the superior sagittal suture that divides the parietal bones. The horizontal membrane is the double layered tentorium cerebellum, which anchors anteriorly at the clinoid processes of the sphenoid bone, and posteriorly at the occiput, at the internal occipital protuberance and along the transverse sinuses, and at the petrous portion of the temporal bone at the sigmoid sinus. The junction between the occiput and the sphenoid bone (the sphenobasilar synchondrosis) has always been considered the midline fulcrum point of the cranium, where the skull has the ability to flex and extend. However, the sphenobasilar synchondrosis fuses at about the age of 20 and loses the ability to flex and extend. Note too, that while all the other cranial bones involved in motion have membrane attachments at their motion points, the sphenobasilar synchondrosis becomes a fused junction without any membranous attachments across that joint.

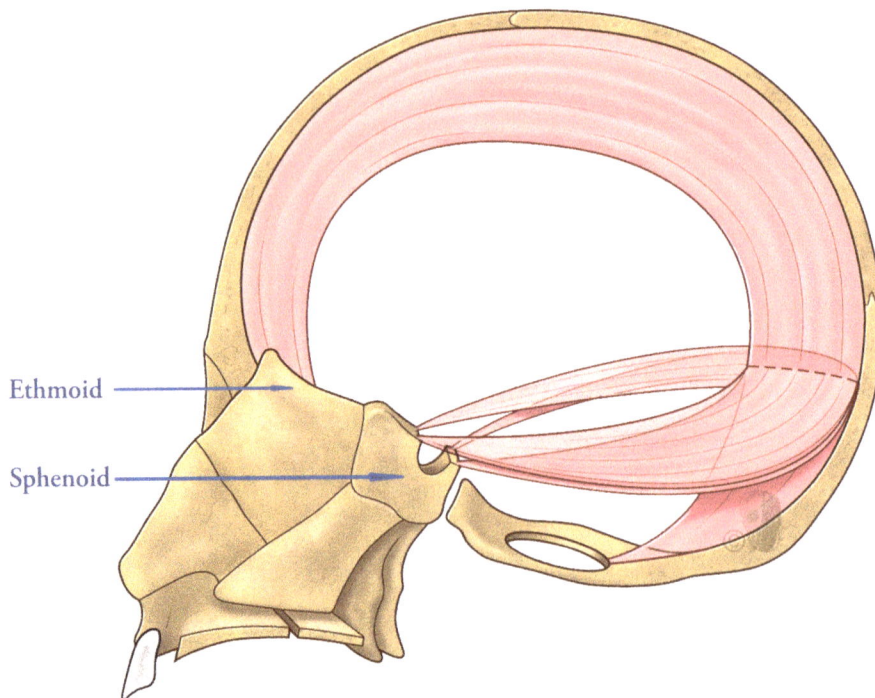

Ethmoid

Sphenoid

Figure 4.2 Reciprocal Tension Membranes: Ethmoid–sphenoid fulcrum

ANTERIOR POLE

The internal dynamics of cranial function and cranial motion have been misunderstood and poorly identified for many years. The sphenobasilar synchondrosis has historically been responsible for cranial motion, but when this junction fuses at around the age of 20, it ceases to become a functional component. The anterior and posterior poles are the more dynamic and functional structures that are responsible for membrane integrity. The anterior pole is the crista galli of the ethmoid bone, which anchors the anterior part of the falx cerebri. The posterior part of the falx cerebri anchors at the internal occipital protuberance and the straight sinus. From the straight sinus, the falx cerebelli – the continuation of the falx cerebri – attaches and continues vertically to anchor at the posterior part of the foramen magnum, while encapsulating the occipital sinus at the posterior margin.

The ethmoid bone articulates posteriorly with the body of the sphenoid, and inferiorly with the anterior border of the vomer. The inferior surface of the vomer, in turn, articulates with the superior plate of the maxilla. Dr Mark Pick explains the ethmoid–sphenoid junction in his book, *Cranial Sutures*:

> Slightly gouged to fill the ethmoid's medial condylar surface, the sphenoid's medial
> socket extends to the posterior margin of the ethmoid's cribriform plate. The
> sphenoid's lateral articular surfaces are positioned posteriorly deeper into the

suture's articular seam; they repeatedly display scooped out condylar pockets that appear to function as rocking surfaces for the adjacent pseudo-condylar projections of the ethmoid. Because of its condylar configurations anteroposterior rocking is the primary mode of motion. However, the pliability of the ethmoid's membranous osseous nature also appears to sanction transverse or multidirectional oblique gliding.

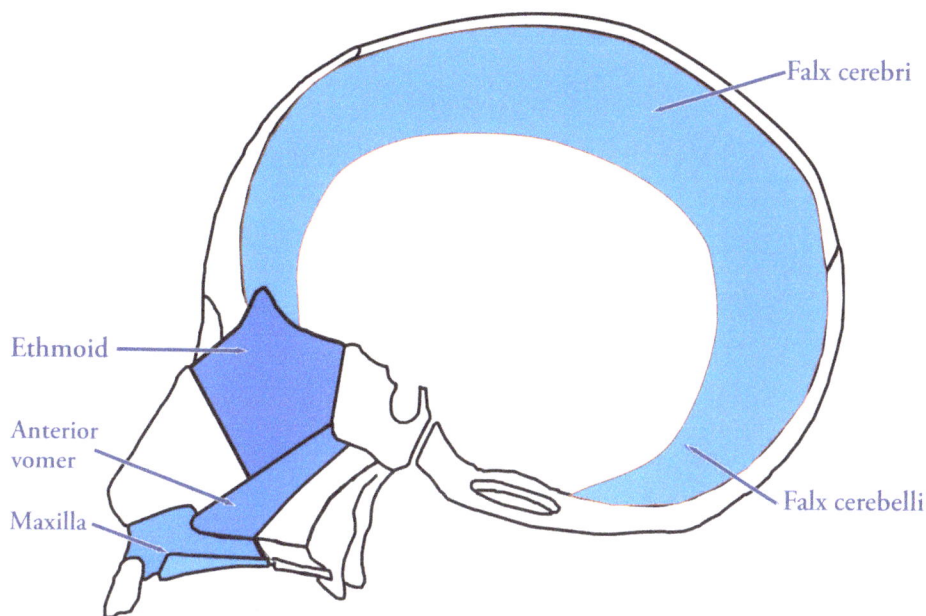

Figure 4.3 Anterior Pole: Ethmoid, falx cerebri, vertical component

POSTERIOR POLE

The posterior pole is the body of the sphenoid, which anchors the tentorium cerebellum at the anterior and, posteriorly, the clinoid processes which surround the sella turcica. There are two layers of membrane that make up the tentorium. The superior layer, as an extension of the falx cerebri, attaches to the anterior clinoids, while the lower layer, an extension of the falx cerebelli, attaches to the posterior clinoids. The attachments of the tentorium at the clinoid processes form the fourth cranial membrane, also a horizontal membrane, the diaphragma sella. This is a small dual membrane that surrounds and supports the hypophyseal stalk of the pituitary.

The anterior body of the sphenoid articulates with the posterior aspect of the ethmoid, while the inferior body of the sphenoid articulates with the superior aspect of the vomer. The posterior body of the vomer runs adjacent to the pterygoid plates of the sphenoid, while the inferior aspect of the vomer articulates with the superior plate of the palatines. So the palate comprises of two maxillae and two palatines, which are joined sagittally at the intermaxillary and interpalatine sutures, and coronally at the palatomaxillary suture. These four bones are activated by respiration, and in turn, through the palate, activate the vomer, and both the anterior and posterior portions, which then activate the ethmoid and the sphenoid. Using the palate as a contact point, the ethmoid and sphenoid are brought into synchronous function, facilitating movement on the vertical and horizontal dural membranes. These actions are also brought about by tongue thrust and swallowing.

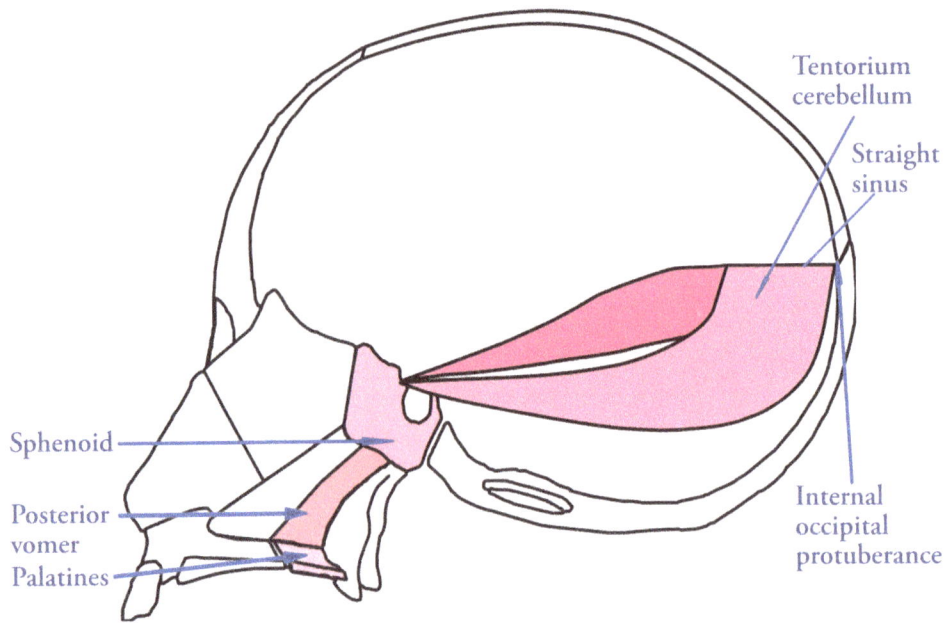

Figure 4.4 Posterior Pole: Sphenoid, tentorium, horizontal vector

Anterior and Posterior Pole

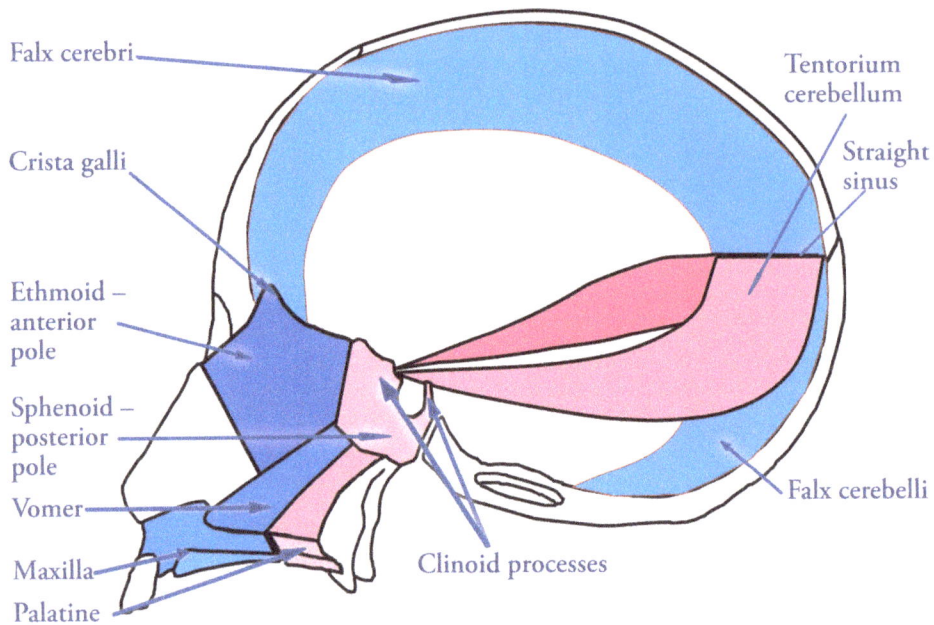

Figure 4.5 Anterior and Posterior Poles: Hinge suture between the ethmoid and sphenoid

The combined effect of the RTM and their anchor points within the cranium provide the cranium with a pulse, rhythm and cranial motion. Cranial motion is a part of cranio sacral function/rhythm, a part of diaphragmatic respiration and cardiovascular activity. All these rhythms and pulses allow for brain activity (thought, memory, concentration and processing), blood in through the circle of Willis and out through the venous sinuses. On the peripheral boundaries of the cranial RTM are venous sinuses that collect ischaemic blood from the brain. This is removed through the superior and inferior sagittal sinuses (falx cerebri) to the confluence of the sinuses along the transverse sinuses, and sigmoid sinuses (tentorium cerebellum) into the internal jugular vein. For this drainage system to work, all the vessels (venous sinuses) need to be open, fully dilated and straight. If the dural membranes are taut, fully expanded and at their maximum surface tension, then the venous sinuses will drain efficiently. When the cranial membranes become distorted the membranes become crimped, warp the venous sinuses and reduce the flow and drainage capability. Cranial homoeostasis depends on all the components maintaining the membrane system to be symmetric, the dynamics within (endosteum) and without (periosteum), the skull balanced, and the fluid ebbing and flowing (entering and exiting) in equal volume.

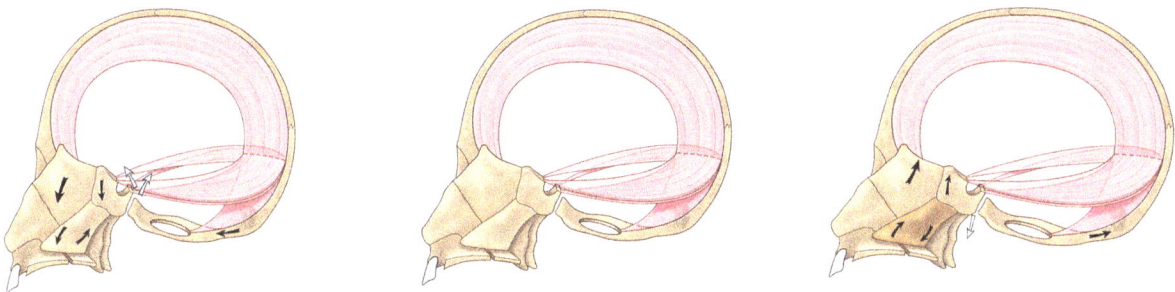

Figure 4.6 (left) Cranial Flexion; (centre) Cranial Neutral; (right) Cranial Extension

CRANIAL FLEXION

Cranial flexion occurs during respiration – the inhalation phase. The falx cerebri and the falx cerebelli arch in a superior inferior direction, tightening the superior and inferior sagittal sinuses and the occipital sinus, pulling on the straight sinus and opening the confluence of the sinuses. The tentorium cerebellum is pulled together at the anterior and posterior anchor points – the sphenoid, the occiput and the temporal bones – tightening the transverse and sigmoid sinuses and the internal jugular vein. While the diaphragma sellae becomes contracted between the anterior and posterior clinoid processes, constricting the hypophyseal stalk at the hypophyseal plexus and activating the hypothalamus.

Anteriorly, the activity of the vomer follows the external rotation of the maxillae and the internal rotation of the palatines, pulling the ethmoid bone inferiorly, while the sphenoid body moves superiorly. This ensures that the ethmoid and sphenoid bodies move in opposite directions, activating membrane dynamics – the anterior and posterior poles.

CRANIAL NEUTRAL

Cranial neutral shows all the RTM in asymmetric and balanced position. The vertical membranes separate the left and right brain, and left and right cerebellum. The horizontal membranes separate the brain from the cerebellum. The ethmoid and sphenoid bones lie in juxtaposition, supported by the vomer which, in turn, lies on the superior surfaces of the maxillae and palatine bones.

CRANIAL EXTENSION

Cranial extension occurs during respiration – the exhalation phase. The falx cerebri and the falx cerebelli flatten in a superior inferior direction, relaxing the superior and inferior sagittal sinuses and the occipital sinus, pulling on the straight sinus and relaxing the confluence of the sinuses. The tentorium cerebellum is relaxed at the anterior and posterior anchor points – the sphenoid, the occiput and the temporal bones – loosening the transverse and sigmoid sinuses and the internal jugular vein. While the diaphragma sellae becomes relaxed between the anterior and posterior clinoid processes, freeing the hypophyseal stalk at the hypophyseal plexus, pumping the hypothalamus.

Anteriorly, the activity of the vomer follows the internal rotation of the maxillae and the external rotation of the palatines, allowing the ethmoid bone to move superiorly, while the sphenoid body moves inferiorly. This ensures that the ethmoid and sphenoid bodies moves in opposite directions activating the membrane dynamics – the anterior and posterior poles.

Parachutes

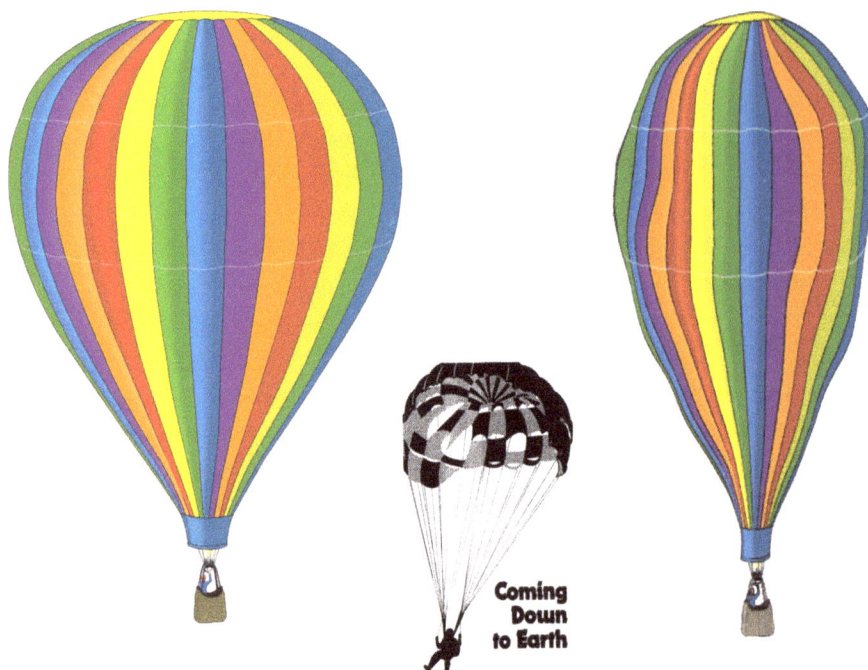

Figure 4.7 Parachutes

Figure 4.7 shows how all the ropes pulling on the parachute canopy are required to bring the parachutist to earth safely. If there is a malfunction with the canopy, caused by asymmetric rope activity, then air will escape from the canopy and it will collapse, creating a loss of resistance for the parachutist. In the same way all the RTM need to be symmetric and have the same amount of pull on the membranes if homoeostasis is to be maintained. Changes in these dynamics will add to stasis and malfunction physiologically. Some use a plumb line to define the vertical aspects of the spine and look carefully at the horizontal levels including angles at the head, the shoulder and pelvis. Changes in these dynamics will disrupt stasis and cause physiological malfunction.

DURAL MEMBRANE INNERVATION

Branches of the trigeminal, vagus and the first three cervical spinal nerves and branches from the sympathetic trunk pass to the dura. The dura contains numerous sensory endings, they are sensitive to stretching that can result in debilitating headaches. Stimulation of the sensory endings of the trigeminal nerve above the level of the tentorium cerebellum, produces referred pain to an area of skin on the same side of the head. Stimulation of the dural endings below the level of the tentorium produce pain referred to the back of the neck and the back of the scalp, along the distribution of the greater occipital nerve.

ATLAS SUBLUXATION

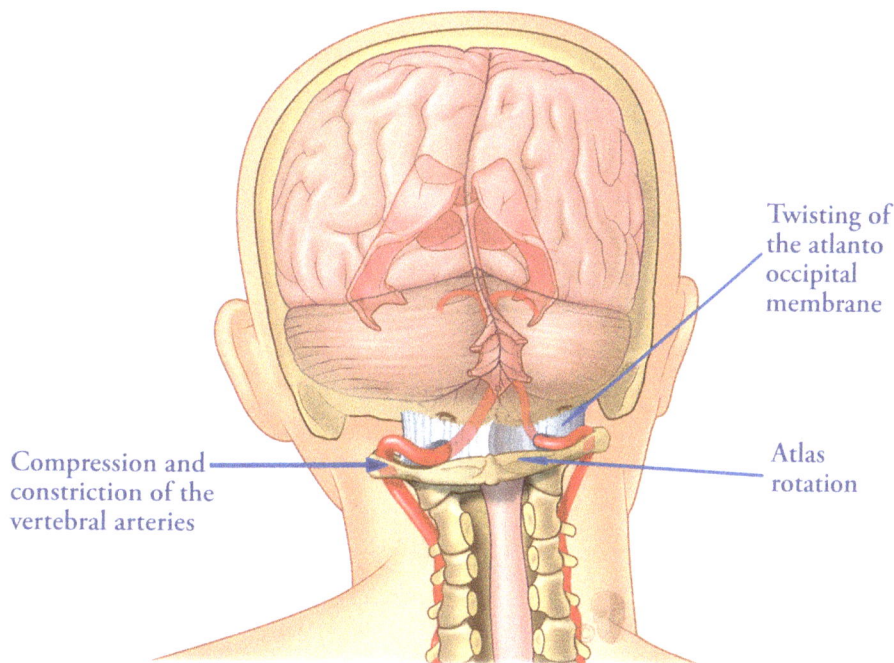

Figure 4.8 Atlanto-Occipital Membrane Atlas Distortion

When assessing the causes of an atlas subluxation one has to consider where this primary lesion has emerged. Due to irregularities of the atlas and the axis in relation to the occiput, subluxation of the upper cervical spine is influenced by a number of factors. Between the atlas and the occiput is the atlanto-occipital membrane, housing the vertebral venous plexus, part of the auxiliary plexus that runs the length of the spinal column. It also protects two vertebral arteries and the carotid arteries flowing into the circle of Willis that, in turn, feeds the brain with oxygenated blood. In the transverse processes of the atlas vertebra are the two vertebral foramena through which vertebral arteries emerge and form a sigmoid flexure before penetrating the atlanto-occipital membrane, negotiating the vertebral venous plexus and entering the foramen magnum.

Birth trauma involving forceps, ventouse or caesarean, as a result of the foetal head presenting incorrectly, can bring enormous torsion to the atlanto-occipital junction and subluxate the atlas, changing the juxtaposition of the atlanto-occipital membrane, altering the apertures and circumferences of the carotid and vertebral arteries, and denuding the flow of arterial blood into the circle of Willis.

Subluxations to the upper cervical spine can also occur as a result of whiplash injuries sustained throughout life and from a very early age. These might be innocuous falls, head bumps and skeletal misalignments which accumulate and add further torsion to the atlas.

Finally, once the dentition comes to fruition, and irregularities into this formation are established, the TMJ becomes congested, with the mandibular condyle compressing the retrodiscal tissue. The trigeminal nerve becomes compromised, and their nuclei react, particularly the trigeminal ganglion and the trigeminal spinal nuclei, which lie in the spinal cord adjacent to C1, C2 and C3. This reaction will always create an atlas subluxation, as the atlas and axis attempt to balance the occipital condyles on the lateral masses of the condyles of the atlas. Malocclusions will change the lateral and medial pterygoid muscles that attach the mandibular condyles of the mandible to the medial and lateral plates of the pterygoid plates and change the alignment of the sphenoid bone. The superior orbital fissures, between the greater and lesser wings of the sphenoid, provide a pathway for several cranial nerves including CN II, CN III, CN IV, the trigeminal nerve CN V and CN VI. Atlas subluxations as a result of malocclusions render this type of subluxation as a secondary or tertiary problem. This presents the chiroprator with a huge challenge since continual adjustment to the atlas as a primary cause will bring no resolution, unless the malocclusion is resolved.

VASCULAR SYSTEM

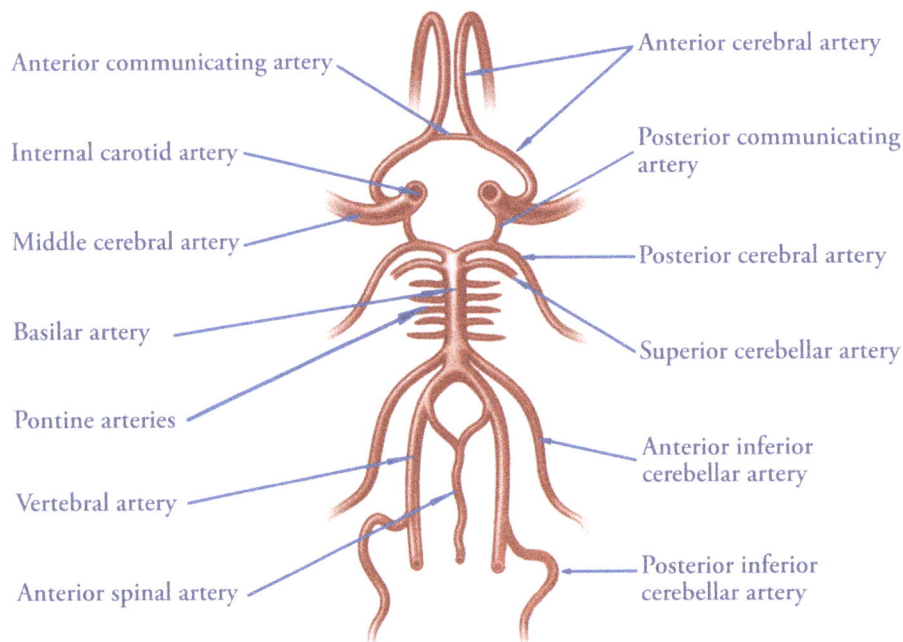

Figure 4.9 Circle of Willis

The heart pumps oxygenated arterial blood through the carotid and vertebral arteries into the circle of Willis, a large reservoir at the base of the brain, which feeds the brain through the anterior and posterior communicating arteries. This blood is then circulated through the brain, servicing the frontal, parietal, occipital and temporal lobes, as well as the highly vascular tela choroidea of the two lateral, third and fourth ventricles. The tela choroidea are part of invaginated pia mater which form the choroid plexuses of the four ventricles to produce CSF.

Once the arterial blood has divested itself of oxygen the blood becomes ischaemic and is then collected through the venous sinus system. This system includes the inferior and superior sagittal sinuses converging at the confluence of the sinuses, where it is then diverted through the transverse and sigmoid sinuses to the internal jugular vein. The anterior inferior aspects of the brain, namely the cavernous and intercavernous sinuses, drain through the superior and inferior petrosal sinuses, to the transverse and sigmoid sinuses, to the internal jugular vein. Ischaemic blood is also moved through the basilar plexus into the vertebral venous plexus, draining through the foramen magnum.

This drainage of ischaemic blood out of the brain should normally balance the inflow of arterial blood from the circle of Willis, maintaining the balance of intracranial pressure. However, with the advent of cranio fascial torsion, the membranes of the brain, the falx cerebri, the falx cerebelli and the tentorium cerebelli, become distorted and inhibit efficient and optimum drainage. This results in a pressure differential between the arterial blood in and the ischaemic blood out of the brain and creates an excess of intracranial pressure. This phenomenon is discussed in detail in Part IV, Cranio Vascular Dynamics.

CRANIAL NERVES

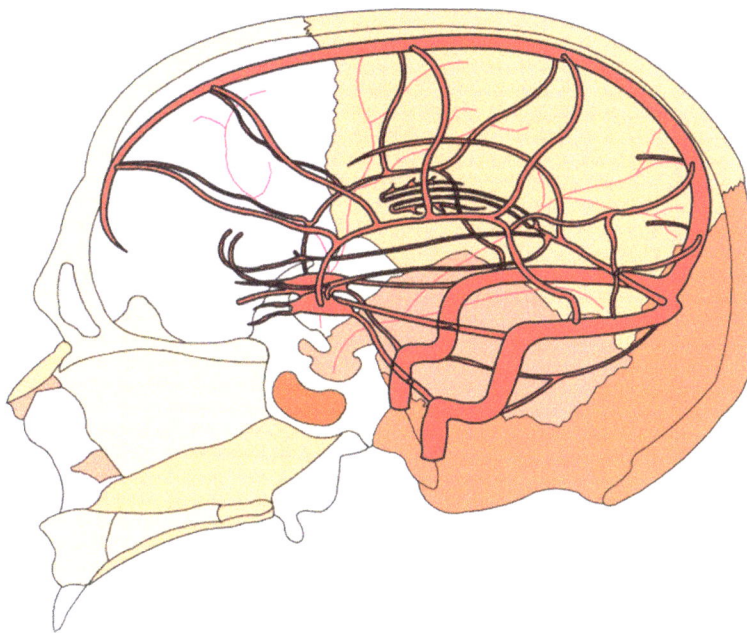

Figure 4.10 Venous Sinus System

Each one of the 12 pairs of cranial nerves exit from their nuclei through the fascia (dural meninges) that line the surface of the brain and the apertures leaving the cranium.

The sensory cranial nerves (CN) I and II – olfactory and optic – have their nuclei in the diencephalon, while CN VIII's – vestibulocochlear – is in the pons.

The motor cranial nerves are III, IV, VI, XI and XII – oculomotor, trochlear, abducens, spinal accessory and hypoglossal.

Sensory cranial nerves and hypoglossal are formed in an homologous column; III and IV are found in the midbrain; VI in the pons; and XI and XII in the medulla.

The mixed cranial nerves are V, VII, IX and X – trigeminal, facial, glossopharyngeal and vagus. Embryologically these are derived from neural crest cells, from the first pharyngeal arch (the trigeminal), from the second pharyngeal arch (the facial), from the third pharyngeal arch (the glossopharyngeal), and from the fourth pharyngeal arch (the vagus). Because these nerves are all generated embryologically at the same time and from neural crest cells, they all intimately connect and reflex together.

Cranial Nerve Nuclei

The cranial nerve nuclei follow early embryological development, with cranial nerves I and II having their nuclei in the diencephalon. Cranial nerves III and IV have their nuclei in the midbrain. Cranial nerves V, VI, VII, VIII and IX have their nuclei in the pons, and cranial nerves X, XI and XII have their nuclei in the medulla. The sensory components of the mixed cranial nerves V, VII, IX and X have their nuclei in the pons and medulla.

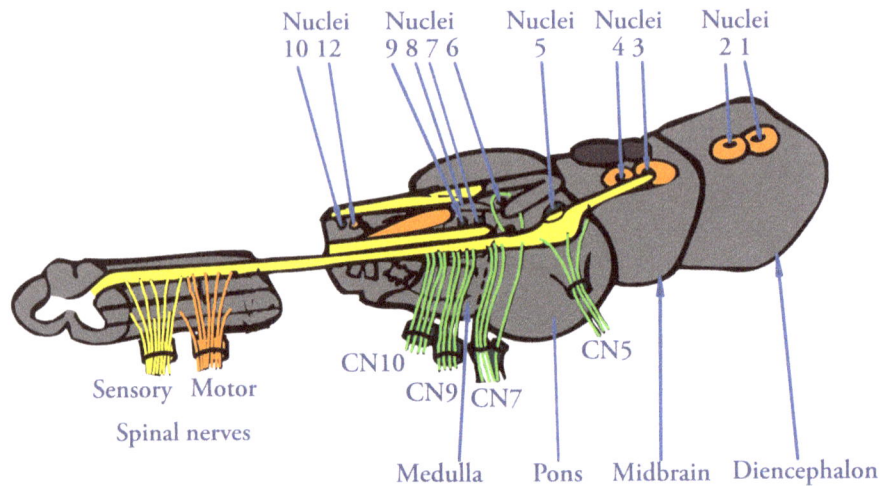

Figure 4.11 Cranial Nerve Nuclei

Sensory Cranial Nerves

When one looks at cranial nerves I, II, and VIII (the sensory nerves, although they originate from the diencephalon and the pons), cranial nerve I is controlled by the crista galli of the ethmoid bone, cranial nerve II goes through the optic canal of the sphenoid bone, and cranial nerve VIII goes through the internal acoustic meatus of the temporal bone.

In fascial development, the 'anterior pole' is controlled by the ethmoid bone, while the 'posterior pole' is controlled by the sphenoid. The anterior pole controls the falx cerebri and the falx cerebelli, while the posterior pole primarily controls the tentorium cerebellum and the diaphragma sellae. These sensory nerves are protected by different cranial bones, ensuring that if there is minimal damage to either anterior or posterior pole there will at least be some survival mechanism for one or two of the sensory nerves, by compensation through other cranial plates.

Motor Cranial Nerves

These are similar to the motor nerves. Cranial nerves III, IV and VI, the oculomotor, the trochlear and the abducens, are the motor nerves that control eye movement and the ocular muscles that ensure the eyeball can move up, down, left, right and obliquely.

Cranial nerve XI is the spinal accessory that controls the upper trapezius and the SCM muscle, which keeps the head in an erect position and enables the neck to turn from side to side. Cranial nerve XII, the hypoglossal, controls the tongue and the ability to suckle.

In the first few months of life the only thing an infant can do is look, move its head from side to side, defecate, urinate, cry, grip and suckle. These basic elements of survival are in fact the basic motor components that allow the brain to set down a template for early facilitation of motor function, a vital function for the cranial motor nerves. Until the human body is able to sit up and walk and bear weight, these are really the only motor muscles the body will use.

Mixed Cranial Nerves

The motor and sensory components of the mixed cranial nerves V, VII, IX and X (cranial nerves V and X – the trigeminal and vagus – control the cranial meninges). Cranial nerves III, VII, IX and X all have autonomic fibres that are parasympathetic. The parasympathetic component of the oculomotor acts as a pupil constrictor, and to ciliary muscles of the lens for near vision. The parasympathetic division of CN VII, the facial nerve, causes lacrimation and supplies the submandibular and sublingual salivary glands. In CN IX the parasympathetics go to the parotid gland and in CN X, the parasympathetics go to the heart, lungs and digestive system up to the splenic flexure, taste from the epiglottis and pharynx, sensation from the pharynx, posterior meninges and the region near the ear, the aortic arch, chemoreceptors (measuring oxygen tension in the blood) and baroreceptors (stretch receptors).

Pharyngeal Arches – Fourth Week

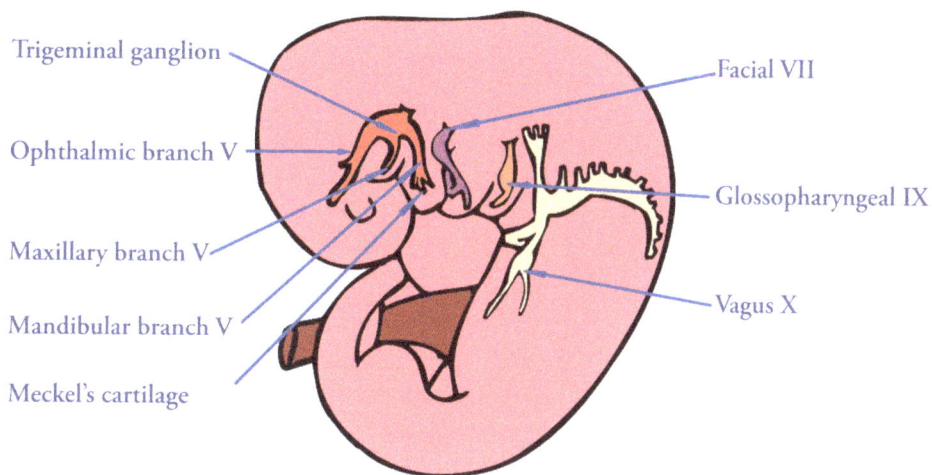

Figure 4.12 Fourth Week Cranial Nerve Development in the Pharyngeal Arches

Neural crest cells originate in the neuroectoderm of the fore-, mid-, and hindbrain regions and migrate into the pharyngeal arches. These arches appear in the fourth and fifth weeks of development. Each pharyngeal arch carries its own cranial nerve.

The trigeminal supplies the first pharyngeal (branchial) arch. Meckel's cartilage develops here, along with the premaxilla, maxilla, zygomatic bone, part of the temporal bone, the bones of the middle ear, and the mandible.

The cranial nerve for the second pharyngeal arch is the facial nerve. The cartilage of the second pharyngeal arch gives rise to the stapes, the styloid process of the temporal bone, the stylohyoid ligament and the upper part of the hyoid bone, and the muscles of facial expression.

The third pharyngeal arch produces the glossopharyngeal nerve, the lower part of the body of the hyoid and the stylopharyngeal muscle.

The fourth pharyngeal arch is supplied by the superior laryngeal branch of the vagus nerve (thyroid and constrictors of the pharynx) and the sixth arch by the recurrent laryngeal branch of the vagus (intrinsic muscles of the larynx).

The four pairs of mixed cranial nerves are the 'survival nerve group':

- Trigeminal nerve moves the mandible to locate and find the nipple
- Facial nerve latches on to the nipple and seals the lips around it

- Glossopharyngeal nerve pushes the tongue on to the nipple and presses the nipple on the palate
- Vagus nerve extracts, swallows and digests the milk, removes the nutrition for the body, defecates and removes the waste, while maintaining heart and lung function.

These four pairs of mixed cranial nerves appear at the pharyngeal arches on day 23 of embryological development. The other cranial nerves appear only in week 6.

Cranial Nerves and Cranial Bones

Each pair of cranial nerves leaves its nuclei and proceeds to exit the cranial vault. All these apertures are found within the cartilaginous part of each individual cranial bone (as opposed to the membranous component) and offer the strongest support to the cranial nerves as they traverse through the bony aperture. Given the complexity of the cranial plates and skull, together with the internal web of membranes, it would seem that brain function was designed to have duplicate and triplicate fail-safe relays. Built into this complicated system are 'communicators' and 'junction box fuses' that can be brought into play when there is a breakdown in both function and transmission of information from source to end organ. White matter is made up of three different types of fibre:

Commissural fibres

These fibre bundles run from right to left and vice versa connecting the two cerebral hemispheres – each fibre connecting to the same area in the opposite hemisphere.

Association fibres

These are white fibres that run between the front and the back of the brain in each hemisphere.

Projection fibres

These are white fibres deep within the subconscious core that project up into conscious cortical areas – where our subconscious emotions enter our consciousness.

These fibres cover the entire brain, bringing information from the front to the back and vice versa, and from side to side. When a breakdown occurs these fibres create new pathways to process information. If one segment breaks down another segment will redistribute the information load to other tissues.

Sensory input to the brain is vital and the three main sensory organs (eyes, ears and mouth), feed the limbic system (hippocampus, amygdala and fornix) with sensory information so the body can differentiate where it is in time and space. If the temporal area is damaged, sensory information can still be received through nose, mouth, skin and proprioceptive joints within the body. This also applies to the other temporal bone, so that the body may generally compensate, adapt and continue as before, but less efficiently. In the same way, the structure of the brain, developed embryologically from the three primary vesicles, contains many safeguards to ensure normal neurological transmission is optimised as much as is physiologically normal and possible.

Trigeminal Nerve

The ophthalmic and maxillary divisions of the trigeminal nerve are purely sensory. The mandibular division is the mixed component, having both a motor nucleus (masticator nucleus, which is located in the mid pons and innervates all the masticatory muscles) and a sensory nucleus. The sensory nucleus of the trigeminal nerve is the largest of the cranial nerve nuclei. It extends from the midbrain, caudally through the pons, to the spinal cord as far as the third cervical segment. The trigeminal nucleus has three subnuclei, starting in the mesencephalon with the mesencephalic nucleus. This carries proprioceptive information providing reflex control for bite, tooth contact, hard palate, TMJ capsule and occlusal planes. The pontine trigeminal nucleus in the pons is concerned with sensation from the face. The nucleus of the spinal tract, which merges with the dorsal grey matter of the spinal cord, is primarily concerned with perception of pain, temperature and touch.

Branches of the trigeminal nerve

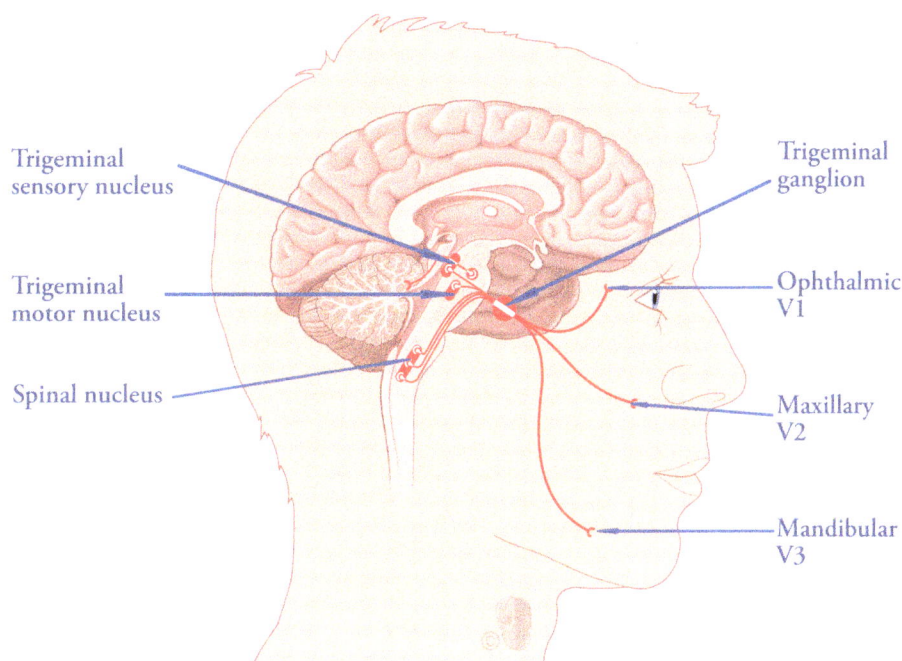

Figure 4.13 Branches of the Trigeminal Nerve and Nuclei

It is worth noting the sensory components of the trigeminal nerve that affect the cranial fascia:

- Ophthalmic VI – meningeal branch to the tentorium cerebellum
- Maxillary V2 – meningeal branch to the middle and anterior cranial fossae
- Mandibular V3 – meningeal branch to the middle and anterior cranial fossae
- C1, C2 and C3 innervate the posterior fossa through the ascending branches of the upper cervical nerves.

Trigeminal – Cranial Fascia

The trigeminal nerve provides sensory innervation to the face and should be distinguished from the facial nerve that controls the muscles of facial expression. The trigeminal nerve also has a small branchial branch motor root, which travels within the mandibular division and is responsible for controlling the muscles of mastication and some other small muscles. The trigeminal nerve also provides touch and pain sensation for the nasal sinuses inside the nose, mouth and anterior two-thirds of the tongue. In addition, pain sensations from the super tentorial (above the tentorial dural mater) are supplied by the trigeminal nerve, while dura of the posterior fossa is innervated by cranial nerve X, the vagus and the upper cervical nerve roots.

Periodontal Membrane

NB When corrections are made for CFD and stabilising the descending cranial major, the correction is made through the sensory portion of the ophthalmic and maxillary divisions of the trigeminal nerve. In a normal occlusion, when the bite is symmetric, simultaneous and of the same bilateral pressure, the periodontal membranes within the alveolus of the individual teeth in the four quadrants are stimulated together through the mandibular and maxillary branches of the trigeminal nerve. The occlusal reaction affects the sensory branches into the anterior and middle cranial fossae.

It should be noted that the upper soft palate is innervated by the recurrent laryngeal nerve, which arises from the vagus nerve anterior to the subclavian artery. When testing takes place for the dominant brain side, having the patient say 'aah' activates the meningeal branch of the vagus nerve and the side of the palate that pulls up highest, indicates the ipsilateral side of the dominant brain while the other side appears to be more flaccid.

CONCLUSION

Reciprocal Tension Membranes (RTM)

The falx cerebri, the falx cerebellum, the tentorium cerebelli and the diaphragma sellae are the RTM that support the brain and attach it to the various bones of the cranium. They also support the venous sinus system, the drainage mechanism for the brain.

Anterior Pole

The anterior pole of the falx cerebri attaches to the crista galli of the ethmoid bone anteriorly, and the straight sinus and the internal occipital protuberance posteriorly. The falx cerebellum, an extension of the falx cerebri, attaches to the straight sinus and at the foramen magnum, along the occipital sinus posteriorly.

Posterior Pole

The posterior pole of the tentorium cerebelli attaches to the anterior and posterior clinoid processes of the sella turcica of the sphenoid body anteriorly, and the straight sinus and the internal occipital protuberance, posteriorly.

Cranial Flexion – Extension

Motion of the RTM in flexion and extension mode, as the body goes from inhalation to exhalation.

Dural Membrane Innervation

Branches of the trigeminal, vagus and the first three cervical spinal nerves and branches from the sympathetic trunk pass to the dura.

Atlas Subluxation

The upper cervical spine, because of the irregularities of the atlas and the axis in relation to the occiput, is influenced by a number of factors resulting in subluxation. Birth trauma involving forceps, ventouse or caesarean, as a result of the foetal head presenting incorrectly, can bring enormous torsion to the atlanto-occipital junction and subluxate the atlas, changing the juxtaposition of the atlanto-occipital membrane. Subluxations to the upper cervical spine can also occur as a result of whiplash injuries sustained throughout life and from a very early age. Finally, once the dentition comes to fruition, and irregularities in this formation are established, the TMJ becomes congested with the mandibular condyle, compressing the retrodiscal tissue, and the trigeminal ganglion becomes compromised, creating stress in the trigeminal spinal nucleus resulting in an atlas subluxation.

Vascular System

The vascular system is an irrigation system with blood flowing into the brain and venous blood exiting the brain. This has to be maintained for homeostasis.

Cranial Nerves

Each one of the 12 pairs of cranial nerves exit from their nuclei, through the fascia (dural meninges) that lines the surface of the brain and each of the apertures leaving the cranium.

- Cranial nerve nuclei
- Sensory cranial nerves

- Motor cranial nerves
- Mixed cranial nerves
- Pharyngeal arches
- Cranial nerves and cranial bones
- Trigeminal nerve

Sensory Cranial Nerves

CN I, II, and VIII are sensory nerves, although originating from the diencephalon and the pons. CN I is controlled by the crista galli of the ethmoid bone, CN II goes through the optic canal of the sphenoid bone and CN VIII goes through the internal acoustic meatus of the temporal bone.

Motor Cranial Nerves

The motor nerves are cranial nerves III, IV, VI, XI and XII. CN III, IV and VI, the oculomotor, the trochlear and the abducens, are the motor nerves that control eye movement and the ocular muscles which ensure that the eyeball can move up, down, left, right and obliquely.

Mixed Cranial Nerves

The mixed cranial nerves are the motor and sensory components of CN V, VII, IX and X responsible for the motor and sensory functions of head, neck, thorax and abdomen.

Pharyngeal Arches – Week 4

Neural crest cells originate in the neuroectoderm of the fore-, mid-, and hindbrain regions and migrate into the pharyngeal arches. These arches appear in weeks 4 and 5 of development. Each pharyngeal arch carries its own cranial nerve.

Cranial Nerves and Cranial Bones

Each pair of cranial nerves leaves its nuclei and proceeds to exit the cranial vault. As with the cranial nerve nuclei, cranial nerves come from various brain components, delineated by their embryological development.

Trigeminal Nerve

The ophthalmic and maxillary divisions of the trigeminal are purely sensory. The mandibular division is a mixed component, having both a motor nucleus (masticator nucleus, located in the mid pons and innervates all the masticatory muscles), and a sensory nucleus.

Trigeminal – Cranial Fascia

The trigeminal nerve provides sensory innervation to the face and should be distinguished from the facial nerve that controls the muscles of facial expression.

Periodontal Membrane

Innervated through the sensory portion of the ophthalmic and maxillary divisions of the trigeminal nerve.

CHAPTER 5

CHANGES IN BRAIN FROM DISTORTED CFD

MAJOR BRAIN COMPONENTS

The major brain components that cross the midline between the left and right brain and lie under the inferior sagittal sinus require communications between both sides of the brain, their sensory input and responses in order to process the information gathered in each part of the brain. These components include:

- Pituitary – the master endocrine gland of the body controls all the endocrine glands, including thyroid, thymus, pancreas, adrenal and ovaries/testes
- Optic chiasma – which relays messages through the optic nerve and the peripheral margins, across the brain to the occipital lobe where the visual centres are located
- Corpus callosum – which integrates and processes intellectual material from both left and right parts of the brain and interconnects these cerebral hemispheres. When deficient, this process of integration is retarded and can produce dyslexic behavioural issues. This has nothing to do with intellectual potential, but is a processing deficit
- Lateral ventricles – producing CSF crosses the midline in its circulation through the interventricular foramen of Monro, into the third ventricle through the aqueduct of Sylvius, into the fourth ventricle. The third and the fourth ventricles lie in the midline of the brain and their circulation and distribution is affected by changes in the midline structures. Further distribution of CSF from the fourth ventricle is facilitated through the apertures of Luschka and Magendie into the cisterns of the brain, and into the cisterna magnus, the cisterna pontis and the cisterna interpeduncularis (cisterna basalis).

There is also CSF movement into the central canal, which follows the spinal cord to its termination at S2, and is an extension of the ventricular system of the spinal cord.

The commissary of the fornix joins the fornix in its distribution from the limbic system and connects the olfactory cortices and association cortices of the temporal lobe.

The limbic system controls emotional and behavioural dynamics, takes sensory input from the ophthalmic, auditory and visual centres, and is the psychological centre of the brain.

The fornix fimbria is the major pathway of the hippocampus, providing information in short-term memory to other parts of the limbic system and cortical association areas for further processing, or to be laid down as long-term memory.

The thalamus – the junction box of the brain, where the main concentration of nuclei exists and where administration of the brain takes place – relays information from the brainstem to the cortex and between cortical regions.

The hypothalamus regulates appetite, thirst, sexual drive and autonomic neuroendocrine functions.

The basal ganglia are the neuronal cell bodies deep within the white matter. These are groups of paired brain nuclei that play a crucial role in the integration and organisation of coordinated motor activity. When integrated with the cerebellum the basal ganglia turn the derived conscious activity into reality.

The brainstem – the medulla oblongata often just referred to as the medulla – is the lower half of the brainstem continuous with the spinal cord. Its upper part is continuous with the pons. The medulla contains the cardiac, respiratory, vomiting and vasomotor centres dealing with heart rate, breathing and blood pressure.

The pons is identified by the anterior surface of the brainstem by transverse fibres that continue at the internal surface of the middle cerebellar peduncles. The posterior surface of the pons forms the transverse half of the floor of the fourth ventricle called the rhomboid fossa. The two sides of the pons are framed by the middle cerebellar peduncles; the inflow tracts from the cerebrum to the cerebellum. All these structures identified in the pons are involved in motor function.

All these aforementioned structures lie within the midbrain. Changes in their status by cranio fascial torsion will produce physiologic changes compromising their function and their optimum potential for transmitting specific neurological information. These cranio fascial alterations are felt from both a cranial and a spinal standpoint, altering the effects to the autonomic, central and peripheral nervous systems. These changes through the midline of the brain can occur at birth, but are certainly exacerbated by physical, emotional and chemical influences on the body throughout life. These dynamics are essentially part of human physiology and cannot be ignored from a clinical standpoint. Unfortunately, only a minority of practitioners are aware of the problems caused by asymmetric torsion as outlined in the text and in general we ignore these problems at our peril.

This is where the defined health of the human body comes under scrutiny and it is imperative that exposure of this type of malfunction should be further explored. Our understanding of this phenomenon, although so basic in its appearance, is the underlying reason for 'dis-ease' in many patients that confront us on a daily basis. Please do not underestimate the importance of this chapter.

Ascending/descending

For many years, confusion arose as a result of a lack of understanding what constituted a major force within the body. Dentists were working with teeth, their restoration and position within the 'jaw-to-jaw' relationship but were ignoring skeletal biomechanics and the effect on the cranium and its postural affects. Chiropractors were focused on skeletal and spinal column subluxations without addressing the dental cranial aspects. As a result, both were ignoring the importance of defining a major causative and aetiological agent.

Research into ascending/descending dynamics was carried out by Dr Jean-Pierre Meersseman, and substantiated by Dr Piet Seru, and was defined according to the structures relating to the stomatognathic system. Their findings indicated that descending majors related to stomatognathic system dysfunction, while ascending majors related to issues that were not of the stomatognathic aetiology.

STOMATOGNATHIC SYSTEM

The stomatognathic system plays an important role in postural control. It is a functional unit characterized by several structures: skeletal components (maxilla and mandible), dental arches, soft tissues (salivary glands, nervous and vascular supplies), and the TMJ and masticatory muscles. These structures act in harmony to perform different functional tasks (e.g. to speak, to break food down into small pieces, to swallow). In particular, the TMJ makes muscular and ligamentary connections to the cervical region, forming a functional complex called the 'cranio cervico-mandibular system'. The extensive afferent and efferent innervations of the stomatognathic system are reflected in the extensive representation of the orofacial district in the motor and sensory areas of the cerebral cortex.

Numerous anatomical connections between the stomatognathic system's proprioceptive inputs and nervous structures are implicated in posture (cerebellum, vestibular and oculomotor nuclei, superior colliculus). If the proprioceptive information of the stomatognathic system is inaccurate, then head control and body position may be affected. In addition, the myofascial system plays an important role in posture, and treatment of muscular-skeletal disorders is associated with TMJ disorders, occlusal changes, and tooth loss.

Loading the muscles of mastication immediately changes the periosteal torsion which, in turn, pulls the sutures and the endosteum, and cranio fascial drag results. The cranio fascial drag will immediately change the RTM at the anterior and posterior poles, creating pressure on the cerebral hemispheres and the cerebellum. The spontaneous torque and cranial fascial reaction will produce a fascial distortion right throughout the body, through the cranial cavity, thoracic cavity, diaphragm, abdomen, pelvic floor and upper and lower extremities. The descending cranial major (or the stomatognathic major) is a chiropractic nightmare, and a high percentage of chiropractic patients present with descending cranial majors, or cranio fascial dynamic torsion. The cranial effect of the lockdown of the sutural system of the cranium also means that there is a reduction of CSF movement into the perivascular spaces of the membranous system and the brain goes into shut down, or starvation mode.

The RTM will become distorted, in turn distorting the cerebral and cerebellar hemispheres. In turn, the tentorium will change the position of the sphenoid at the anterior/posterior clinoid processes, the petrous portion of the temporal bone, the sphenobasilar synchondrosis, the occiput, foramen magnum and jugular foramen. This affects cranial nerves II, III, IV, V, and VI through the optic canal and the sphenoid superior orbital fissure, cranial nerves VII and VIII through the internal auditory meatus, cranial nerves IX, X, and XI through the jugular foramen, and cranial nerve XII through the hypoglossal canal. Malocclusions disturb the trigeminal nerve and in particular the sensory branches that emanate into the anterior and middle cranial fossae (meningeal branches of the mandibular and maxillary division of the trigeminal nerve). Jamming the skull also produces restriction at the jugular foramen, affecting the sensory part of the vagus nerve that controls the posterior fossa, again resulting in pain and neurological dysfunction.

When one discusses an ascending major, one is talking in terms of anything that does not involve the stomatognathic area. This largely takes care of most of the biomechanical, spinal and pelvic dysfunctions that chiropractors deal with daily. Treatment of the ascending major therefore, would necessitate balancing a sacroiliac lesion, a lumbosacral lesion, a bilateral sacroiliac fixation, rotation of the pelvic girdle, spinal subluxations and extremity irregularities. This is what chiropractors do best.

However, the chiropractor is now able to correct cranio fascial torsion, reducing neurological interference, reinstating the horizontal and vertical components of the falx cerebri, the falx cerebelli and the tentorium cerebellum and balancing the brain.

Chiropractic understanding of descending stomatognathic problems can now use 'brain-balancing' techniques to reverse a descending cranial major into an ascending major. To a large degree this negates the necessity of dental intervention, both orthopaedically and orthodontically, which is an enormous blessing for most patients.

Dentists have, for a long time, been using energy driven appliances, both fixed and moveable, to a point where orthopaedic appliances will actually change the format and structure of the maxilla–mandibular relationship, externally rotate internal maxillae and vice versa, and artificially introduce dynamic vectors into the skull, which may or may not be of benefit. The chiropractic cranial approach to brain balancing and stabilising the trigeminal and vagus nerves, stimulating CFD, and removing fascial drag is done in a manner where the body is assessed and corrected immediately.

Fixed orthopaedic and orthodontic appliances introduce vectors into the skull, which are reinforced 24 hours of the day for the duration of the treatment.

Those vectors are manmade and, although they are assessed using modern technology, the author defies any functional orthodontist/orthopaedist to be able to drive the vectors required in the skull through fixed appliance to the degree the body needs. Once the work of the fixed appliance has been completed, the arch of the maxilla, its relationship with the vomer, and the vomer's relationship with the ethmoid and sphenoid bones can be permanently changed.

NERVES OF THE UPPER AND LOWER TEETH

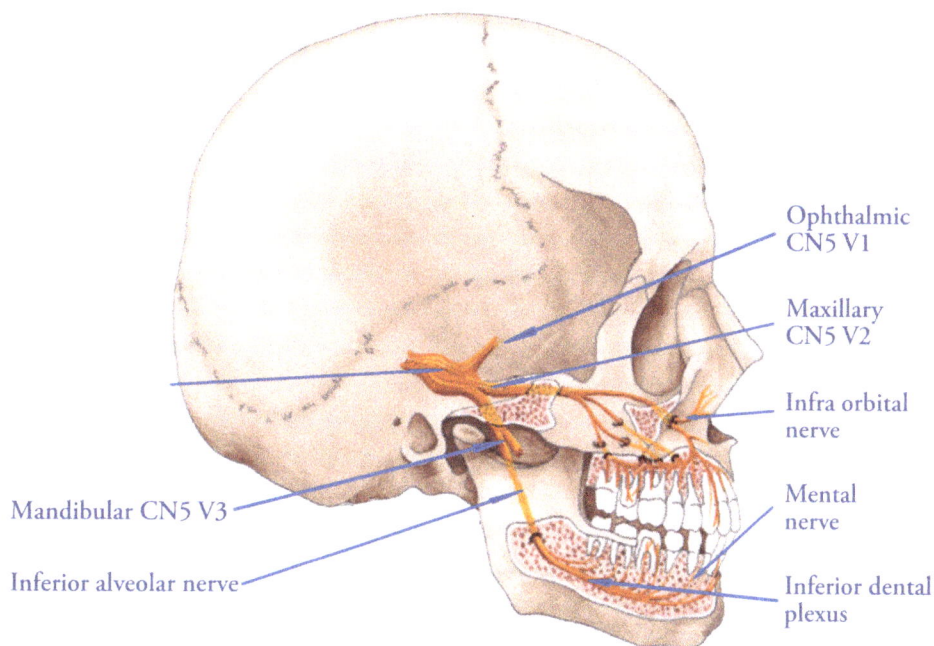

Figure 5.1 Nerves of the Upper and Lower Teeth

The lateral view of the skull shows the trigeminal complex in its relationship to the mandible and the maxillae. The ophthalmic division of the trigeminal feeds up into the lateral margins of the face over the pterion; the greater wing of the sphenoid, the maxillary division which feeds into the upper arch of the maxillae through the infra orbital nerve and inserts into all eight sockets of the alveoli. The mandibular division of the trigeminal nerve feeds into the lower jaw, into the inferior alveolar nerve and into the eight sockets of the alveoli. The mental nerve feeds into the mandibular ramus and towards maturity is heavily invested in the root of the wisdom tooth. All three divisions of the trigeminal nerve feed into the trigeminal ganglia that lies adjacent to the TMJ. From the trigeminal ganglia, the trigeminal nerve feeds up into the mesencephalic nucleus (midbrain), the pontine nucleus (pons) and the spinal trigeminal nucleus (medulla) in the upper cervical spine.

The anatomy of the canine tooth that is embedded in the alveolus, shows the crown of the tooth covered in enamel under which lies the dentin, surrounding the pulp cavity which contains the artery and the nerve for that tooth. Cementum surrounds the root of the tooth where peri alveoli ligaments secure the tooth within the socket and insert it into the bone of the jaw. At the root of the tooth is the apical foramen which allows the passage for the artery and the nerves.

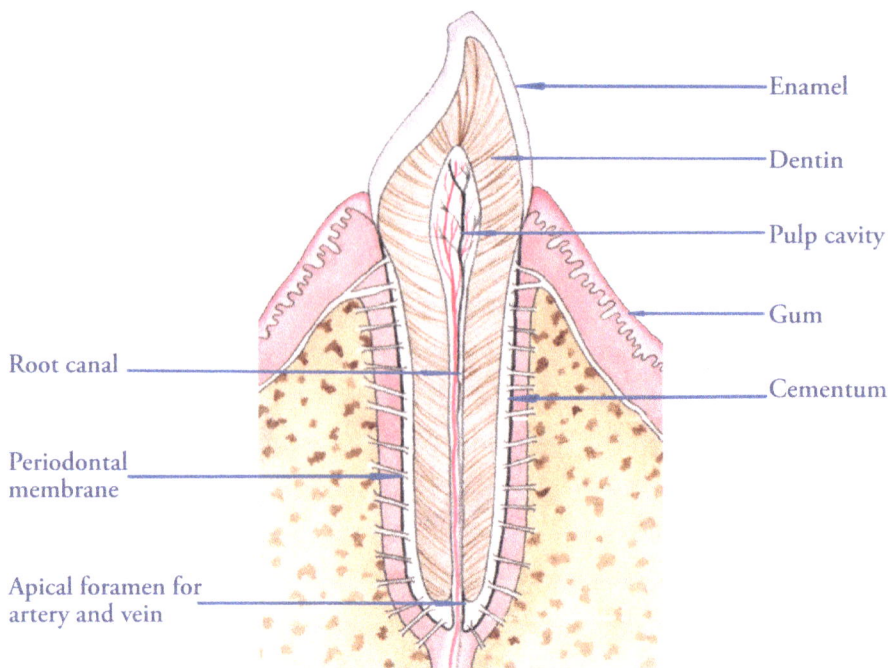

Figure 5.2 Tooth: Longitudinal section

NORMAL OCCLUSION

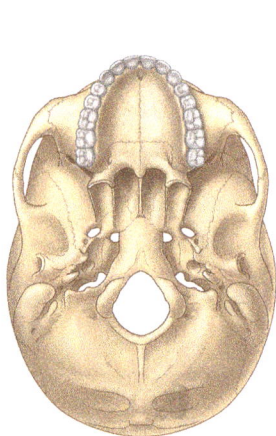

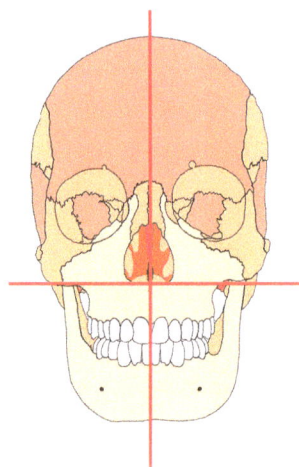

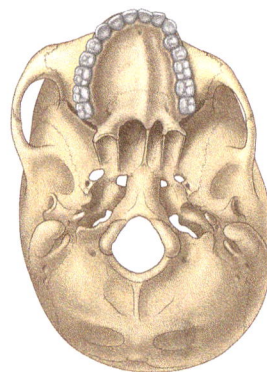

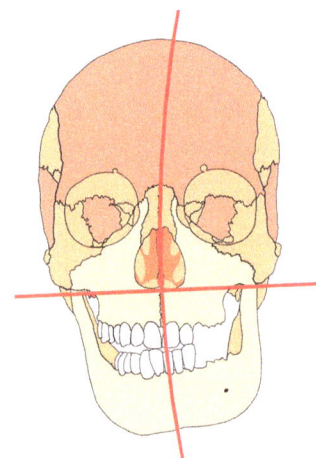

Figure 5.3 Normal Occlusion: Normal bite   *Figure 5.4 Malocclusion: Abnormal bite*

In a normal occlusion when the bite is symmetric, simultaneous and of the same bilateral pressure, the periodontal membranes within the alveolus of the individual teeth in the four quadrants are stimulated together through the mandibular and maxillary branches of the trigeminal nerve. The occlusal reaction also affects the trigeminal sensory branches into the anterior and middle cranial fossae. Each tooth is reflexed to a dedicated organ and a muscle, and each tooth fits into the alveolus and attaches to the periodontal ligament. The periodontal ligament that is part of the periodontal membrane is developed from mesodermal cells of the dental sac. This is a derivation of mesenchyme, which is of neural crest origin and forms the dental papilla. The dental papilla gives rise to the dentin and pulp of the tooth, while the enamel develops from the enamel organ that is derived from ectoderm. The upper jaw is controlled

74

by the maxillary branches of the trigeminal nerve while the lower jaw is controlled by the mandibular branches of the trigeminal nerve. The jaw is supported by the canine, two bicuspids or premolars, two molars and a wisdom tooth in each quadrant. The canine of both the lower and upper jaw disclude the teeth from coming into contact when the mandible moves in a lateral or anterior direction, while the lateral and medial incisors are used purely for cutting and barely contact the upper incisor.

According to Dr Willi May the human body swallows between 800 and 1,000 times a day. Observations made by Dr May suggest that each time one swallows, the teeth come into occlusion. Each time the teeth come into occlusion cranial stability is achieved and the stomatognathic structures remain balanced. A normal balanced occlusion means that the maxillary and mandibular teeth come into contact symmetrically, simultaneously and with equal pressure on all the contact teeth and within the buccal and lingual cusps of those individual teeth.

MALOCCLUSION

A malocclusion occurs when the maxillary and mandibular teeth come together asymmetrically, out of synchrony and with uneven pressure. The malocclusion changes the maxillary/mandibular relationship and will create stomatognathic dysfunction, either at the teeth edge or within the TMJ, reducing dental stability and increasing neurological dysfunction. The malocclusion will create irritability through the mandibular and maxillary branches of the trigeminal nerve. This, in turn, will counterbalance and compensate by increasing muscle load on one or several of the mastication muscles (masseter, buccinator, lateral and medial pterygoid and temporalis) all of which are controlled and innervated by the mandibular/motor branch of the trigeminal nerve.

Malocclusions also affect the mandibular condyle relationship within the mandibular/glenoid fossae. The internal pterygoid muscle is attached to the condylar head of the mandible. The external pterygoid muscle is attached to the ramus of the mandible. This dysfunctional relationship affects the internal and external pterygoid muscles attaching to the internal and external pterygoid plates of the sphenoid bone. The torsion created by these muscles on the pterygoid plates will pull and distort the sphenoid bone and, in turn, distort the horizontal membrane – the tentorium cerebellum – the venous sinuses and, consequently, drainage through the internal jugular vein.

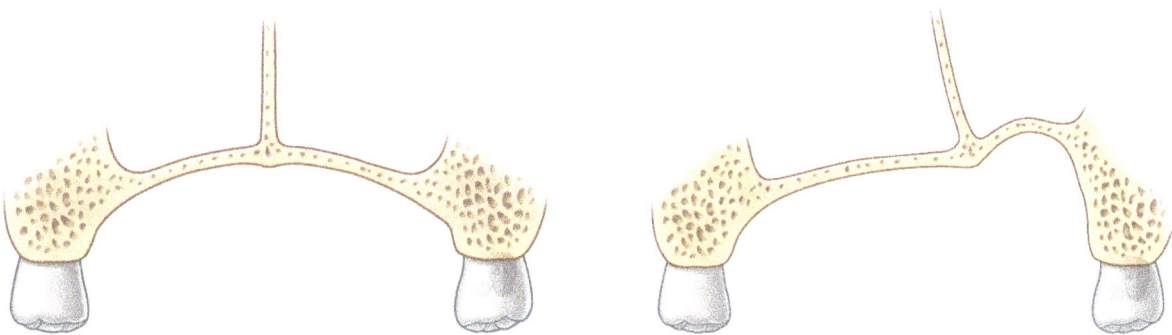

Figure 5.5 (left) Class 1 Maxilla: Bilateral maxillae flexion
Figure 5.6 (right) Torqued Maxilla: Right maxilla flexion and left maxilla extension

Cranio fascial Distortion

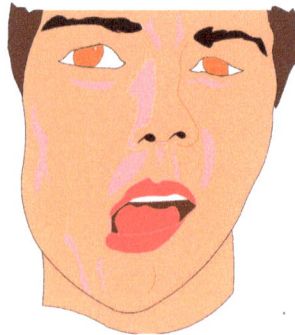

Figure 5.7 Cranio Fascial Distortion Expression: Abnormal bite

When looking at a patient's facial profile, one must observe any lack of symmetry. One will notice a large eye and a smaller eye, indicating the tilt and rotation of the sphenoid. The sphenoid supports the orbits of the eye, behind which lies the superior orbital fissure housing the cranial nerves that move the eyes. When the sphenoid moves posterior on the left, it pulls the eyeball posterior with it, giving the impression of a smaller orbit and a smaller eye. Conversely, when the right sphenoid moves anteriorly, it will pull the ocular orbit forward giving the impression of another larger orbit and the eye will appear anterior. This is the result of cranio fascial distortion – a counterclockwise torque. Notice also the nasal septum will move to the left towards an internally rotated maxilla. The mandible will tend to deviate to that side, as the TMJ will move posterior on the left as the temporal bone follows the depressed sphenoid and moves the temporal bone posteriorly external rotation. Notice in Figure 5.7 that the mandible moves to the right, although the discussion has described the mandible moving to the left. The variance in mandibular deviation will only be evident when the patient is asked to open the mouth slowly. One will also notice the high externally rotated frontal bone on the right following the large ocular orbit. The left frontal bone will be internally rotated and follow the smaller ocular orbit. Smooth coupling in the cranium is discussed in Chapter 6.

DESCENDING MAJOR STRESS

Major stressors involved in the stomatognathic area are usually driven by the position of the teeth, their malocclusion position and the loss of dentition found in the patient.

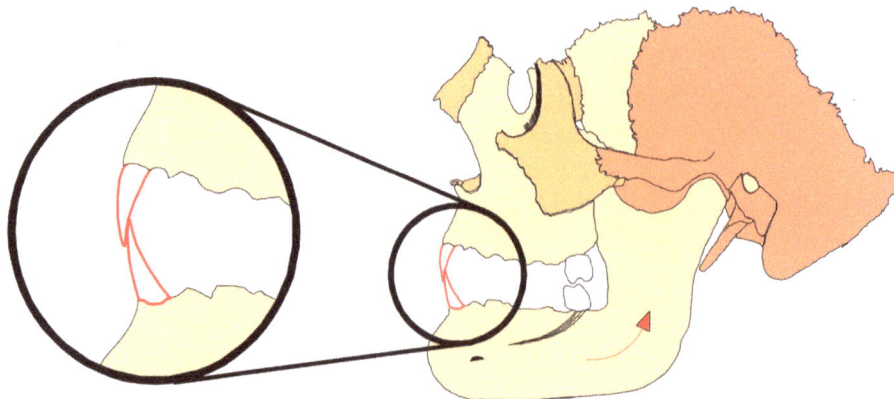

Figure 5.8 Incisal Interference

Incisal interference occurs when the medial and lateral incisors of the maxilla contact the lower medial and lateral incisors on occlusion, forcing the mandible into a retrusive of position, jamming the retrodiscal tissue at the posterior aspect of the TMJ. The position the mandible finds itself in will depend on which maxillary incisors contact the lower mandibular incisors.

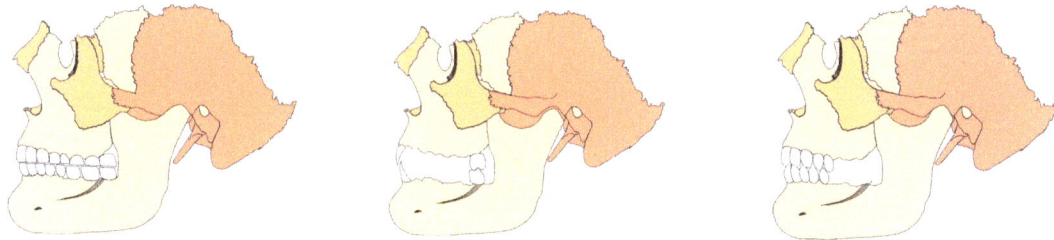

Figure 5.9 (left) Loss of Vertical: Bruxing; (centre) Loss of Dentition: No lower dental support; (right) Loss of Posterior Support

Loss of vertical occurs when the posterior teeth have worn out or have been intruded over the years and result in incisal interference. The loss of vertical is measured from the top of the mandibular condyle to the roof of the mandibular/glenoid fossa. Sometimes this loss of vertical can be measured in millimetres.

Loss of dentition as a result of dental extractions results in the loss of vertical and posterior support, again resulting in incisal interference and disturbance to the TMJ.

Loss of posterior support indicates extractions of the wisdom teeth (number 8) or the molars (numbers 6 and 7) which again results in incisal interference as the entire masticating surface of the occlusion is forced anterior. The solution would indicate either dental implants or a dental bridge that would reinstate the posterior support, increase the vertical, remove congestion from the TMJ and allow the incisors to assume their normal relationship with the maxillary and mandibular incisors.

Crossbites will occur when the mandible deviates either to the left or to the right, contacting the maxillary teeth, usually at the canines or the incisors – producing a unilateral crossbite. A bilateral crossbite occurs when the class II maxilla is too narrow to be accommodated in a normal occlusal manner, resulting in contacts with the mandible on the lingual aspect of the teeth – usually in a couple of places. The bilateral crossbite can also occur when the posterior mandibular teeth are intruded lingually and prevent normal maxillary mandibular occlusion.

Edge to edge occlusion occurs when a class III malocclusion is attempted orthodontically, to change to a class I, in an attempt to expand the upper arches of the maxilla and force the incisors anteriorly and out of contention with the incisors of the mandible. This will often fail, as the orthodontics are carried out in an immature mouth, and with future growth and development the attempted class I will end up as an edge to edge malocclusion.

All these major stressors will invariably not be controlled or corrected by cranial adjustments and dental intervention will have to be implemented to recreate the status quo.

DESCENDING MINOR STRESS

The minor stresses, which include mandibular deviation, premature contacts and deviant tongue movement, are usually corrected by stabilising the pelvis, spine and cranial membranes whereby normal muscle control is implemented.

Mandibular deviation can result with abnormal torsion and spasm of the internal and external pterygoid muscles whose contact on the mandibular condyles and the pterygoid plates of the sphenoid can change the balance of the sphenoid bone, the tentorium, and the temporal and occipital bones.

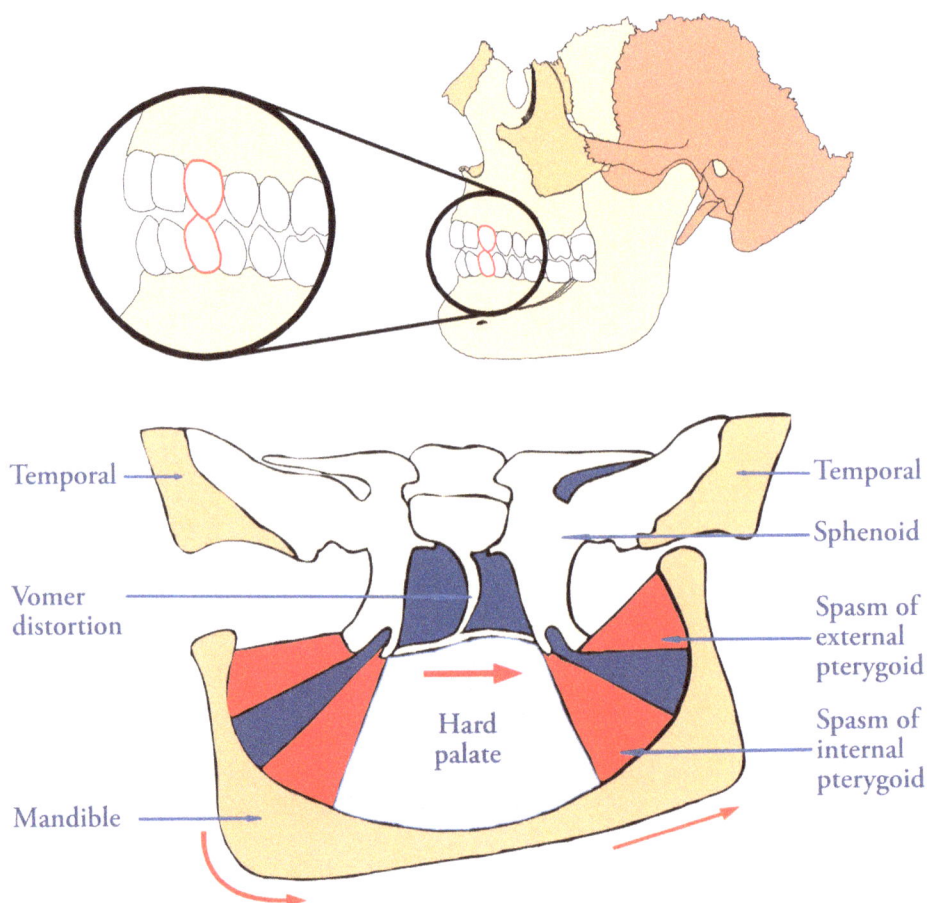

Figure 5.10 Minor Stress: (top) Premature contact; (bottom) Temporomandibular joint dysfunction

Premature contact occurs when there is a contact and slip of the occlusal surface, usually at the canines (number 3) or the premolars (numbers 4 and 5), creating an incomplete occlusion and disruption to the TMJs.

Deviant tongue movements can be changed by many factors within the stomatognathic system. Retraining of the deviant tongue with myofascial exercises and stabilising the rest of the stomatognathic system will usually resolve the tongue issues and reduce this minor stress.

These three minor stresses can all be corrected by cranial adjustments and usually do not involve dental intervention. It is in the interests of the patient that cranial and skeletal adjustments be maximised, before any other form of dental application is applied. Early intervention of dental procedures will usually complicate the ability of the stomatognathic system to compensate and adapt fully and can produce prolonged and unnecessary dental treatment. Remember that dental intervention changes the original format of the occlusion and thereby the natural stomatognathic position, and when achieved can change the dynamics irrevocably and forever. This means that if the dental intervention is incorrect, going back to the baseline is not an option and can result in years of trial and error to try and reinstate the original dynamics. Dental intervention when necessary, and if accurately applied by a knowledgeable dentist who understands the dynamics of the spinal and cranial physiology, can make beneficial changes to the occlusion and ultimately to the stomatognathic system and reinstate a healthy outcome to the patient.

ASCENDING MAJOR

In most cases, the correction of cranio fascial torsion will allow the system – the central nervous system – to increase its tolerance and its ability to compensate and adapt. The stomatognathic system will then be stabilised and the parameter checks will be neutralised.

If none of the parameters change then the problem is not part of the stomatognathic system and can then be labelled as an ascending major. The utilisation of these parameter checks and the assessment of the ascending/descending major using the Meersseman Test in the presence of cranio fascial torsion, is absolutely vital in the clinical appraisal of one's patient.

The stomatognathic system is primarily run by the trigeminal nucleus – the largest nucleus in the brain – and there are many neurological implications. Not using this knowledge and application will not only defer the correct treatment plan but could also prevent the patient from recovering.

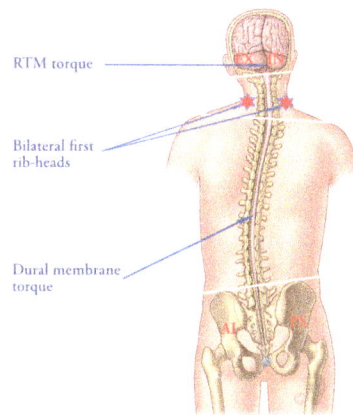

Figure 5.11 Bilateral Sacroiliac Rotation: A to P motion

In essence, ascending majors will involve dysfunctional components of a foot lock, ankle bone displacement, knee problems involving the medial and lateral meniscus, hip dysplasia or degenerative changes within the acetabulum, and pelvic derangements. These will include dural torque, sacroiliac ligamentous disruption and a lumbar sacral disc prolapse. The latter two are biomechanical dysfunctions that bring about imbalance to the pelvic girdle. Lumbosacral disc prolapse, if acute, will require immediate resolution, particularly if the signs and symptoms indicate immediate attention. This means that although a descending major is obvious, the disc issue may be a priority in the short term, followed by the descending major. This requires a full clinical assessment and clinical decisions have to be a priority in order to achieve a good clinical outcome.

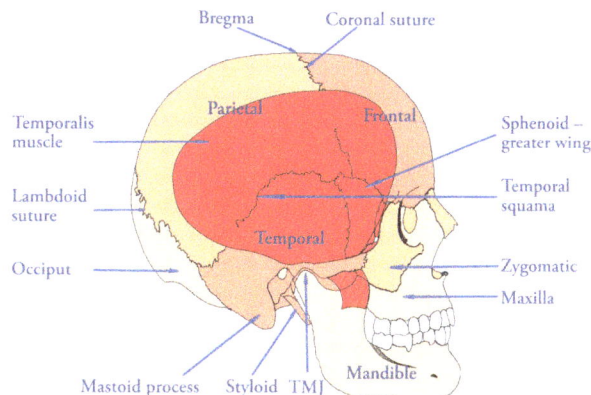

Figure 5.12 Normal Temporomandibular Joint: The temporalis covers all the sutures of the lateral cranium

MUSCLES OF MASTICATION

Apart from the buccinator muscle, all the muscles of mastication are controlled by the motor part of the mandibular branch of the trigeminal nerve:

- Temporalis muscle is innervated by a nerve supply from the deep temporal branches of the anterior trunk of the mandibular nerve
- Masseter muscle's nerve supply is the masseteric nerve from the anterior trunk of the mandibular division of the trigeminal nerve
- Internal pterygoid muscle's nerve supply is the medial pterygoid nerve of the mandibular division of the trigeminal nerve
- External pterygoid muscle's nerve supply is the lateral pterygoid nerve of the anterior trunk of the mandibular division of the trigeminal nerve
- Buccinator muscle's nerve supply is the buccal branches of the facial nerve.

To assess and correct cranial fascial dynamics one has to use indicators to fully evaluate the problem.

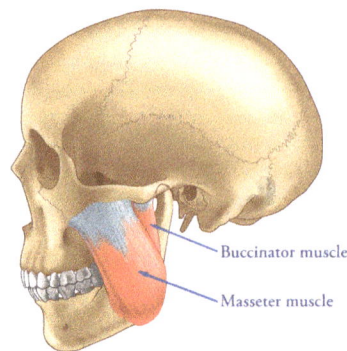

Figure 5.13 Muscles of Mastication: (left) Masseter muscle; (right) buccinator muscle

VISUAL INDICATORS

As cranial fascial distortion alters the internal dynamics of the skull, changes also take place in the external features of the skull and more apparent changes become more obvious. When noted in a clinical environment these characteristics will show exactly how the skull has changed and one is able to extrapolate how the internal mechanics are malfunctioning. As the skull bones become the anchor points for the dural membranes, changes in their position will affect how the brain is balanced within the cranium and how the arteries and veins become more inhibited in their physiologic function. Attention will be drawn to the effects created by internal and external frontal bone changes and their linkage to internal and external temporal bone alterations (see Chapter 6).

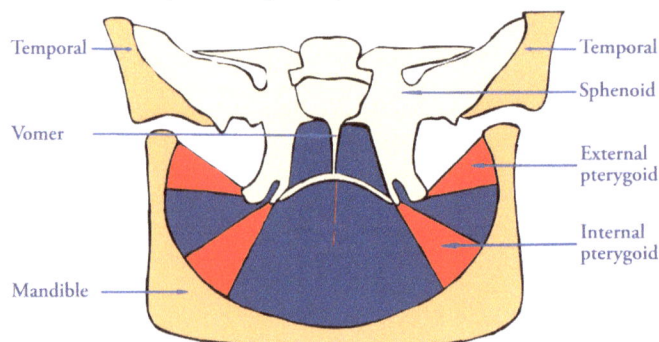

Figure 5.14 Spheno Temporomandibular Relationship

CONCLUSION

Major Brain Components

The major brain components that cross the midline between the left and right brain and lie under the inferior sagittal sinus require communication between both sides of the brain, their sensory input and responses in order to process the information gathered in each part of the brain.

Ascending/Descending Majors

Research into ascending/descending dynamics was carried out by Dr Jean-Pierre Meersseman and substantiated by Dr Piet Seru, and was defined according to the structures relating to the stomatognathic system. Their findings indicate that descending majors related to stomatognathic system dysfunction, while ascending majors related to issues that were not of the stomatognathic aetiology.

Stomatognathic System

The stomatognathic system is a functional unit characterised by several structures: skeletal components (maxilla and mandible), dental arches, soft tissues (salivary glands, nervous and vascular supplies), and the TMJ and masticatory muscles.

Nerves of the Upper and Lower Teeth

All three divisions of the trigeminal nerve feed into the trigeminal ganglia that lies adjacent to the TMJ.

Normal Occlusion

In a normal occlusion when the bite is symmetric, simultaneous and of the same bilateral pressure, the periodontal membranes within the alveolus of the individual teeth in the four quadrants are stimulated together through the mandibular and maxillary branches of the trigeminal nerve.

Malocclusion

A malocclusion occurs when the maxillary and mandibular teeth come together asymmetrically, out of synchrony and with uneven pressure. The malocclusion changes the maxillary/mandibular relationship and will create stomatognathic dysfunction either at the teeth edge, or within the TMJ, reducing dental stability and increasing neurological dysfunction.

Descending Major Stress

Major stressors involved in the stomatognathic area are usually driven by the position of the teeth, their malocclusion position and the loss of dentition found in the patient.

Descending Minor Stress

The minor stresses, which include mandibular deviation, premature contacts and deviant tongue movement are usually corrected by stabilising the pelvis, spine and cranial membranes whereby normal muscle control is implemented.

Ascending Major

If none of the parameters change then the problem is not part of the stomatognathic system and can then be labelled as an ascending major.

Muscles of Mastication

- Temporalis
- Masseter
- Internal pterygoid
- External pterygoid
- Buccinator.

Visual Indicators

As cranial fascial distortion alters the internal dynamics of the skull, changes also take place on the external features of the skull and more apparent changes become more obvious.

CHAPTER 6

CRANIAL DISTORTION PATTERNS

CRANIAL SMOOTH COUPLING

As pelvic and spinal changes take place, with the pelvis moving into a rotational position, the pectoral girdle will shift to balance and accommodate the motion of the pelvis. Head posture likewise will move to accommodate balance and position to maintain a gravitational force of equilibrium. With smooth coupling, as discussed in earlier chapters, the horizontal planes of the pelvis, spine and cranium will move in such a fashion as to accommodate roll (a horizontal accommodation), pitch (a vertical accommodation) and yaw (a combination of the two). These are aeronautical terms which best describe a plane in flight, and how it maintains its height and direction when other vectors are in force.

Non-smooth coupling occurs when the skeletal components are damaged (as in the form of a disc prolapse through trauma) and the pelvis, spine and cranium will adapt in any way possible to remain upright. When one changes one dynamic in a smooth coupling, the rest of the structure will accommodate and bring about a simple resolution to the problem, that is, if the pelvic girdle rotates and one hip moves anterior and the other hip moves posterior, then by bringing the pelvis into balance and levelling the horizontal plane, the pectoral girdle and the cranium will follow suit and acquire stability. This will not occur in a non-smooth coupling.

When discussing the cranial vault and the coupling effect each bone has on another, the same premise of smooth and non-smooth coupling exists. Smooth coupling in the cranium will usually result in an uncomplicated birth process and the torque effect of the torsional pressures applied by that process will allow that cranium to shift into a clockwise or counterclockwise torsional rotation. If, however, trauma at a later stage in life is applied, then the smooth coupling may become a non-smooth coupling and create irregular patterns and cranial dysfunction.

Smooth cranial coupling in a counterclockwise torque can be identified as follows: starting at the right external frontal, followed by a right external maxilla, then crossing that line to create a left internal maxilla and the left internal frontal. The sphenoid now comes into consideration and the greater wing of the sphenoid becomes depressed as the left temporal bone goes into external rotation. The left occiput follows the external temporal and becomes externally rotated. Crossing the midline, the right occiput now becomes internally rotated and pulls the left temporal bone into internal rotation. The junction point of the occiput being pulled by the internal right temporal pushes the right greater wing of the sphenoid into an elevated position. The effect of this internal rotation will cause a closing effect on the jugular foramen at the junction of the right occiput and the right temporal bone.

A clockwise torsion of the cranium will be the exact opposite of what has been described. In order not to confuse the reader, counterclockwise torsion will be discussed as the basic format in this book. Counterclockwise torque appears in most instances, as the normal birth presentation is a left occiput anterior which follows with the mother's usual pelvic position as a right external (posterior ileum) and a left internal (anterior ileum). This endorses the birth process as a clockwise function but the uterine-vagina forces produce a counterclockwise torsion on the infant. Bear in mind that at 32 weeks the foetal head, being heavier than the rest of the body, inverts and becomes lodged in the pelvic canal with the aforementioned mother's pelvic position, creating a torque that is consistent with the last few weeks of pregnancy. This established position also accounts for the same torsional affects being applied to an infant born as an emergency caesarean. Elective caesareans at 38–39 weeks mean that the foetal head probably does not undergo the same torsional forces as the foetus that goes to full term and why these infants have fewer cranial distortions.

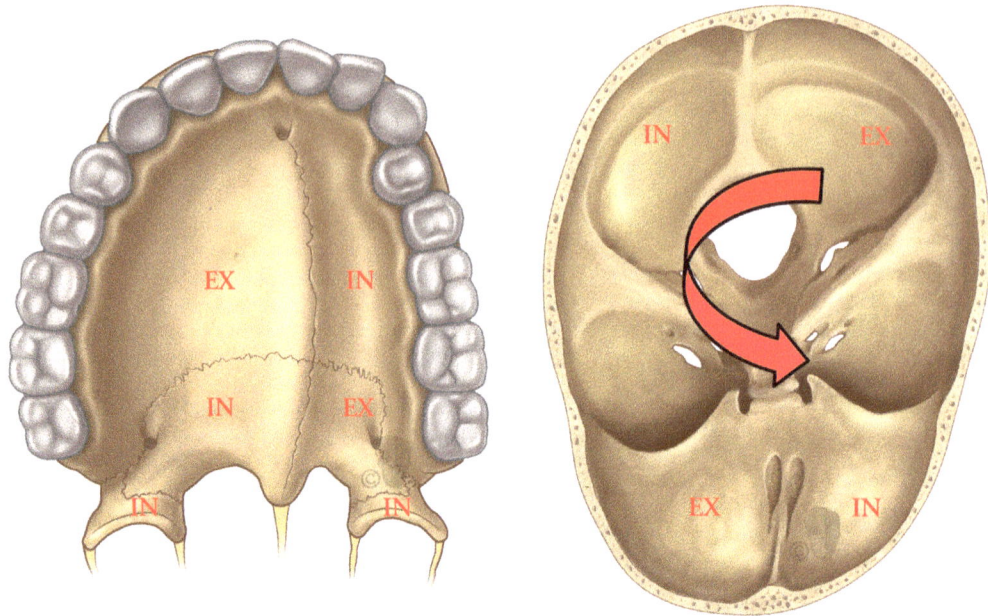

Figure 6.1 Counterclockwise Torque: At right, elevated greater wing of sphenoid

SMOOTH COUPLING COUNTERCLOCKWISE TORQUE

When the head is rotated to the left and both feet are rotated to the right and the bilateral arm test is positive, this is a smooth coupling with a counterclockwise pattern and the following cranial configuration will be observed:

- Right frontal external
- Right maxilla external
- Left maxilla internal
- Left frontal internal
- Left depressed greater wing of the sphenoid
- Left temporal external
- Left occiput external
- Right occiput internal
- Right temporal internal
- Right elevated greater wing of the sphenoid.

The superior and inferior views of the skull and the inferior view of the maxilla show the smooth counterclockwise torque configurations of the various skull bones. The IN/EX denotations as depicted on the cranial bones not only show the internal and external rotation of the bones, but also indicate the phases of inhalation and exhalation that the patient has to perform when the corrections are being made. When correcting an internal rotation lesion (an extension lesion), the bone must be taken into external rotation (flexion) while the patient inhales. When correcting an external rotation lesion (a flexion lesion), the bone must be taken into internal rotation (extension) while the patient exhales. This is the standard procedure for correcting cranial lesions and must be adhered to rigorously if one is to achieve the optimum result. The correction phase of the IN not only shows the internal lesion, but also indicates to the doctor the inhalation phase of respiration that needs to be applied in performing the correction. In the same way, the correction phase of the EX not only shows the external lesion, but indicates to the doctor the exhalation phase of respiration that needs to be applied in performing the correction.

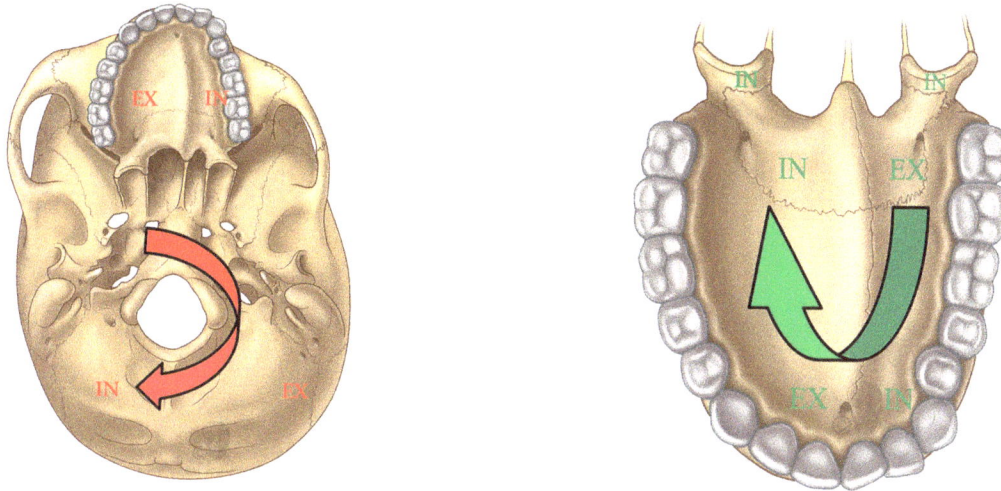

Figure 6.2 (left) Counterclockwise Torque; (right) Clockwise Correction

In terms of cranial correction, one must understand that the dural meningeal system and the endosteum are firmly adhered to the internal surface of the cranial bone, while the periosteum and muscle layers are adherent to the external surface of the cranial bone. So, in fact, the cranial correction that one is trying to achieve is directly affecting the membrane system, which is the ultimate objective. The venous sinus system is intimately interwoven within the membrane system, so while correcting cranial lesions, one is effectively making the drainage of the brain more efficient, reducing swelling, inflammation and constriction of the vessels. This stabilises the homeostatic function of blood volume into the brain, equal to the blood volume leaving the brain.

SMOOTH COUPLING CLOCKWISE TORQUE

If there is a positive reaction to the head in a right rotation position, with both feet rotated to the left, then it is a smooth coupling with a clockwise pattern and the following cranial configuration will be observed:

- Left frontal external
- Left maxilla external
- Right maxilla internal
- Right frontal internal
- Right depressed greater wing of the sphenoid
- Right temporal external
- Right occiput external
- Left occiput internal
- Left temporal internal
- Left elevated greater wing of the sphenoid.

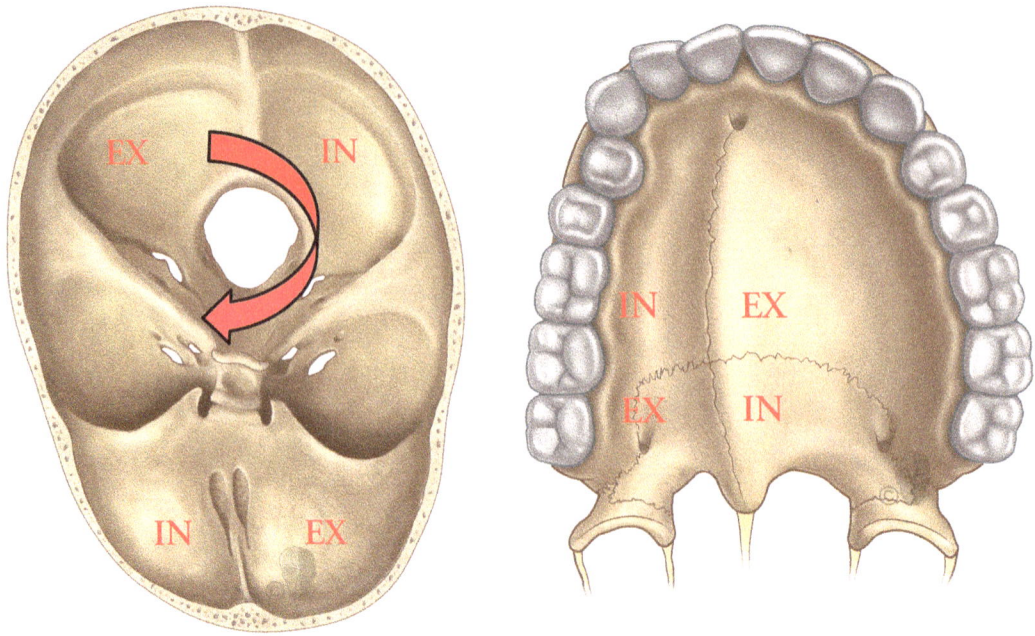

Figure 6.3 Clockwise Torque

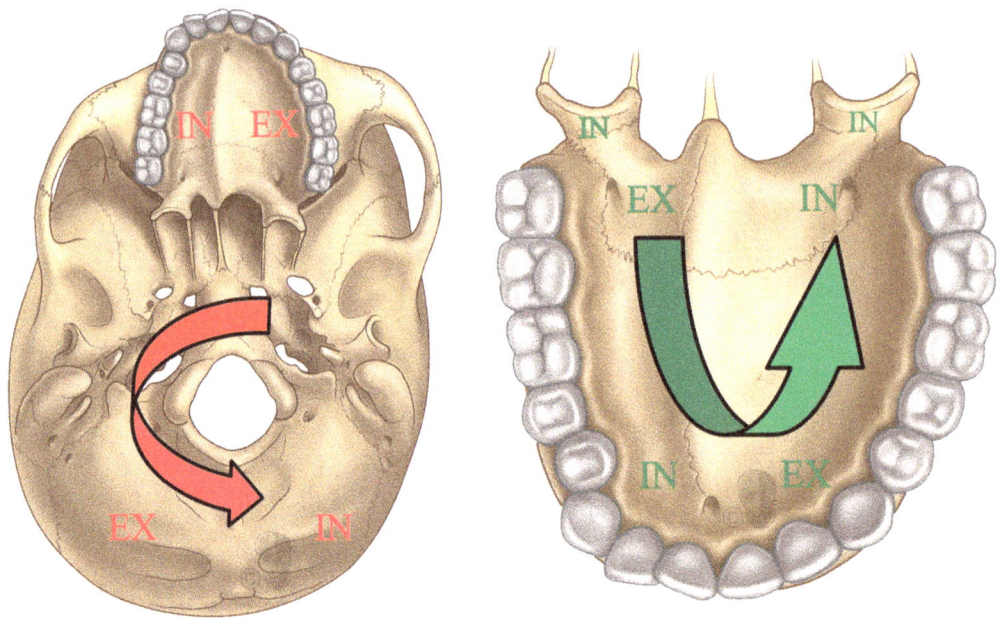

Figure 6.4 (left) Clockwise Torque; (right) Counterclockwise Correction

EXTERNAL FRONTAL INDICATORS

When looking at cranial distortions, the same effects of smooth coupling are had by taking a rectangular box and pressing the two opposite corners towards one another, thereby creating a shape where the two corners that are compressed together result in a much smaller diagonal than between the uncompressed sides. The compressed sides would indicate internal rotation and the uncompressed sides would indicate the external rotational dimensions. This, in essence, occurs when the cranial vault undergoes torsional pressures. The right would complement the external occiput/temporal on the left, creating a larger dimension than the internal frontal, and on the left and the internal occiput/temporal on the right.

Following the smooth coupling effect on the cranium, notice the pronounced external frontal bone, the elevated greater wing of the sphenoid and the large ocular orbit. As the sphenoid bone is elevated the superior orbital fissure opens and allows clear passage for all the vessels and nerves. The sphenoid moves anteriorly as it elevates, bringing the pterygoid plates anteriorly and tightening the internal and external pterygoid muscles that attach to the condyle of the mandible, pulling the mandible from right to left. The elevation of the external frontal produces the external rotation of the maxilla and causes a malocclusion with the two right dental quadrants. The nasal bones follow the external maxilla.

The facial expressions produced by the external frontal produce a 'startled look' as the eye is larger and pushed forward by the greater wing of the sphenoid. This is the eye that concentrates and is alert. The external frontal bone when looked at from the side produces a 'ski slope' appearance. The external maxilla produces a flat cheek and gives the effect of the face being almost wedge-shaped from right to left.

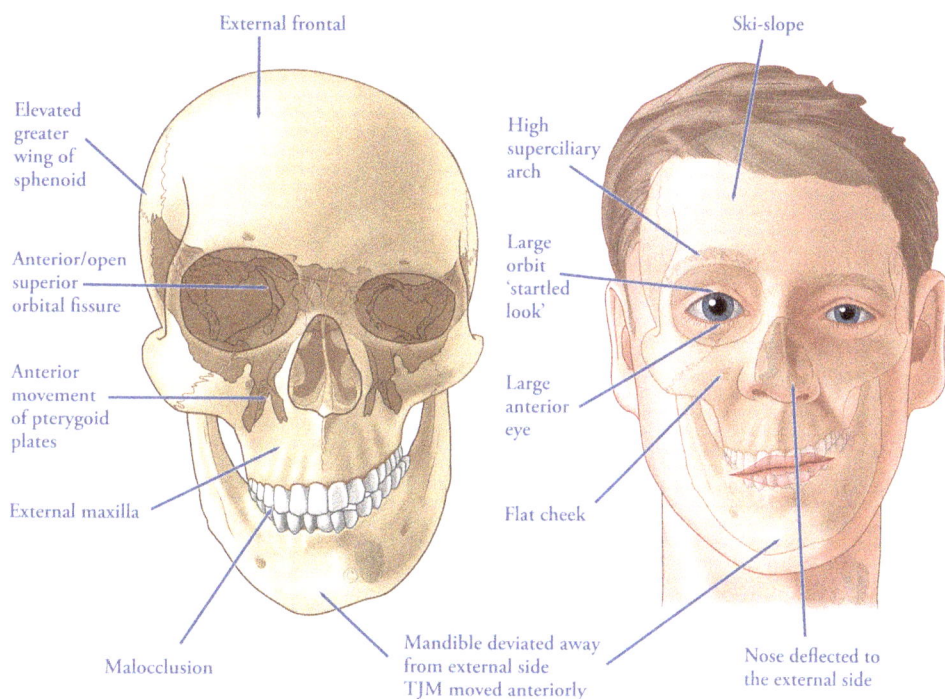

Figure 6.5 External Frontal Indicators

INTERNAL FRONTAL INDICATORS

Internal frontal indicators show a depressed frontal bone which, when looked at from the side, shows the 'ski jump' culminating on the low superciliary arch. The small ocular orbit compresses the superior orbital fissure and a posterior inclination of the greater wing of the sphenoid, and a posterior movement of the pterygoid plates. These cranial plate movements follow the external temporal bone and the external occiput, where the tentorium is stretched to its maximum at the transverse sinus between the confluence of the sinuses (occiput) and the petrosal ridge (temporal bone). The maxilla appears more pronounced on this internal maxilla side – a high cheek – and has the effect of creating a crossbite malocclusion.

Internal frontal

Depressed greater wing of sphenoid

Superior orbital fissure closes

Pterygoid plates move posteriorly

Internal maxilla

Crossbite

Mandible deviates to the internal side
Posterior TMJ

Ski-jump

Low superciliary arch

Smaller orbit smaller posterior eye

High cheek

Labial crease pronounced

Teeth worn

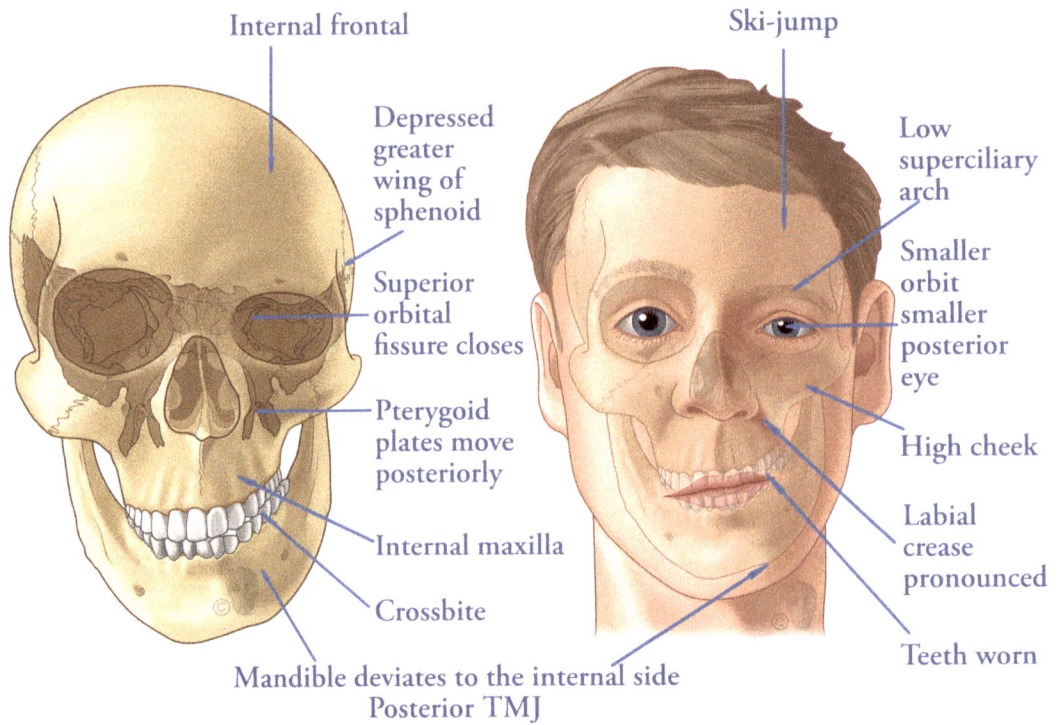

Figure 6.6 Internal Frontal Indicators

EXTERNAL TEMPORAL INDICATORS

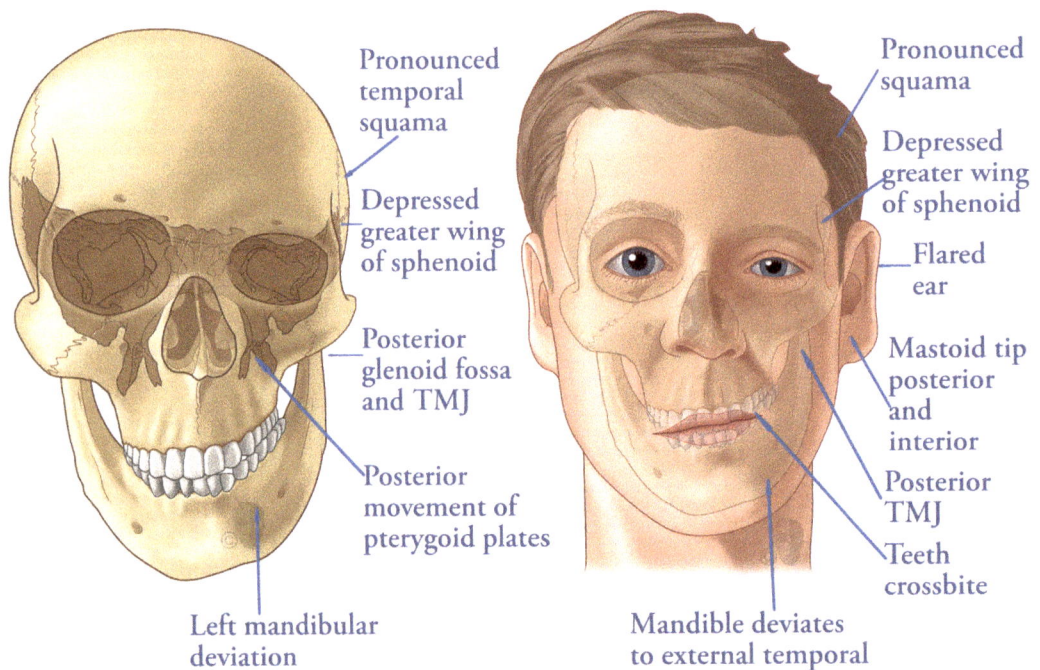

Pronounced temporal squama

Depressed greater wing of sphenoid

Posterior glenoid fossa and TMJ

Posterior movement of pterygoid plates

Left mandibular deviation

Pronounced squama

Depressed greater wing of sphenoid

Flared ear

Mastoid tip posterior and interior

Posterior TMJ

Teeth crossbite

Mandible deviates to external temporal

Figure 6.7 External Temporal Indicators

These are the left temporal indicators which lie adjacent to the left external occiput. As was outlined in the smooth coupling indicators, the greater wing of the sphenoid becomes depressed following the external temporal. The temporal squama becomes more pronounced as the mastoid tip moves medial and anterior, taking the TMJ posterior (the glenoid fossa). Notice how the sphenoid drops to the left and the posterior, closing the superior orbital fissure and restricting the apertures for the cranial nerves and vessels. The pterygoid plates are also moved posterior, pulling on the pterygoid muscles and deviating the mandible posterior to the left, as the right pterygoid plates move anterior and superior relative to one another. This causes a malocclusion on the two left dental quadrants as they are occluded, creating a possible crossbite and incisal interference. The nasal septum deviates towards the external frontal, pulling the left maxilla into internal rotation and restricts the left upper palate, resulting in congestion of the left upper dental quadrant giving the appearance of a high cheek.

The facial view of the external temporal immediately shows the constriction of the left ocular orbit pulling the eye posterior as a result of the left internal frontal – the low superciliary arch. In infants, and in particular in newborns, this eye always appears weepy and red as a conjunctivitis and does not appear to focus or concentrate. This symptom is brought about by the weak medial rectus muscle (CN III). The ear flares on the external temporal as a result of the left temporal squama. The left labial crease is more pronounced as a result of the left internal maxilla and together with the left frontal internal gives the face a compressed appearance.

INTERNAL TEMPORAL INDICATORS

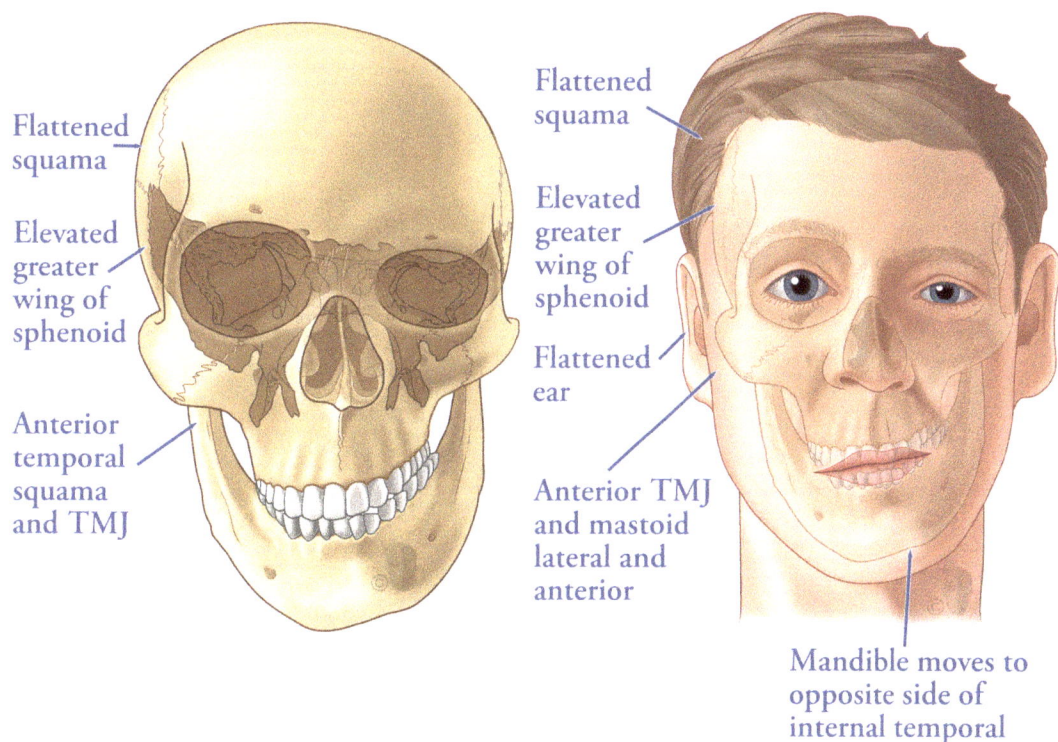

Flattened squama

Elevated greater wing of sphenoid

Anterior temporal squama and TMJ

Flattened squama

Elevated greater wing of sphenoid

Flattened ear

Anterior TMJ and mastoid lateral and anterior

Mandible moves to opposite side of internal temporal

Figure 6.8 Internal Temporal Indicators

The right internal temporal appears with the flattened wing of the sphenoid pulling the eye anterior and opening the superior orbital fissure. The ocular orbit appears larger on the right external frontal and with a high superciliary arch the eye appears larger and more engaging. The internal temporal moves the glenoid/mandibular fossa anterior and opens the TMJ, giving the ear a flattened appearance. The pterygoid plates move anterior, lengthening the pterygoid muscles, and release the right mandibular condyle which has the effect of creating a malocclusion on the right upper and lower dental quadrants.

The facial view of the right internal temporal shows the flattened squama, the high superciliary arch and the very pronounced open eye. It also shows the open wedge appearance of the face primarily as the mandible deviates to the left with the external temporal bone and the flat cheek of the right external maxilla.

NORMAL SKULL

The superior view of the skull shows the cranial floor with the frontal bone, the temporal bone and the occiput surrounding the foramen magnum. The occipital bone meets the temporal bone at the petrous portion of the temporal bone and provides the anchor point for the tentorium cerebellum, the internal auditory meatus (which carries the acoustic and the facial nerves) and the jugular foramen – the aperture that allows passage of the glossopharyngeal, the vagus and spinal accessory nerves and the internal jugular vein. The petrous portion of the temporal bone is an extension of the ridge and groove of the transverse sinus of the occipital bone. The occipital fossa provides the bed for the occipital lobes of the brain; the temporal fossa provides the bed for the temporal lobes; and the frontal fossa provides the bed for the frontal lobes.

The intracranial dural membranes (the RTM) have specific anchor points in the cranial vault. The falx cerebri has its anchor point in the crista galli of the ethmoid bone and the tentorium cerebelli has its anchor point in the petrous portion of the temporal bone. The falx cerebelli has its anchor point at the internal occipital protuberance and at the foramen magnum, and the diaphragma sellae has its anchor point at the anterior and posterior clinoid processes of the sphenoid bone.

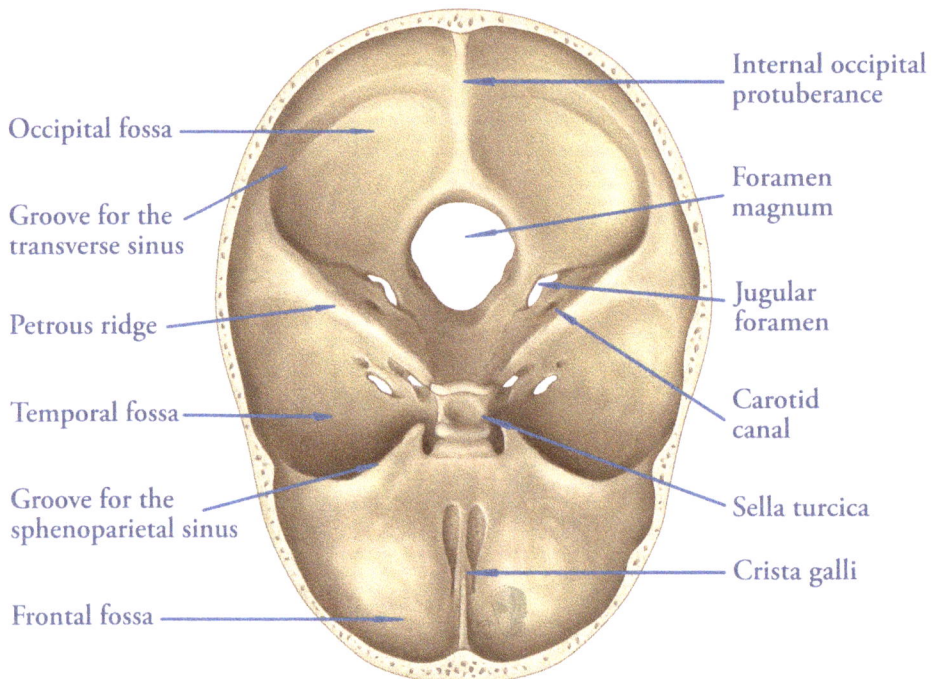

Occipital fossa

Groove for the transverse sinus

Petrous ridge

Temporal fossa

Groove for the sphenoparietal sinus

Frontal fossa

Internal occipital protuberance

Foramen magnum

Jugular foramen

Carotid canal

Sella turcica

Crista galli

Figure 6.9 Textbook Skull

BALANCED MAXILLA

Intra-oral corrections are made primarily at the roof of the mouth, the palate. The bones that make up the palate are representative of the anterior cranial plates. The hard palate is represented by the two maxillae and the two palatine bones separated by the cruciate suture.

The maxillae are representative of the frontal bone that at birth is made up of two parts separated by the metopic suture, which usually fuses by the age of two; these are separated by the intermaxillary suture.

The two palatine bones are representative of the ipsilateral temporal bones and are separated by the interpalatine suture.

The two hamuli or pterygoid plates are located posterior to the palatine bones and are part of the sphenoid bone. The medial pterygoid plate is found bilaterally medial to the wisdom tooth (number 8) and a ¼ inch posterior. The pterygoid plates are also the insertion points for the internal and external pterygoid muscles.

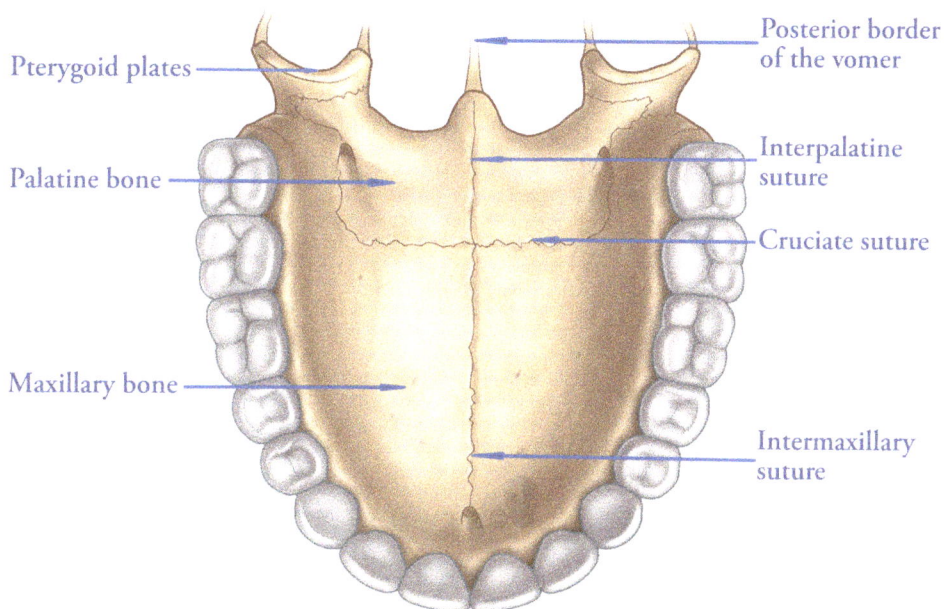

Figure 6.10 Textbook Maxillae

NORMAL OCCLUSION

The inferior view of the mouth in Figure 6.11 shows the two maxillae in external rotation and the teeth that come from those two arches. The medial and lateral incisors, the canines, the premaxillary, the molars and the wisdom teeth are the full complement of the maxillae.

Posterior to the maxillae are the two internally rotated palatines, which abut the two pterygoid plates. The mandibular teeth are in the same configuration and occlude with the maxillary teeth, with the buccal cusps of the mandibular teeth occluding with the inter-cusp position of the maxillary teeth, providing an overlap of the maxillary teeth over the mandibular teeth. This occlusal configuration represents a class I occlusion.

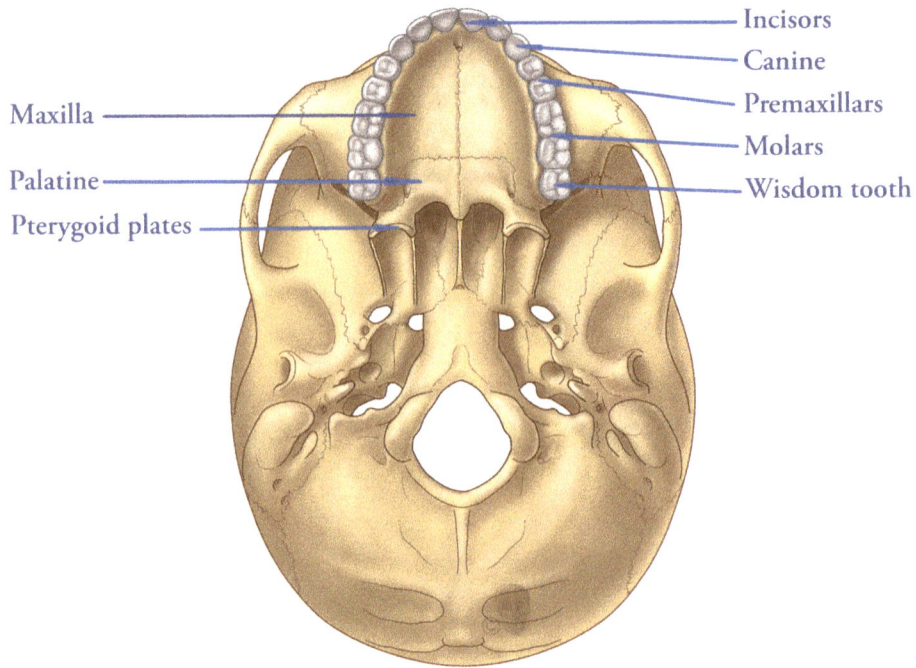

Incisors
Canine
Maxilla
Premaxillars
Molars
Palatine
Wisdom tooth
Pterygoid plates

Figure 6.11 Textbook Occlusion

NORMAL EYES

In normal circumstances, both eyes should be on an even plane, both orbits the same size and both eyes should be alert and focused. Structurally, the sphenoid should be level, both vertically and horizontally, the superior orbital fissures will then be open, allowing full neurological and arterial access to the vessels that pass through them.

The cranial nerves that control the eyes are in full control of any orbital movement, including the medius rectus muscles when orbital convergence is required. Muscles should not fatigue. The optic nerves should transmit evenly to the optic chiasma and to the visual fields in the occiput.

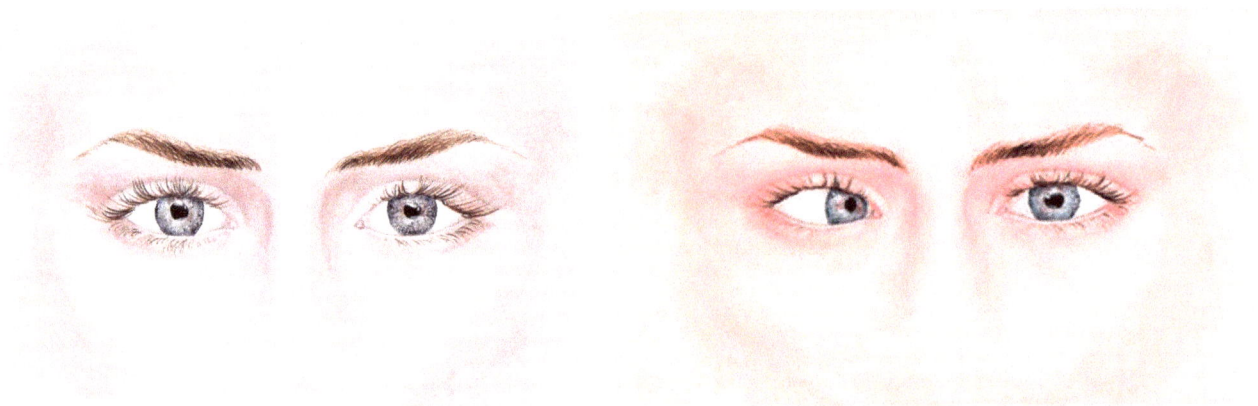

Figure 6.12 (left) Normal Ocular Function; (right) Poor Ocular Convergence

POOR OCULAR CONVERGENCE

It is important for the chiropractic doctor to identify the dominant eye, generally seen on the external frontal side, usually with a larger orbit and a more direct looking eye. Dominant eye tests will illustrate whether the left or the right eye is dominant. Identification of the dominant brain is done by asking the patient to cough while looking at the uvula of the soft palate and watching whichever side moves superiorward when the patient activates the uvula by saying 'aah'. This is activated by the vagus nerve, and the side that pulls highest indicates the dominant brain side. This will usually be on the contralateral side to the dominant eye.

Tests for eye convergence are done using the oculomotor nerve, cranial nerve III and identifying the weak or fatigued medial rectus muscle. Remember, the medial rectus muscle has a homologous partner on the ipsilateral side with the multifidus muscle, which extends from C2 down to the sacrum. The dominant brain side will usually be on the external temporal, external occipital side, and will usually be opposite the jugular foramenal compression area. For example, one can see a dominant eye on the right with an external right frontal bone; a dominant brain on the left, the contralateral side, with an external temporal and an external occipital bone. Jugular foramenal compression will be on the right jugular foramen, usually on the internal temporal/internal occiput side. The non-dominant eye will be the left eye, weak medial rectus muscle will be on the left side, with poor convergence (convergence insufficiency). The multifidus muscle will be ipsilateral to the medial rectus and will therefore appear to be hypotonic on the left side of the spine.

DETERMINATION OF DOMINANT BRAIN

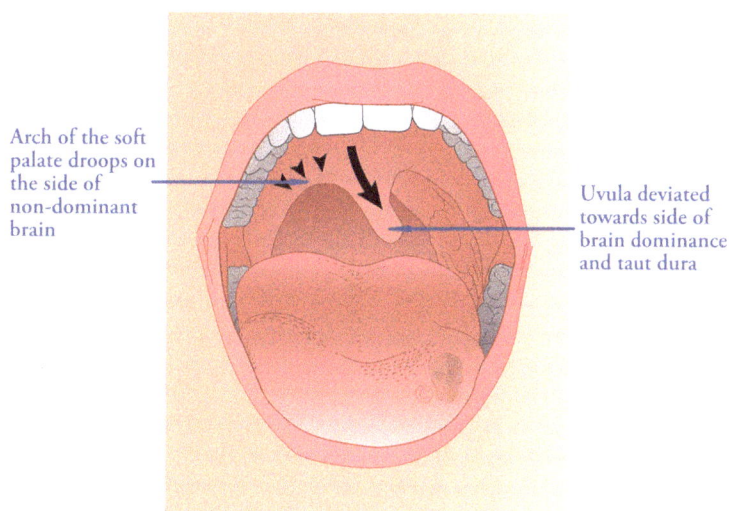

Arch of the soft palate droops on the side of non-dominant brain

Uvula deviated towards side of brain dominance and taut dura

Figure 6.13 Determination of Dominant Brain

The dominant brain is evident on the external occiput/external temporal and the depressed greater wing of the sphenoid side, whereas the non-dominant brain appears to be on the internal occiput/internal temporal and the elevated greater wing of the sphenoid side. In the majority of cases one sees the former pattern as occurring the most, which produces a left external occiput, left external temporal, right internal occiput and right internal temporal. This gives rise to a dominant left brain and dominant right eye, usually rendering the person right-handed.

If one does a test for the dominant eye in the case we have just mentioned, the dominant eye will be on the right external frontal side of the skull, primarily because there is more room for that right eye to develop. With the larger external frontal dimension, the sphenoid greater wing will be elevated on the right and the superior orbital fissure will not be distorted – this produces an alert and dominant eye. The left eye, on the other hand, is very much the submissive partner and the non-dominant eye; smaller internal frontal, depressed greater wing of sphenoid and distortion superior orbital fissure. Dominant eye tests will show that the right eye is dominant.

Therefore, the dominant right eye dominates the left brain. The left brain produces a right-handed dominance and makes sure that the left sensory/motor functions of the cerebral hemispheres dictate more effectively into the right hand and right foot.

Scientific observations have shown that in a person with a dominant right eye, the right leg has a shorter gait than the left leg and the right arm travels less than the left arm, bearing in mind that the right external ilium also appears on the relative short leg side.

MULTIFIDES MUSCLES

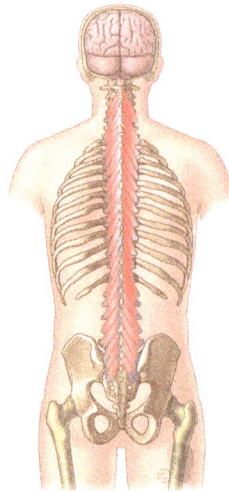

Figure 6.14 Multifides Muscles

The medius rectus muscle has a homologous partner on the ipsilateral side with the multifidus muscle, which extends from C2 down to the sacrum. The multifidus muscles start at the sacral bone at the base of the spine and extend up to the axis. The muscles feature multiple insertion points along the spine, specifically into the spinous process of each vertebra. These series of muscles are further divided into two groups that include the superficial muscle group and the deep muscle group. The multifidus muscles help to take pressure off the vertebral discs so that our body weight can be well distributed along the spine. Additionally, the superficial muscle group keeps our spine straight, while the deep muscle group contributes significantly to the stability of our spine.

The weak medius rectus muscle occurs on the non-dominant eye. The reason that there is poor convergence on the non-dominant eye is that the counterclockwise cranial torque and fascial distortion gives rise to a torsion on the oculomotor nerve, which fatigues the muscle on recurrent convergence activity until it no longer performs as it should. The sphenoid has moved posterior and inferior, closing the superior orbital fissure and pulling the left internal maxilla with it. Applying fixed braces to the upper arch on this individual results in locking the maxillae, keeping the sphenoid posterior and inferior and disallows any compensation to movement in the skull. The result can activate the multifidus muscles in a weakened area of the spine causing it to buckle under these dynamics and produce a scoliosis. This problem needs to be monitored carefully when applying fixed braces to the upper arch under any circumstances – particularly in adolescence.

INDICATORS FOR ANTERIOR AND POSTERIOR POLES

The frontal/maxilla bones of the skull are intimately and directly related to the crista galli of the ethmoid bone – the anchor point of the falx cerebri – by the vomer, and therefore represents the anterior pole, and are denoted by IN. Similarly the temporal/occiput are directly linked to the sphenoid – the anchor point for the tentorium cerebellum – by the basilar portion of the occiput and the petrous portion of the temporal bone, and represent the posterior pole and are denoted by EX.

The vomer is the lynchpin of the entire cranial membrane system. The action that it exerts and the dynamics that it employs creates the viability of cranial physiology as explained earlier.

The sphenoid bone provides the anchor point for the membranes – the tentorium and the diaphragma sellae around the sella turcica, in the body of the sphenoid – and also provides the leverage by which the membrane's tautness can be controlled and the vector provided by the medial and lateral pterygoid plate that is activated through the mouth at the hamulus. Disengaging the pterygoid plates allows the posterior pole to correct itself.

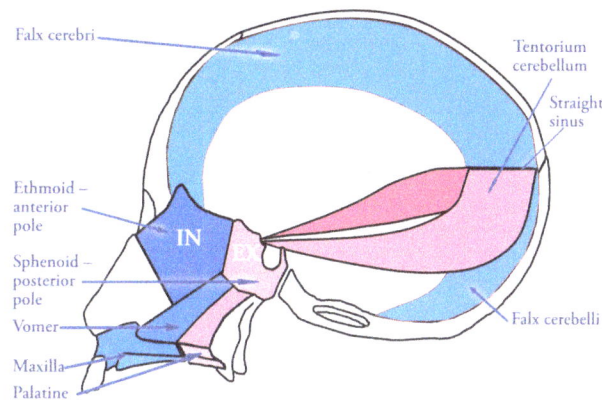

Figure 6.15 Anterior and Posterior Poles

ADULT SKULL

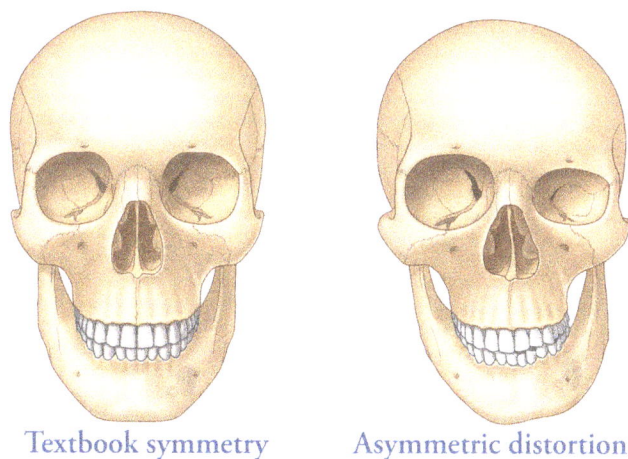

Textbook symmetry   Asymmetric distortion

Figure 6.16 Adult Skull: (left) Textbook symmetry, (right) asymmetric distortion

The adult skull on the left in Figure 6.16 shows symmetry in all its aspects. The bilateral external rotation of the frontal bones gives two large ocular orbits with both eyes level and on the same plane. This produces bilateral greater wings of the sphenoid on the same level and subsequently the pterygoid plates are evenly disposed, with even tension on both pairs of the internal and external pterygoid muscles allowing the mandible to swing symmetrically within the glenoid/mandibular fossae. This produces a bilateral externally rotated maxillae and a class I occlusion.

The adult skull on the right shows a counterclockwise cranial distortion, producing a large ocular orbit on the right side with a large dominant eye and the low superciliary arch on the left side with a posterior non-dominant eye. Both these eyes follow the right external frontal and the left internal frontal. The greater wings of the sphenoid slope to the left side of the skull, producing an internal temporal on the right and an external temporal on the left. The right pterygoid plates on the right side follow the anterior sphenoid that is elevated, while the left pterygoid plates move posterior and the sphenoid becomes depressed. The right external maxilla and the left internal maxilla produce a malocclusion when closing on the opposite arches of the mandible that is pulled to the left and posterior. This counterclockwise distortion has been emphasised in this book, as the majority of distortions follow this pattern.

NORMAL SKELETAL BALANCE

Normal skeletal balance is observed with level head, level shoulders and a level pelvis. The spine is vertical and the cranium maintains a level posture, allowing the brain and spinal cord to function at optimal potential. The TMJs are level and neurologically balanced with the sacroiliac joints of the pelvis.

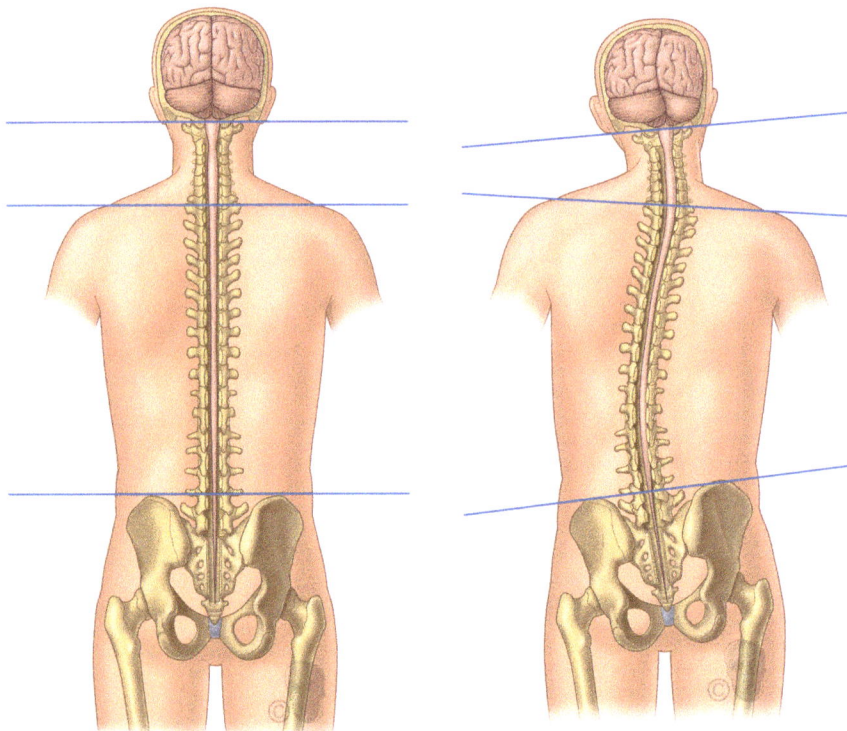

Figure 6.17 (left) Normal Skeletal Balance; (right) Dural Meningeal Torque

DURAL MENINGEAL TORQUE

Dural meningeal torque occurs when, in this instance, the right ileum moves posterior and external, while the left ileum moves anterior and inferior. This produces a relatively short leg on the right as the trochanteric head is elevated while the relative long leg on the left ileum is depressed. Both sacroiliac joints become torqued as both the inferior and superior interosseous ligaments surrounding the sacroiliac joints are put under strain as the sacrum realigns itself within the rotated pelvis. The lines indicating the level of the head, the shoulders and the pelvis show that this is a smooth coupling. There is reciprocal movement between the right internal temporal bone, which moves in relation to the left internal ileum, and the left external temporal bone, which moves in relation to the right external ileum. The TMJs move in an equal and opposite direction of their opposing sacroiliac joints. Both the TMJ and the sacroiliac joint are highly proprioceptive. As the level of the head follows the level of the pelvis, the brain supported by the dural meninges – the falx cerebri, the falx cerebellum and the tentorium cerebellum – become distorted, changing the position and physiology of the cranial organs, as well as the arterial and venous circulation of the brain. The torque of the spinal cord means that all 24 pairs of spinal nerve roots also become torqued and interfere with normal nerve transmission, and the vertebrae of the spinal column become subluxated. This type of posture produces neurological dysfunction and has central symptomatology – the central organs controlled by the parasympathetic and sympathetic nervous systems.

Sacroiliac strain

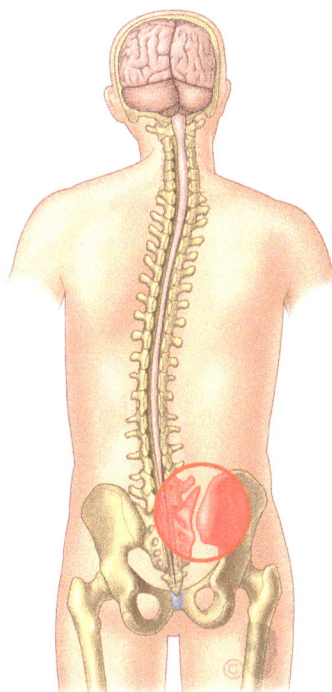

Figure 6.18 Sacroiliac Strain

As the torsion on the superior and inferior interosseous ligaments increases, the weight-bearing sacroiliac joints become strained and stretched, creating a sacroiliac lesion – in this instance usually on the right side, which corresponds to the left congested TMJ as the mandible deviates to the left. This can produce a descending major as the malocclusion directly impinges on the stomatognathic system. If this is the case the malocclusion has to be addressed to balance the stomatognathic system. If the sacroiliac joint is the ascending major then the weight-bearing joint has to be corrected. As a result of the sacroiliac joint instability the latissimus dorsi pulls at T6 (pancreas), C4 (phrenic nerve to the diaphragm) and its attachment at the anterior head of the humerus, depressing the shoulder girdle and implicating the shoulder (rotator cuff), elbow and wrist (carpal tunnel). On the opposite side (left) the upper trapezius muscle pulls on the mastoid, distorting the TMJ and its relationship with the condyle of the mandible, affecting the vestibular mechanism – both balance and hearing. The right temporalis muscle becomes stretched as a result of the left deviating mandible and adds to the complication of the TMJ, producing headaches, trigeminal neuralgia and tic douloureux, basically changing the trigeminal ganglia and its nerve complex. The spinal nucleus adjacent to C1, C2 and C3 can, with trigeminal dysfunction, create a malocclusion and subluxate C1 and possibly C2.

Below the waist the inguinal ligament becomes distorted, affecting the sartorius and gracilis muscles which insert into the medial aspect of the knee, disrupting the medial meniscus, while on the opposite leg (left) the tensor fasciae latae (TFL) pulls into the lateral aspect of the left knee. Both these consequences change the gait and ultimately challenge the ankle and the foot. This posture produces weight-bearing changes and has lateral symptomatology. This is a biomechanical weight-bearing lesion.

LUMBAR SACRAL LESION

If the sacroiliac lesion is not corrected the weight-bearing lesion becomes exacerbated and the patient starts to become antalgic, affecting the L5/S1 disc. As the spinal scoliosis deteriorates, the disc becomes swollen, prolapses and can rupture. The posture of this patient starts to appear as a non-smooth coupling. This is always indicative of a lumbosacral disc lesion, usually representative of a sciatic involvement. The head follows the shoulder and the antalgic lean becomes evident and is diagnostic in regard to the type of disc lesion. When the body leans away from the side with sciatica, the lesion is a lateral disc bulge appearing external to the spinal canal. If the body leans toward the side with sciatica, this is a medial disc bulge that can be more difficult to resolve because the disc bulge lies within the intervertebral foramen at the source of the nerve root. If the body is bent forward, the disc prolapse is pressing on the theca, representing a central disc prolapse and, depending on the severity, may be resolved or surgical intervention may be necessary.

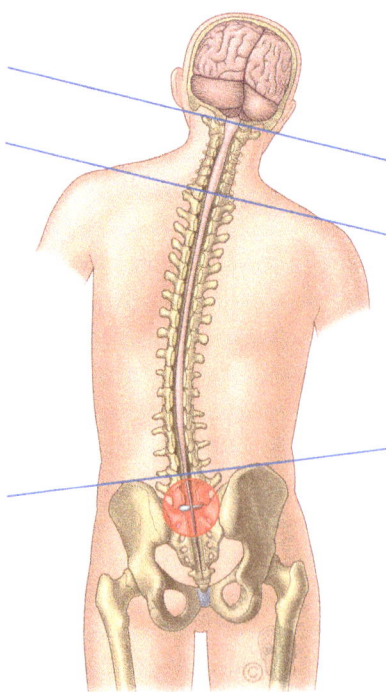

Figure 6.19 Lumbar-Sacral Disc Lesion

Another possible cause of a lumbar disc lesion could be an ongoing presence of an atlas subluxation, as L5 and the atlas have a Lovett Brother relationship. The compensation and adaptation at the atlas become compromised and L5 will subluxate accordingly, eventually leading to a disc prolapse and antalgia.

As L5 and T9 (adrenal) are part of the subluxation pattern, many older patients – particularly men – undergo chronic adrenal exhaustion, which means they are constantly utilising their mineral reserves stored in muscles, ligaments and tendons, resulting in a weakened musculoskeletal system. At the pinnacle of this adrenal exhaustion, usually brought about by a period of excessive stress, T9 can no longer cope and the L5 disc prolapses. Resolution of this type of lesion can be achieved by a change in lifestyle, chiropractic care and the use of mineral supplements.

CRANIAL NERVE EXAMINATION

Cranial Nerve I – Olfactory Nerve

The olfactory system is made up of the olfactory epithelial bulb and tract. The olfactory epithelium is located in the roof of the nasal cavity and extends on to the nasal conchae and the nasal septum. This is a special sensory nerve (special afferent) and the olfactory tract exits through the foramen of the cribriform plate of the ethmoid. It has its nuclei in the diencephalon and its function is sensation of smell.

Cranial Nerve II – Optic Nerve

This is a special sensory nerve (afferent somatic). It has its nuclei in the lateral geniculate nucleus of the diencephalon. Light entering the pupils travels to the back of the eye and passes through the retina to the rods and cones. The information received by the rods and cones is transmitted down the optic nerve track, through the optic foramen on the lesser wing of the sphenoid, to the optic chiasma, through the lateral geniculate nucleus and finally to the occipital lobe.

Cranial Nerve III – Oculomotor Nerve

This nerve has two components. The first is the visceral motor (general visceral efferent) and provides the parasympathetic supply to constrictor pupillae and ciliary muscles via the ciliary ganglion. It has its nucleus in the nucleus of Edinger Westphal in the rostral midbrain and exits from the cranium through the superior orbital fissure of the sphenoid bone. It facilitates the contraction and accommodation of light through the pupil. The second component is the somatic motor (general somatic efferent) that supplies the levator palpebrae superioris, superior rectus, medial rectus, inferior rectus and the inferior oblique muscles of the eye. It has its nucleus in the oculomotor nucleus situated in the rostral midbrain. It exits through the superior orbital fissure of the sphenoid bone and is responsible for ocular movement.

Cranial Nerve IV – Trochlear Nerve

This is a somatic motor (general somatic efferent) nerve and supplies the superior oblique muscle of the eye. It has its nucleus in the trochlear nucleus of the midbrain and exits through the superior orbital fissure of the sphenoid bone.

Cranial Nerve V – Trigeminal Nerve

The trigeminal nerve has two components. The sensory component (somatic afferent) innervates the sensory branches of the ophthalmic, maxillary and mandibular nerves to the skin and mucous membranes of the face and head, external aspects of the tympanic membrane and the meninges of the anterior and middle cranial fossae. It has its nucleus in the trigeminal sensory nucleus situated in the pons and the various branches of the trigeminal nerve exit through three separate foramena. The ophthalmic division exits through the superior orbital fissure of the sphenoid bone, the maxillary division through the foramen rotundum of the greater wing of the sphenoid and the mandibular division through the foramen ovale of the greater wing of the sphenoid.

The second component is the motor component (visceral efferent) that controls muscles of mastication (the temporalis, masseter and pterygoid), the tensor tympani, the tensor veli palatini, the mylohyoid and the anterior belly of the digastric. It has its nucleus in the trigeminal motor nucleus situated in the pons and exits through the foramen ovale situated in the greater wing of the sphenoid. Its function is mastication, to open and close the mouth, move the jaw from side to side.

Cranial Nerve VI – Abducens Nerve

This is a somatic motor nerve (somatic efferent) which supplies the lateral rectus muscle of the eye. It has its nucleus in the abducens nucleus situated in the pons and exits through the superior orbital fissure of the sphenoid bone. Its function is to move the eyeball in lateral directions.

Cranial Nerve VII – Facial Nerve

This nerve has four components. The sensory component (somatic afferent) supplies the skin of the concha of the auricle – the small area of skin behind the ear – and supplies the wall of the acoustic meatus and external tympanic membrane. It has its nucleus in the spinal trigeminal nucleus of the rostral medulla and exits through the internal acoustic meatus of the temporal bone. It displays sensitivity to the external ear reflex and the external ear and mastoid region.

The second component is visceral sensory and receives impulses from the anterior two-thirds of the tongue and the hard and soft palates. It has its nucleus in the nucleus solitarius of the rostral medulla and exits through the internal acoustic meatus along the petrotympanic fissure of the temporal bone. Its function is to taste.

The third component is a visceral motor (visceral efferent) and stimulates the lacrimal, submandibular and sublingual glands, as well as the mucous membranes of the nose and hard and soft palates. It has its nucleus in the superior salivatory nucleus in the rostral medulla and exits through the internal acoustic meatus of the temporal bone. Its function is for glandular secretion, salivation and crying.

The fourth component is a motor (visceral efferent) and supplies the stapedius, the stylohyoid, posterior belly of the digastric muscles, muscles of facial expression, including the buccinator, platysma and occipitalis muscles. It has its nucleus in the facial nucleus of the pons and exits through the internal acoustic meatus of the temporal bone. It is responsible for facial expression, smiling and closing eyelids.

Cranial Nerve VIII – Acoustic/Vestibulocochlear

This is a sensory nerve (special afferent) and receives auditory information from the cochlea and balance information from the semicircular canals in the organ of Corti. It has its nucleus in the vestibulocochlear nucleus in the medulla and exits through the internal acoustic meatus of the temporal bone through the medial geniculate nucleus to the temporal cortex. Its function is hearing and balance.

Cranial Nerve IX – Glossopharyngeal Nerve

This nerve has four components. The first component is a motor (visceral efferent) and supplies the striated muscles of the stylopharyngeus. It has its nucleus in the nucleus ambiguus of the medulla and exits at the jugular foramen of the occiput. Its action is swallowing.

The second component is motor (visceral efferent) and supplies the optic ganglion and stimulates the parotid gland. It has its nucleus in the nucleus salivatorius in the rostral medulla and exits through the jugular foramen of the occiput. It is responsible for glandular secretions and salivation.

The third component is sensory (special afferent) for taste on the posterior one-third of the tongue. It has its nucleus in the nucleus solitarius in the medulla and exits through the jugular foramen of the occiput. Its function is taste.

The fourth component is a general sensory (general somatic afferent) which provides the sensitivity of the external ear, posterior one-third of the tongue, the tympanic nerve and the carotid sinus. It has its nucleus in the nucleus solitarius of the medulla and exits through the jugular foramen. Its function is taste.

Cranial Nerve X – Vagus Nerve

This is comprised of four components. The first is a motor (visceral efferent) to the pharynx, tongue, larynx, and tensor veli palatini. It has its nucleus in the nucleus ambiguus in the medulla and exits through the jugular foramen of the occiput. Its function is swallowing and elevating the palate.

The second component is visceral motor (visceral efferent) to the glands of the pharynx and larynx and the thoracic and abdominal viscera. It has its nucleus in the dorsal motor nucleus of the medulla, exits through the jugular foramen of the occiput and its function is to stimulate secretions to the gastric glands.

The third component is the somatic sensory (somatic afferent) from the skin behind the ear and in the external acoustic meatus. It has its nucleus in the spinal trigeminal nucleus of the medulla, exits through the jugular foramen of the occiput and its function is sensitivity to touch.

The fourth component is visceral sensory (visceral afferent) from the larynx, trachea, oesophagus and thoracic and abdominal viscera. It has its nucleus in the nucleus solitarius of the medulla, exits through the jugular foramen of the occiput and its function is to taste, swallow and talk.

Cranial Nerve XI – Spinal Accessory Nerve

It is a motor (visceral efferent) nerve that supplies function to the SCM and the trapezius muscle. It has its nucleus in the lateral part of the anterior grey column of the upper five or six segments of the spinal cord, approximately in line with the nucleus ambiguus, enters through the foramen magnum and exits through the jugular foramen of the occiput. Its function is to turn the head and lift the shoulders.

Cranial Nerve XII – Hypoglossal Nerve

This is a somatic motor (somatic efferent) nerve which supplies the intrinsic and extrinsic muscles of the tongue. It has its nucleus in the hypoglossal nucleus of the medulla and exits through the hypoglossal foramen of the occiput. Its function is to move the tongue.

CONCLUSION

Cranial Smooth Coupling
- See diagrams

Smooth Coupling Counterclockwise Torque
- Right frontal external
- Right maxilla external
- Left maxilla internal
- Left frontal internal
- Left depressed greater wing of the sphenoid
- Left temporal external
- Left occiput external
- Right occiput internal
- Right temporal internal
- Right elevated greater wing of the sphenoid

Smooth Coupling Clockwise Torque

- Left frontal external
- Left maxilla external
- Right maxilla internal
- Right frontal internal
- Right depressed greater wing of the sphenoid
- Right temporal external
- Right occiput external
- Left occiput internal
- Left temporal internal
- Left elevated greater wing of the sphenoid

External Frontal Indicators

- See diagrams

Internal Frontal Indicators

- See diagrams

External Temporal Indicators

- See diagrams

Internal Temporal Indicators

- See diagrams

Normal Skull

- See diagrams

Balanced Maxilla

- See diagrams

Normal Occlusion

The inferior view of the mouth shows the two maxillae in external rotation and the teeth that come from those two arches. The medial and lateral incisors, the canines, the premaxillary, the molars and the wisdom teeth are the full complement of the maxillae.

Normal Eyes

In normal circumstances, both eyes should be on an even plane, both orbits the same size and both eyes alert and focused. The medial rectus muscles will move evenly as there is no cranial torque.

Poor Ocular Convergence

The convergence of the eyes is controlled by the medius rectus muscles. As the brain moves into a counterclockwise torque, the right medial rectus follows the torque and maintains convergence, while the left medial rectus has to move in a clockwise direction against the torque and weakens, leaving the left eye unable to converge.

Determination of Dominant Brain

The dominant brain is evident on the external occiput/external temporal and the depressed greater wing of the sphenoid side, whereas the non-dominant brain appears to be on the internal occiput/internal temporal and the elevated greater wing of the sphenoid side.

Multifides Muscle

The medius rectus muscle has a homologous partner on the ipsilateral side with the multifidus muscle, which extends from C2 down to the sacrum. The multifidus muscle starts at the sacral bone at the base of the spine and extends up to the axis. The muscle features multiple insertion points along the spine, specifically into the spinous process of each vertebra.

Indicators for Anterior and Posterior Poles

The frontal/maxilla bones of the skull are intimately and directly related to the crista galli of the ethmoid bone (the anchor point of the falx cerebri) by the vomer, and therefore represent the anterior pole, and are denoted by IN.

Similarly the temporal/occiput are directly linked to the sphenoid (the anchor point for the tentorium cerebellum), by the basilar portion of the occiput and the petrous portion of the temporal bone, and represent the posterior pole and are denoted by EX.

Adult Skull

The adult skull shows symmetry in all its aspects. There is bilateral external rotation of the frontal bones giving two large ocular orbits with both eyes level and on the same plane. This produces bilateral greater wings of the sphenoid on the same level and subsequently the pterygoid plates are evenly disposed, with even tension on both pairs of the internal and external pterygoid muscles, allowing the mandible to swing symmetrically within the glenoid/mandibular fossae. This produces a bilateral externally rotated maxillae and a class I occlusion.

Normal Skeletal Balance

Normal skeletal balance is observed with level head, level shoulders and a level pelvis. The spine is vertical and the cranium maintains a level posture, allowing the brain and spinal cord to function at optimal potential. The TMJs are level and neurologically balanced with the sacroiliac joints of the pelvis.

Dural Meningeal Torque

Dural meningeal torque occurs when, in this instance, the right ileum moves posterior and external, while the left ileum moves anterior and inferior. This produces a relatively short leg on the right as the trochanteric head is elevated, while the relative long leg on the left ileum is depressed. Both sacroiliac joints become torqued as both the inferior and superior interosseous ligaments surrounding the sacroiliac joints are put under strain as the sacrum realigns itself within the rotated pelvis.

Sacroiliac Strain

As the torsion on the superior and inferior interosseous ligaments increases, the weight-bearing sacroiliac joints become strained and stretched, creating a sacroiliac lesion – in this instance usually on the right side, which corresponds to the left congested TMJ as the mandible deviates to the left.

Lumbar Sacral Lesion

If the sacroiliac lesion is not corrected, the weight-bearing lesion becomes exacerbated and the patient starts to become antalgic, affecting the L5/S1 disc. As the spinal scoliosis deteriorates, the disc becomes swollen, prolapses and can rupture. The posture of this patient starts to appear as a non-smooth coupling.

Cranial Nerve Examination

The notes for the cranial nerves give a full description of the nerves and their function.

THE DISLOCATED BRAIN

PART II

CRANIAL PHYSIOLOGY

AND DYNAMICS

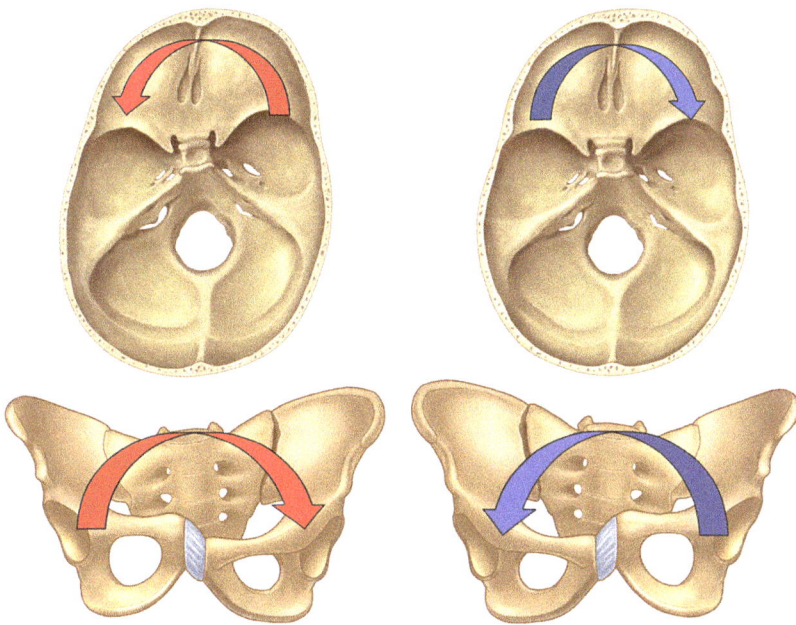

CONTENTS PART II

ILLUSTRATIONS PART II

INTRODUCTION TO PART II

The purpose of this cranial module is to introduce the subject of craniopathy to healthcare workers who are not familiar with the workings and functioning of the cranium. The brain constitutes 80% of the central nervous system (CNS) that lies above the atlas vertebra. The importance of understanding the cranial function and interdependence of the brain components with cranial physiology is paramount to achieving the end goal.

The spinal cord changes at the foramen magnum, to become the pia mater (innermost covering of the brain), the arachnoid mater (second covering of the brain) and the dura mater, which separates into the meningeal dura (covers the brain and incorporates the entire vascular irrigation system) and the endosteal dura (covers the internal surface of the cranium).

The periosteal dura covers the external surface of the cranium (the considerations for this undertaking the membrane component – the reciprocal tension membranes).

CHAPTER 1

INTERNAL DYNAMICS OF THE CRANIUM

The reciprocal tension membrane (RTM) components include:

- Falx cerebri – vertical component separating cerebral hemispheres
- Falx cerebelli – vertical component separating the cerebellar hemispheres
- Tentorium cerebelli – horizontal component, separating the cerebrum from the cerebellum
- Diapragma selli – horizontal component lying in the sella turcica

These membranes support, protect and separate the brain components to ensure that the brain retains homeostasis.

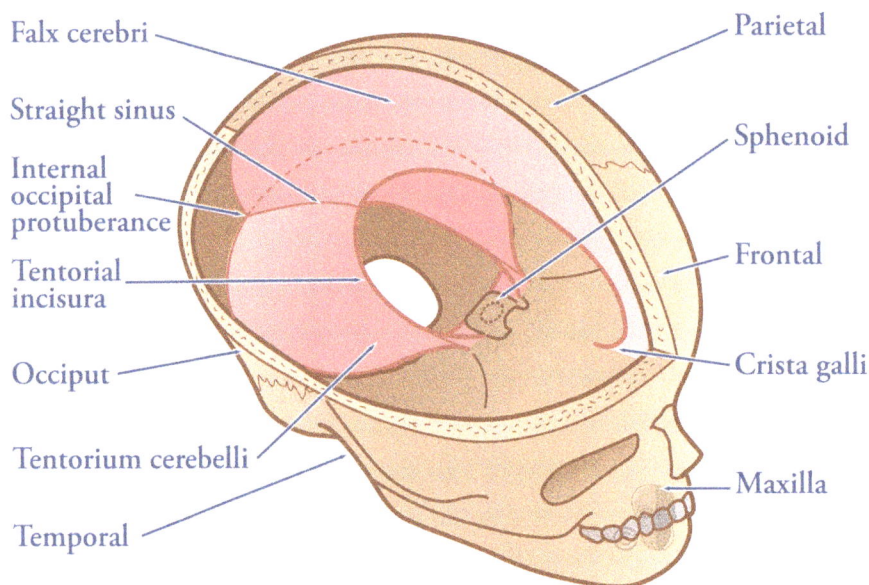

Figure 1.1 Pictorial View of the Reciprocal Tension Membranes

The vascular component includes all the vessels that make up a unique 'irrigation system' within the brain, balancing arterial inflow and venous outflow. To create homeostasis the irrigation system has to allow blood volumes into the brain equal to blood volumes flowing out of the brain. Of note are the reciprocal arrangements the cranium has with the pelvis, and how they influence each other:

- Temporomandibular joint (TMJ) and its reciprocation with the opposite sacroiliac joint
- Muscle attachments from the spine and their insertions into the cranium, and their applied forces to cranial membrane forces in abeyance to Newton's Law that 'each action has an equal and opposite reaction'.

The central brain components include the:

- Ventricular system – production and circulation of cerebrospinal fluid (CSF)
- Cingulate gyrus
- Supracallosal gyrus
- Corpus callosum
- Fornix
- Caudate nucleus
- Hippocampus formation and the amygdala.

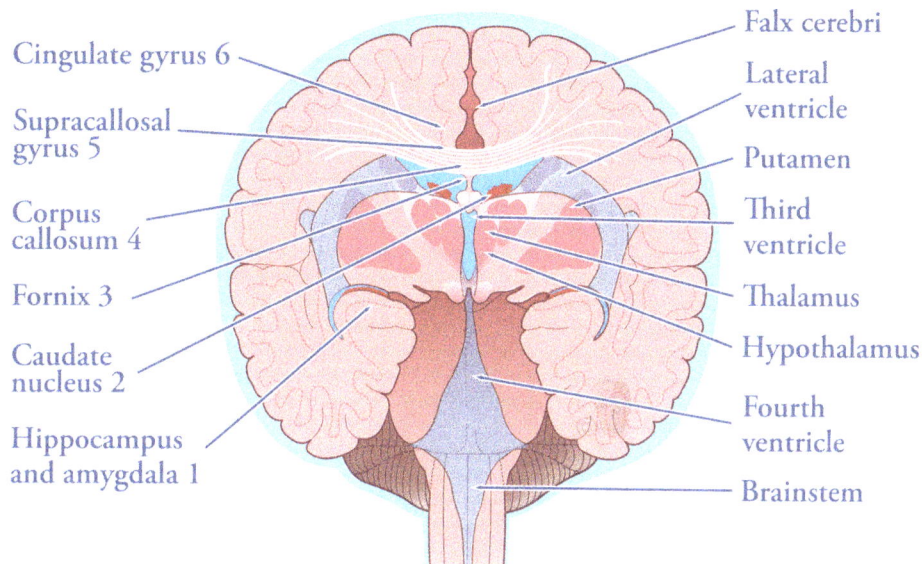

Figure 1.2 Ventricular System Lift Shaft

They are influenced by the intracranial membranes.

The central neurological pathways and conduits:

- Thalamus
- Hypothalamus
- Midbrain
- Pons
- Cerebral peduncles
- Cerebellar peduncles
- Medulla oblongata.

These components are all covered in cranio fascial dynamics (CFD) sections in this book that discuss the various traumatic forces applied to the brain, with their resultant consequences.

CRANIAL OSTEOLOGY

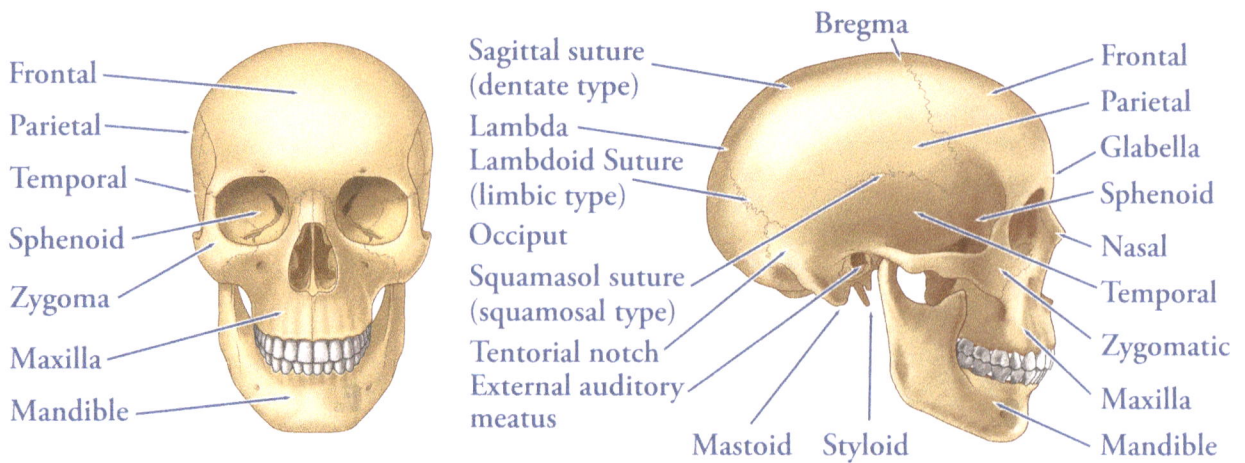

Frontal

Parietal

Temporal

Sphenoid

Zygoma

Maxilla

Mandible

Sagittal suture (dentate type)

Lambda

Lambdoid Suture (limbic type)

Occiput

Squamasol suture (squamosal type)

Tentorial notch

External auditory meatus

Bregma

Frontal

Parietal

Glabella

Sphenoid

Nasal

Temporal

Zygomatic

Maxilla

Mandible

Mastoid   Styloid

Figure 1.3 Anterior and Lateral Views of the Cranium: Bones and sutures

The cranium is made up of the following bones, either in pairs or as single bones, and the final alignment depends on their embryological development:

- Occipital bone (1)
- Parietal bones (2)
- Frontal bone (1)
- Sphenoid bone (1)
- Temporal bones (2)
- Mandible (1)
- Nasal bones (2)
- Palatine bones (2)
- Maxillary bones (2)
- Vomer (1)
- Ethmoid bone (1)
- Ossicles, internal bones of the ear found in the internal auditory meatus (6).

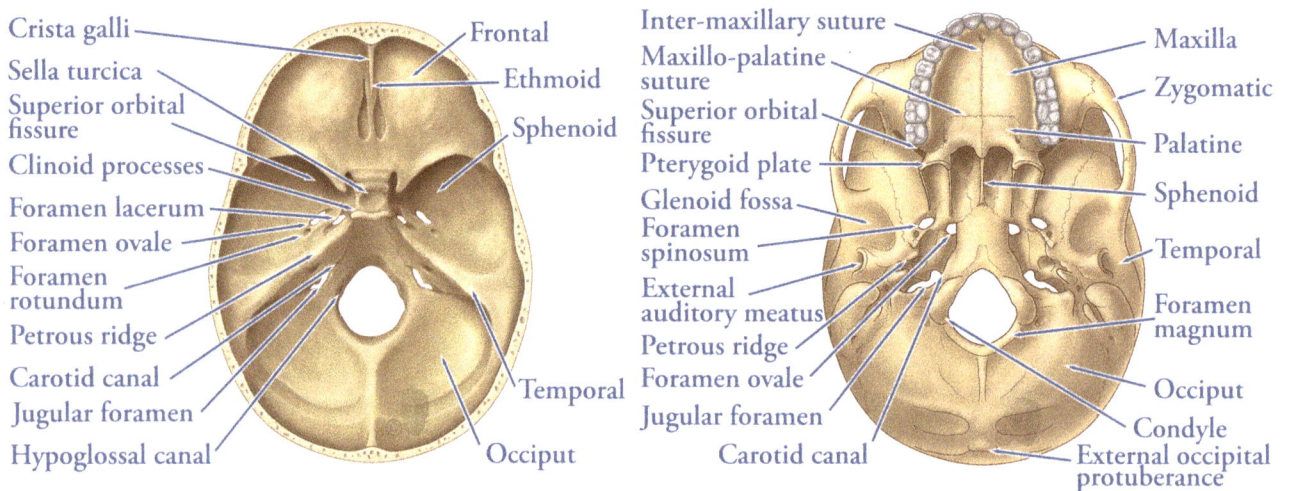

Crista galli

Sella turcica

Superior orbital fissure

Clinoid processes

Foramen lacerum

Foramen ovale

Foramen rotundum

Petrous ridge

Carotid canal

Jugular foramen

Hypoglossal canal

Frontal

Ethmoid

Sphenoid

Temporal

Occiput

Inter-maxillary suture

Maxillo-palatine suture

Superior orbital fissure

Pterygoid plate

Glenoid fossa

Foramen spinosum

External auditory meatus

Petrous ridge

Foramen ovale

Jugular foramen

Carotid canal

Maxilla

Zygomatic

Palatine

Sphenoid

Temporal

Foramen magnum

Occiput

Condyle

External occipital protuberance

Figure 1.4 Superior View of Internal Cranium; Inferior of View of Cranium

CARTILAGINOUS AND MEMBRANOUS BONE

Each bone is made up of either cartilaginous bone, which later becomes bone, or membranous bone, which remains as membrane throughout life. Some bones have both cartilaginous and membranous bone embryologically, but change to their defined status in adult life. Cartilaginous bone is found in the cranial floor, creating robust apertures for nerve and vascular pathways, and provides a strong structural foundation for the cranium. Membranous bone is found in the upper parts of the cranium, the side walls, roof and squama, allowing for more flexibility and adaptation in growth and development.

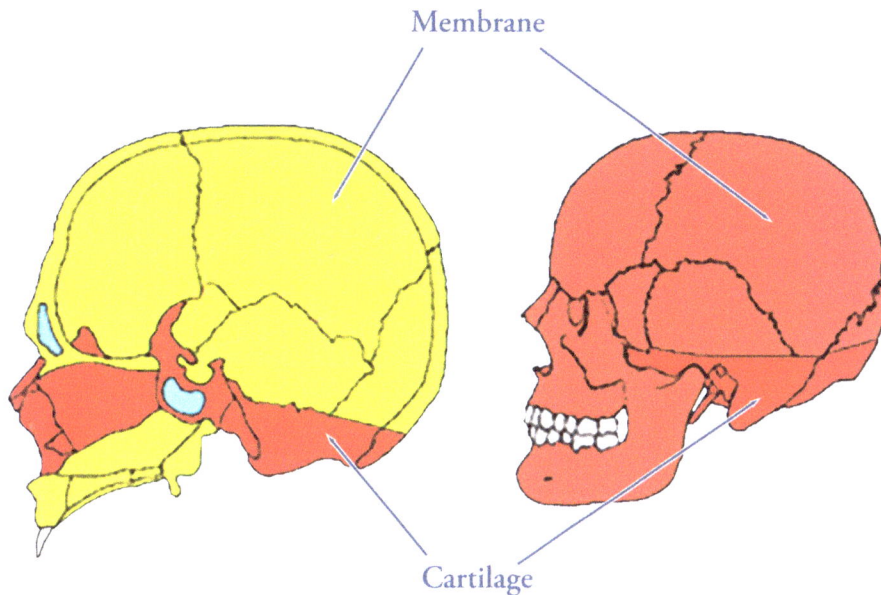

Membrane

Cartilage

Figure 1.5 Ossification of Cranium in Membrane and Cartilage

FORAMENAL APERTURES IN THE CRANIUM FLOOR

These are the apertures pertaining to the various bones making up the cranial floor and the vessels that penetrate these openings.

Sphenoid bone

Superior orbital fissure contains:

- Oculomotor nerve III
- Abducens nerve VI
- Ophthalmic nerve V branch 1 of trigeminal
- Trochlear nerve IV
- Superior ophthalmic vein.

Foramen rotundum contains:

- Maxillary nerve V branch 2 of trigeminal.

Foramen ovale contains:

- Mandibular nerve V branch 3 of trigeminal.

Foramen spinosum contains:

- Middle meningeal artery
- Middle meningeal vein
- Meningeal branch of mandibular nerve V branch 3 of trigeminal.

Temporal bone

Foramen lacerum, located between the sphenoid and the apex of the petrous portion of the temporal bone, contains:

- Greater petrosal nerve (parasympathetic)
- Deep petrosal nerve (sympathetic).

Carotid canal contains:

- Internal carotid artery.

Jugular foramen contains:

- Glossopharyngeal nerve IX
- Vagus nerve X
- Spinal accessory nerve XI
- Internal jugular vein.

Occipital bone

Hypoglossal canal contains:

- Hypoglossal nerve XII.

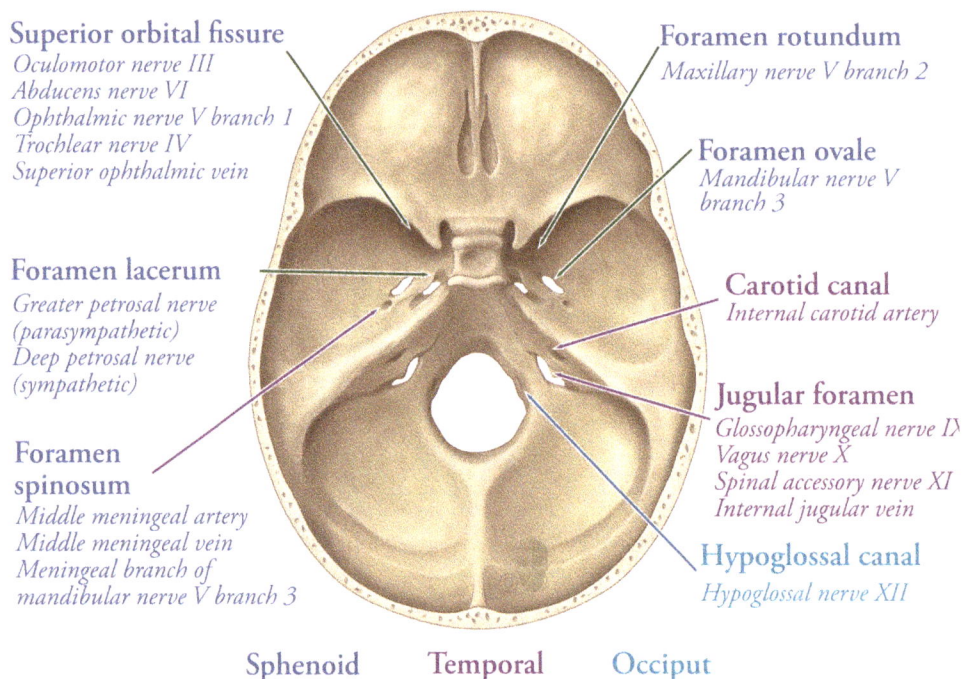

Superior orbital fissure
Oculomotor nerve III
Abducens nerve VI
Ophthalmic nerve V branch 1
Trochlear nerve IV
Superior ophthalmic vein

Foramen rotundum
Maxillary nerve V branch 2

Foramen ovale
Mandibular nerve V branch 3

Foramen lacerum
Greater petrosal nerve (parasympathetic)
Deep petrosal nerve (sympathetic)

Carotid canal
Internal carotid artery

Jugular foramen
Glossopharyngeal nerve IX
Vagus nerve X
Spinal accessory nerve XI
Internal jugular vein

Foramen spinosum
Middle meningeal artery
Middle meningeal vein
Meningeal branch of mandibular nerve V branch 3

Hypoglossal canal
Hypoglossal nerve XII

Sphenoid   Temporal   Occiput

Figure 1.6 Foramenal Apertures in the Floor of the Cranium

CHAPTER 2

CRANIAL OSTEOLOGY

OCCIPITAL BONE

Embryologically the occiput is made up of four sections:

a. Basilar portion, joins the body of the sphenoid at the sphenobasilar synchondrosis – *ossified in cartilage*

b. Two condylar portions are found between the basilar portion and the occipital squama, and provide the articulation with the lateral masses of the atlas. The hypoglossal canal receives the hypoglossal nerve (CNXII) – *ossified in cartilage*

c. Occipital squama attaches anteriorly to the condylar portions, and joins the temporal bone at the occipito-mastoid suture, and the parietals at the lambdoid suture – *ossified in membrane*.

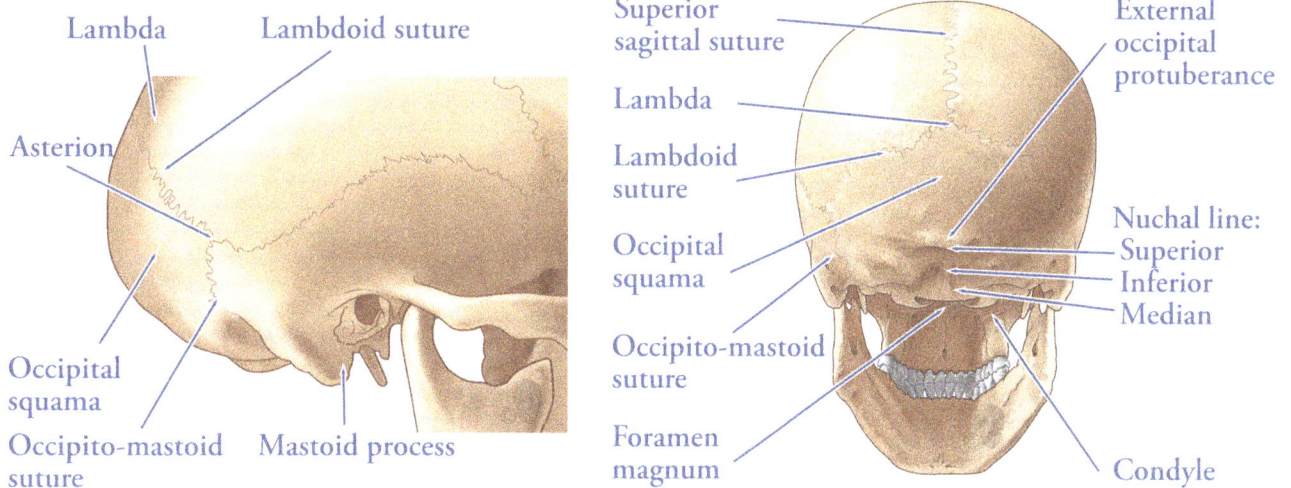

Figure 2.1 Occipital Bone

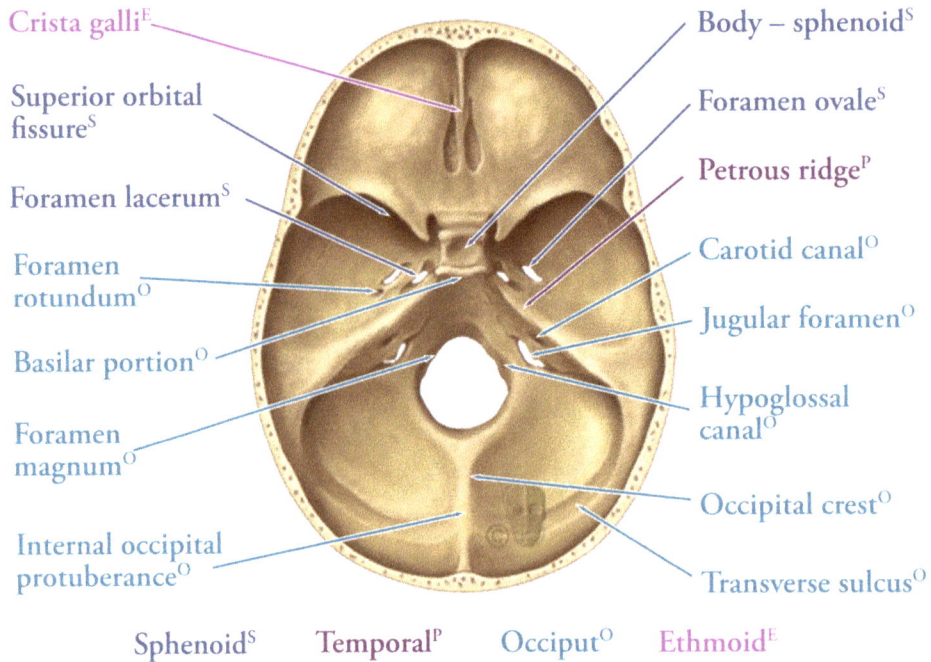

Crista galli[E]
Superior orbital fissure[S]
Foramen lacerum[S]
Foramen rotundum[O]
Basilar portion[O]
Foramen magnum[O]
Internal occipital protuberance[O]

Body – sphenoid[S]
Foramen ovale[S]
Petrous ridge[P]
Carotid canal[O]
Jugular foramen[O]
Hypoglossal canal[O]
Occipital crest[O]
Transverse sulcus[O]

Sphenoid[S]   Temporal[P]   Occiput[O]   Ethmoid[E]

Figure 2.2 Anatomy of Superior View of the Cranium

The occipital bone has a trapezoid outline and is rather cup-like in shape. It is pierced by a large oval aperture, the foramen magnum, through which the cranial cavity communicates with the vertebral canal. The curved expanded plate posterior to the foramen magnum is the squama. On the external part of the squama is the external occipital protuberance, the anchor point for the ligamentum nuchae. Adjacent and lateral to the external occipital protuberance is the superior nuchal line, which is the attachment to the trapezius muscle medially and the sternocleidomastoid (SCM) muscle laterally. On either side, lateral to the foramen magnum, are the two occipital condyles where the lateral masses of the atlas articulate. Anterior to the foramen magnum is the basilar portion of the occiput. The basilar portion of the occiput articulates with the sphenoid bone forming the sphenobasilar synchondrosis. The internal occipital protuberance lies on the internal surface of the occipital squama, which is the functional anchor point for the tentorium cerebelli and the falx cerebelli. Indentations in the internal surface of the squama provide for the transverse sinuses, the sagittal sinus and the straight sinus.

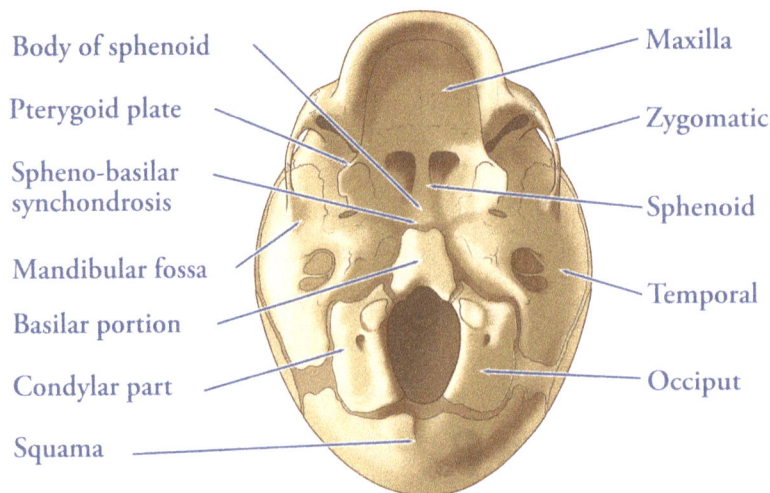

Body of sphenoid
Pterygoid plate
Spheno-basilar synchondrosis
Mandibular fossa
Basilar portion
Condylar part
Squama

Maxilla
Zygomatic
Sphenoid
Temporal
Occiput

Figure 2.3 Inferior View of Infant Skull

Significance in CFD

The occiput is part of the sacro-occipital pump mechanism. The external surface of the occiput provides a thick horizontal eminence to which the erector spinae muscles attach – the superior nuchal line. These muscles also attach to the sacrum and provide a direct connector to the occiput. When the occiput flexes, so does the sacrum, providing the pump action that draws CSF from the fourth ventricle, down the central canal of the spinal cord, towards the sacral bulb. On exhalation this process is reversed, thus completing the sacro-occipital pump mechanism.

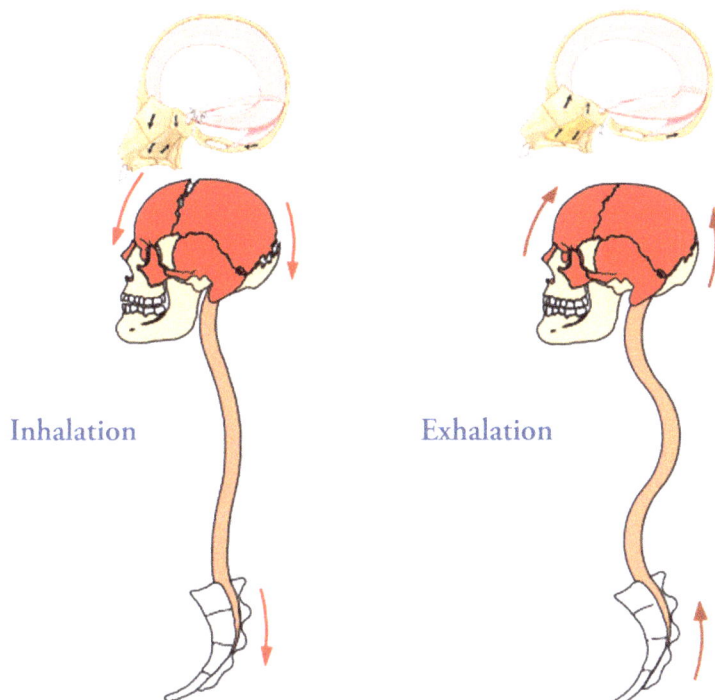

Inhalation   Exhalation

Figure 2.4 Reciprocal Tension Membranes in Diaphragmatic Respiration

The inner surface of the occiput provides a horizontal groove as an extension of the internal occipital protuberance for the transverse sinus and the sigmoid sinus (encapsulated by the tentorium cerebelli) to anchor securely to this horizontal membrane, interwoven into the endosteal dura. This opposes the superior nuchal line and the tough insertion of the erector spinae muscles into the periosteal dura. These two dural membranes are a continuation of each other – fascia.

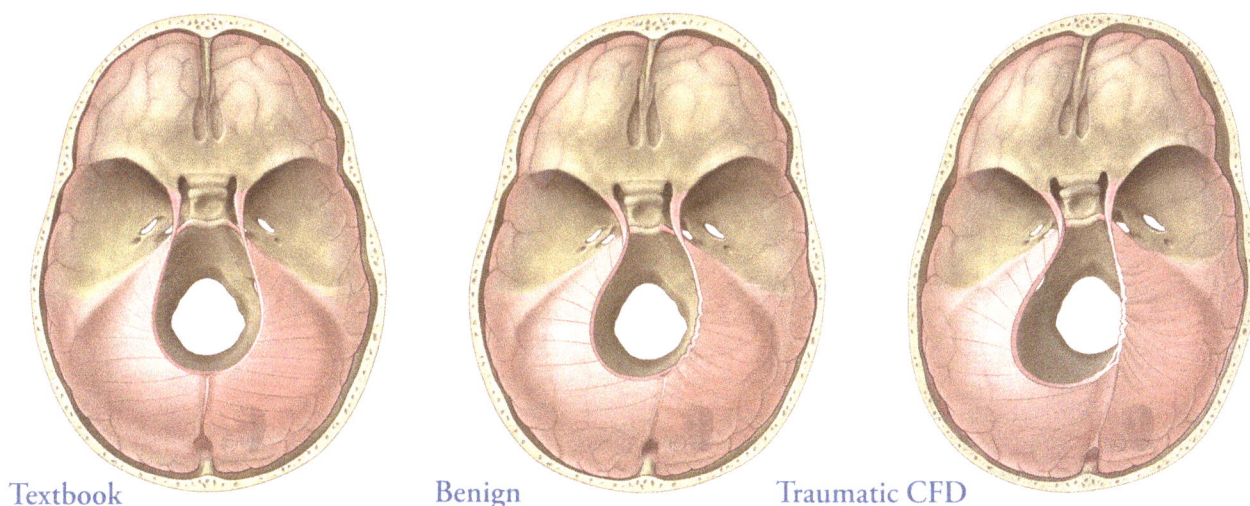

Textbook   Benign   Traumatic CFD

Figure 2.5 Tentorium Cerebelli Attachments to the Occiput

117

The tentorium cerebelli (internal occiput) lies in opposition to the erector spinae muscles (external occiput) and acts in accordance with Newton's Laws – each action has an equal and opposite reaction. When the sacrum moves out of balance, that affects the erector spinae muscles, which in turn changes the occiput at the superior nuchal line. This warps the occiput, changing the robust insertion of the tentorium cerebelli and the encapsulated transverse and sigmoid sinuses, potentially changing the drainage potential of the brain.

Similarly, the effect of brain trauma will create a torque of the RTM, and the reverse process ensues. Cranio fascial distortion has a potential to disrupt the sacro-occipital pump, CSF circulation and brain drainage – major factors in retained homeostasis.

Similarly, a change to the basilar portion of the occiput in young people (prior to the ossification of the sphenobasilar synchondrosis) will have a disruption to the synchondrosis with cranio fascial distortion, where the dural fascia changes the position of the sphenoid body (the anterior pole of the tentorium cerebelli). This has ramifications in the posterior insertion of the tentorium cerebelli, at the internal occipital protuberance and the groove of the transverse and sigmoid sinuses, with the erector spinae muscles and the sacrum challenging Newton's Laws.

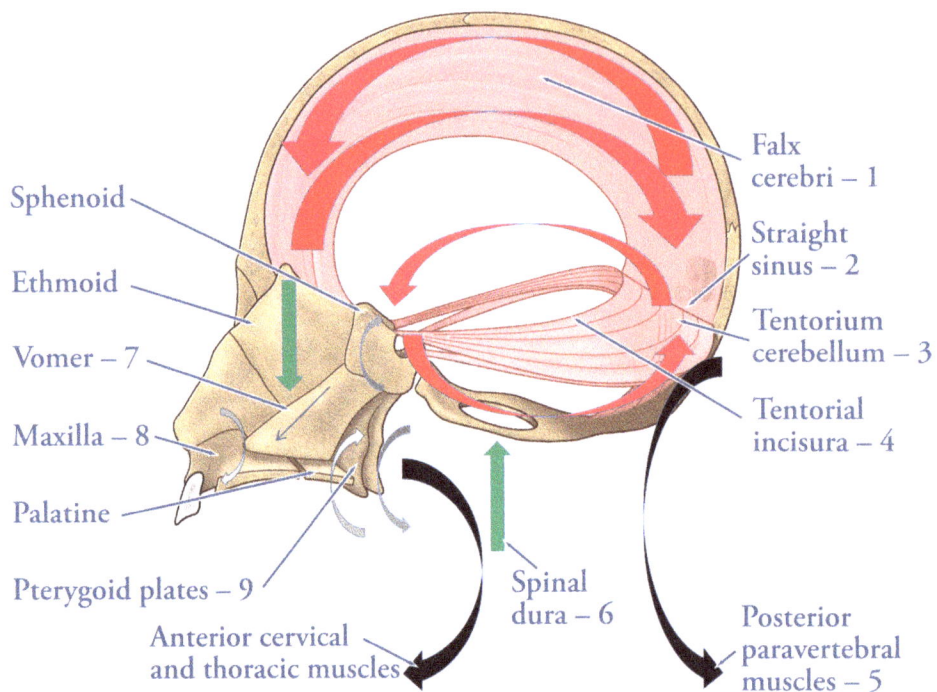

Figure 2.6 Newton's Second Law: F = ma, each force has an equal and opposite reaction

After ossification takes place at the sphenobasilar synchondrosis, this junction no longer has the ability to flex and extend independently, while changes to either bone – the sphenoid or the occiput – will be more critical to cranial stability.

The petrous portion of the temporal bone will also be affected as changes to either the sphenoid or occiput will adversely affect the temporal bone's balance to the external musculature temporalis, buccinator, masseter, internal and external pterygoid muscles.

Also affected are the mandibular fossa (mandibular deviation) the internal acoustic meatus (facial and acoustic nerves), the petrous portion (the encapsulation of the superior petrosal vein by the lateral tentorium cerebelli anchor point) and the jugular foramen (vagus and spinal accessory nerves and the internal jugular vein), foramen lacerum, carotid canal and the foramen ovale.

TEMPORAL BONE

Embryologically, the temporal bone is made up of three parts:

a. The squama – *ossified in membrane*
b. The petromastoid portion– *ossified in cartilage*
c. The tympanic ring– *ossified in membrane*

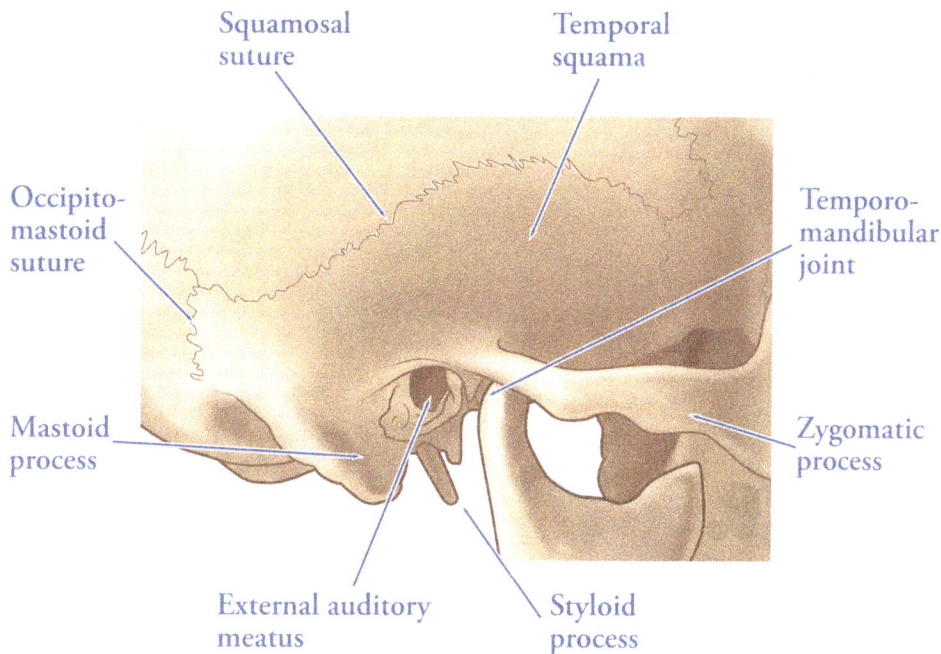

Figure 2.7 Temporal Bone

Osteology

The temporal squama is concave when viewed from the interior and provides the lateral wall of the cranium. The petrous portion of the temporal bone provides the lateral anchor point for the tentorium cerebelli, encapsulating the superior petrosal sinus, and provides the axis of rotation for temporal motion. The petrous portion also houses the internal auditory meatus, the tympanic membrane and the ossicles.

The apex of the petrous portion provides the anterior or internal opening for the carotid canal, and forms the posterolateral margin of the foramen lacerum.

The jugular foramen is part of the posterior margin of the petrous portion, and is formed by the adjacent border of the occiput.

The squama also contributes to the formation of the zygomatic process and the mandibular or glenoid fossa, together with the condyle of the mandible, forms the temporomandibular joint.

Carotid canal contains:

• Internal carotid artery

Jugular foramen contains:

• Glossopharyngeal nerve, 9
• Vagus nerve, 10
• Spinal accessory nerve, 11
• Internal jugular vein

Significance in CFD

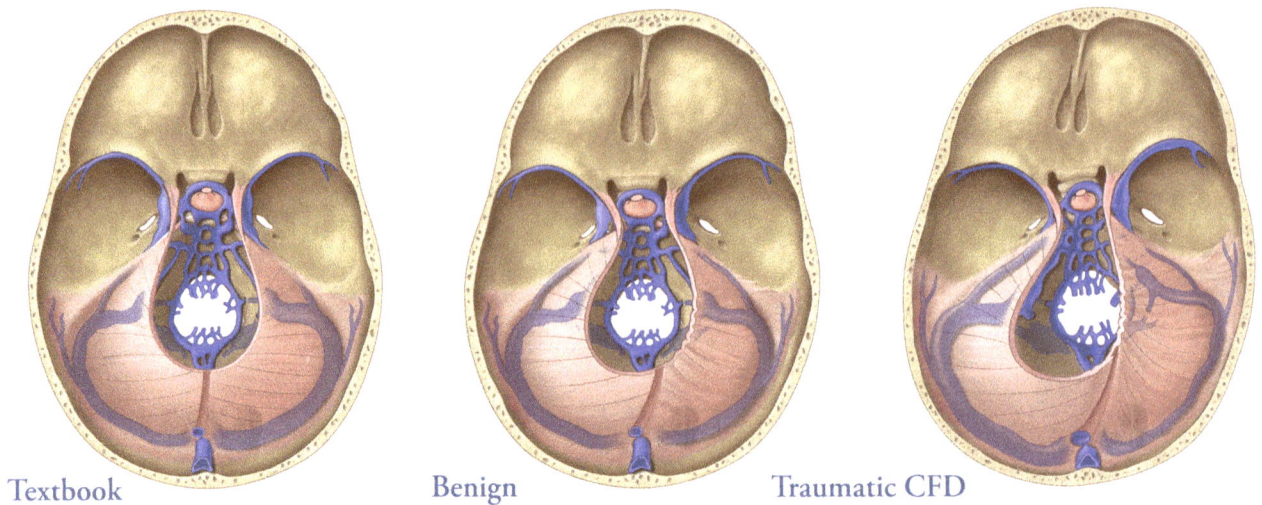

Textbook　　　　　Benign　　　　　Traumatic CFD

Figure 2.8 Cranial Floor Venous Drainage

The lateral anchor points, at the petrous portion of the temporal bone, for the tentorium cerebelli, encapsulating the superior petrosal sinus – allowing temporal brain drainage.

The tentorial incisura interference in both diaschisis and necrotic traumatic forces, largely influences the endosteal and meningeal dura when the temporal bone goes into internal rotation, as it will congest the apertures of the temporal bone on that side.

The right internal rotation of the temporal bone causes closing of the carotid canal and the jugular foramen.

The temporomandibular joint and its reciprocation with the opposite sacroiliac joint become focal issues when one or other is weakened by its complementary fascia.

SPHENOID BONE

Embryologically the sphenoid is made up of 5 parts:

a. body of the sphenoid – *ossified in cartilage*
b. lesser wings (2) of the sphenoid – *ossified in cartilage*
c. greater wings (2) of the sphenoid – *ossified in membrane*

Osteology

The sphenoid is the central bone of the cranium and the most important from a functional standpoint. It is situated at the base of the skull, anterior to the temporal and basilar parts of the occiput. It is divided into a median portion or body, the greater and two lesser wings extending outwards from the side of the body, and two pterygoid processes which project from its inferior surface. On the superior surface of the body is the sella turcica, which provides the fossa for the pituitary gland. Anterior and posterior to the sella turcica are the anterior and posterior clinoid processes, which are the anchor points for the diaphragma sellae and the anterior pole of the tentorium cerebelli. Anterior to the sella turcica is the chiasma groove, in which the optic chiasma lies.

The pterygoid processes are especially important targets for cranial corrections.

120

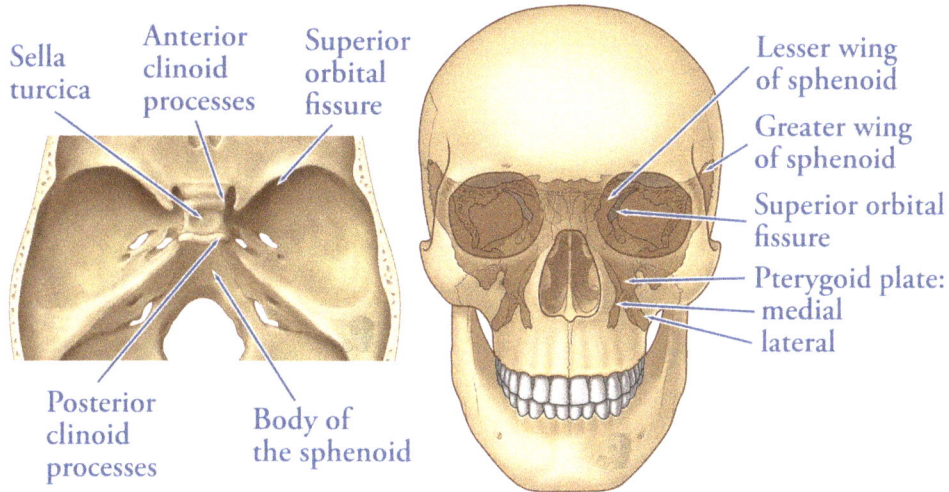

Figure 2.9 Sphenoid Bone

Significance in CFD

Focusing on the central bone of the cranium, given counterclockwise torque the right greater wing moves anterior and superior, while the left greater wing moves posterior and inferior. This gives rise to a larger ocular orbit on the right, although the right eye is comfortably accommodated, the left orbit becomes smaller, retruding the eye and compressing it. This results in poor ocular convergence on the left medial rectus muscle, innervated by the oculomotor nerve (CN III).

That warping action pulls the mandibular fossa relatively posterior in relation to the right mandibular fossa, causing left mandibular deviation on translation, resulting in a crossbite and a malocclusion. The pterygoid plates are an inferior extension of body of the sphenoid and are made up of the external/lateral pterygoid plate, which anchors the external pterygoid muscle, and the hamulus or internal/medial pterygoid plate, which anchors the internal pterygoid muscle. Both these muscles attach to the mandible and create lateral and protrusive movement of the mandible, and are thus influenced by torsional movement of the sphenoid.

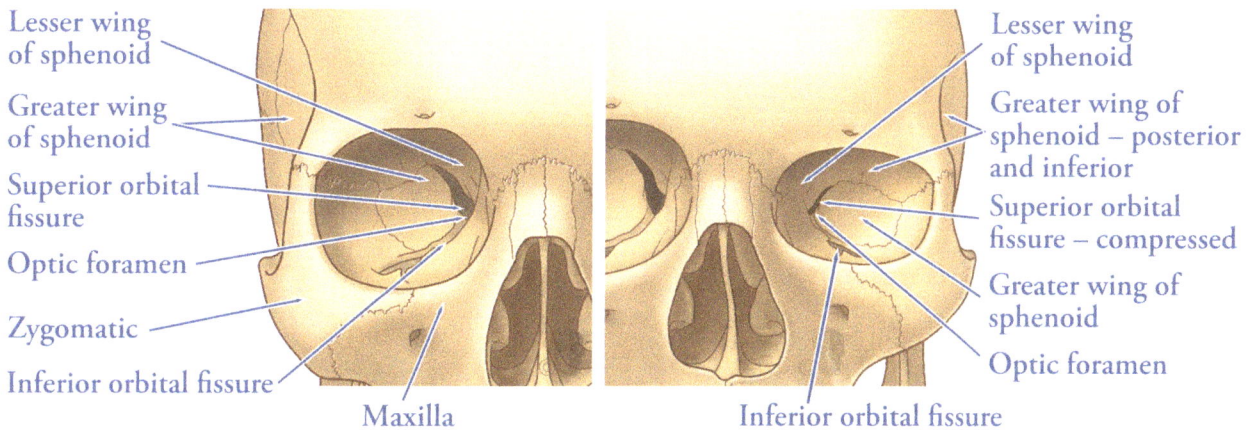

Figure 2.10 Ocular Orbits: Textbook right orbit; Distortion of left orbit

As the greater wings on the right move anterior and superior, the superior orbital fissure lying between the greater and lesser wings, opens up, while on the left, the superior orbital fissure closes down. This has huge implications to the vessels that pass through the superior orbital fissure. These vessels, both neurological and vascular are:

- Oculomotor nerves, 3
- Abducens nerves, 4
- Ophthalmic nerves, 5, branch 1 of trigeminal
- Trochlear nerves, 6
- Superior ophthalmic vein.

The optic foramen lying just medial to the superior orbital fissure, carrying the optic nerve (CN II), comes under the same influence, closing down on the left and opening up on the right.

The cavernous sinuses, both left and right, and the intercavernous sinus, surround the body of the sphenoid, resulting in a torque of these sinuses when the sphenoid twists. The largest vessel traversing the cavernous sinuses is the internal carotid artery. When this becomes distorted in the left cavernous sinus it then exits and travels superior to join the circle of Willis, possibly accounting for the high incidence of aneurysms at that junction.

The optic chiasma lies at the anterior of the sphenoid body and above the cavernous sinuses on the anterior wall of the sella turcica, (superior to the pituitary, inferior to the hypothalamus) and so comes under the direct influence of sphenoid torque.

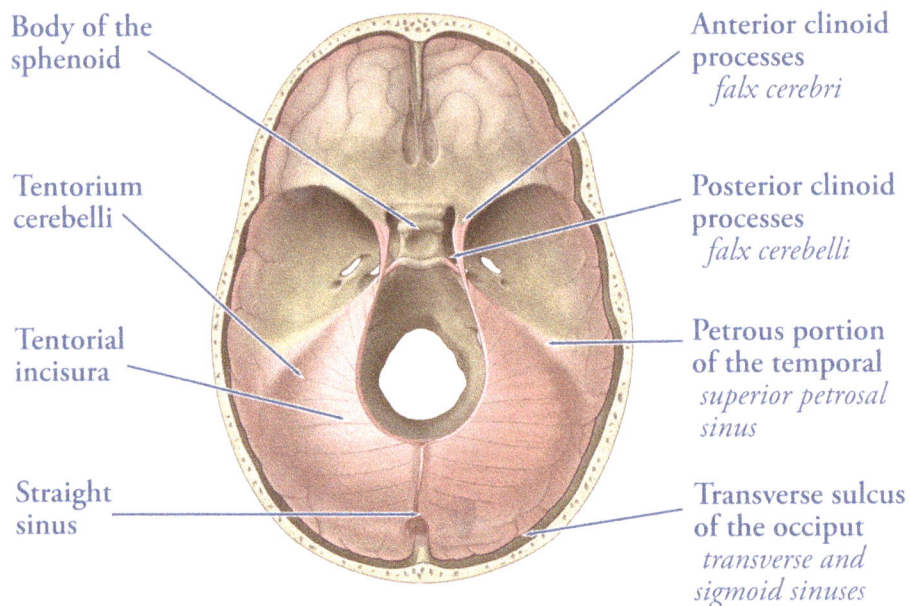

Body of the
sphenoid

Tentorium
cerebelli

Tentorial
incisura

Straight
sinus

Anterior clinoid
processes
falx cerebri

Posterior clinoid
processes
falx cerebelli

Petrous portion
of the temporal
*superior petrosal
sinus*

Transverse sulcus
of the occiput
*transverse and
sigmoid sinuses*

Figure 2.11 Superior View of the Cranium: Tentorium cerebelli attachments

The body of the sphenoid seats the sella turcica, in which the pituitary lies, attached to the hypophyseal stalk. This penetrates the diaphragma sellae, the horizontal dural membrane that attaches to the anterior and posterior clinoid processes.

These processes also provide the anterior anchor points to the tentorium cerebelli, the two-layered, main horizontal dural membranes that separate the brain from the cerebellum.

- The lower layer of the tentorium cerebelli is made up of the dura supplied from the falx cerebelli, the inferior vertical dural membrane. This attaches to the occipital groove of the occiput, encapsulating the occipital sinus and has a common border superiorly with the straight sinus, inserting at the posterior clinoid process of the sella turcica

- The upper layer is an extension of the vertical dural membrane, the falx cerebri, which separates the left and right cerebral hemispheres also encapsulating the superior sagittal sinus superiorly (the anterior superior drainage vessel) and the inferior sagittal sinus inferiorly (the anterior inferior drainage vessel). It has a common border at the internal occipital protuberance, the straight sinus, with the tentorium cerebelli and the falx cerebelli. From the straight sinus the tentorium cerebelli anchors at the anterior clinoid processes of the sella turcica.

The most important aspect of the tentorium cerebelli is the tentorial incisura. This is a division of the tentorium cerebelli at the anterior aspect of the straight sinus, forming the two sheaths of the tentorium cerebelli that separate and envelope the central core components of the brain penetrating through the tentorial incisura. These are the ventricular system, the midbrain, the pons and the medulla oblongata.

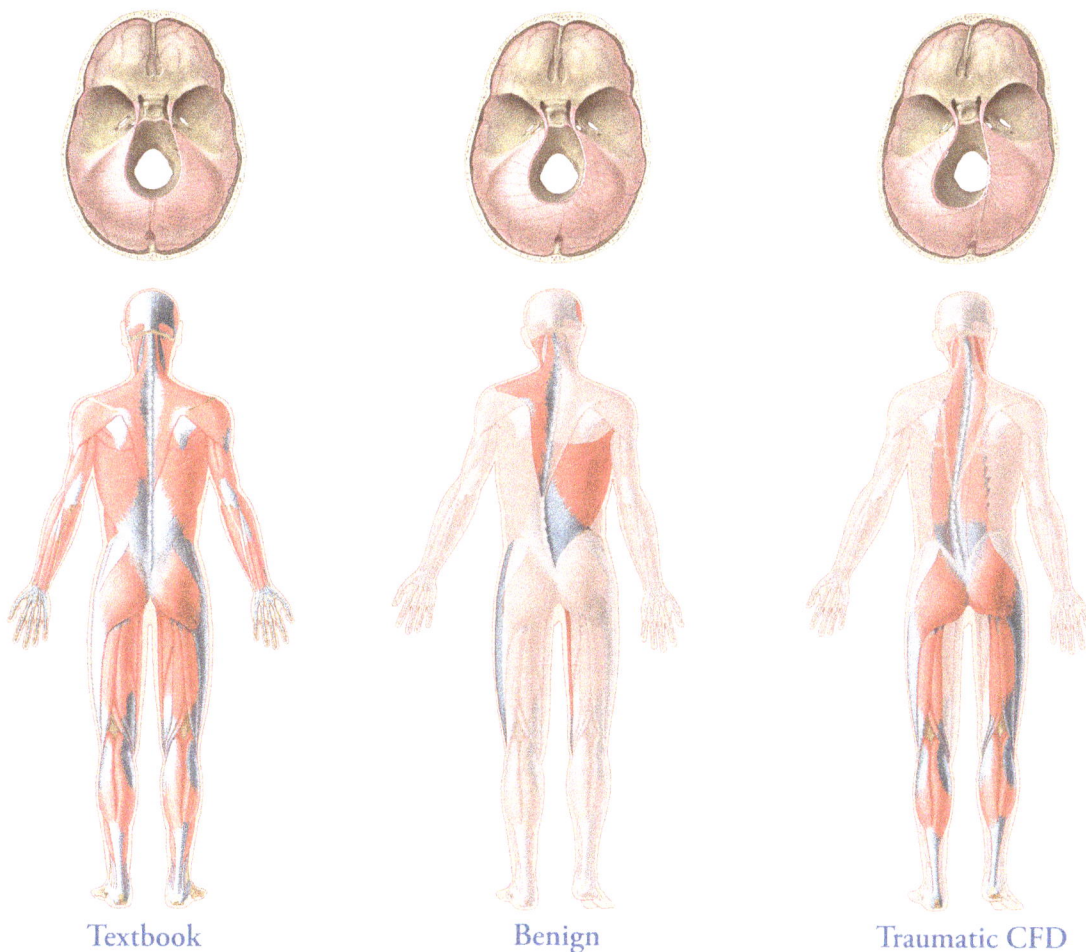

Textbook   Benign   Traumatic CFD

Figure 2.12 Reciprocal: Tentorial incisura and erector spinae muscles (also see Figure 2.8)

The posterior border of the tentorium cerebelli at the posterior aspect of the straight sinus, anchors into the transverse sulcus of the occipital bone. This encapsulates the transverse sinus and the sigmoid sinus before draining into the internal jugular vein then exiting the cranium through the jugular foramen.

The lateral aspect of the tentorium cerebelli attaches to the petrous portion of the temporal bone, encapsulating the superior petrosal sinus before it joins the sigmoid sinus.

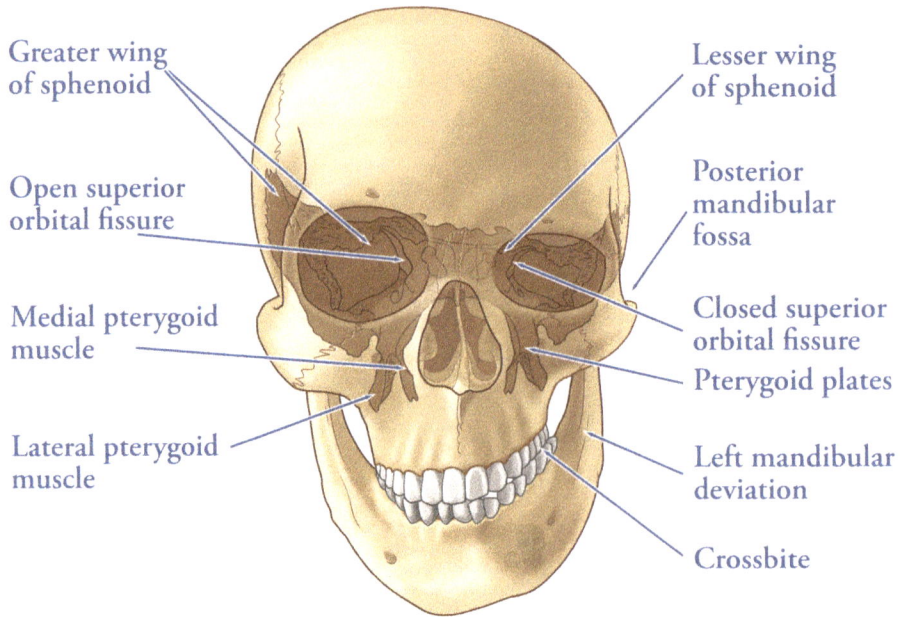

Figure 2.13 Traumatic CFD of the Sphenoid

These anchor points of the tentorium cerebelli, anteriorly, posteriorly and laterally, are the most significant elements of brain drainage, with the sphenoid bone playing a critical role. The tentorial incisura is also possibly the most influential membrane in the cranium, where it plays a hugely significant role in central brain homeostasis.

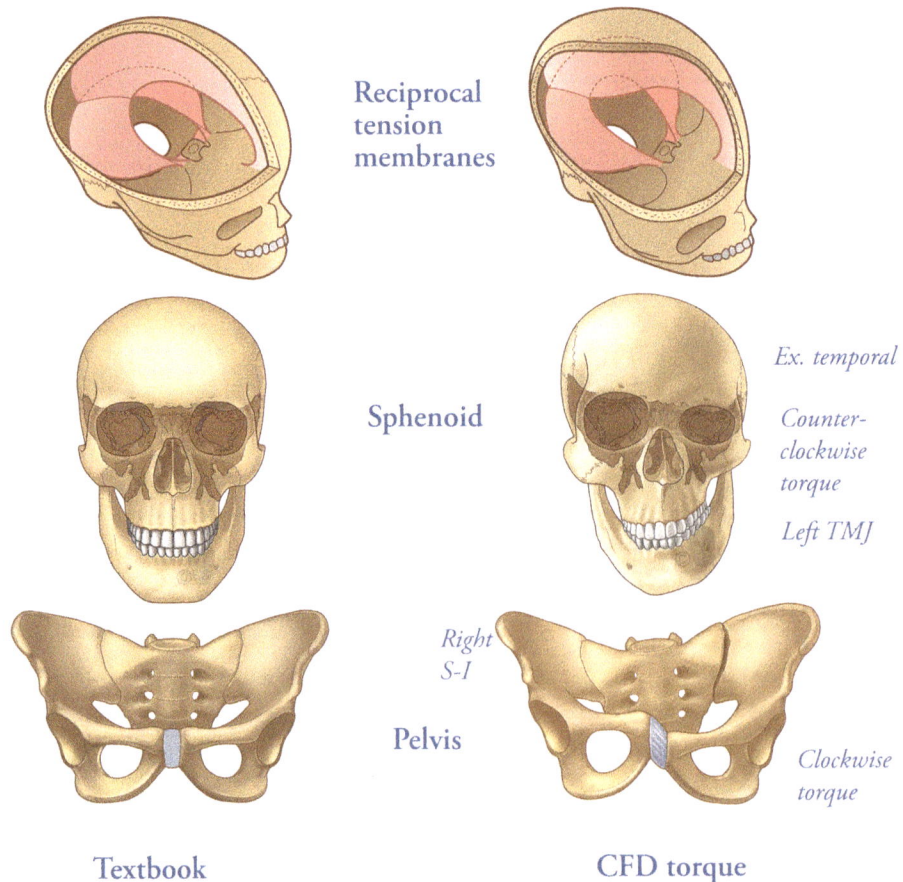

Figure 2.14 Cranio–Pelvic Reciprocity

Note that the greater wings of the sphenoid are contact points for the practitioner to control the sphenoid bone in various cranial movements, either by single hand (thumb and little finger) or using a single contact, depending on the width of the hand. Being the central controlling bone of the cranium, the greater wings can be used to control most aspects of misalignment within the cranium.

PARIETAL BONE

This is a paired bone that covers the parietal lobes and forms the roof of the calvarium. Embryologically the parietal bones are *ossified in membrane*.

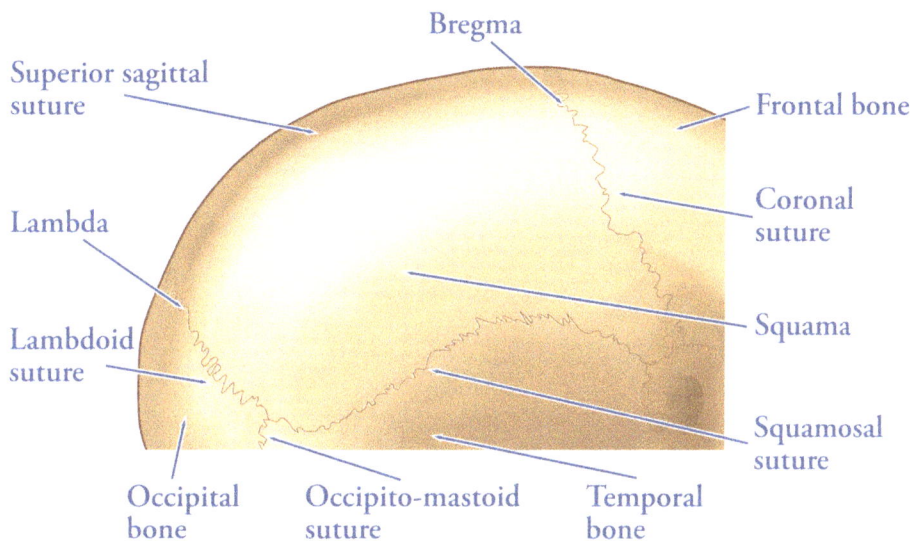

Figure 2.15 Parietal Bone

The important coronal suture separates the frontal bone from the two parietals. Parietal bones form the sides and roof of the cranium and are both concave in shape when viewed from the interior and ossified from membrane. The two parietal bones are divided by the important superior sagittal suture.

On the inferior surface of the superior sagittal suture lies the superior sagittal sinus. The temporal ridge sits on the external surface of the squama, below which anchors the very strong temporalis muscle. The parietal bones articulate with the temporal bones at the squamosal suture and with the occiput at the lambdoid suture – the asterion. The point of contact anteriorly with the greater wing of the sphenoid, the temporal and the frontal bone, is known as the pterion.

Significance in CFD

The bregma and the lambda are the points of the anterior fontanelle and the posterior fontanelle, respectively. They represent the attachments internally for the superior sagittal sinus, and are points of reference in cranial scanning where, if positive, indicate a disruption to the superior sagittal sinus, or possibly the attachment or a twist of the vessel.

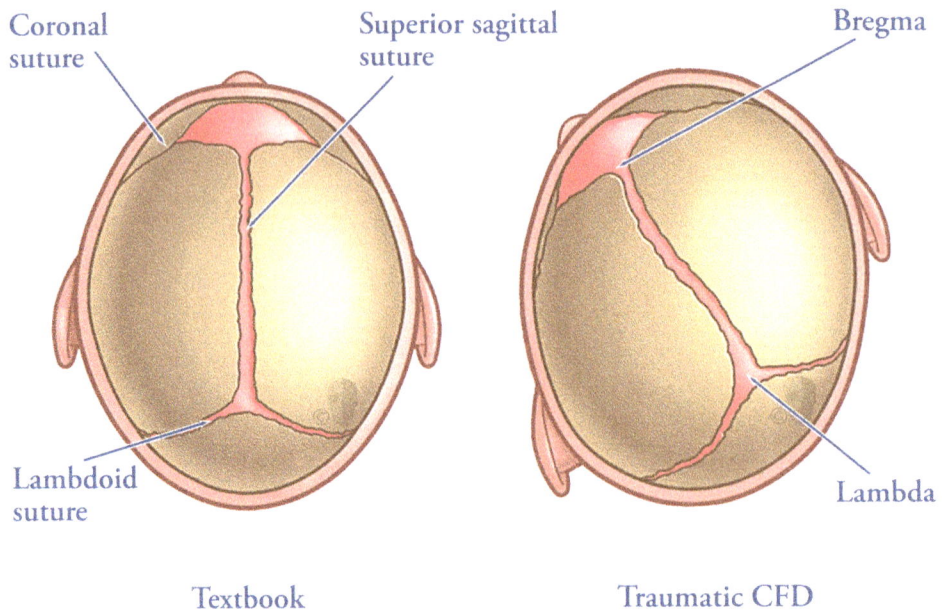

Coronal suture
Superior sagittal suture
Bregma
Lambdoid suture
Lambda

Textbook

Traumatic CFD

Figure 2.16 Superior View of Infant Parietal Bones

FRONTAL BONE

Embryologically the frontal bone is *ossified from membrane*.

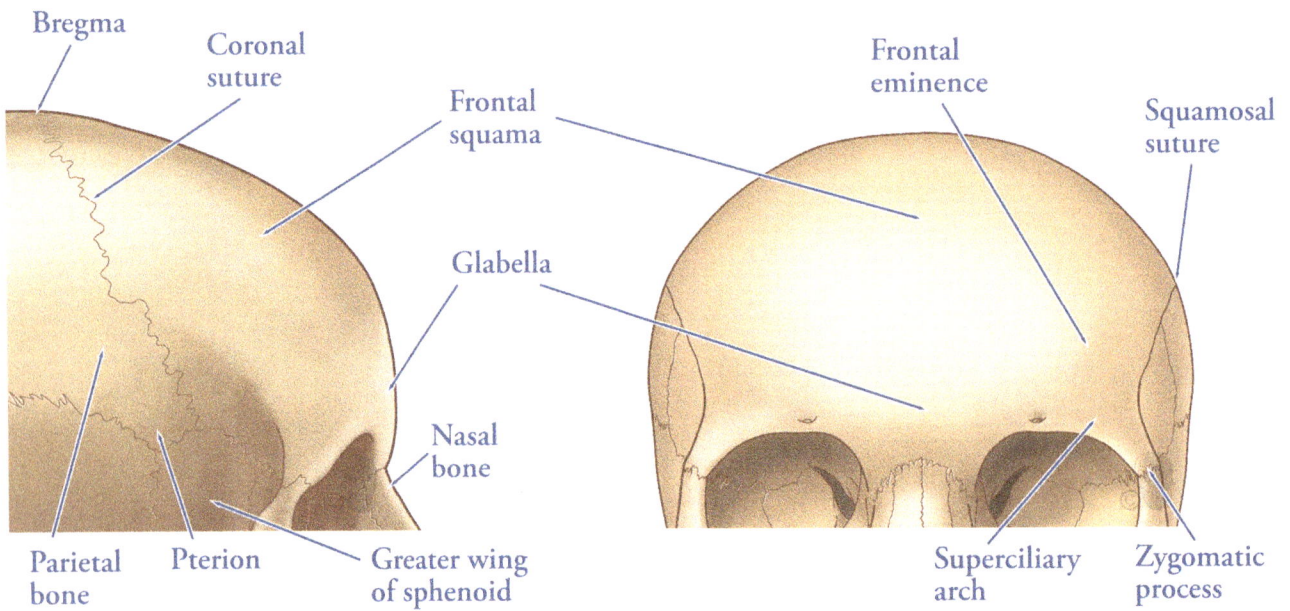

Bregma
Coronal suture
Frontal squama
Frontal eminence
Squamosal suture
Glabella
Nasal bone
Parietal bone
Pterion
Greater wing of sphenoid
Superciliary arch
Zygomatic process

Figure 2.17 Frontal Bone

This consists of two portions: the concave portion being the squama corresponding with the forehead; and an orbital or horizontal portion which is involved in the formation of the roofs of the orbital and nasal cavities. In infancy the squama is separated by the metopic suture, which may persist throughout life, however, it usually disappears and forms the frontal surface of the glabella. The internal surface of the frontal bone at the metopic suture forms part of the anchor point of the superior sagittal sinus. The frontal eminences which appear on either side of the squama above the supraciliary arch are landmarks that are often identified in cranial problems.

Significance in CFD

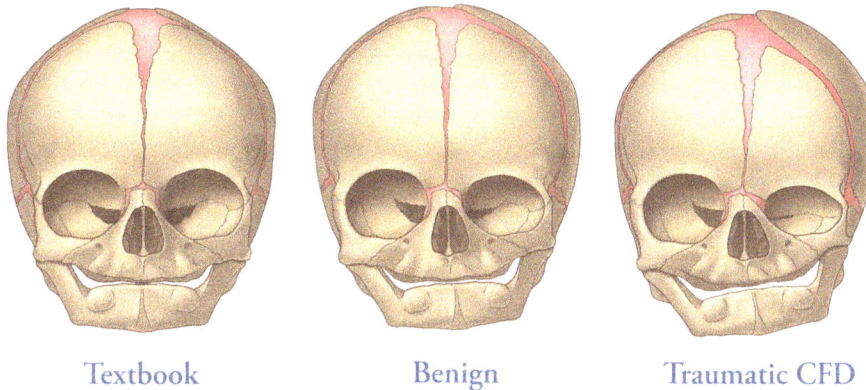

| Textbook | Benign | Traumatic CFD |

Figure 2.18 Anterior View of Infant Cranium: Shows frontal bone separated by metopic suture

The supraciliary arches form the roof of the ocular orbit and are supported anteriorly and medially by the maxillary process. The anterior lateral support is the zygomatic bone attaching to the frontal bone process. The posterior part of the ocular orbit is made up of the sphenoid bone, posteriorly, the lacrimal, ethmoid and palatine bones, medially.

The frontal, parietal and occipital bones form a groove for the superior sagittal sinus, and in cranial scanning the glabella, bregma and lambda are isolated as reference points to indicate the status of the superior sagittal sinus.

The state of the ocular orbit in a counterclockwise torque will give rise to an enlarged right orbit and a smaller restricted left orbit. Similarly, the right frontal eminence will be more pronounced on the right externally rotated frontal bone (opposing the left externally rotated occipital bone) and less pronounced on the left internally rotated frontal bone (corresponding to the right internally rotated occipital bone).

ZYGOMATIC OR MALAR BONE

Embryologically *ossified in membrane*. The frontal bone forms the prominence of the cheek, part of the lateral wall and floor of the orbit and part of the temporal and intra-temporal fossa. It presents a malar, orbital and temporal surface. It is the locknut bone of the cranium, and articulates with the maxilla, frontal and temporal bones. This is a paired bone.

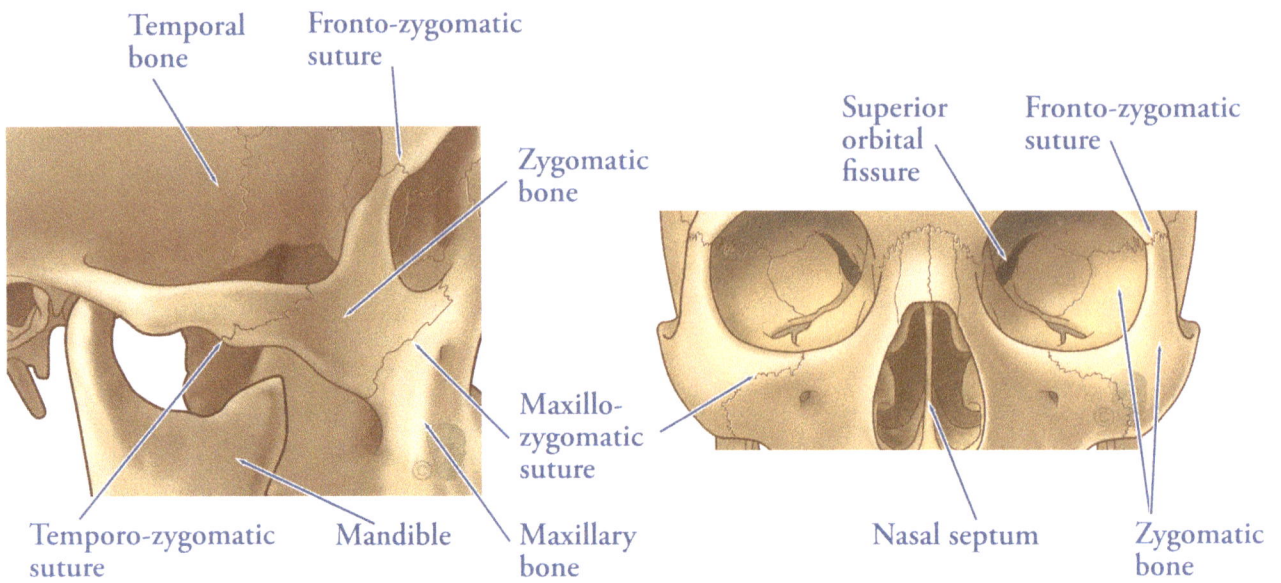

Figure 2.19 Zygomatic Bone

Significance in CFD

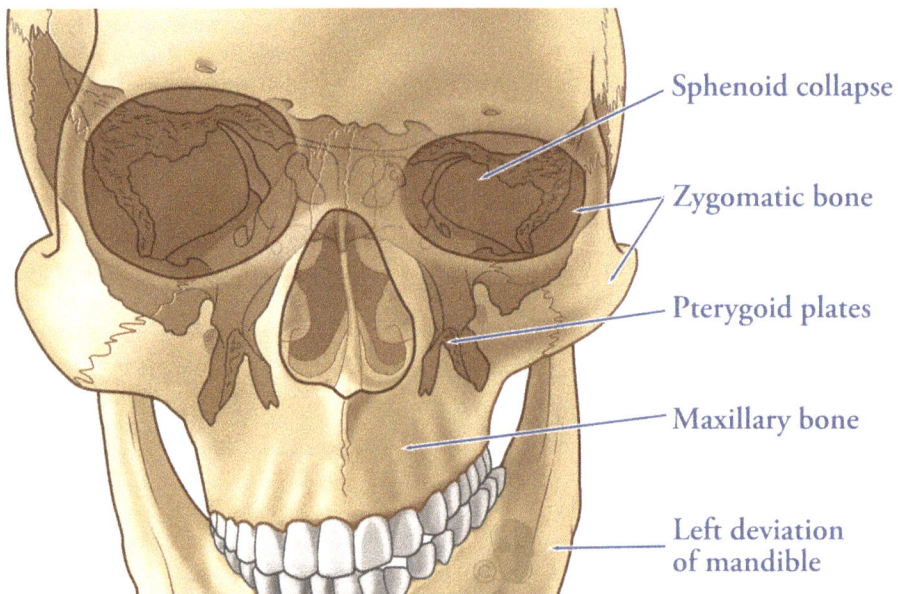

Figure 2.20 Zygomatic with Traumatic CFD

The zygomatic bone is the locknut on the face, and will need to be taken into consideration when cranial adjustments are being made to the maxillae, frontal and temporal bones, especially decongesting the TMJs.

MAXILLARY BONES

Embryologically the maxillary bones are *ossified in membrane*.

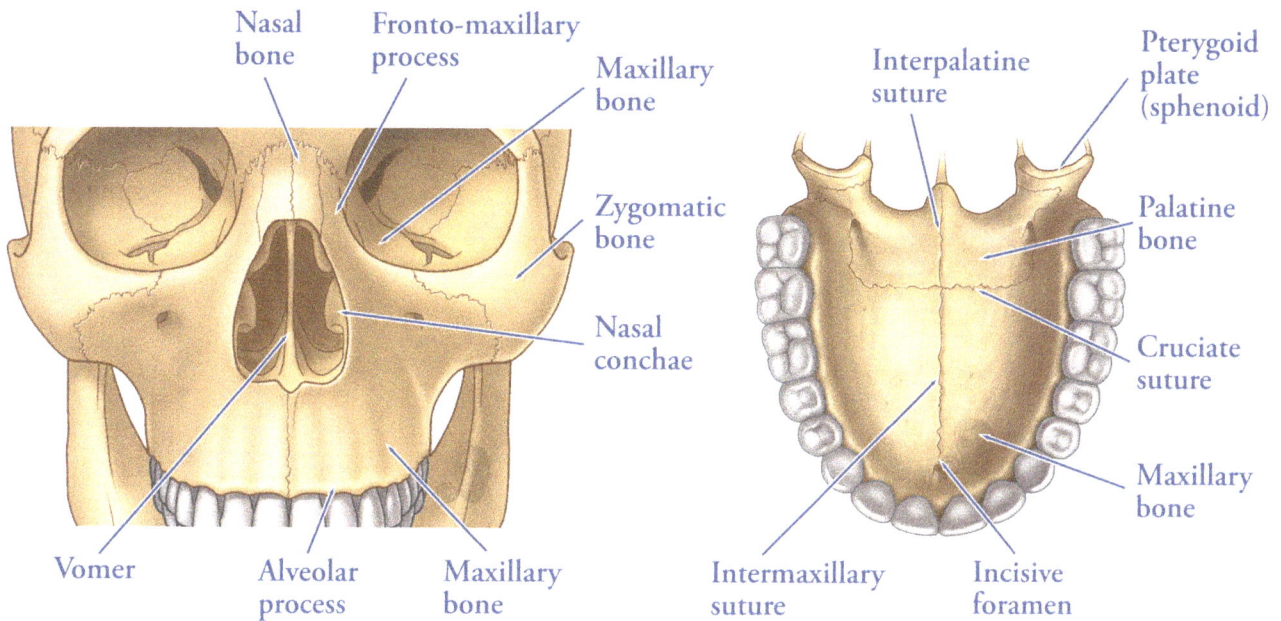

Figure 2.21 Maxillary Bones

The maxillae are the largest bones of the face, excepting the mandible, and form, by their union, the whole of the upper jaw. Each exists by forming the boundaries of four cavities: the roof of the mouth; the floor and lateral wall of the nose; the floor of the orbit and maxillary sinuses. It also enters into the formation of two fossae – the infratemporal and pterygoid palatine – and the two fissures, the inferior orbital and the pterygo-maxillary. Each bone consists of a body and four processes: frontal bone, frontal, alveoli and palatine.

Significance in CFD

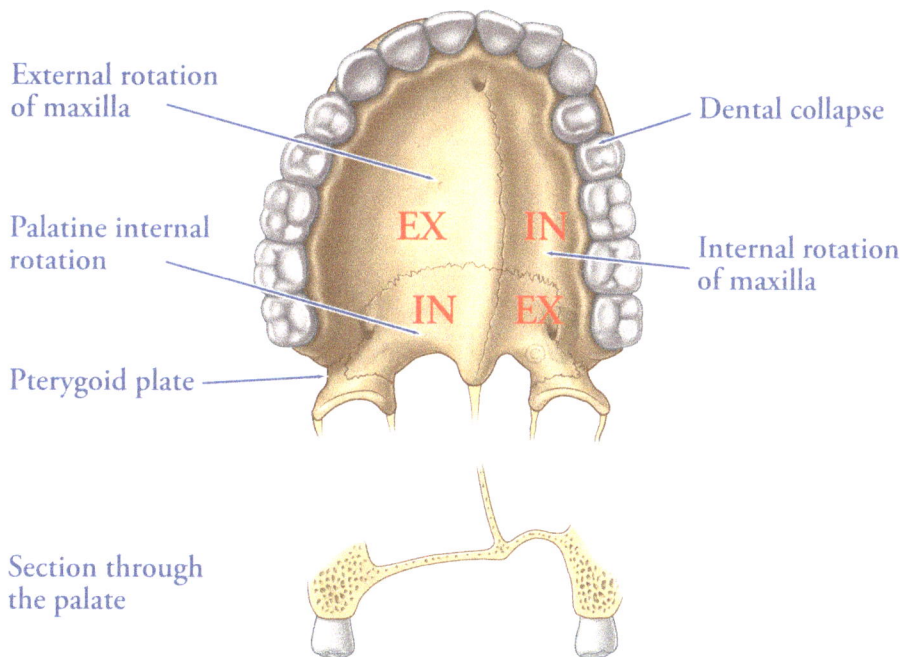

Figure 2.22 Counterclockwise Torque of Maxilla

The maxillary bones are the major external contact points in de-torquing the cranium, while the roof of the maxillary bones is used to augment drainage of the cavernous sinuses.

Specific details regarding occlusion and relationship with the mandible in a 'jaw to jaw' occlusion is studied in further chapters. The 'neurologic tooth' also reflects the state of the alveolus, from both maxillary and mandibular points of view. Tooth to tooth contact occurs about 1,500 times a day. This includes mastication and swallowing. The tooth to tooth contact is significant in that an electric circuit is established to define each tooth contact, initially with the trigeminal ganglion and ultimately with the brain. When this is missing, aberrant tooth behaviour ensues, changing the profile and posture of the tooth within the alveolus, and affects the periodontal ligament and the trigeminal ganglion.

The maxillary teeth and gums also play a big part in the stomatognathic system, involving the trigeminal (CN V), the facial (CN VII), glossopharyngeal (CN IX) and vagus (CN X) nerves. Disruption to this neurological stability has many consequences.

NASAL BONES

These are two small oblong bones placed side by side to form, by their junction, the bridge of the nose. Each bone is ossified from membrane overlying the anterior parts of the cartilaginous nasal capsule.

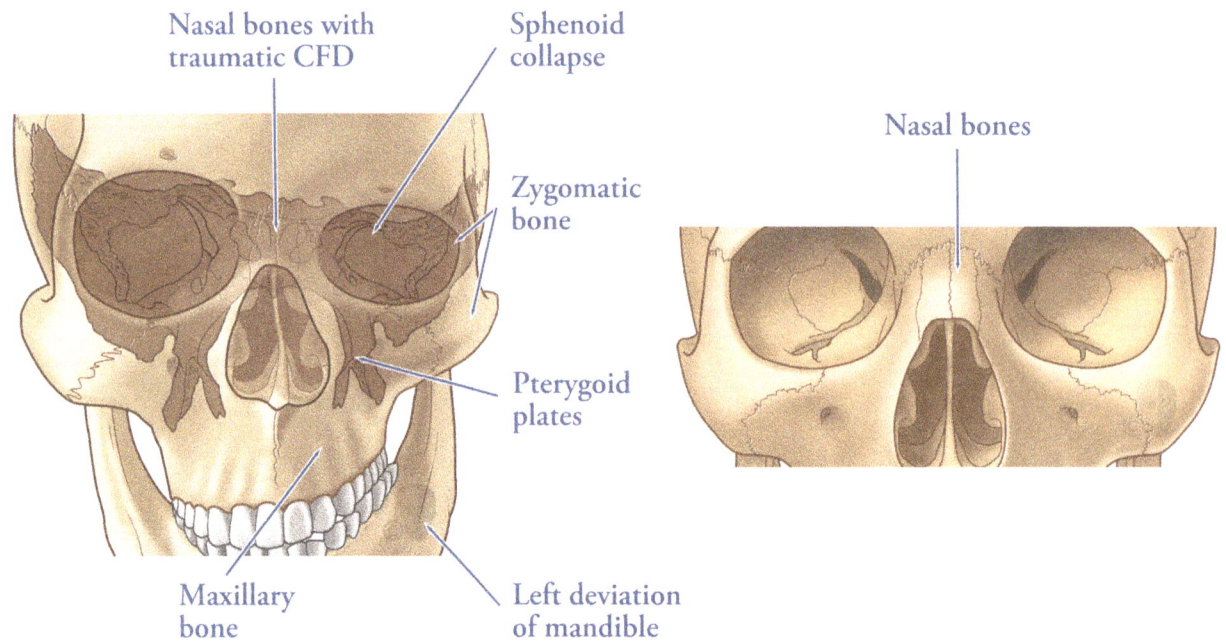

Figure 2.23 Nasal Bones

MANDIBLE

The mandible contains the lower teeth and consists of the horizontal portion, the body and two perpendicular portions, the rami, which join the body nearly at right angles. The mandible is ossified from fibrous membrane. The condyles of the mandible articulate with both temporal bones in the mandibular fossae. The right and left halves of the mandible fuse during the first postnatal year.

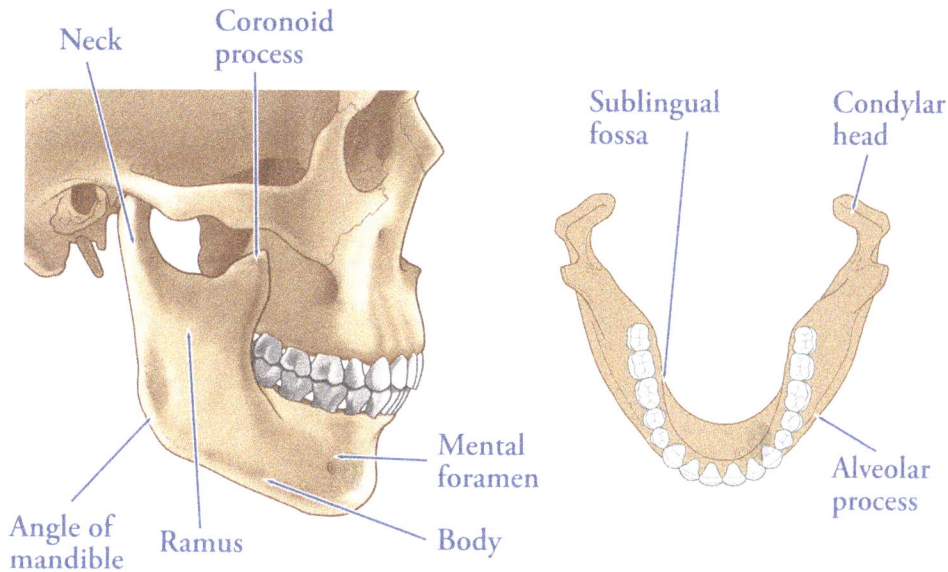

Figure 2.24 Mandibular Bone

Significance in CFD

Specific details regarding occlusion and relationship with the mandible, in a 'jaw to jaw' occlusion will be gone into further detail in further chapters. The 'neurologic tooth' also reflects the state of the alveolus, from both maxillary and mandibular points of view. Tooth to tooth contact comes into being about 1,500 times a day. This is including mastication and swallowing. The tooth to tooth contact is significant in that an electric circuit is established to define each tooth contact. When this is missing, aberrant tooth behaviour ensues changing the profile and posture of the tooth within the alveolus, and affects the periodontal ligament.

The mandibular teeth and gums also play a big part in the stomatognathic system, involving the trigeminal (CN V), the facial (CN VII), glossopharyngeal (CN IX) and vagus (CN X) nerves. Disruption to this neurological stability has many consequences.

The mandible is used in intra-oral cranial adjustments to achieve mandibular decongestion of the TMJ.

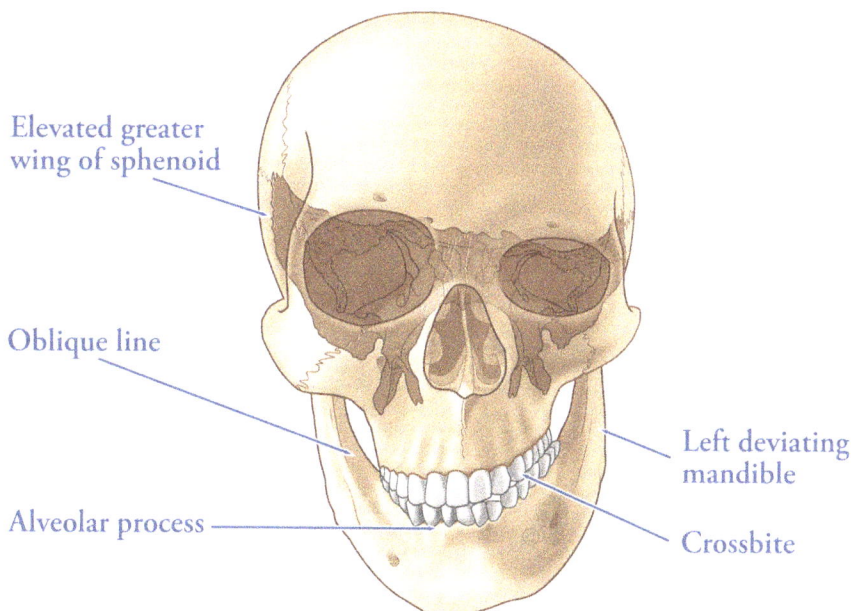

Figure 2.25 Mandible with Traumatic CFD

VOMER

Embryologically, the body of the vomer is *formed from membrane, while the attachments to the various bones on the peripheral borders are generated in cartilage.*

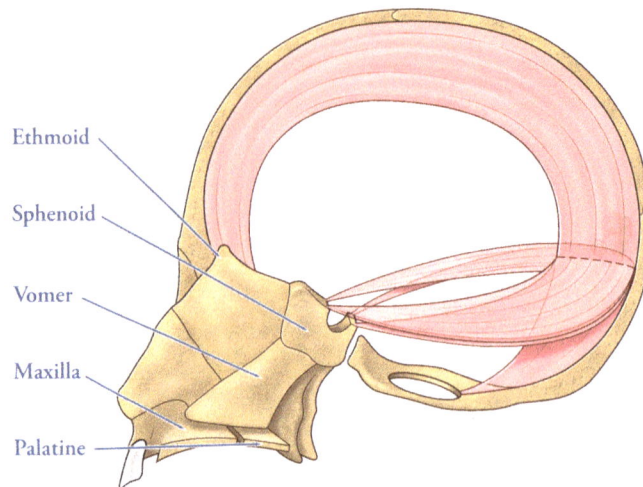

Ethmoid

Sphenoid

Vomer

Maxilla

Palatine

Figure 2.26 Reciprocal Tension Membranes and the Vomer: Ethmoid–sphenoid fulcrum

The vomer is a perpendicular, plough-shaped membrane, that attaches at its superior border with the ethmoid, posterior superior border to the body of the sphenoid bone, while the posterior border inferiorly attaches to the palatine bone posteriorly and the maxilla in the anterior posterior aspect. It acts like a tarpaulin pulling the ethmoid towards the maxilla, while the sphenoid pulls the palatine towards itself, as though the sheet pulls the four bones in different directions. The crucial point about the vomer is that it can only pull, as a tarpaulin can between two points, but has no ability to push as it would collapse.

Significance in CFD

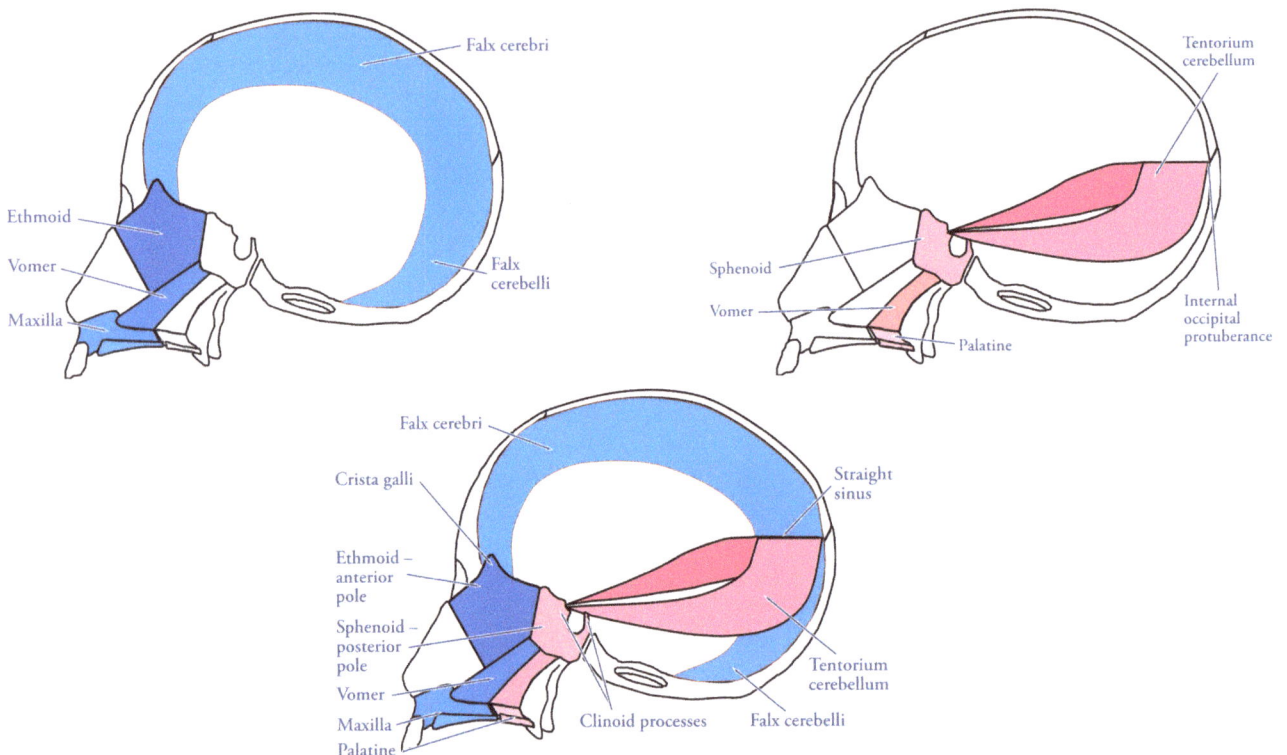

132

Figure 2.27 (top left) Anterior Pole; (top right) Posterior Pole; Anterior and Posterior Poles

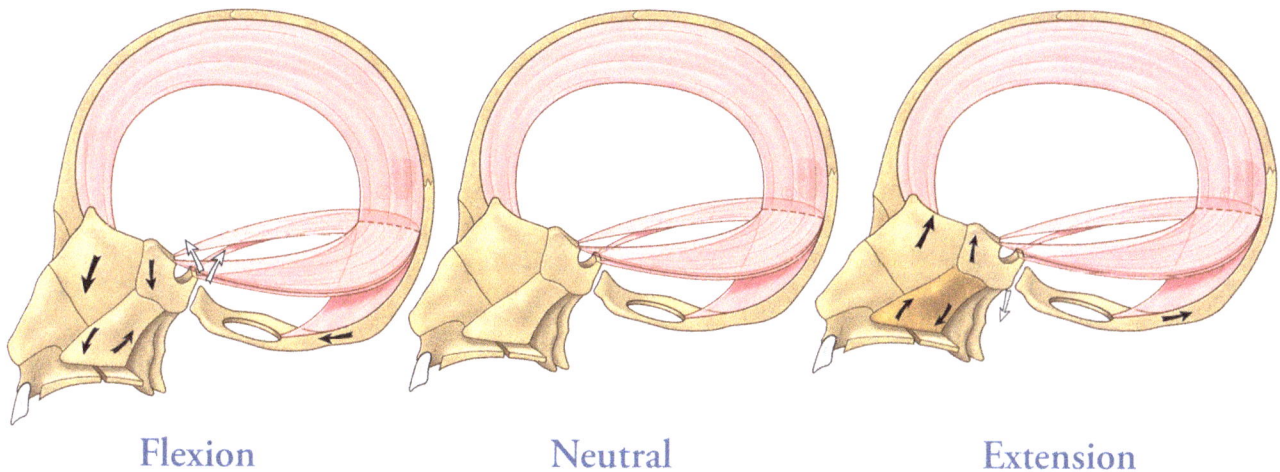

| Flexion | Neutral | Extension |

Figure 2.28 Respiration Phases of the Cranial Membranes

The vomer acts as a vertical vector within the cranium, and is an extension in respect of dynamics to the falx cerebri and falx cerebelli. The frenulum of the under surface of the tongue is another vertical vector. The action of the vomer is to activate the ethmoid and sphenoid bone in unison with the maxillae and the palatines. The crista galli on the superior aspect of the ethmoid is the anchor of the anterior pivot, while the inferior aspect is the common, superior border of the vomer. During inhalation the anterior part of the vomer is pulled inferior by the maxillae going into external rotation, while the ethmoid and crista galli (the anterior pole) are also pulled inferior, tightening the falx cerebri and the falx cerebelli. The tentorium cerebelli now flexes at its anchor point, at the clinoid processes of the sphenoid body (posterior pivot), pulling with it the sphenoid, which activates the posterior vomer and the inferior border attached to the palatines. In essence, this creates flexion/extension of the sphenobasilar synchondrosis in a young pre-ossification subject (ossification of the sphenobasilar synchondrosis can occur between the ages of 17 and 25). After the ossification has taken place the flexion and extension will move to the junction of the ethmoid/sphenoid junction – the anterior and posterior poles.

SACRUM AND ILIA IN DIAPHRAGMATIC RESPIRATION

The sacrum lies in between the ilia of the pelvis. The ilia reciprocate with the temporal bones in a linear diaphragmatic respiration, so that the sacrum flexes with inhalation and extends in exhalation. This motion is accepted as long as the pelvis is linear and balanced, and the two sacroiliac joints are stable, and the interosseous ligaments are balanced and stable. The bilateral motion of the external temporal bones will create a bilateral external rotation of the ilia, and vice versa. When the occiput flexes on inhalation, the sacrum flexes, creating the sacro-occipital pump mechanism that assists in movement of CSF, up and down the spinal cord and the cisterns. This linear diaphragmatic respiration also creates a linear motion of the ventricular system into flexion and extension, promoting the movement of CSF from the two lateral ventricles, the third ventricle and the fourth ventricle, and the motion of CSF through the two lateral apertures of Lushka, the medial aperture of Magendie and the spinal canal. This discussion is about linear diaphragmatic respiration.

Cardiovascular respiration brings an entirely different, additional and superimposed dynamic to cranial respiration, and is discussed in detail further on.

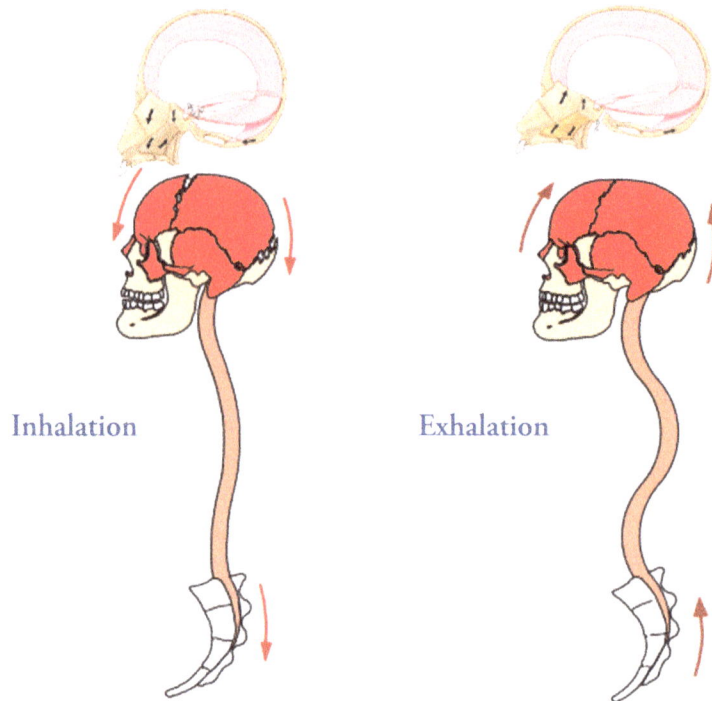

Inhalation   Exhalation

Figure 2.29 Reciprocal Tension Membranes in Diaphragmatic Respiration

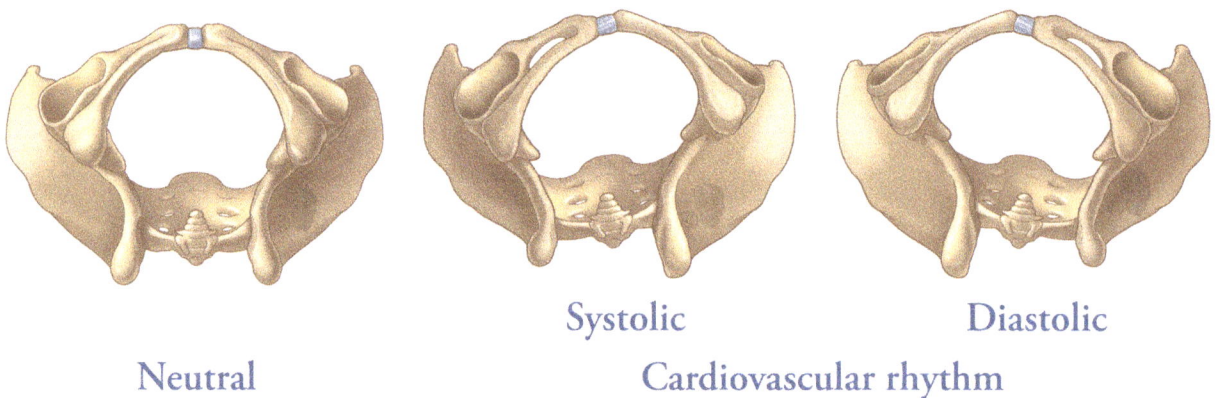

Systolic   Diastolic

Neutral   **Cardiovascular rhythm**

Figure 2.30 Sacral Function with Cardiovascular Rhythm

Significance in CFD

The sacro-occipital pump mechanism plays a significant role in the movement of CSF. When the pelvis is balanced and symmetrical, diaphragmatic and cardiovascular impulses drive the CSF from the sacral bulb in the sacral body, up the spinal cord, towards the cisterns of the brain for reabsorption through the arachnoid granulation into the superior sagittal sinus. Once traumatic CFD is introduced, the pump mechanism becomes compromised and the sacral pump mechanism fails in its optimum function to drive CSF flow. The pelvis may have external and internal rotation, the sacrum consequently locks, inducing sacroiliac failure to the neurological weight-bearing ability. Stagnation of CSF ensues in the cord, the cisterns and the ventricles. Hence the importance to remove the CFD torque at the cranial and pelvic levels.

CHAPTER 3

CRANIAL MOTION

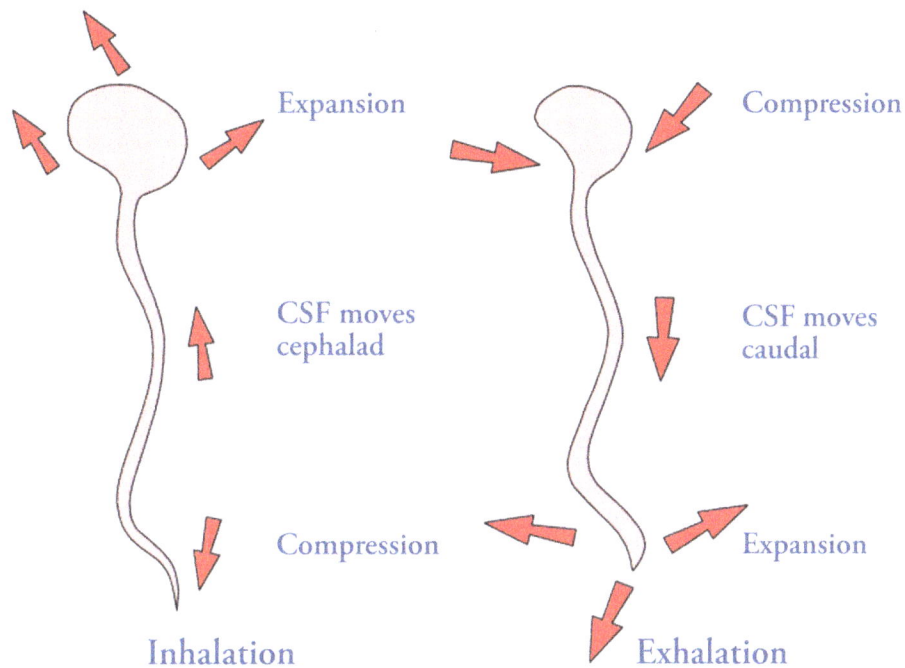

Figure 3.1 Movement of Cerebrospinal Fluid with Diaphragmatic Respiration

CRANIAL MOTION

The cranium is a bony cavity which protects and supports the core of the central nervous system – the brain. The support mechanism comes in the form of the RTM (see Figure 1.1). These separate the cerebral hemispheres from the cerebellum and, in turn, divide each of the cerebral and cerebellar hemispheres from one another. These RTM anchor to various internal structures of the skull and are part of the dynamic dural meningeal system. The system respirates through the cardiovascular system (at 68–72 pulses a minute) and the diaphragmatic respiratory system (at 18–20 pulses a minute) and the cranial rhythmic impulse (CRI; at 8–14 pulses a minute).

The cardiovascular impulse creates a counterclockwise motion of the brain as a result of the larger vessels and greater volume of venous blood draining the brain. This is the rhythmic component of the cranial impulse and corresponds with the linear motion of the diaphragmatic respiratory impulse. In the opinion of the author, when these two pulses coincide, it produces the CRI that is discussed by other authorities as a separate CRI. The inherent motion of this system depends on the sutural system of the skull, each suture defining the separate and distinct motion of each of the cranial bones and the reciprocal motion of the sacrum. Cranial technique is therefore not a question of moving the osseous components of the skull, but rather allowing the dural meningeal system to find its level of optimum homeostatic function through membranous balancing to provide production, circulation and absorption of CSF to be constant throughout the system. Correction is made through the muscles of the fingers directing motion and letting respiration move the cranial components through the dura, as well as intra-oral correction of the RTM attachments through the mouth.

The normal rhythm of life is expressed by the term "primary sacral respiration" and the recognition that a healthy cranium cannot exist in a sick or distorted body. The pelvis and its sacral divider is as important to health and neural flow as is the cranium and its contents. Life begins with inhalation, putting the dural meningeal system into a state of flexion, resulting in external rotation of the cranial bones and the pelvis. Life ends (death) with exhalation, dural meningeal extension and internal rotation of the cranial bones and pelvis.

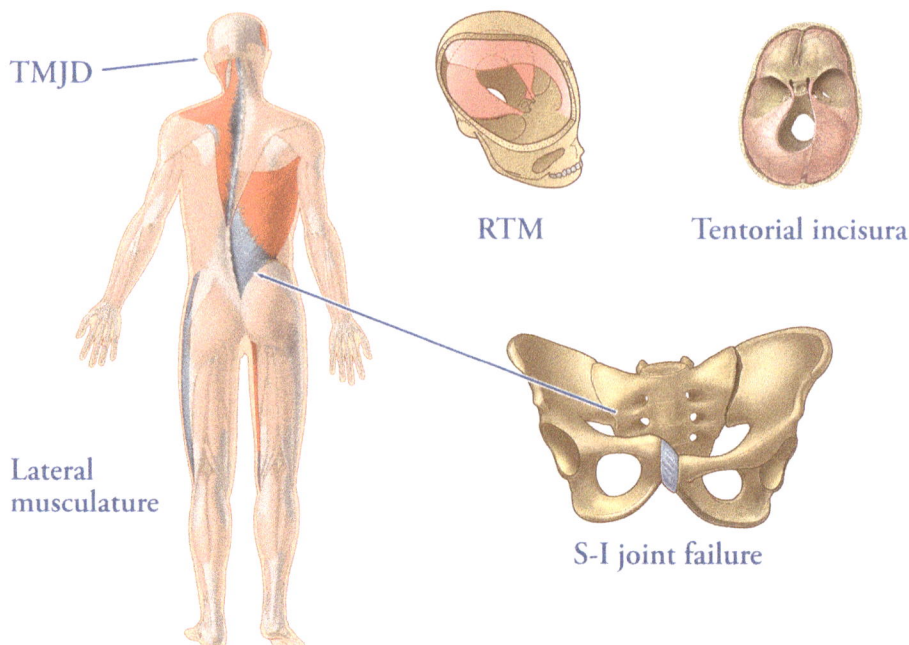

TMJD

RTM   Tentorial incisura

Lateral
musculature

S-I joint failure

Figure 3.2 Traumatic CFD Results in Cranio Pelvic Failure: Stagnation of CSF

One of the intricate factors in cranial mechanics is the locking mechanism of the sphenoid bone in relation to all cranial and facial bones, except the mandible. The sphenoid bone (the central bone of the skull) can subluxate other cranial components and, as such, is the mechanism used to correct these structures. This is either through the anterior or posterior hard palate, which influences the vomer affecting the sphenoid, or through the leverage of the medial and lateral pterygoid plates (the hamulus). The mandible and its junction with the maxillae at the inter-cusp contact of the upper and lower teeth forms the largest and most dynamic suture in the skull. Malocclusions at this sutural level will have a profound and devastating effect on cranial motion and function.

The cranial sutural system is the chief source of cranial pathologies, for when a suture loses its mobility, all structures underlying that particular fixed area must suffer from blood loss or congestion, from tissue swelling and expansion and, finally, from tissue fibrosis. Cranial motion is essential to cranial function. The brain substance must be constantly revitalised, the CSF must move and circulate through the ventricular system and the spinal cord to maintain homeostasis.

Scientific Evolution of Cranial Motion

> Viola Fryman, on 13 May 1963, made the first successful recording of skull motion
> and found it to be between .0005 and .001 of an inch.

Among other researchers who have demonstrated cranial motion are Michael and Retzlaff who demonstrated cyclic cranial bone displacement of 5 to 7 cycles per minute.

Tettambel et al. demonstrated skull motion independent from simultaneous pulse and respiration recordings, revealing CRIs.

Baker's further study of the maxillary teeth showed .0276 inch movement between the second molars and, after several months of occlusal equilibration, his conclusion was that the skull bones moved along these sutures.

Silverman demonstrated changes in occlusion resulting from pressure on various parts of the skull.

Girton et al. demonstrated in the 1930s the concept of a sacroelectrical phenomena above the scalp, of waves between 5 to 8 cycles per minute.

These are among some of the many documented pieces of evidence that demonstrate cranial bone motion. A more detailed account of research into cranial motion can be found in David Walther's *Applied Kinesiology* (Vol II).

OSSIFICATION OF THE SKULL

The inferior view shows the base of the skull and outlines the membranous and cartilaginous areas.

The anterior end of the ethmoid bone, the lesser wings and the body of the sphenoid, the basal portion of the occiput, the condylar area of the occiput and the petrous portion of the temporal bones, are all ossified from cartilage. The cartilaginous ossification of these bones form the apertures through which the twelve pairs of cranial nerves exit from the cranium. The squama of the frontal bone, the greater wings of the sphenoid, the squama of the temporal bones, the squama of the occiput and the two squama of the parietal bones form most of the ossified membranous areas. These membranous areas of the superior part of the cranium allow for more flexible mobility than their counterparts on the floor of the cranium.

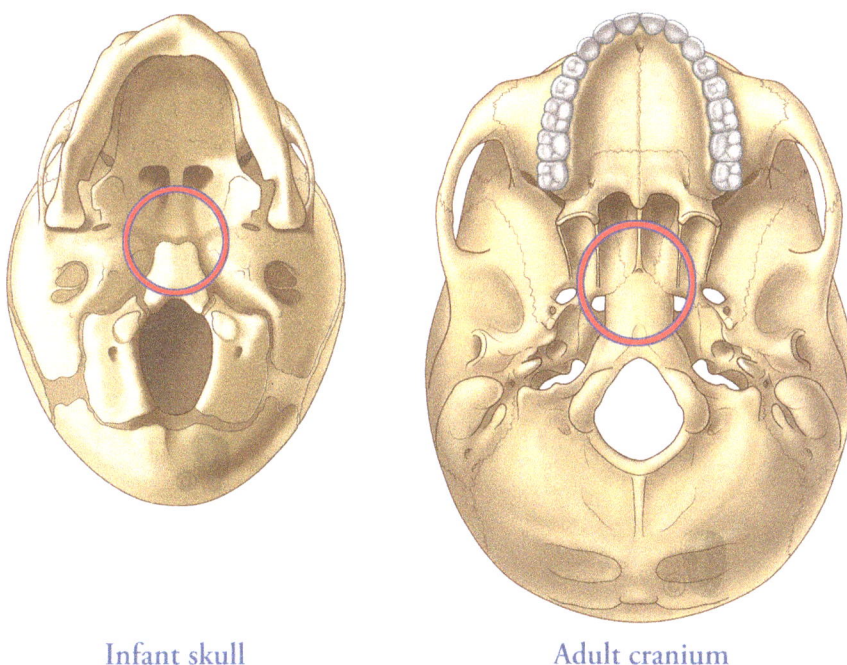

Infant skull   Adult cranium

Figure 3.3 Ossification of the Cranium: Note the ossification result of the sphenobasilar synchondrosis

The sagittal section shows the membranous and cartilaginous areas of the cranium. Note again the floor of the cranium is made of cartilage where the apertures for the twelve pairs of cranial nerves exit, apart from the maxillary and mandibular branches of the 5th cranial nerve – the trigeminal – which exit through the foramen rotundum and ovale respectively. These are found in the membranous area of the greater wing of the sphenoid. The superior orbital fissure is surrounded by the greater wing of the sphenoid (generated from membrane) and the lesser wing of the sphenoid (generated in cartilage).

This view depicts the membranous and cartilaginous areas. Note the rounded concave squama areas, when viewed internally, of the occiput, parietal, frontal and temporal bones which form the membranous areas.

THE LOVETT BROTHER RELATIONSHIP

Or the Resistance Plus Contraction Factor (R Plus C Factor) Lateral View

The Lovett Brother Relationship (R plus C factor) means that there is a paired reciprocity between the skeletal structures (i.e. atlas and fifth lumbar work together, axis and fourth lumbar work together, third cervical and third lumbar etc.). When the fifth lumbar moves out of position or subluxates, there will be compensation at the level of the atlas. If the fourth lumbar moves there will be compensation at the level of the axis and so on. This paired reciprocity also exists within the pelvis, where the ilium has paired reciprocity with the temporal bone, the sacrum with the occiput, and the coccyx with the sphenoid.

Note the similarity in shape of the occipital squama and the sacrum, the concave inner curves which, incidentally, provide intrabone flexion and extension. The two temporal bones rotate in equal and opposite directions to the ilia. The temporal and ilia are similar in shape and movement. In this regard, note the sacroiliac joint and its counterpart the occipito-mastoid suture.

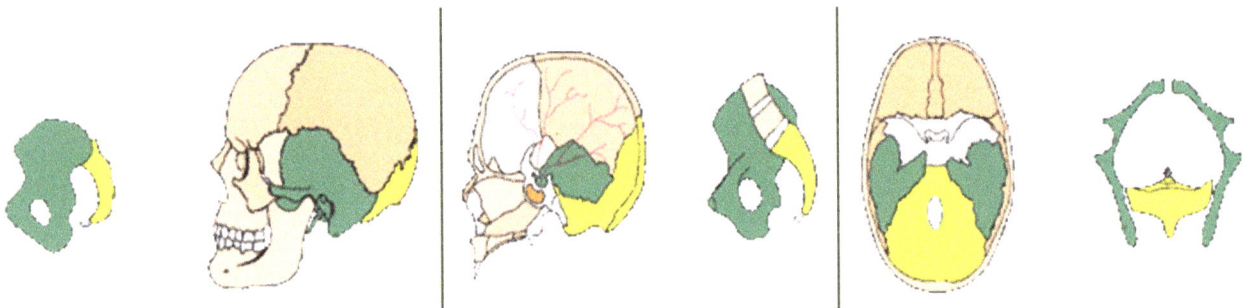

Figure 3.4 Lovett Brother Relationship
Green – ilium and temporal bone reciprocate; yellow – sacrum and occiput reciprocate

The mid-sagittal section of the skull shows the occiput, sacrum, temporals and the ilia. Notice the coccyx and its reciprocal bone the sphenoid. Also note the sphenobasilar synchondrosis of the sphenoid and occiput and the sacro-coccygeal junction – both free junctions, until ossification takes place in puberty or later.

In the superior views of the base of the skull and the pelvic floor, note the position of the ilia to their reciprocal bones, the squama of the temporal bones, the occipital squama and the sacral body, and the sphenoid bone and the coccyx.

CHAPTER 4

DIAPHRAGMATIC RESPIRATION

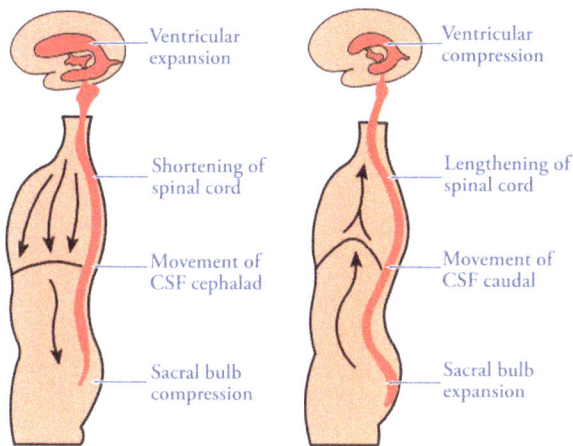

Figure 4.1 Diaphragmatic Respiration

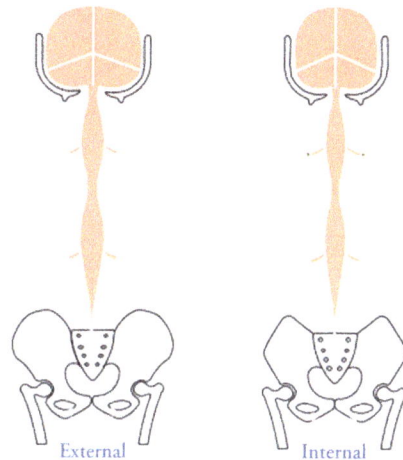

Figure 4.2 Rotation of the Temporals and Ilia

When describing diaphragmatic respiration, one has to understand that this is a linear activity, created by a linear dynamic – the diaphragm. The lungs are a central bilateral structure, and with the diaphragmatic influence the motion is one of inhalation and exhalation, contraction and expansion of the lungs, with air moving in and out of the lungs in a symmetric motion. With inhalation and exhalation, the diaphragm moves in a linear motion and all the examples of this motion are discussed below. With this linear activity, there is a bilateral mirroring of all the supportive skeletal structures, equally responding to bilateral function. The other dynamic is the cardiovascular pulse, which is the brain drainage component, moving blood from the brain, to the left side of the body, to the heart, then to the right side to the liver, and then back to the left to the heart, through the lungs and back to the body and the brain. This movement consists of a helical motion, which is where the rhythmic pulse comes into being. The combination of the linear and the rhythmic create the cranial motion discussed below.

The cycle of diaphragmatic respiration starts in the neutral position. As air is inhaled into the lungs the diaphragm is depressed, pushing the abdominal organs into the pelvic floor, externally rotating both ilia and flattening the lumbar lordosis. This has an effect of compressing the sacral bulb (dural arachnoid sac) forcing CSF into the cephalad, as the spinal cord shortens as a result of more dural membrane being pulled into the cranium to facilitate cranial expansion. At the same time as inhalation takes place the ventricles of the brain expand, allowing the choroid plexuses of the ventricles to secrete CSF into the ventricles.

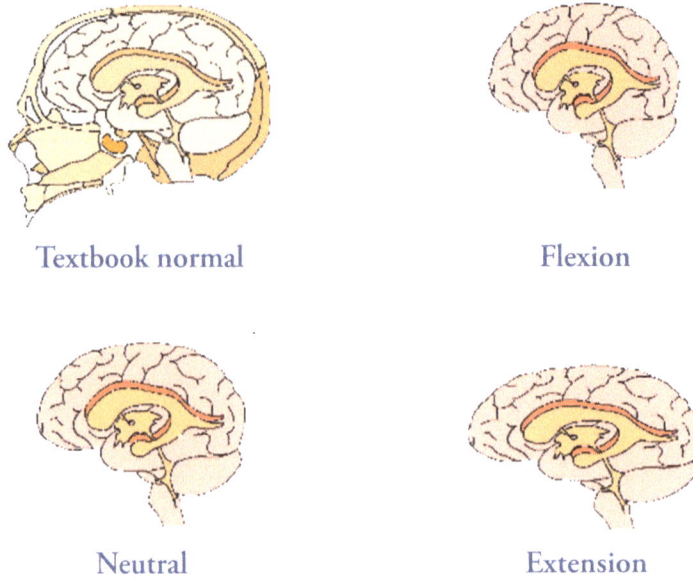

Figure 4.3 Respiration of the Ventricular System

While the brain expands to facilitate the ventricles, the cisterns on the peripheral area of the brain become compressed, forcing CSF up towards the superior sagittal sinus for reabsorption, through the arachnoid granulation. After the peak of inhalation the cycle returns through neutral to the exhalation phase.

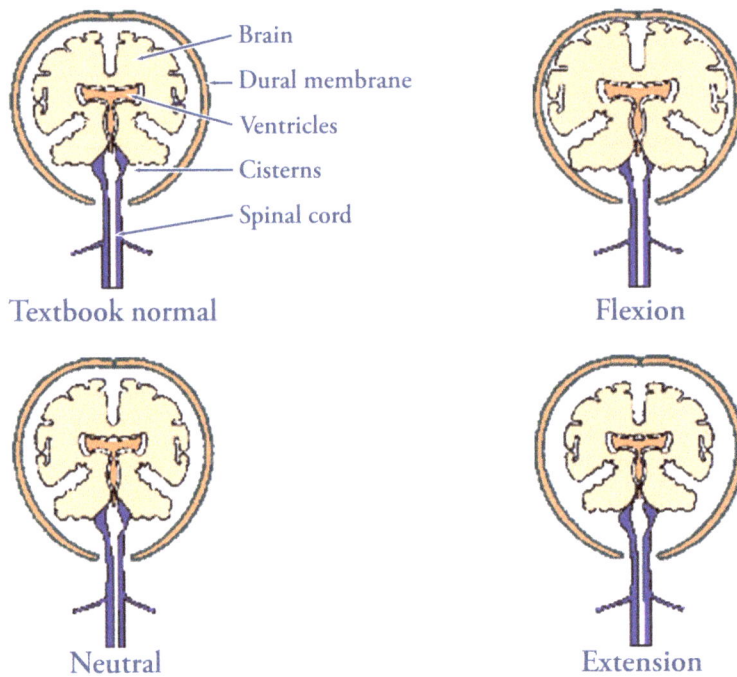

Figure 4.4 Respiration of the Cisterns

In the exhalation phase, air is released out of the lungs allowing the diaphragm to relax, the abdominal organs return to their normal position, the ilia become internally rotated, the lumbar lordosis returns and the sacral bulb expands, and the spinal cord lengthens as the cranial dura is released from the cranial compression. At the same time the ventricles compress, forcing CSF out of the two lateral, third and fourth ventricles in a caudal direction. The brain in turn contracts, allowing the peripheral cisterns to expand and absorb CSF. Once the exhalation phase has peaked the cycle will move back into the neutral position.

CRANIAL FLEXION AND EXTENSION

Lateral View of the Cranium

Showing the ethmoid, frontal, sphenoid, temporal and occipital bones.

Cranial flexion and extension follows the sphenobasilar synchondrosis and the result is a symmetric type of motion produced by diaphragmatic respiration. On inhalation the frontal, temporal and occipital bones go into bilateral external rotation as a result of sphenobasilar flexion. In diaphragmatic respiration, as the body inhales, the A to P diameter of the skull decreases, the lateral dimension increases, moving the skull into a full flexion position of maximum lateral expansion with minimal anterior to posterior (A to P) compression. The frontal temporal and occiput move into bilateral symmetric external rotation. As the sphenobasilar synchondrosis moves through the neutral position, then into the exhalation phase, the lateral dimension of the skull decreases significantly and the A to P dimension increases.

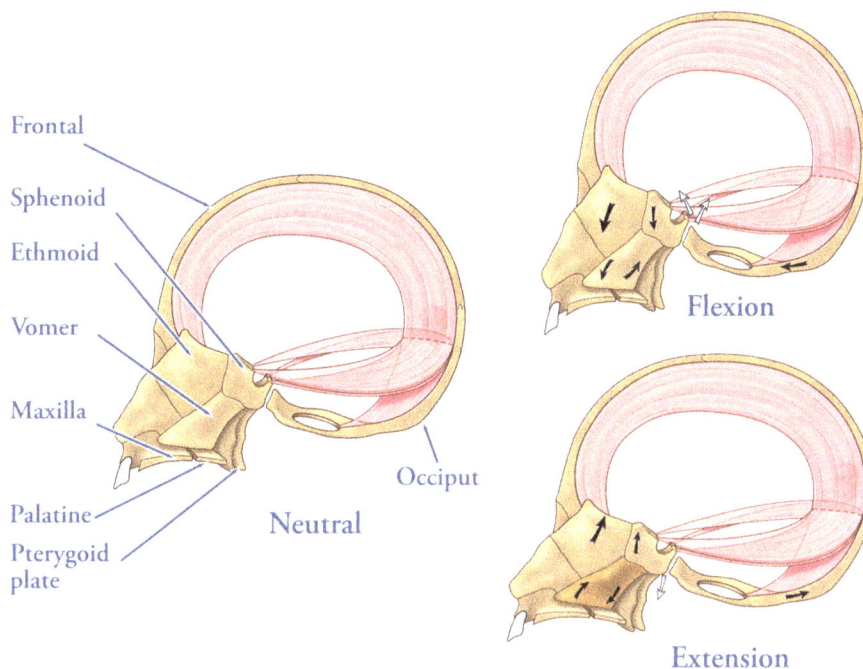

Figure 4.5 Cranial Vault Respiration Stages

On the extension phase of the sphenobasilar synchondrosis, the skull reaches maximum A to P expansion and lateral compression. The frontal, temporal and occipital bones move into bilateral symmetric internal rotation. This is the extension phase of the sphenobasilar synchondrosis. As the body leaves exhalation towards the neutral position, the lateral and anteroposterior dimensions return to a neutral position.

The sagittal view of the cranium showing the sphenobasilar synchondrosis and other related bones.

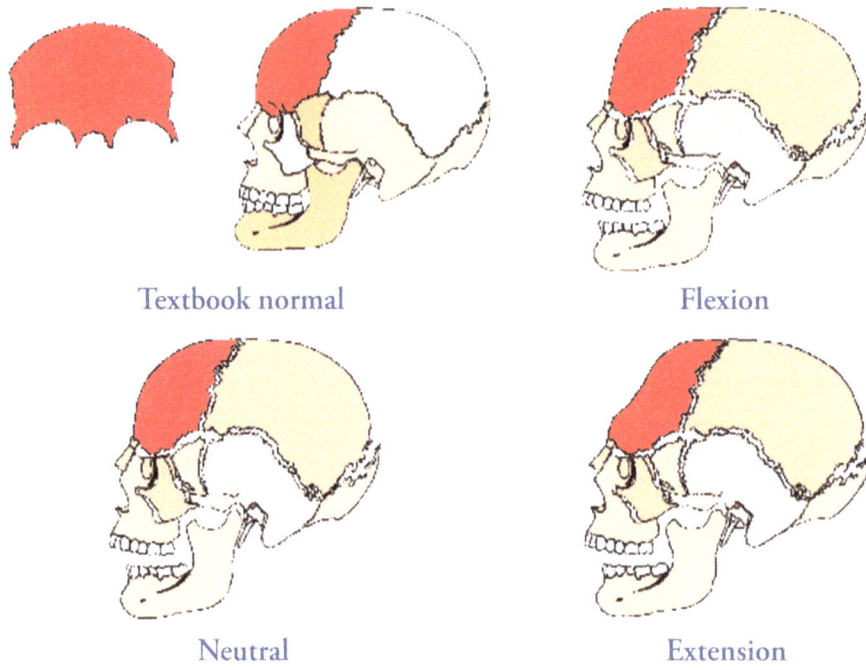

Textbook normal

Flexion

Neutral

Extension

Figure 4.6 Frontal Bone Respiration Stages

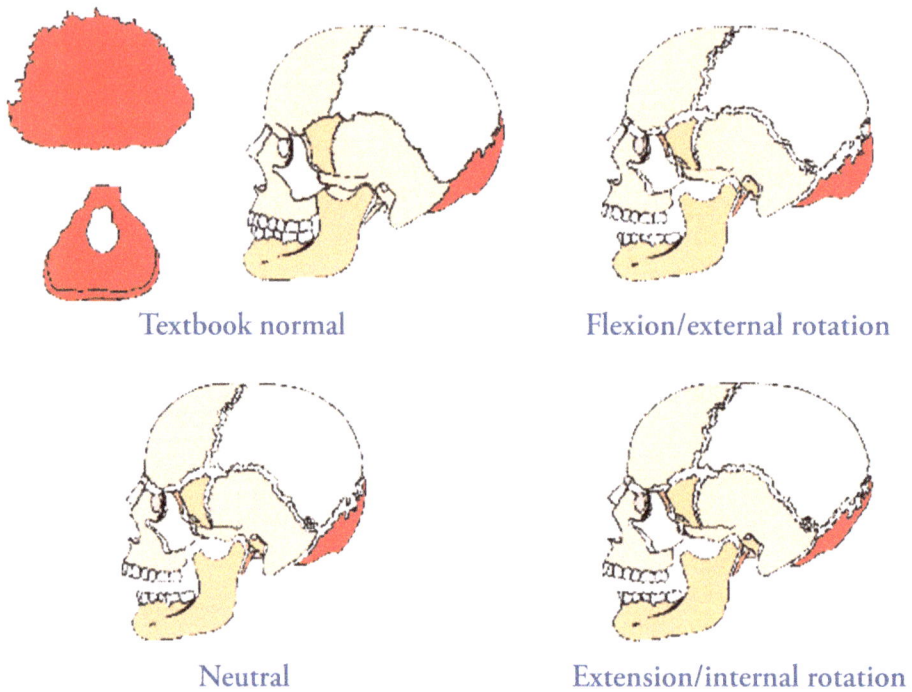

Textbook normal

Flexion/external rotation

Neutral

Extension/internal rotation

Figure 4.7 Occipital Bone Respiration Stages

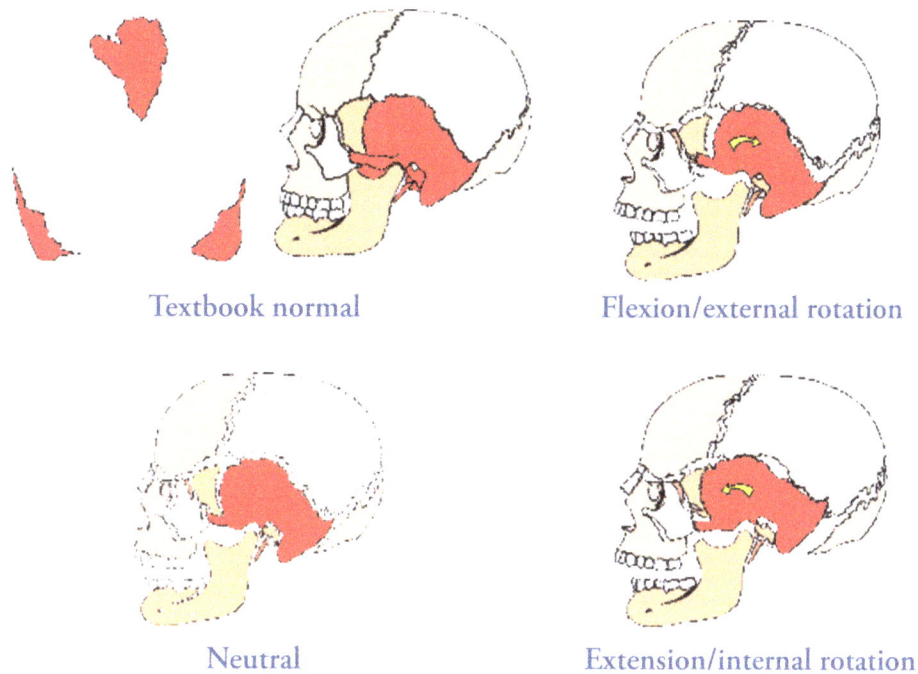

Textbook normal	Flexion/external rotation
Neutral	Extension/internal rotation

Figure 4.8 Temporal Bone Respiration Stages

On inhalation the sphenobasilar mechanism goes into a state of flexion, the anterior posterior diameter of the skull decreases while the superior to inferior dimension increases. On the exhalation phase the cranium goes into a more elongated position where the anterior posterior diameter increases, the superior to inferior dimension decreases, while the sphenobasilar synchondrosis goes into an extension phase. The full respiratory range shows the sphenobasilar mechanism going into flexion on inhalation, through neutral and into extension on exhalation then returning to neutral.

Posterior View of the Cranium

Viewing the posterior of the cranium from a neutral position. On inhalation the lateral aspect increases while the superior inferior diameter increases, taking it to the peak of inhalation/flexion then returning through neutral to the exhalation or extension phase where both the lateral and superior to inferior dimensions decrease totally, returning to a neutral phase.

Increase in the lateral dimension as well as the superior to inferior dimension on the inhalation phase of the sphenobasilar synchondrosis. A decrease in the lateral dimension as well as the superior to inferior dimension on the exhalation phase of the sphenobasilar synchondrosis.

RECIPROCAL TENSION MEMBRANES (RTM)

The RTM (falx cerebri, falx cerebelli, tentorium cerebelli and the diaphragma sellae) are the vertical and horizontal components of the support and balancing dynamics of the cranium. The RTM also support the brain drainage system (superior and inferior sagittal sinuses, the transverse and sigmoid sinuses and the internal jugular veins). In diaphragmatic respiration, as is indicated by the graphics, the inhalation and exhalation phases of respiration are linear and dynamic. This is very different to the cardiovascular phase in drainage which provides/facilitates a counterclockwise direction driven by the increased volume of venous blood through the internal jugular veins.

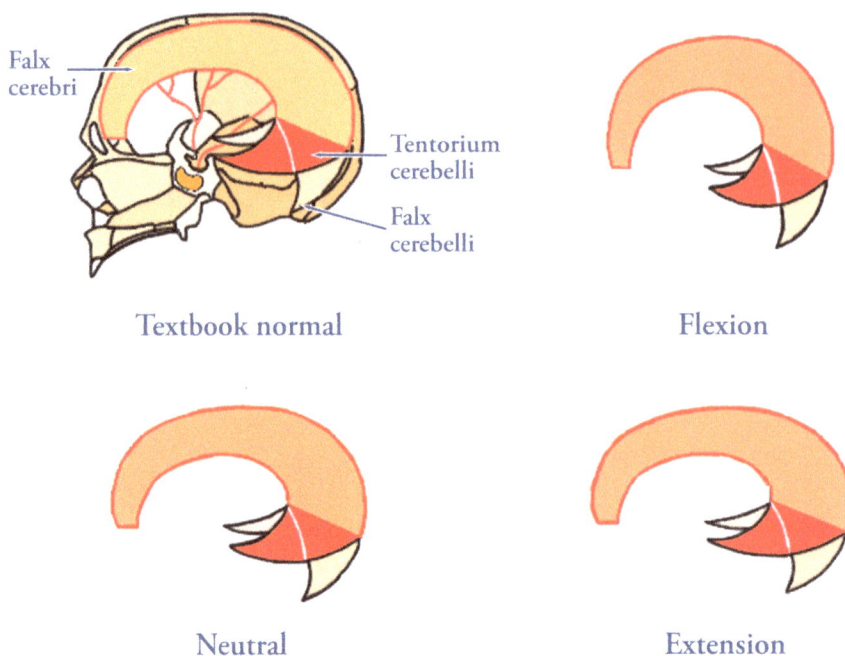

Figure 4.9 Respiration of the Reciprocal Tension Membranes

The RTM are superimposed within the cranium and leading from the neutral phase into the inhalation or flexion stage, the A to P diameter decreases as the superior to inferior diameter increases. It returns to the neutral position, then into the exhalation or extension phase, where the A to P diameter increases and the superior to inferior diameter decreases.

With diaphragmatic respiration, the sphenobasilar synchondrosis goes into flexion on inspiration, moving the RTM into flexion with a diminished A to P dimension and an increased superior to inferior dimension, and increased lateral dimension with bilateral external rotation of the temporals. On expiration the sphenobasilar synchondrosis goes into extension, moving the RTM into extension, increasing the A to P dimension and decreasing the superior to inferior dimension and lateral dimension.

BRAIN AND VENTRICLES

As the neutral position changes into a phase of inhalation or flexion, the ventricular components shorten in an A to P diameter and increase on a superior to inferior diameter. The entire brain and ventricles expand at this point of the cycle, with the ventricles filling with CSF from the choroid plexuses. At the peak of the flexion stage the A to P diameter has decreased, the superior to inferior diameter has increased, and the lateral dimension increases to a maximum. This is slowly reversed, moving towards the neutral position of the cyclic stage and as exhalation takes place the A to P diameter increases and the superior to inferior diameter and lateral dimension decreases. The ventricles are now being compressed, moving CSF out of the ventricular system caudal towards the sacral bulb. At the peak of exhalation the A to P diameter is greater, and the superior to inferior diameter and lateral dimension decrease to a minimal.

The flexion or inhalation phase expands the ventricles, diminishing the A to P dimension and increasing the superior to inferior dimension. The extension or exhalation phase compresses the ventricles, increasing the A to P dimension and decreasing the superior to inferior dimension.

VENTRICULAR AND CISTERN RESPIRATION

A sagittal view of the skull shows the two lateral ventricles, the third ventricle and the fourth ventricle, the brain and spinal cord. The peripheral area between the brain and cranium forms the cisterns which, with diaphragmatic respiration, forms a cranial pump, sucking CSF into the cisterns on exhalation and forcing CSF towards the sagittal sinus on inhalation.

Ventricular expansion on inhalation causes the brain to enlarge and compress the cisterns on the lateral borders of the skull, thereby pushing CSF cephalad through the sub-arachnoid space to the absorption point of the arachnoid granulation at the superior sagittal sinus. From the inhalation phase follows the neutral position into the exhalation phase. The exhalation phase causes ventricular compression, allowing the brain to compact while the cisterns enlarge, drawing CSF from the surrounding tissue and spinal cord.

The CSF will remain in this area until it is pumped to the sagittal sinus on the next phase of inhalation. At the end of exhalation or the extension phase the process is repeated.

VENOUS SINUS SYSTEM

The venous sinus system is entirely encapsulated by dural membrane and is devoid of valves, allowing a free flow of blood through the entire system, primarily influenced by pressure gradient. This is apparent with the added complexity of cranio fascial distortion, where the vessels of the venous sinus system can be stretched, compressed or twisted, delaying the capability of drainage potential.

The venous sinus system is superimposed within the cranium, going from the neutral phase into the inhalation phase the A to P dimension decreases, as the superior to inferior dimension and the lateral dimension increases, returning to neutral, before going into the exhalation phase, where the A to P diameter increases, and the superior to inferior diameter and the lateral dimension decreases, going back into neutral position.

The flexion or inhalation phase decreases the A to P dimension of the venous sinus system and increases the superior to inferior dimension. On the exhalation or extension phase the venous sinus system A to P dimension increases and the superior to inferior dimension decreases.

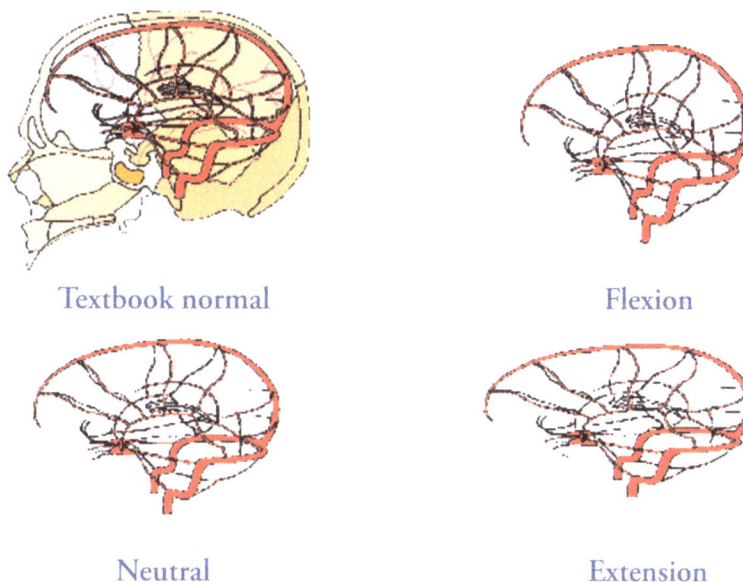

Textbook normal

Flexion

Neutral

Extension

Figure 4.10 Respiration of the Venous Sinus System

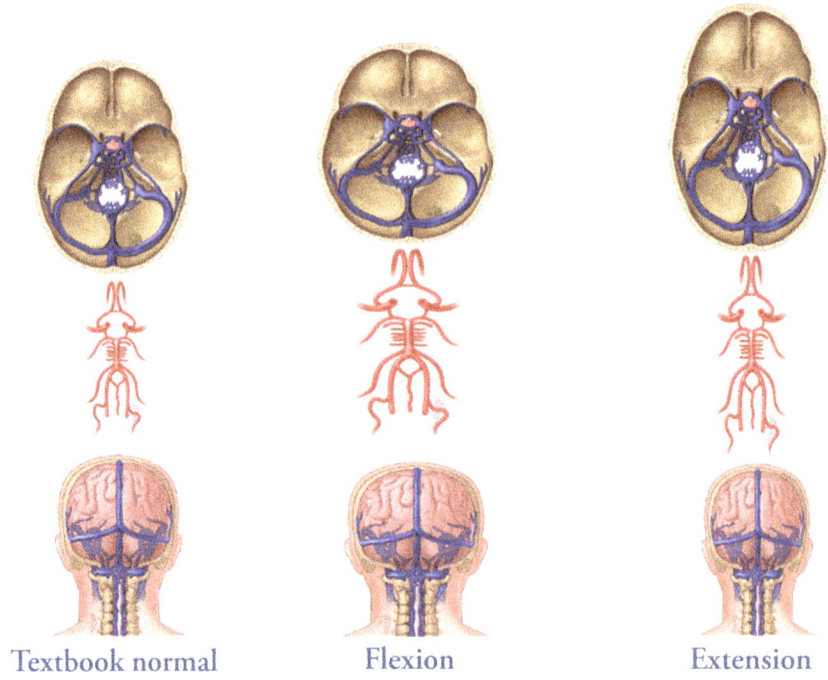

Figure 4.11 Vascularisation with Diaphragmatic Respiration

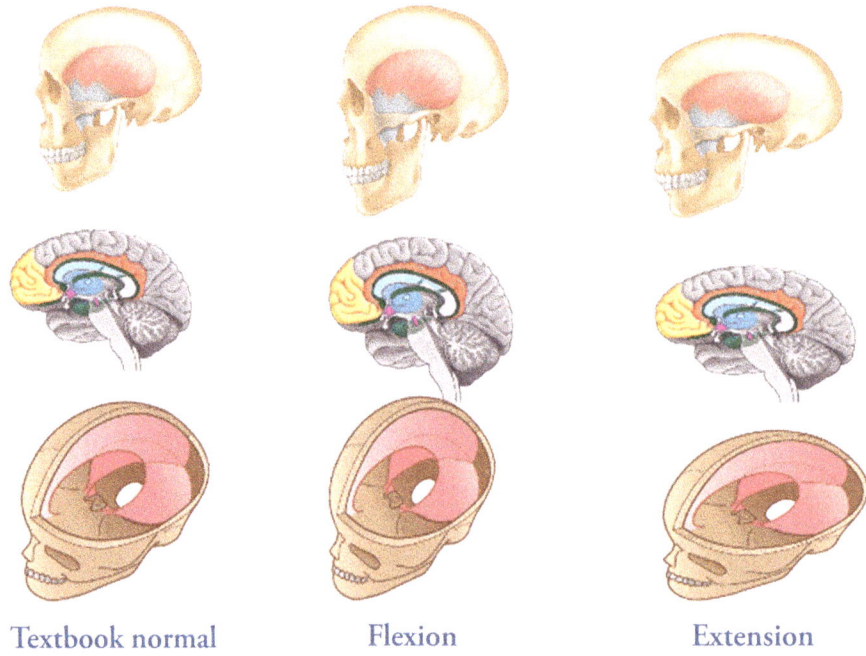

Figure 4.12 Diaphragmatic Respiration Phases

CHAPTER 5

CARDIOVASCULAR RHYTHMIC IMPULSE

As discussed in Chapter 3, cardiovascular drainage is responsible for a counterclockwise motion of the brain from about 32 to 35 weeks of foetal development. This is created by the larger drainage vessels on the right side of the brain – the superior sagittal sinus and the right transverse sinus. There is also a greater volume of venous blood drained from the right side of the brain, giving a propensity for the brain to move in a counterclockwise direction, in a rhythmic pulsing motion. This rhythmic motion accompanies the linear motion of the diaphragmatic respiration, meaning that the brain is in constant linear A to P motion, as well as a constant counterclockwise motion (returning to a clockwise motion between the cardiac beats). While the cranium is driven in a counterclockwise direction, the pelvis is driven in a reciprocal clockwise direction in order to maintain balance and stability. If both were driven in the same direction, one would fall over, balance and stability would fail and the sacro-occipital pump mechanism would be corrupted, leaving the flow of CSF to stagnate and a resultant chaos of the nervous system.

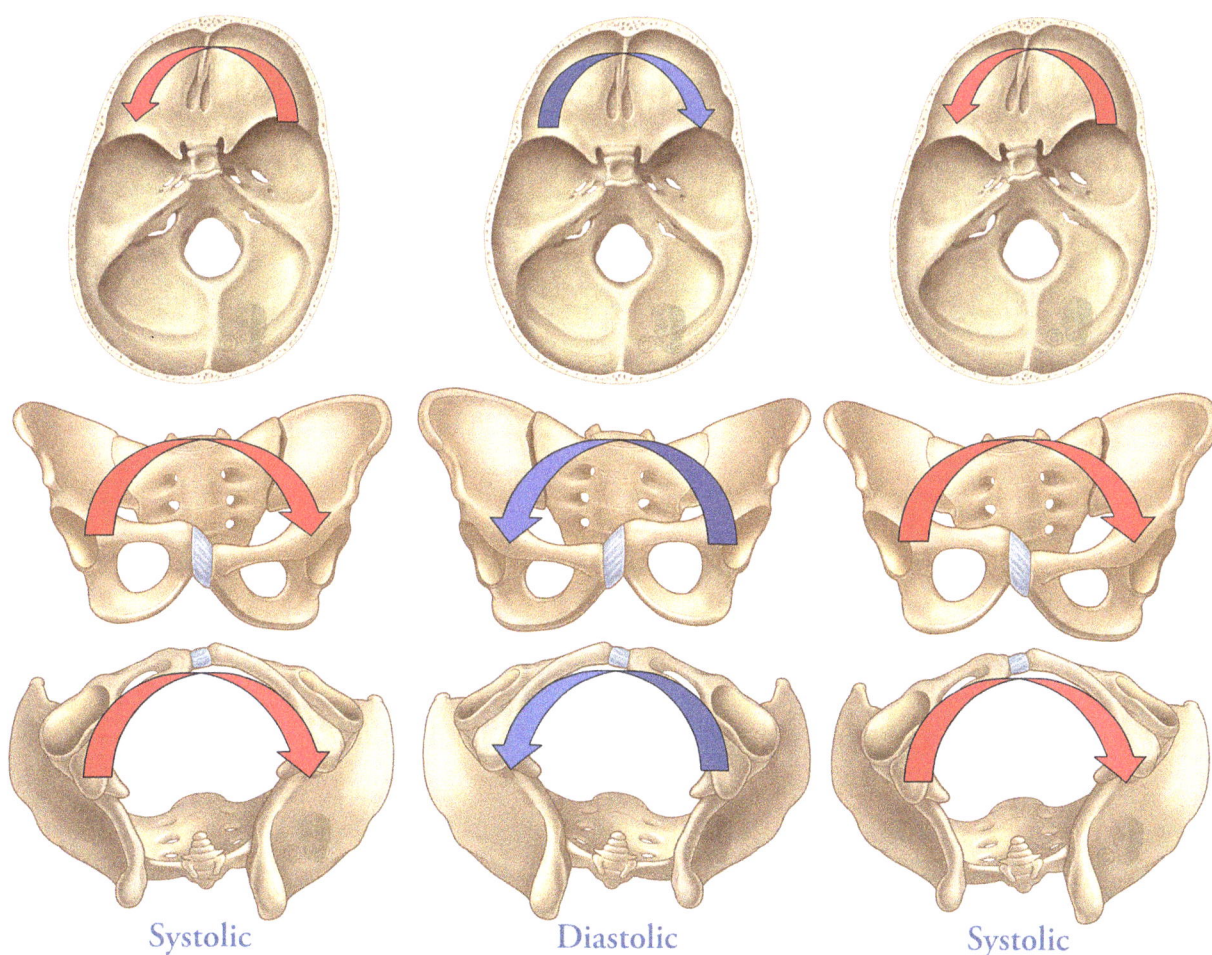

| Systolic | Diastolic | Systolic |

Figure 5.1 Cardiovascular Rhythmatic Respiration – Cranium; (middle and bottom) Sacral Function with Cardiovascular Rhythm – Pelvis: One phase of the heartbeat producing counterclockwise torque

The coincidental or corresponding rhythms mean that between the pulses in this cyclic behaviour, some pulses will coincide at the same time, giving rise to what numerous cranial exponents refer to as the CRI, a third impulse. The author does not agree. Both the diaphragmatic impulse (linear activity) and the cardiovascular impulse (rhythmic activity) are the only plausible dynamics that result in cranial motion. In the historic understanding of this cranial motion, both the diaphragmatic and the cardiovascular motions were assumed to be linear, but *Gray's Anatomy* states that the vessels of drainage and the different volumes concerned clearly indicate that the cardiovascular behaviour is rhythmic, which supports the author's rationale.

Supporting this rhythmic pulse, CFD clearly shows that with the counterclockwise motion of the brain (preceding the growth of cranial plates) the cranium will assume a posture of a right external frontal and a left external temporal/occiput, and a left internal frontal and a coinciding right internal temporal/occiput. The sphenoid, being the central bone of the cranium, pivots and follows the right external frontal by moving the greater wing anterior and superior on the right, while the greater wing on the left follows the external temporal/occiput, and moves posterior and inferior. This in turn allows the RTM to move in a linear direction with diaphragmatic respiration, as well as a rhythmic direction with cardiovascular activity, in ensuring that the optimum drainage potential is reached in a homeostatic environment. These two dynamics also play a reciprocal role in sacral activity, allowing the linear movement of the A to P motion of the sacrum, in diaphragmatic breathing, while allowing the fishtailing activity of the sacrum to be accomplished with the cardiovascular beat.

The same is true for the ilia in responding to bilateral external and internal rotation, reciprocating with the external and internal rotation of the temporal bones, on inhalation and exhalation, while the cranio fascial dynamic allows the reciprocation of the left external temporal rotation with the right ilium in external rotation, while the other temporal and ilia move through internal rotation within the same phase. This activity is a symphonic motion when all the dynamics are in homeostasis.

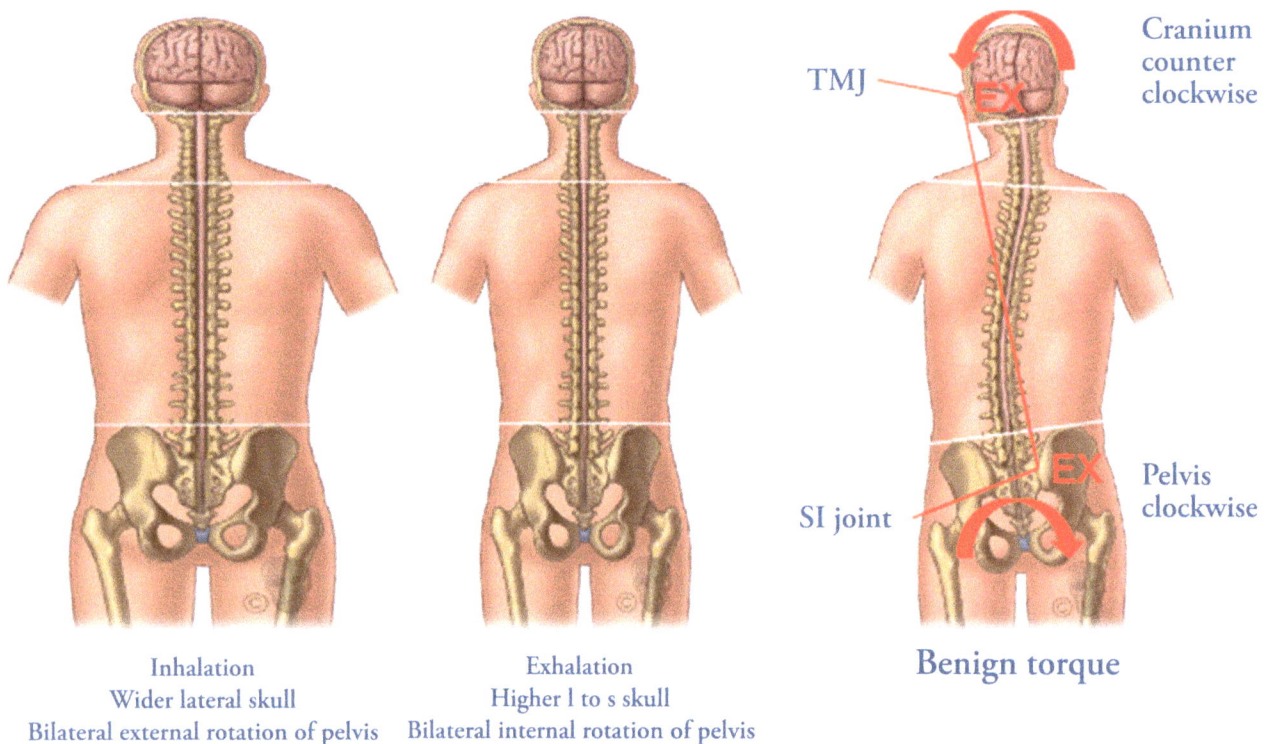

Inhalation
Wider lateral skull
Bilateral external rotation of pelvis

Exhalation
Higher l to s skull
Bilateral internal rotation of pelvis

TMJ

SI joint

Cranium counter clockwise

Pelvis clockwise

Benign torque

Figure 5.2 Reciprocal Dynamic Forces – CFD: Diaphragmatic phases superimposed on cardiovascular phases

TRAUMATIC CRANIO FASCIAL DISTORTION

In the following, selected graphics showing the textbook normal, followed by the benign and the traumatic crano fascial distortion, it must be remembered that the benign counterclockwise distortion is the normal cardiovascular rhythm. This benign counterclockwise motion will not show any clinical signs until it reaches the traumatic CFD stage, by which time the cranial torque has gone beyond the benign stage. For the most part, the benign stage will not reach adulthood, as there are likely to be traumatic incidents in a person's life – as one experiences in a clinical setting – that unfortunately occur within the normal tenets of life. If one considers the invasive encounters one meets in one's life, far removed from any birth intervention, it is not difficult to assume that over a life's span one could escape the traumas of life – physical, emotional, chemical and spiritual – without subjecting our brain core to insult in some way.

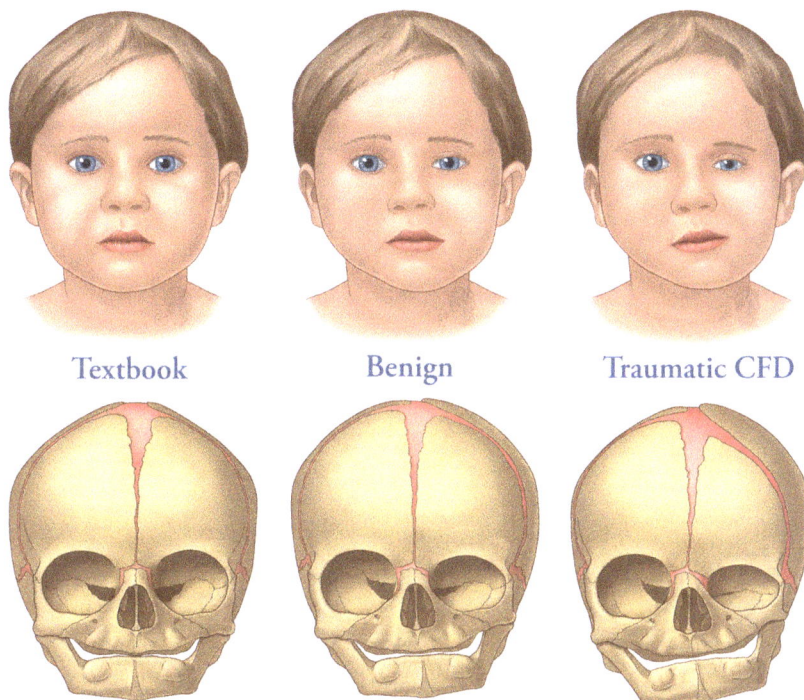

| Textbook | Benign | Traumatic CFD |

Figure 5.3 Cardiovascular Rhythmatic Respiration – Infant Cranium: Shows frontal bone separated by the metopic suture

The three phases of the infant face, from textbook, to benign and then traumatic CFD, indicate how the benign is the major phase of cardiovascular function. The traumatic CFD will usually occur in the prepubescent years of life, while the cranium is still developing, and these superimposed traumas will lead to the diaschisis and necrotic indicators that will be in place as the child grows. For that reason, any necrotic indicators, or mixed indicators as illustrated, will be markers of early traumas to the body. That is the evidence in adulthood of the necrotic, particularly, that the cranium will show the dramatic changes from a diaschisis to a necrotic structural change. It also highlights the evidence of a short leg finding in the left ilium in adulthood, as to the early incidence of a non-smooth result or a total necrotic confirmation of very early trauma.

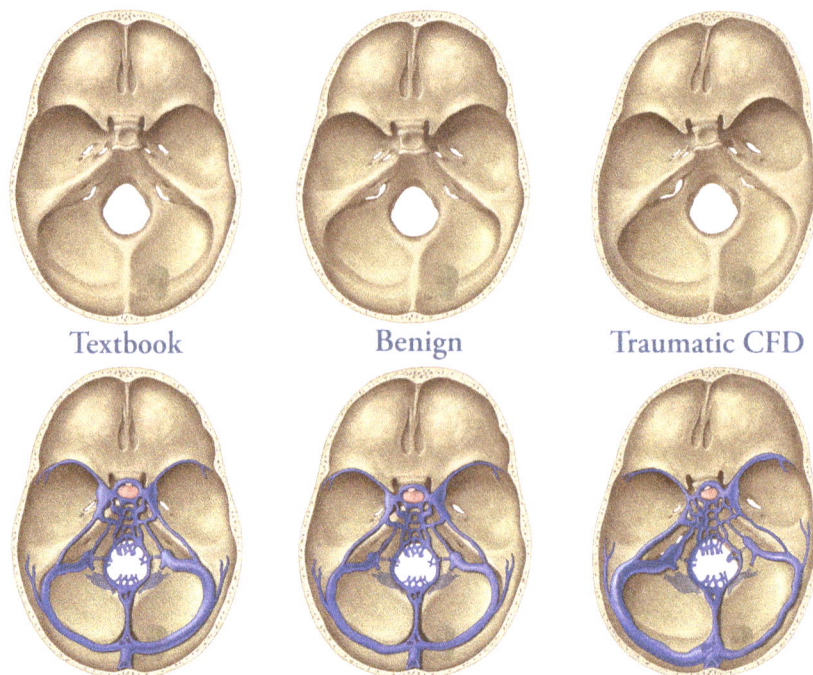

Figure 5.4 Cardiovascular Rhythmatic Respiration – Cranium and Drainage

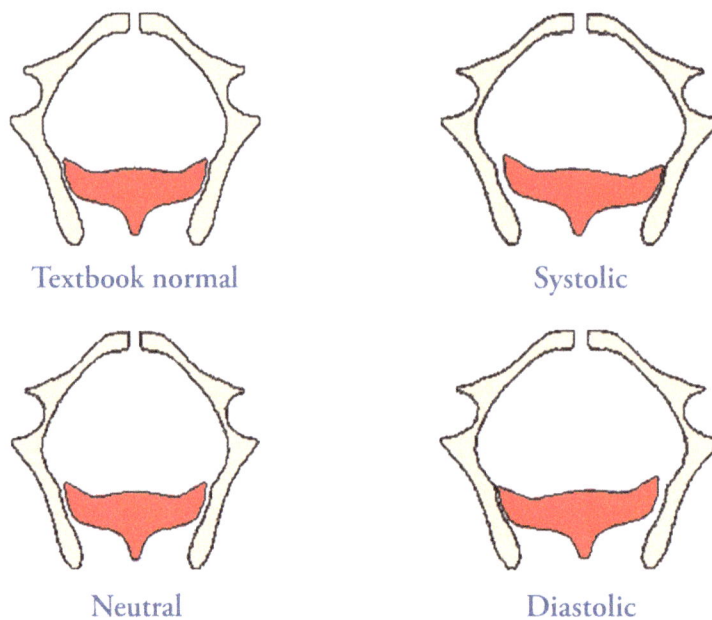

Figure 5.5 Cardiovascular Rhythmatic Respiration – Sacrum

The superior view of the cranium shows the potential drainage facility provided by the benign dynamics and the non-clinical findings as the drainage is influenced by the systolic and diastolic phases . Once the traumatic CFD influences occur, the right internal rotation of the fascia narrows the carotid canal and the jugular foramen, restricting venous drainage through the right internal jugular vein. This then obviously diminishes the propensity of the counterclockwise force on the brain, retards drainage and elevates the chances for aneurysms and stroke potential many years down the line. The left external temporal fascia, while stretched and opening the jugular foramen and the carotid canal, the vessels are smaller than their counterparts on the right, so their potential is inhibited, again leading to drainage failure and resultant fluid retention. The posterior view of the drainage confirms the earlier comments, insomuch as the confluence of the sinuses anatomically drain the superior sagittal sinus contents into the right transverse and sigmoid sinuses, and again, the right internal jugular vein.

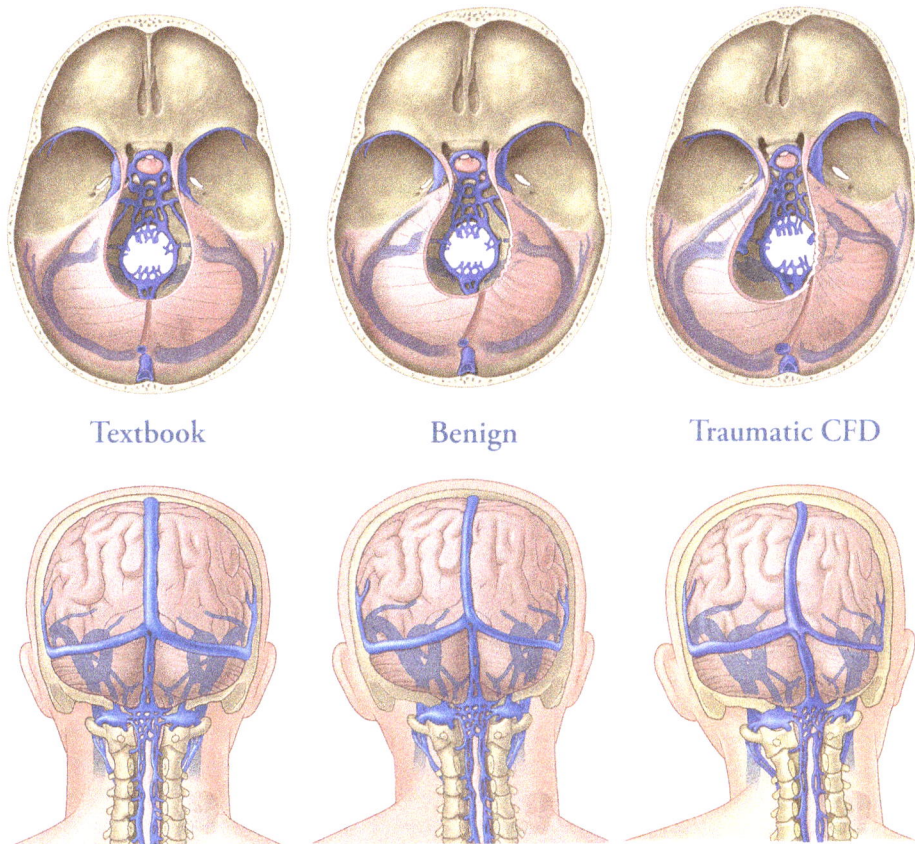

| Textbook | Benign | Traumatic CFD |

Figure 5.6 Cardiovascular Rhythmatic Respiration – Tentorial Incisura

The attachments of the tentorium cerebelli from the body of the sphenoid to the petrous portion of the temporal bone (encapsulating the superior petrosal sinus, draining the cavernous and intercavernous sinuses) and the transverse groove of the occiput (encapsulating the transverse sinus and the sigmoid sinus, draining the superior sagittal sinus), become constricted in the right drainage process by the tentorial cerebelli's distortion through the internal rotation of the right temporal and right occiput. It should also be mentioned here that the tentorial incisura in this traumatic CFD position has a direct influence on the vascular system. The anterior part of the tentorial incisura incorporates the circle of Willis, while the posterior part influences the great vein of Galen and the straight sinus, so when the tentorial incisura is distorted and twisted, it impacts on these arterial and venous vessels, further disrupting the vascular drainage.

The posterior view of the occiput provides the external occipital protuberance and the superior nuchal line, the attachments to the erector spinae muscles coming off the sacrum. These muscles are attached to the external occipital surface, while on the internal surface and opposing them lie the attachments of the transverse and sigmoid sinuses within the occipital groove. Applying Newton's Laws (each action has an equal and opposite reaction), the torque on the tentorium cerebelli directly affects the erector spinae muscles, and vice versa, changing the sacro-occipital pump mechanism externally and the tentorial incisura and the tentorium cerebelli internally – both CSF irrigation and brain drainage.

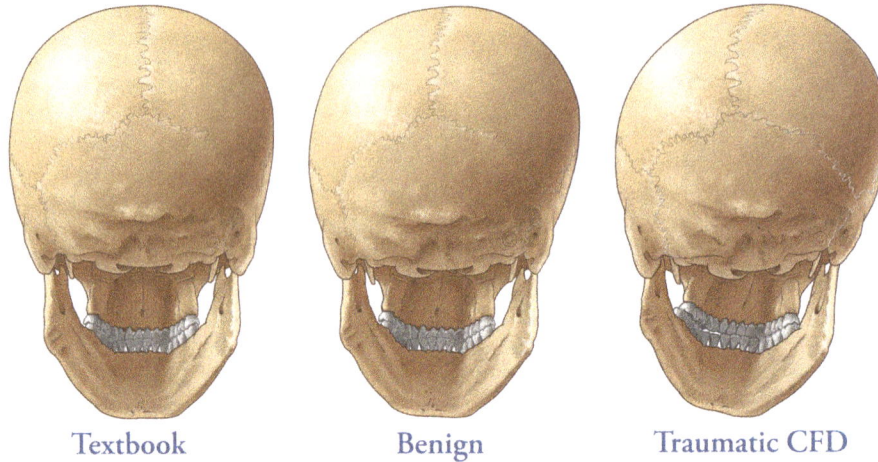

Figure 5.7 Cardiovascular Rhythmatic Respiration – Occiput

The same comments apply to the infant skull, with the added dimension of the immature cranial sphenobasilar junction, which at this early stage of development has not yet ossified, and can therefore influence the jugular foramen, foramen lacerum and the carotid canal (which all lie between the occiput, temporal and sphenoid bones), as well as the foramen magnum and its relationship with the atlanto-occipital membrane (the vertebral arteries penetrate the membrane) and the drainage of the vertebral venous plexus. The anterior pole (falx cerebri) at the ethmoid bone and the posterior pole (tentorium cerebelli) at the sphenoid bone undergo a torque effect, while at their common insertion at the internal occipital protuberance and the straight sinus, the venous drainage is under threat.

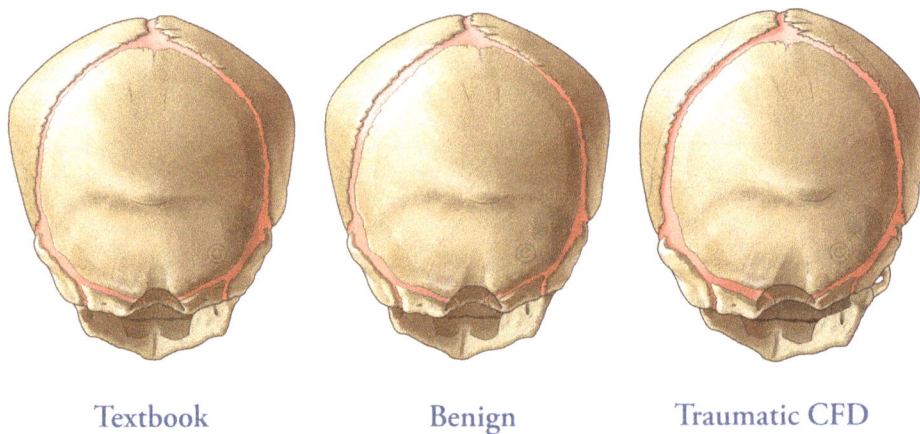

Figure 5.8 Cardiovascular Rhythmatic Respiration – Infant Occiput

These changes to the RTM at the ethmoid, sphenoid and the occiput also affect the spinal dural torque and rotate the pelvis, taking the right ilia into external rotation and the left ilia into internal rotation. When comparing the bilateral internal rotation of the lower extremities, the left foot will internally rotate fully, while the right foot hardly internally rotates at all. This is a pathognomonic sign of cranio fascial distortion within the cranium, and will always be found on traumatic CFD.

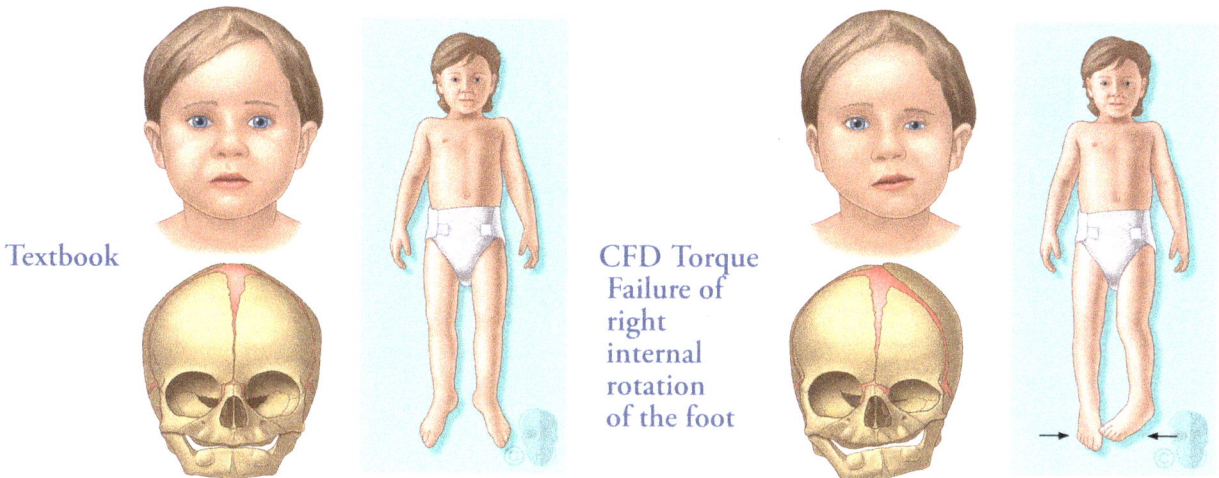

Textbook

CFD Torque
Failure of
right
internal
rotation
of the foot

Figure 5.9 Infant Cranio Fascial Distortion

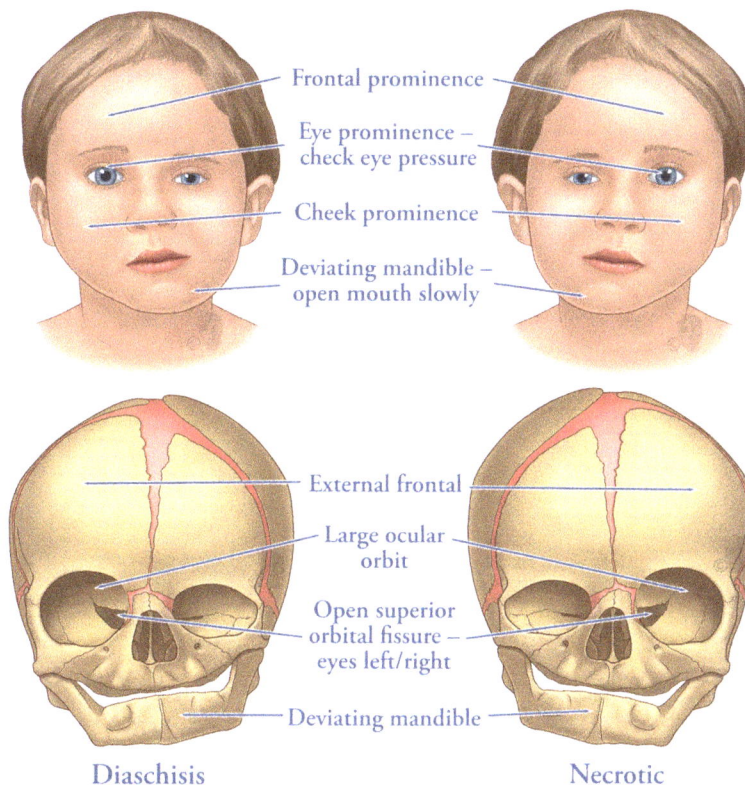

Frontal prominence

Eye prominence –
check eye pressure

Cheek prominence

Deviating mandible –
open mouth slowly

External frontal

Large ocular
orbit

Open superior
orbital fissure –
eyes left/right

Deviating mandible

Diaschisis

Necrotic

Figure 5.10 Facial Recognition for Types of Trauma

Facial recognition plays an important role in assessing the intricacies of diaschisis and necrotic trauma. The large right ocular orbit and the right eye prominence, coupled with the external right frontal bone, suggests a diaschisis trauma and is linked to the left deviating mandible. External pressure on both eyes to compare their relative resistance will confirm the status of the more prominent anterior eye. If the large ocular orbit is present with the large eye on the left, then suspect a necrotic trauma.

Benign – no clinical findings

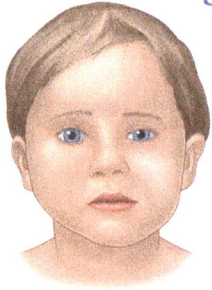

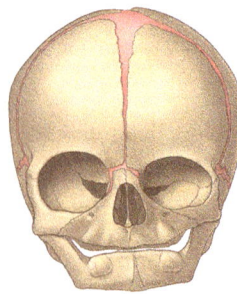

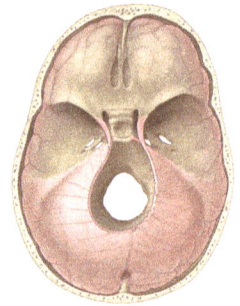

Traumatic CFD – clinically active

Eye
prominence –
eyes left and
eyes right
significant

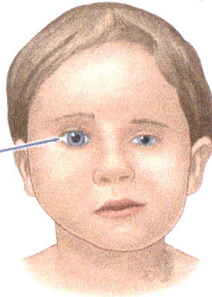

Larger ocular
orbit –
facial
observation

Deviation of
mandible –
open mouth
slowly

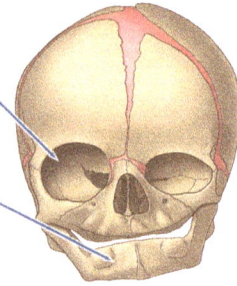

Tentorial
incisura –
jugular
foramen
positive

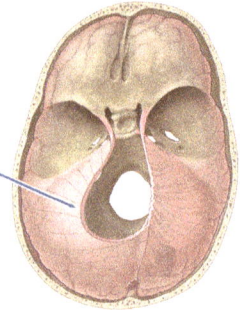

Figure 5.11 Benign vs Traumatic CFD

The turgid left eye and the mandibular deviation to the right may confirm these initial findings. Further testing of the internal rotation of the feet will be confirmation of the necrotic trauma. Both these instances will, if all the findings agree, be classified as 'smooth patterns' in both diaschisis and necrotic. However, when all the classic indicators do not match up, and there are varied diaschisis and necrotic markers, always follow the diaschisis treatment protocols in the first instance, as the counterclockwise motion of the brain is still the original dynamic.

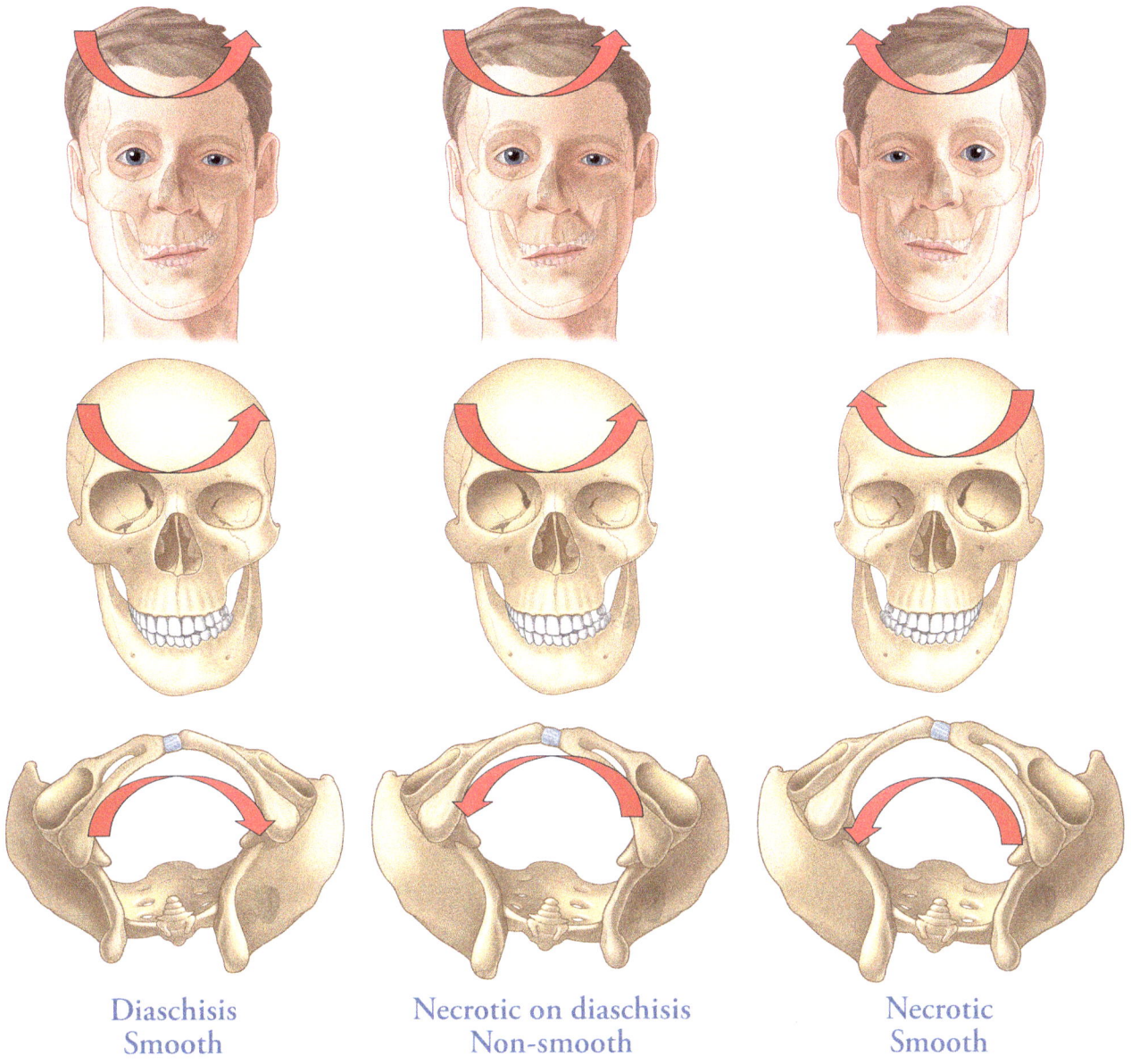

**Diaschisis
Smooth**

**Necrotic on diaschisis
Non-smooth**

**Necrotic
Smooth**

Figure 5.12 Smooth and Non-smooth Patterns with Diaschisis and Necrotic

CHAPTER 6

MUSCLES AND FASCIAL ATTACHMENTS

TO THE CRANIUM

The muscles and dural attachments to the cranium are a significant part of cranial function. There are muscles externally that pair with internal membranes and the magnitude of these forces are vital in creating a stable environment for vascular circulation and drainage. If the indicators for evidence of dural torque and muscle hyper/hypo activity are not removed then consequences will remain.

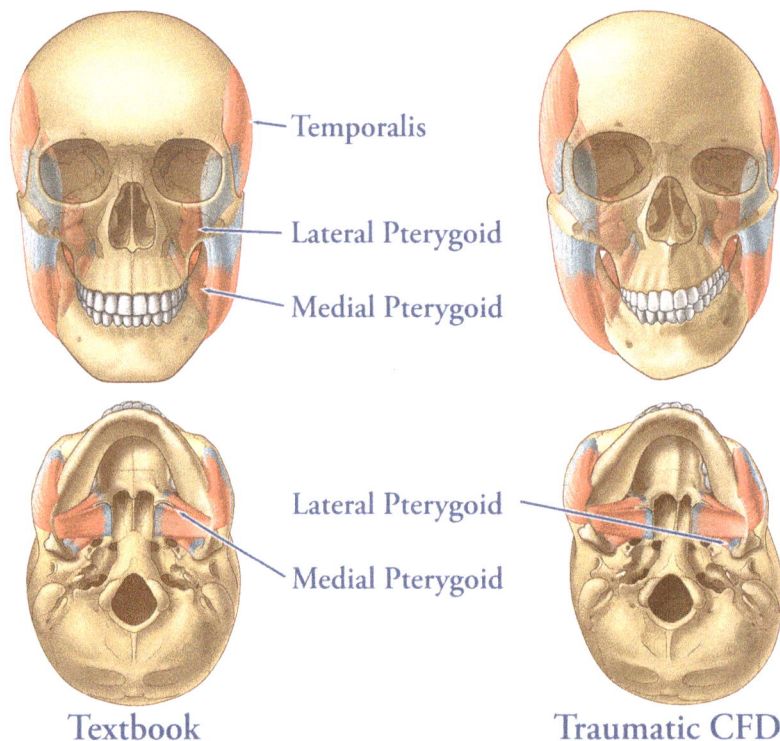

Temporalis

Lateral Pterygoid

Medial Pterygoid

Lateral Pterygoid

Medial Pterygoid

Textbook

Traumatic CFD

Figure 6.1 Muscles Controlling the Mandible

The internal and external pterygoid muscles control the mandibular movement within the mandibular fossa and have a direct influence on jaw to jaw relationship – the occlusion. This relationship is monitored by the trigeminal ganglion, and relies on the relationship with the condyle, the articular disc and the retrodiscal tissue. Temporomandibular joint dysfunction (TMJD) is a breakdown physically of these components and neurologically to the trigeminal ganglia, which in turn will recruit other muscles to obviate the neurological insult – the highest order on the agenda. This will sometimes take precedence over tooth position and inter-cusp relationships, to the detriment of the occlusion. These two muscles come off the pterygoid plates on the inferior surface of the sphenoid bone.

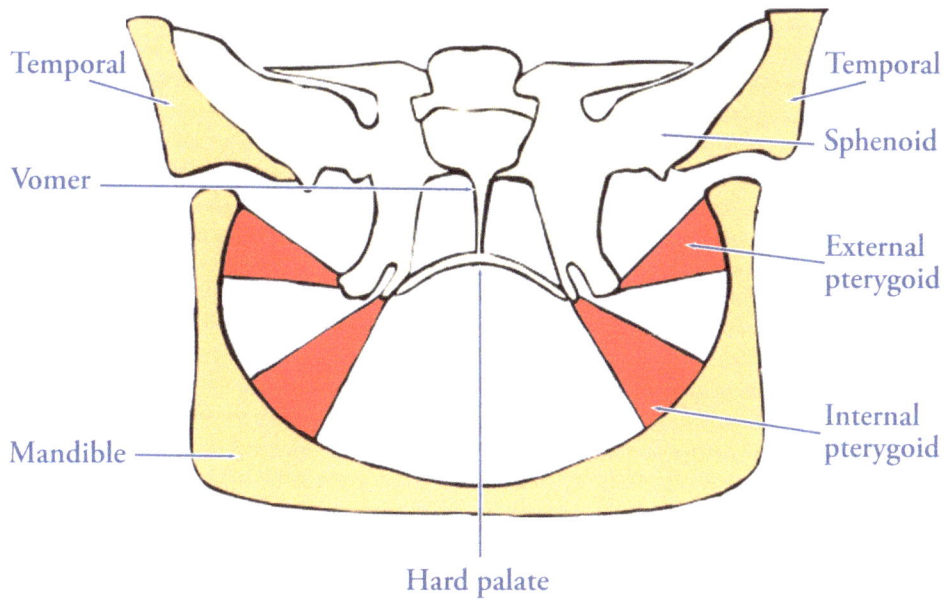

Figure 6.2 Spheno Temporomandibular Muscles

When traumatic CFD takes place and the sphenoid shifts, the muscles will be changed in their attempt to satisfy the occlusion. Tooth to tooth contact happens about 1,500 times a day, with swallowing, chewing and deglutition. This tooth to tooth contact is vital to the neurological balance of the trigeminal nerve complex and the ganglia, through the mesencephalic, pontine and spinal nuclei and the reciprocal sacroiliac joint. This neurological pathway ensures an electric circuit is maintained through the trigeminal ganglion and through the brain. Attempts to change orthodontically or orthopaedically the position of teeth, without addressing the sphenoid, lead to a relapse of the attempted work within a few months. The failure to address the sphenoid will compromise the spinal nucleus, which lies in the upper cervical spine at the levels of C1, C2 and C3 and will always result in a subluxation of the atlas, which in turn distorts the atlanto-occipital membrane and the passage of the vertebral arteries.

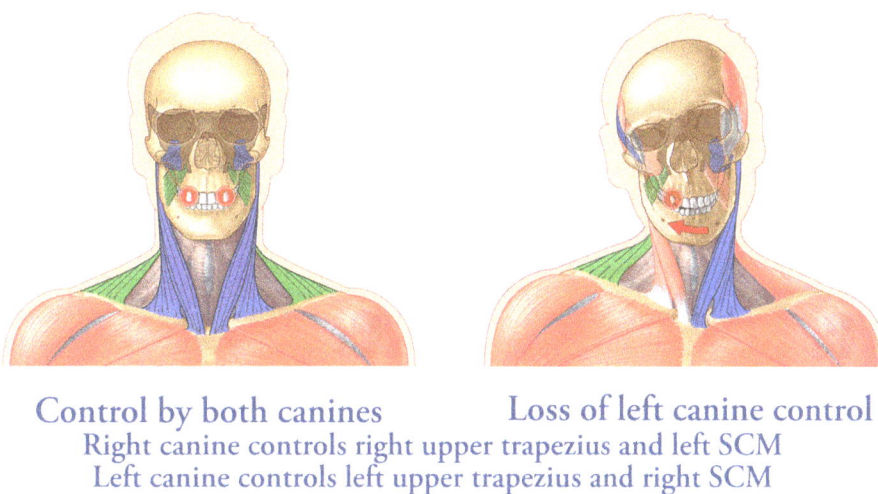

Control by both canines   **Loss of left canine control**
Right canine controls right upper trapezius and left SCM
Left canine controls left upper trapezius and right SCM

Figure 6.3 Upper Trapezius and Sternocleidomastoid Control by Canines

The medial and lateral incisors are embryologically part of the pre-maxilla, which later becomes part of the maxilla. This fusion or ossification takes place about the ninth week in utero. The incisors are thought to be centrally significant in the central core of the vertical dural membranes – the falx cerebri and the falx cerebelli. Contact between the upper and lower incisors is important within the trigeminal ganglion. Losing a central or lateral incisor is thought to change vertical dynamics. The contact is enamel on enamel, and does not influence the position of the mandible, as in incisal interference, whereby on occlusion the maxilla forces the mandible into a retrusive position, into the posterior part of the mandibular fossa.

The canines are formed in each of the alveoli that border the pre-maxillary suture. On contact with one another these teeth provide the circuitry for the ipsilateral upper trapezius and the contralateral SCM muscles. Collectively the canines control lateral motion of the head (trapezius) and rotation (SCM). Failure of one canine not contacting the opposite canine will result in the loss of function to that ipsilateral upper trapezius and the contralateral SCM. That in turn will change the dynamic of the ipsilateral occipital bone and the contralateral SCM – both the lateral and posterior anchors of the tentorium cerebelli. These are subtle changes in the dynamics, but when coupled with traumatic CFD there are consequences.

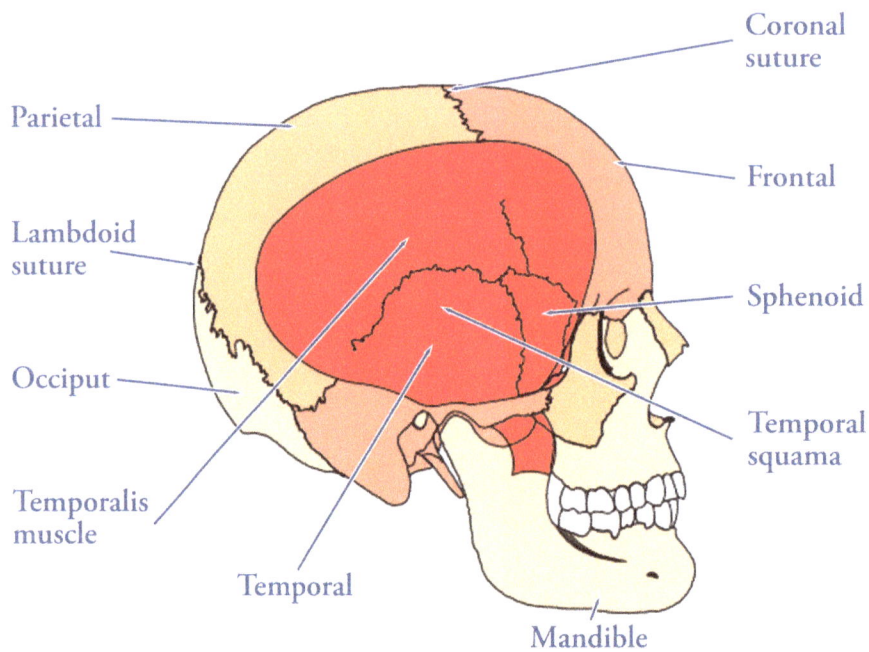

Figure 6.4 Temporalis Muscle

The temporalis is a strong encompassing muscle which covers all the bones of the lateral cranium, either directly or through the periosteal dura, covering the outer surface of the skull. In effect, it can lock the cranium externally when the teeth come together in a full occlusion. It attaches to the coronoid process of the mandible and brings the jaws together. Malocclusions and loss of dentition will reduce the efficacy of the temporalis muscle.

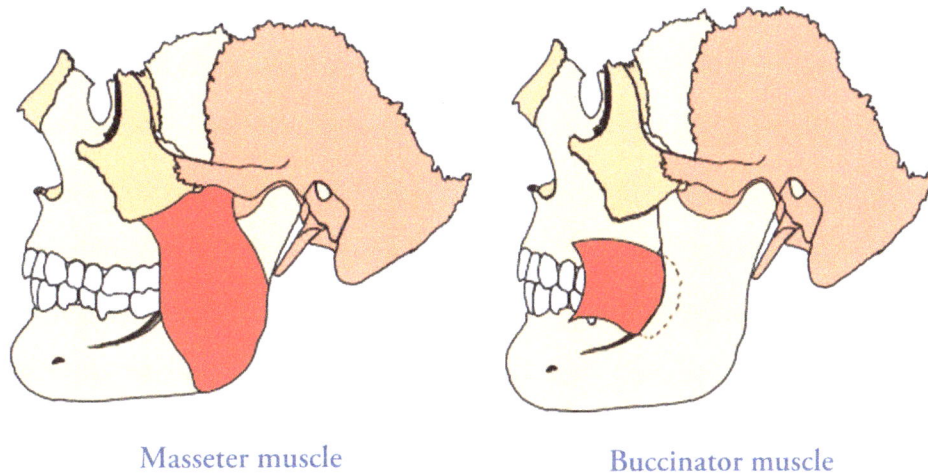

Masseter muscle   Buccinator muscle

Figure 6.5 Muscles of Mastication

The muscles of mastication are the masseter, the temporalis, the internal pterygoid and external pterygoid muscles. The buccinator muscle is classified as an accessory muscle of mastication, due to its role in compressing the cheeks inwards against the molars to aid chewing and swallowing. It is a quadrilateral muscle found in the lateral wall of the oral cavity. The masseter muscle has its origin in the zygomatic arch and maxillary process of the frontal bone bone, and inserts into the angle of the mandible and the inferior half of the lateral surface of the ramus of the mandible. It elevates the jaw.

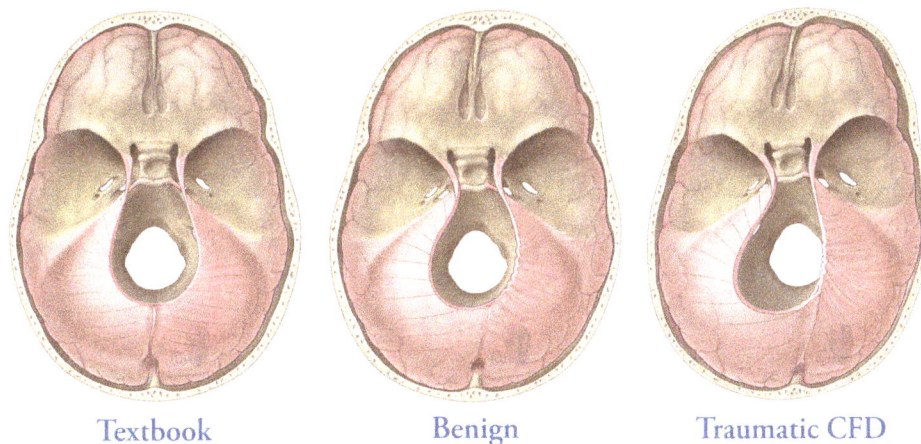

Textbook   Benign   Traumatic CFD

Figure 6.6 Tentorium Cerebelli Attachments to the Occiput and Temporal

The tentorium cerebelli is the horizontal membrane separating the brain from the cerebellum. It has its posterior border along the transverse groove of the occiput, where it encapsulates the transverse and sigmoid sinuses – draining the superior sagittal sinus into the right transverse and sigmoid sinuses and the inferior sagittal sinus through the left transverse and sigmoid sinuses, both draining into their respective internal jugular veins. This represents the anterior and inferior superior drainage of the brain. The lateral border is along the petrous portion/ridge of the temporal bone where it encapsulates the superior petrosal sinus, draining the cavernous and intercavernous sinuses into the sigmoid sinuses and then into the internal jugular veins. Anteriorly, the tentorium cerebelli attaches to the clinoid processes of the body of the sphenoid. The anterior clinoid processes anchor the extension of the falx cerebri, which forms the upper part of the tentorium cerebelli, while the posterior clinoid processes anchor the extension of the falx cerebelli, which forms the lower surface of the tentorium cerebelli.

Between the anterior and posterior clinoid processes lies the sella turcica, which provides the anchor points for the diaphragma sellae – the other small horizontal dural membrane which facilitates the hypophyseal stalk of the pituitary. The posterior anchor point for the falx cerebelli, the falx cerebri and the tentorium cerebelli is the common border of the straight sinus, which drains the inferior sagittal sinus. The tentorial incisura is a dual sleeve separation of the tentorium cerebelli, which starts at the anterior part of the straight sinus and goes around the central core brain organs, enveloping them as a safe passage to the rest of the brain. With traumatic CFD the tentorial incisura inflicts disruption to all the central core brain membranes and their neurological pathways, and in the author's opinion is the most devastating component of the RTM system.

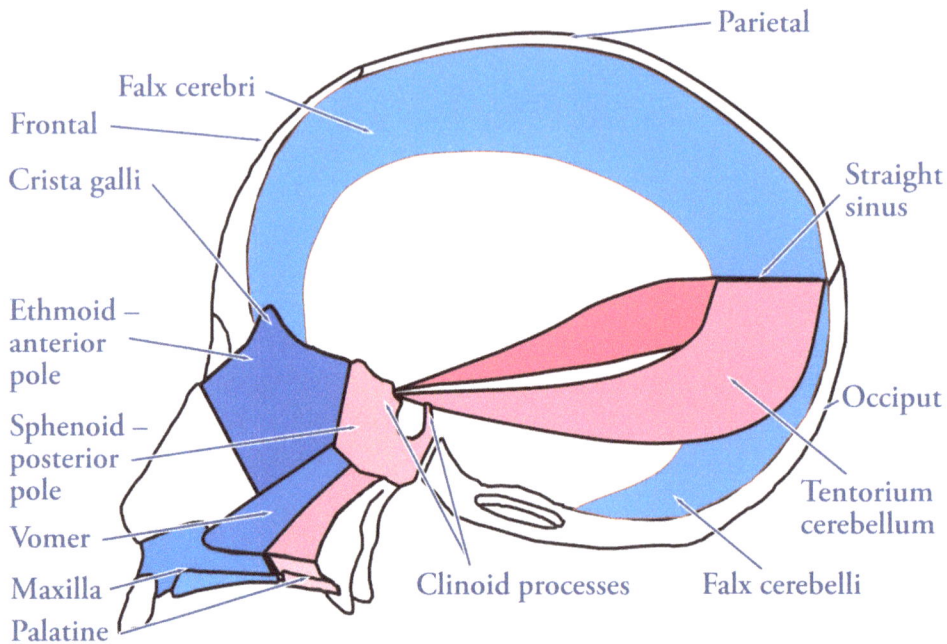

Figure 6.7 Reciprocal Tension Membrane Attachments to Bones: Hinge suture between ethmoid and sphenoid

This graphic is a compilation of the RTM and their anchor points within the cranium. The attachments have all been discussed within this chapter, but for an overall understanding of how the membranes separate, balance and protect the various lobes of the brain, and in particular the function of the vomer within the diaphragmatic and cardiovascular respiration phases see Chapter 2. This balance maintains the ability for the brain to drain, maintains the neurological pathways and conduits, and ensures neurological homeostasis within the body.

CRANIAL RHYTHMIC IMPULSE (CRI)

As far back as the originator of chiropractic, magnetic healer Dr D. D. Palmer, the question of a third cranial impulse, the CRI, has been discussed and theorised over by many prominent craniopaths, chiropractors and others who have brought their hypotheses to the table. All have valid arguments about its origins. I have felt for many years that the two obvious and dynamic pulses found in the body are the diaphragmatic respiratory impulse (a linear motion, at 18 to 20 pulses a minute) and the cardiovascular rhythmic impulse (a rhythmic torqued impulse, at 68 to 72 pulses a minute), and when these impulses are superimposed, they will coincide at points, creating a the third impulse called the CRI. The body produces the two dynamic impulses through normal function of heart and lungs, to my mind, the illusive third impulse must be as dynamic as the other two in maintaining homeostasis.

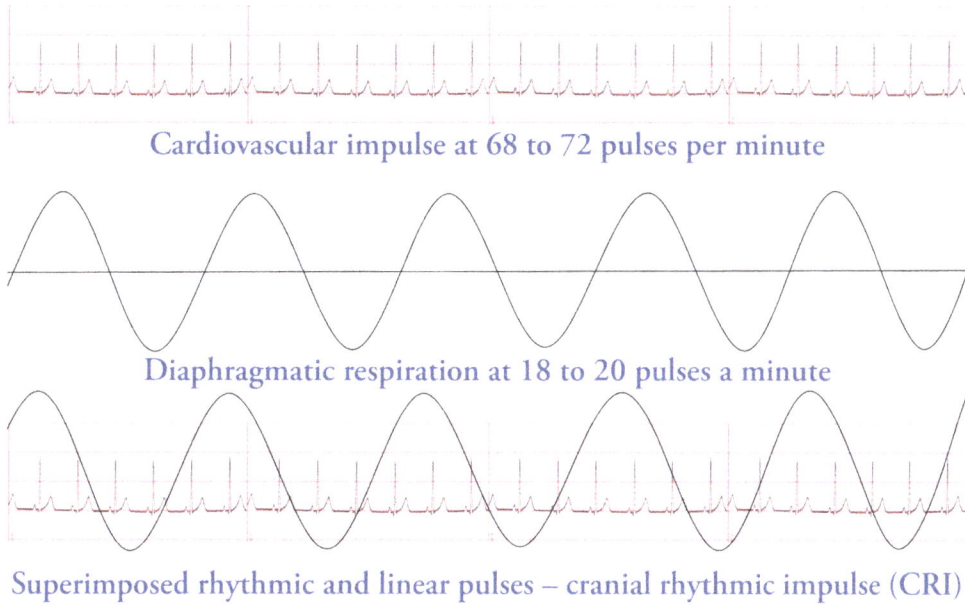

Cardiovascular impulse at 68 to 72 pulses per minute

Diaphragmatic respiration at 18 to 20 pulses a minute

Superimposed rhythmic and linear pulses – cranial rhythmic impulse (CRI)

Figure 6.8 Pulses Evident Within Cranial Function

THE DISLOCATED BRAIN

PART III

CRANIO PELVIC DYNAMICS

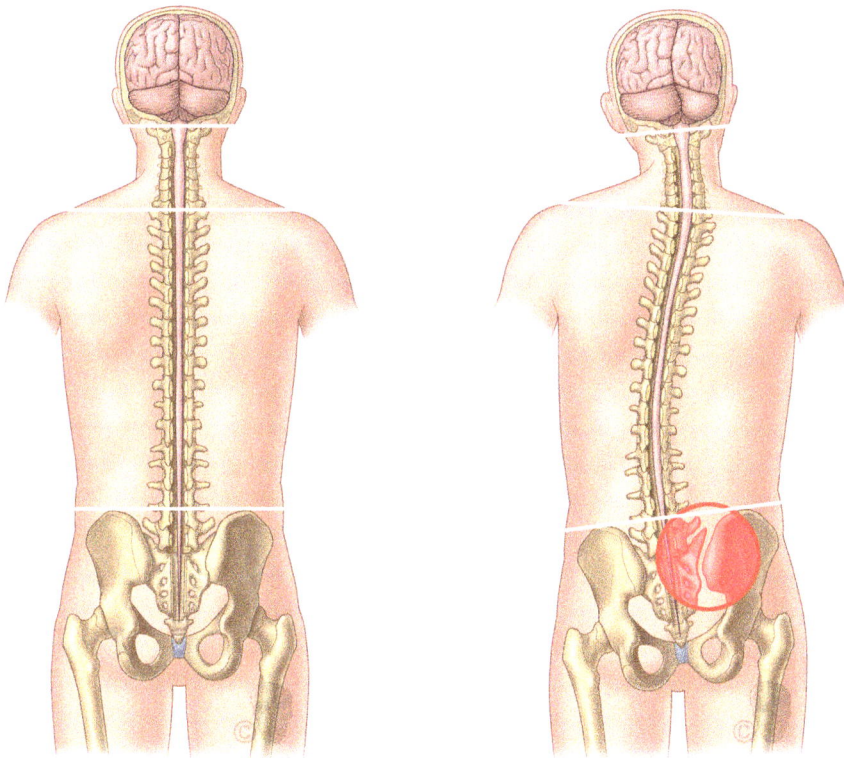

CONTENTS PART III

ILLUSTRATIONS PART III

CHAPTER 1

CRANIO PELVIC DYNAMICS

Cranio fascial dynamics (CFD) as a primary counterclockwise torque produces a left external temporal bone taking with it the external fascia. In addition it will widen the jugular foramen, the carotid canal and the external auditory meatus, and narrow the superior orbital fissure – resulting in poor ocular convergence of the left eye with a compromised oculomotor nerve and a poor, weak and fatigued medial rectus muscle.

The left external temporal bone also reciprocates with the external right ilia, leading to an external right foot that fails to meet in the midline, with the left internally rotated foot, a classic CFD indicator. As a rule the right leg will be relatively shorter than the left, due to the external acetabulum on the right externally rotating the right leg.

Once trauma occurs, a diaschisis force will be superimposed on the cranium which exacerbates the counterclockwise torque, causing the nerve pathways and conduits to stretch and worsening neural transmission.

If, on the other hand, a necrotic force is introduced as a trauma, the resulting superimposed clockwise torque, acts against the original counterclockwise torque, potentially causing nerve pathways and nerve conduits to tear. Depending on the severity of the force, such necrotic trauma may cause damage of varying severity whose long-term effects, if not corrected, can be the precursors to neurological syndromes in years to come. Occasional and possibly accidental head and neck trauma experienced by any individual may be a combination of diaschisis and necrotic forces, which makes the clinical appraisal vital in de-torquing the cranium and, more specifically, the cranial membranes.

A patient presenting the long leg on the right side with the left protrusive eye, the right eye showing poor convergence with the left internal foot restricted, are indicators that warrant careful clinical scrutiny and are dealt with in this book.

THE LOVETT BROTHER RELATIONSHIP OR THE R PLUS C FACTOR

The Lovett Brother Relationship, or the resistance plus contraction (R plus C) factor as described by some authors, is a bio-mechanical reciprocity between the skeletal and cranial structures, in other words, atlas and fifth lumbar work together, axis and fourth lumbar, third cervical and third lumbar. When the fifth lumbar moves out of position or subluxates, there will be a compensation at the level of the atlas. If the fourth lumbar moves there will be compensation at the level of the axis and so on. This reciprocity also exists within the pelvis, where the ilium has paired reciprocity with the temporal bone, and the sacrum with the occiput, hence the name sacro occipital technique. This relationship was first explained by Dr. Major B. DeJarnette in 1946, when he referred to it as the R plus C factor:

> R plus C equals distortion, disease and death. Neutralisation of R plus C equals
>   structural alignment – Health.

The resistance factor (R) is the body's compensation against the contraction factor (C) which produces the distortion. Every muscle movement is a combination of two factors. Contraction, which is the direction of movement, and resistance acting in opposition, that prevents excessive movement, and enables the body to maintain balance in motion. When contraction dominates, distortions may result. When resistance dominates, pain and loss of movement are a consequence. The C factor is contracted and shortened and is the area of muscle spasm. The R factor is generally painful and swollen.

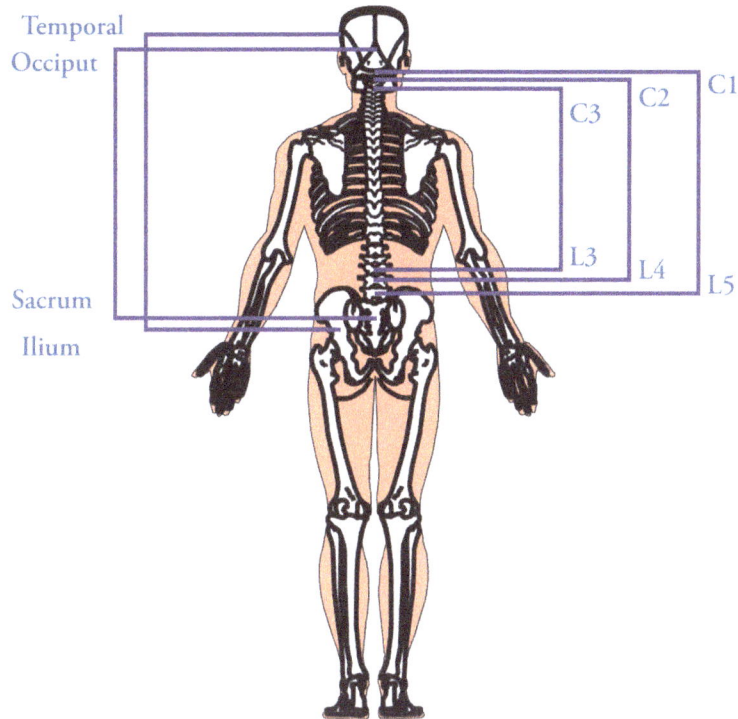

Figure 1.1 Lovett Brother Relationship or the R Plus C Factor: Paired reciprocity of skeletal structures

HAEMODYNAMIC INFLUENCE OF THE CRANIUM

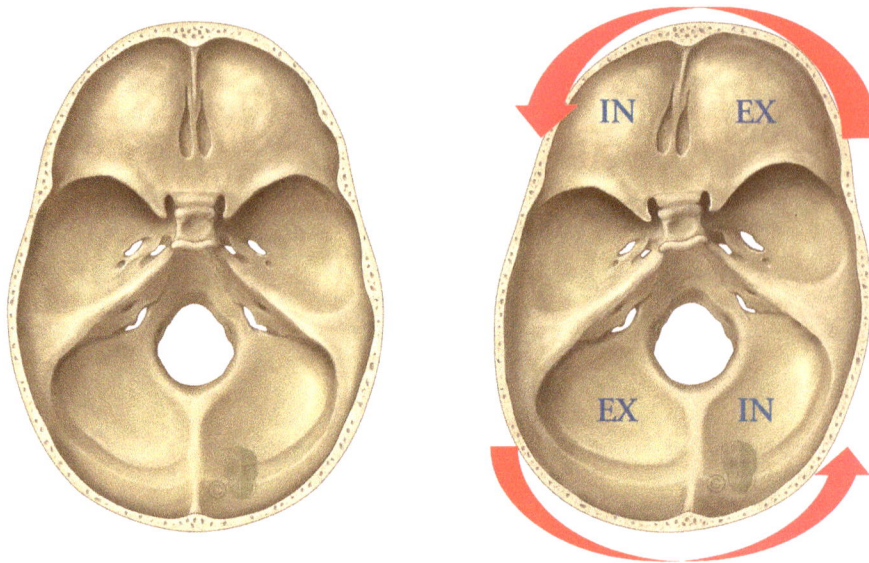

Figure 1.2 Haemodynamic Influence on the Cranium: Textbook symmetry (left), haemodynamic force, counterclockwise torque (right)

Figure 1.2 demonstrates a haemodynamic force producing a greater volume propensity from right to left, creating a counterclockwise torque in the cranium. The subsequently widened blood vessels draining the brain from the right allow a greater volume of fluid to flow right to left. This has occurred in utero.

BALANCED SPINE AND PELVIS

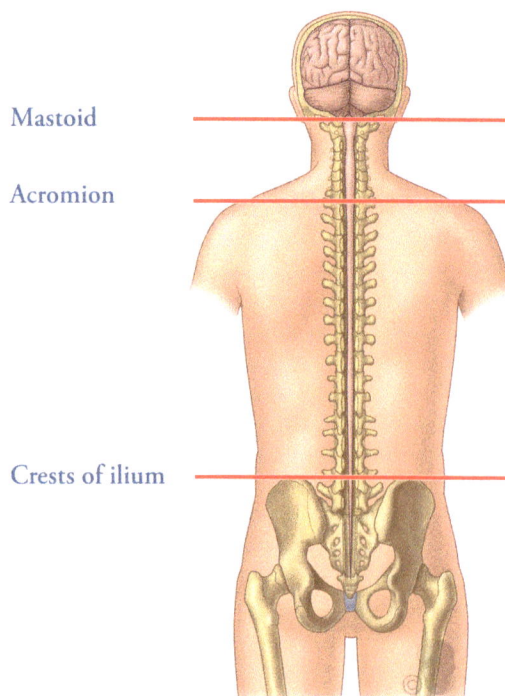

Figure 1.3 Balanced Spine and Pelvis

Vertical and horizontal vectors

    a. In the plumb line or distortion analyser
    b. The vertical lines go through the middle of the spine and bisect the pelvis and the cranium
    c. The horizontal lines go through the mastoids, the acromion processes and the crests of the ilia.

Smooth and non-smooth coupling

    a. Smooth coupling refers to the three horizontal lines going in opposite directions
    b. Non-smooth coupling refers to two or three of the adjacent horizontal lines going in the same direction.

SYMMETRIC BODY MUSCULATURE

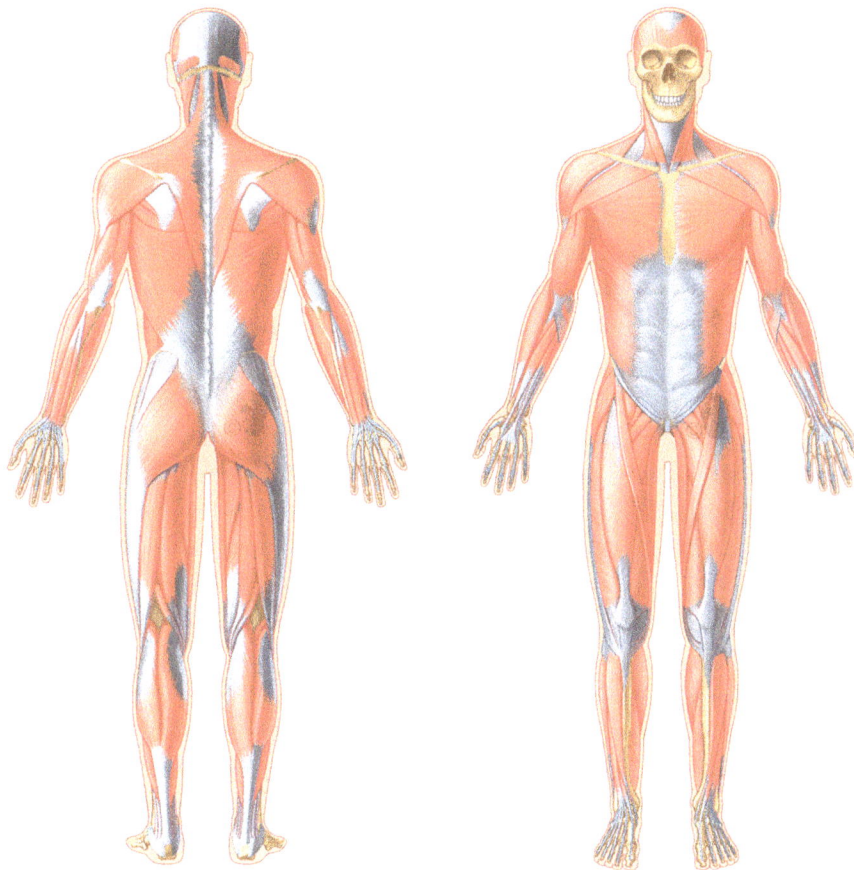

Figure 1.4 Symmetric Body Musculature

The anterior and posterior muscles of the body maintain the system in equilibrium. The anterior muscle groups need to balance the posterior groups in totality to fulfil Newton's Third Law of Motion, which states, 'that for every action there is an equal and opposite reaction'. Once out of the midline, the body will compensate for every motion away from the central midline by using the intricate dynamics of each muscle group, thus homeostasis is maintained.

As the discussion on pelvic dynamics unfolds it becomes apparent that homeostatic influence is always present, while the body will compensate and adapt to the changes, always reinforcing the muscular dynamic to play its part. The fascia, particularly the cranial fascia, has a dynamic on its own, generated as mesenchyme on day 18 of embryological development. It pre-exists all other organs and tissues (except the brain and spinal cord), and its activity is present in utero, defining the foetal form. The muscular and skeletal components are therefore more subservient in their activity, which is why the CFD is so important and rules overall.

BILATERAL SACROILIAC ROTATION

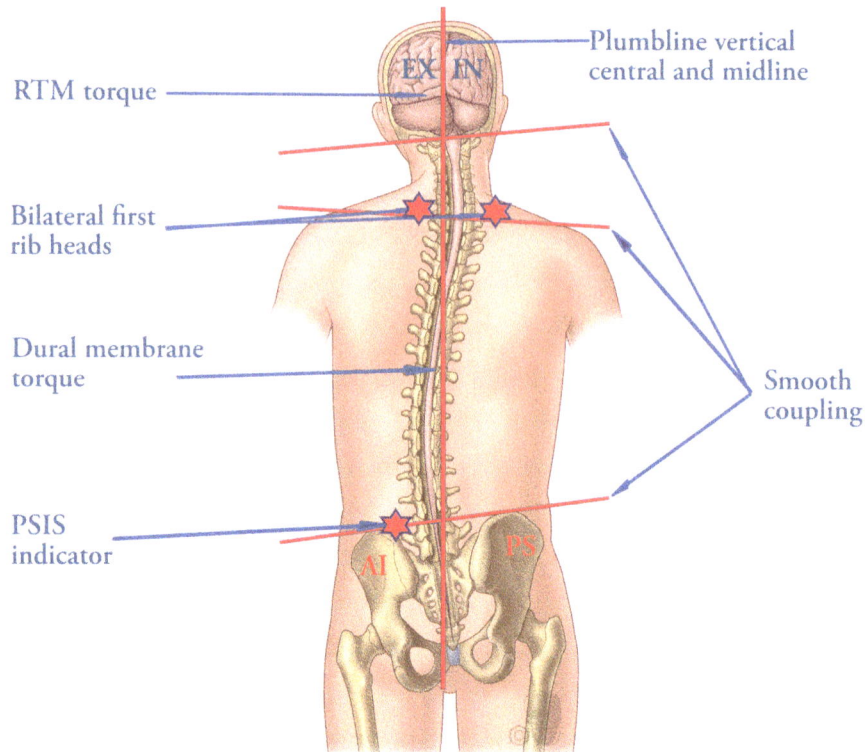

Figure 1.5 Bilateral Sacroiliac Rotation: Dural torque anterior to posterior motion

The first change to the skeletal system occurs with the influence of CFD. The haemodynamic effect of brain drainage, also seen in utero, changes the dynamic forces within the cranium to facilitate the haemodynamic counterclockwise motion of the brain, and supersedes all the other tissues and systems.

The reciprocal tension membranes (RTM) control and balance the brain, separating the left and right hemispheres of the brain, the left and right lobes of the cerebellum, and the brain from the cerebellum:

- Falx cerebri – upper vertical dynamic
- Falx cerebelli – lower vertical dynamic
- Tentorium cerebellum – horizontal dynamic
- Diaphragma sellae – horizontal sella turcica dynamic.

They are made up of the dural meningeal fascia:

- Pia mater– adherent to the brain surface, the meningeal dura
- Arachnoid mater – a layer which provides for the subarachnoid space filled with cerebrospinal fluid
- Dura mater – adherent to the inner surface of the cranium, with head injury, blood collects in the subdural space.

The dural meningeal layer encapsulates the foetal cranial plates which are individual entities – islands of membranous bone – until the later stages of foetal development. At birth there are six fontanelles, which are the inter-membranous centres that allow the brain to grow before they become ossified as sutures at between six and eighteen months. Without the dural constraints controlling the growth, the brain would develop as a perfect sphere. This research explains the influence that dural membranes have on the growth of the cranium.

As the brain grows in a counterclockwise manner it influences the dural membranes so that the islands of membranous bone grow in accordance with the counterclockwise torque engineered by the brain. The outcome of this growth and development is that the cranium is also a counterclockwise orientated osseous structure, with periosteum on the outer surface and endosteum on the inner surface. These two layers originated as the same dural membrane and remain continuous through the sutures, with muscles and fascia attached on the outside and intracranial structures – falx cerebri, falx cerebelli and the tentorium cerebellum – attached on the inside (following Newton's Third Law). This is demonstrated by the fact that the external muscle stresses are complemented and distorted by the internal RTM, altering the brain structure and borders in accordance with Newton's Third Law of Motion.

The outward appearance of the cranium, with the right ocular orbit appearing larger and more anterior than the left ocular orbit which is smaller and posterior, demonstrates just how the cranio fascial dynamic and distortion came about.

The influence of CFD shows the counterclockwise torque of the cranium, with the right occiput and temporal bone becoming more internalised and the left occipital bone and temporal bone becoming more externalised.

The right frontal and maxilla are externalised, while the left frontal and maxilla are more internalised.

The central bone in the cranium is the sphenoid bone which acts as the fulcrum, with the right greater wing moving anterior and superior, while at the other end of the 'see-saw', the left greater wing moves posterior and inferior.

The complexity of the neo-cranial sphenoid, and the occiput and temporal bones is demonstrated by the number of components involved in this important central bone base of the cranium.

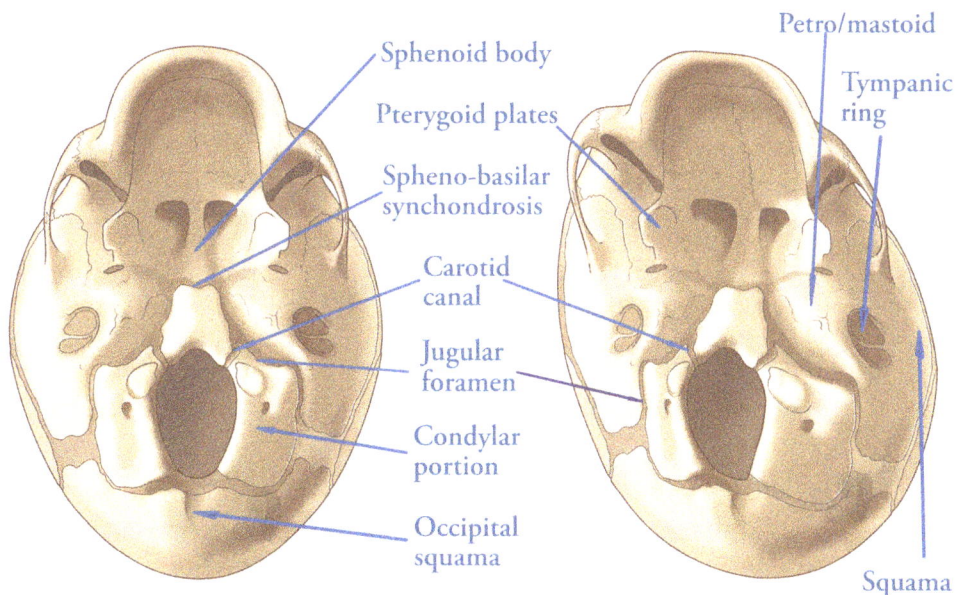

Figure 1.6 Neo-cranial Components: Occiput, temporal and sphenoid bones

The sphenoid has two greater wings generated in membrane, two lesser wings generated in cartilage, and the body – including the pterygoid plates – generated in cartilage. This allows the sphenoid to grow into 'itself' during the growth and development of the benign counterclockwise torque.

The occiput has a number of parts, also allowing it to accommodate the benign counterclockwise torque. It has the basilar portion, which articulates with the body of the sphenoid at the sphenobasilar synchondrosis, which only ossifies at the age of approximately 25. This gives the base of the skull time to construct a strong foundation once the growth and development has been achieved. There are also two condylar portions (generated in cartilage) and the occipital squama (generated in membrane).

The temporal is made up of three components: the squama (generated in membrane); the tympanic ring, which houses the vestibular mechanism (generated in cartilage); and the petrous/mastoid portion. The petrous portion – anchor point for the tentorium cerebellum – is generated in cartilage, as is the mastoid portion – anchor point of the sternocleidomastoid (SCM).

The jugular foramen is found between the occipital-temporal junction, and the carotid canal is found between the sphenoid, occipital and temporal junctions. These osseous membrane bone islands, which assist in the construction of the three cranial bones, perfectly illustrate the sophisticated engineering of the anatomy. Each island is encapsulated by dural membrane becoming the endosteal and periosteal coverings and, as such, providing enormous reinforcement – as in steel rods in concrete – to all the attached components, both inside and outside the cranium.

Figure 1.7 shows the counterclockwise appearance of the cranial floor and the final result of CFD and haemodynamic motion of the brain.

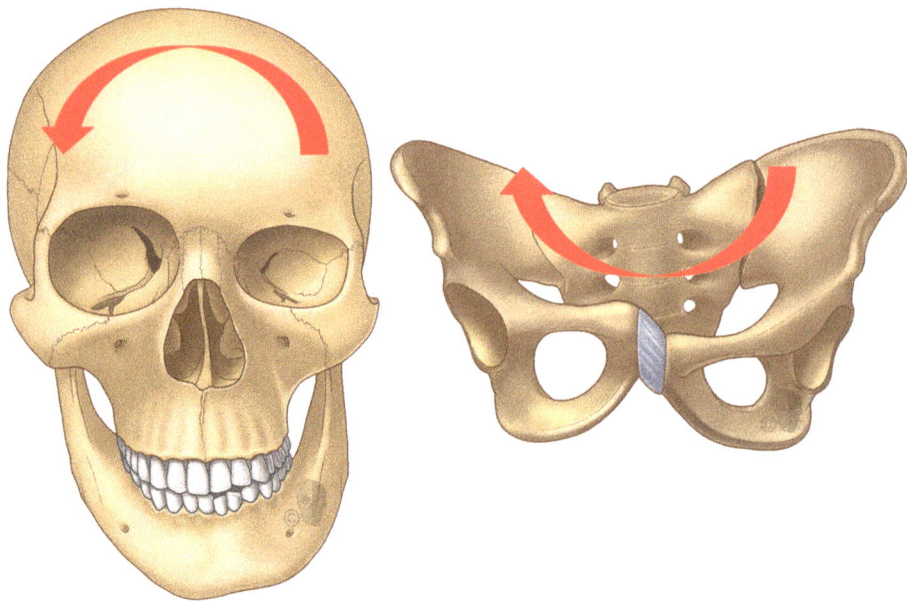

Figure 1.7 Reciprocal Dynamic Forces CFD: Cranium counterclockwise (left); pelvis clockwise (right)

The benign CFD effect on the cranium has a reciprocal effect on the pelvis. To maintain homeostasis, the counterclockwise torque in the cranium becomes the clockwise torque of the pelvis – otherwise we would all fall over!

The left external temporal bone reciprocates with the right external ilium, and the right internal temporal bone reciprocates with the left internal ilium. Both these ilia rotate around the sacrum, creating the clockwise pelvis. The external right ilium produces an elevated superior acetabulum, bringing the right leg into a higher position and externally rotating it – thus when comparing right and left internal rotation of the feet, the right foot remains more externally rotated than the left, which moves more easily into internal rotation. This is a pathognomonic test for traumatic CFD.

The effect of this bilateral sacroiliac rotation is the dural torque that emerges, nominally having an influence on the autonomic nervous system producing – because it is a central issue – central symptomatology.

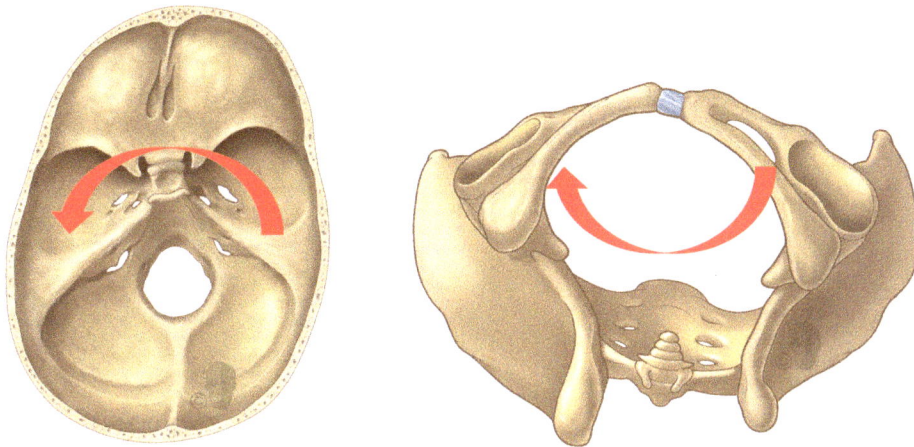

Figure 1.8 Reciprocal Dynamic Forces CFD: Cranium counterclockwise (left); pelvis clockwise (right)

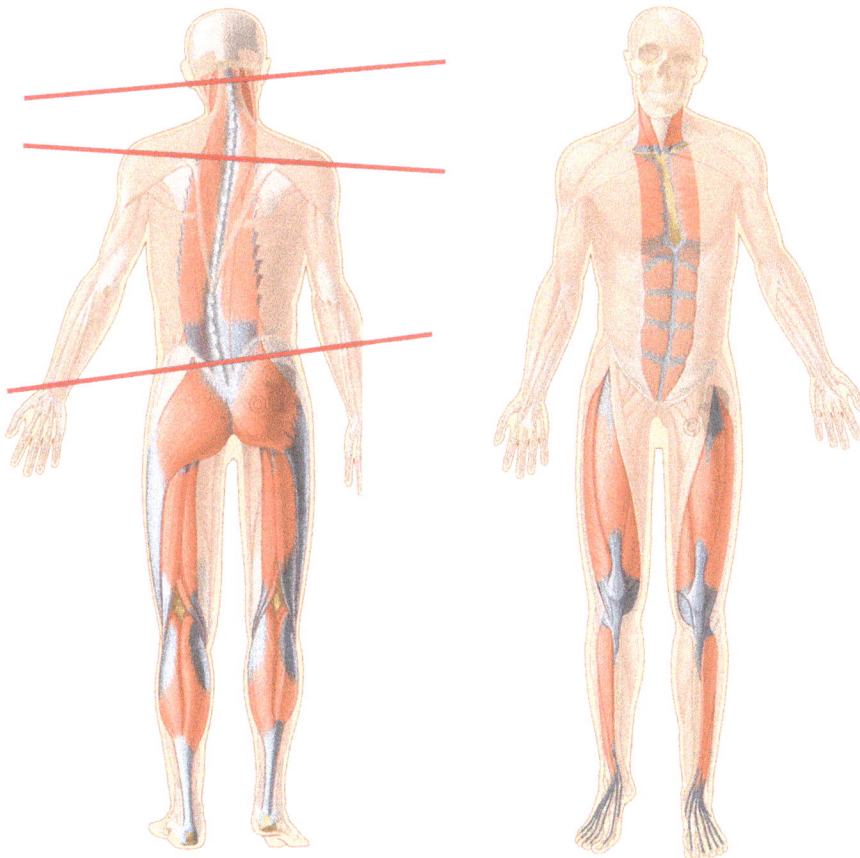

Figure 1.9 Muscle Groups in Bilateral Sacroiliac Rotation: Paravertebral muscles

The introduction to trauma becomes a time of change, from the subtle counterclockwise haemodynamic motion that was introduced in utero, creating a helical motion of venous blood leaving the brain from the venous sinus and ensuring complete drainage and removing as much waste as possible.

The muscle groups in this central lesion comprise all the paravertebral muscles reinforcing the sacrum and the occiput directly, with strong support in the central lower extremities, both anterior and posterior. This characteristic is a strong indicator for the Achille's tendon on the short leg side trying to maintain the body's balance, while heavily influenced by the gastrocnemius, hamstring and gluteal muscles in their clockwise motion. The central support also brings to bear the thoracic inlets, lymph drainage, the diaphragm and the pelvic floor, thus influencing the lungs with breathing, the mediastinal shift for the heart, the diaphragmatic breathing rhythm and capacity, the organs underlying the diaphragm, the liver, gall bladder, the cardiac sphincter of the stomach, the abdominal organs in the abdomen and all the complex intestinal and eliminating organs that rest on the pelvic floor, along with the all-important mesenteric fascia. Prolapses, ruptures and hernias may also occur in this complex knot of organs.

SACROILIAC LESION

This is a boot shaped articulation. The morphology of the sacroiliac joint means it is classified as a joint, as it has nerves and vessels that go through it from side to side. This lesion is not identified on an X-ray and the change in its status is so slight that it is not often considered in clinical assessment. This is probably one of the most overlooked lesions in a clinical appraisal, and why so many people never get relief.

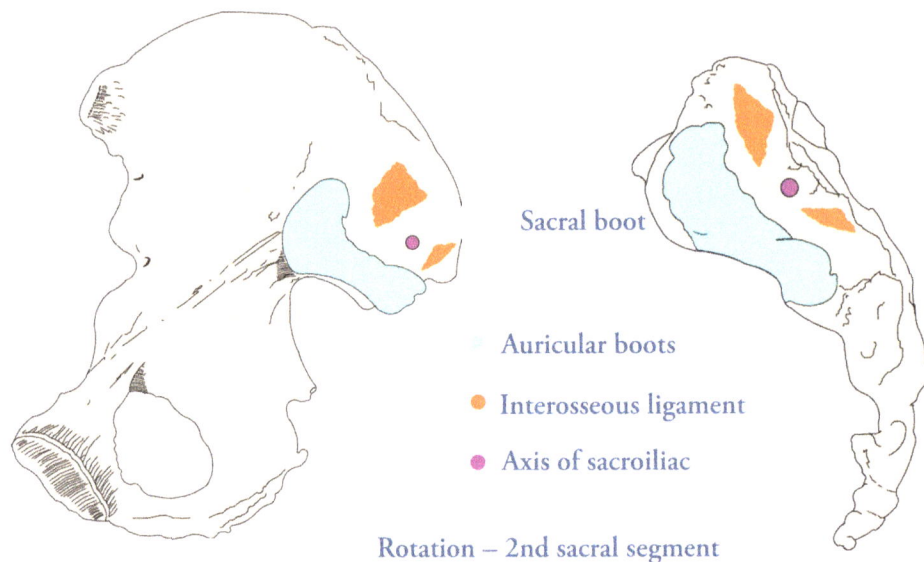

Sacral boot

Auricular boots

● Interosseous ligament

● Axis of sacroiliac

Rotation – 2nd sacral segment

Figure 1.10 Sacroiliac Lesion: Ligamentous failure

- Muscles: there are no muscles or tendons that connect directly through the joint
- Nerve beds: it consists of two nerve beds, one on the sacrum and one on the ilia. These beds have a close adherence when the joint is stable. When the joint is compromised it behaves like an electric plug not put in a socket properly – the light will flicker. When the plug is in place, the light remains bright
- The joint is supported by the superior and inferior interosseous ligaments. This becomes a ligamentous lesion, as the superior and inferior ligaments on the compromised side weaken and fatigue
- Rotation at the joint occurs at the second sacral tubercle, highlighted by the purple dot in Figure 1.11. This rotational pivot point allows the sacrum to flex and extend in reciprocation with the occiput. It will also have some rotational latitude, but there comes a point when the rotation breaks the seal and the joint becomes a lesion.

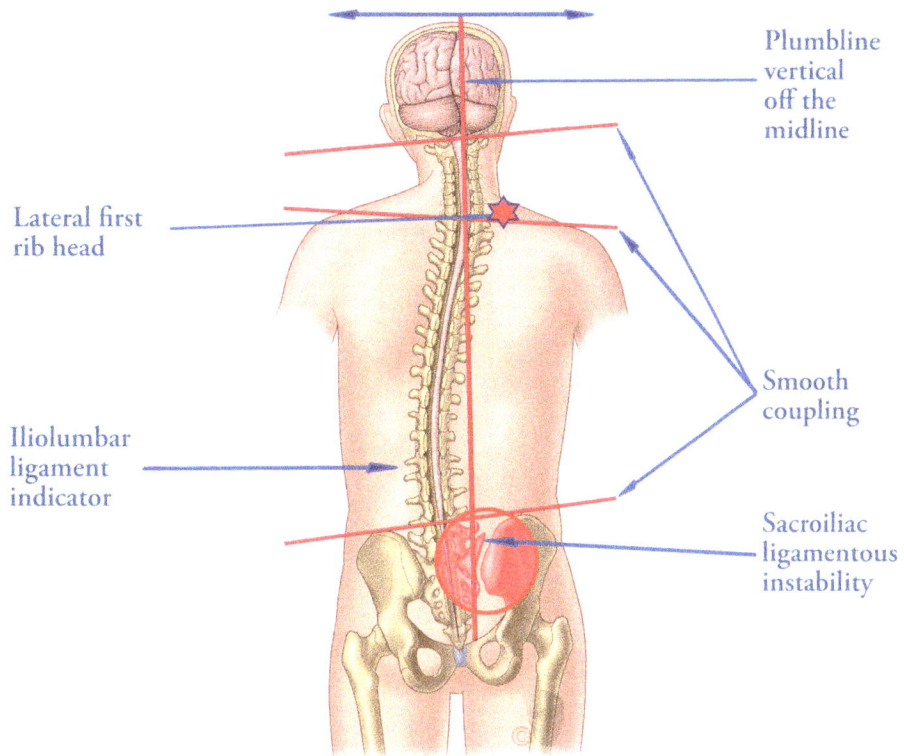

Figure 1.11 Sacroiliac Lesion: Lateral sway

Plumbline
vertical
off the
midline

Lateral first
rib head

Smooth
coupling

Iliolumbar
ligament
indicator

Sacroiliac
ligamentous
instability

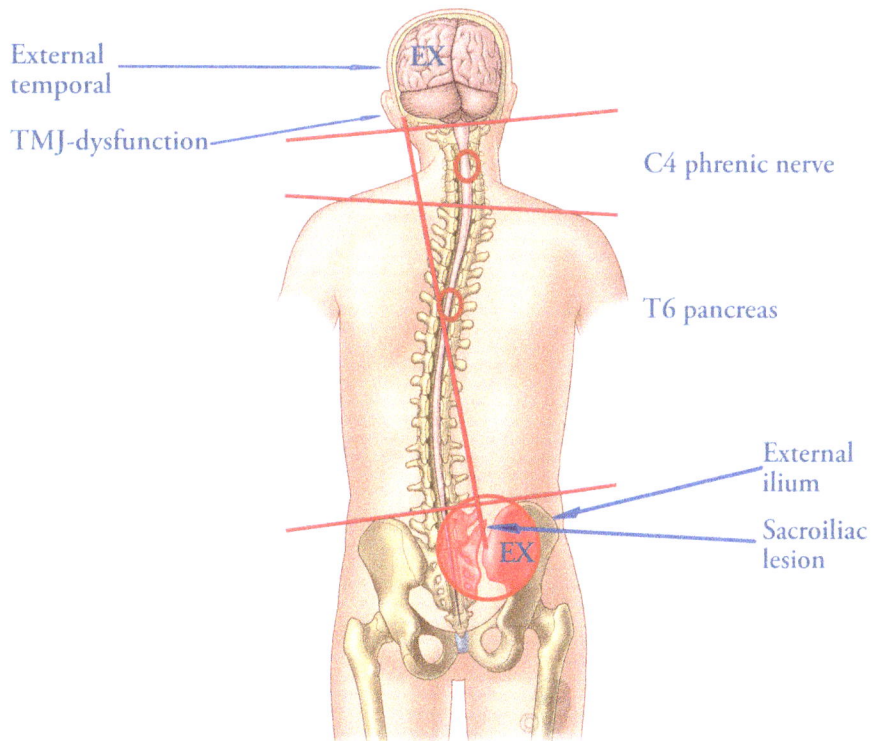

Figure 1.12 Temporomandibular Joint Reciprocates with Sacroiliac Lesion

External
temporal

TMJ-dysfunction

C4 phrenic nerve

T6 pancreas

External
ilium

Sacroiliac
lesion

175

This occurs when the set of interosseous ligaments supporting the sacroiliac joint on the short leg side become stretched and weakened, breaking the neurological seal between the two adjacent nerve beds –the ilia and the sacrum. This causes a loss of neurological integrity between the components of the sacroiliac joint on the short leg side. When this happens, muscle recruitment from adjacent areas takes place.

For argument's sake the discussion will assume a right short leg.

The ipsilateral latissimus dorsi (right) contracts in an effort to support that side of the body, pulling on T6 and the head of the humerus – both insertion points for the latissimus dorsi. T6 is the sympathetic control to the pancreas, which in turn affects C4, the parasympathetic control of the phrenic nerve to the diaphragm.

This in turn contracts the left trapezius muscle inserting into the nuchal line of the occiput opposing the insertion of the tentorium cerebellum at the occipital sulcus, potentially distorting the transverse and sigmoid sinuses on the internal occipital surface and flexing the head to the left. This also twists the straight sinus and compromises the sinus drainage.

This triggers the ipsilateral (right) SCM muscle, rotating and flexing the head left, compromising the brachial plexus, while the contralateral (left) temporalis muscle contracts, pulling the mandible to left side. The reaction from this deviated mandible to the left is a malocclusion, disturbing the left canine contact, which controls the ipsilateral trapezius and the contralateral SCM. This would be a precursor to temporomandibular joint (TMJ) dysfunction, with the condyle compressing the retrodiscal tissue and damaging the articular disc. This would be an ascending scenario.

The reverse situation would apply with traumatic CFD, where the left mandibular deviation would be responsible for loss of canine guidance and contact, implicating the right SCM and the left trapezius muscles. This is a typical descending major, which one would expect with traumatic CFD, and a dental involvement (see Part V, Cranio Dental Dynamics).

MUSCLE GROUPS INVOLVED WITH THE SACROILIAC LESION

Below the sacroiliac joint on the ipsilateral side, the inguinal ligament tightens, affecting the sartorius and gracilis muscles on the short leg side, and the tensor fasciae latae (TFL) on the long leg side.

The muscle groups involved in the sacroiliac lesion are all lateral muscles and have a profound effect on the lower extremities. The right sartorius muscle comes off the right anterior superior iliac spine (ASIS) and inserts into the fascia of the medial knee at the medial meniscus. This becomes displaced and rotates the right femur internally and the right tibia and fibula externally, creating a serious potential knee joint problem. In turn this is exacerbated by the right gracilis muscle which comes off the ischiopubic ramus of the pubic bone and inserts through the medial knee fascia into the upper medial aspect of the tibia, adducting the femur. The peroneus longus lies in the lateral compartment of the lower limb and acts to evert and plantar flex the ankle. Medial knee damage as described will also create a weak and unstable ankle and may represent another weight-bearing problem.

The TFL on the long leg side combines with the tendons of the gluteus muscles to form the iliotibial tract and inserts into the lateral condyle of the tibia. The TFL is a hip abductor. The anterior tibialis partners the TFL and acts to dorsiflex and invert the foot.

The sacroiliac lesion is far-reaching and has multiple joint and limb implications. It should be considered carefully, as most upper and lower extremity problems are treated locally, without taking care of the primary subluxation – the sacroiliac lesion.

This patient will present with a lateral sway and a unilateral rib head.

The lesion is lateral, therefore all the symptomatology will be laterally found.

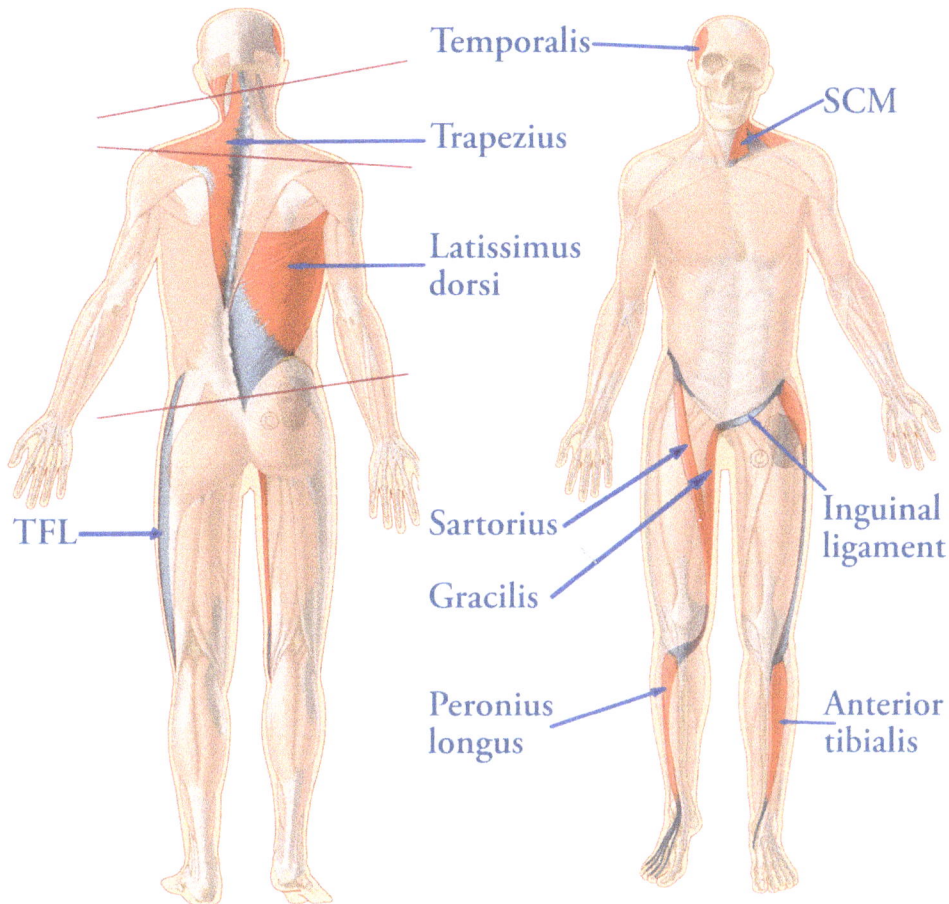

Figure 1.13 Muscle Groups in Sacroiliac Lesion: Lateral muscle groups

CRANIAL IMPLICATIONS AND CONSIDERATIONS

When assessing the equilibrium of the entire skeletal structure, the influence of the muscles and fascial dura need to be considered carefully. One has to understand how the external forces from fascia and muscles on the outside of the skeletal system must complement the internal forces to bring about a homeostatic environment.

Consider the external paravertebral muscle which are connectors from the occiput to the sacrum – central stabilisers when their opposing structures internally adhere to the occipital sulci – opposing the nuchal line of the occiput externally (as mentioned earlier in this chapter).

Now consider the sacroiliac lesion, which is a lateral lesion, and therefore introduces the lateral fascia and musculature. The right sacroiliac lesion recruits the latissimus dorsi – T6 attachment – and the trapezius muscle, overall. More specifically, it involves the upper trapezius muscle which attaches to the medial third of the nuchal line and the external occipital protuberance, the lateral third of the clavicle, the medial aspect of the acromion process and the superior crest of the spine of scapula. The motor nerve supply is the spinal accessory, and the sensory spinal nerves of C3 and C4 – phrenic nerve to diaphragm. Reactive contraction of the trapezius muscle causes flexion of the head and neck, ipsilaterally, and rotation of the neck contralaterally. Internally, this action causes the opposing force to be recruited, namely the transverse and sigmoid sinuses encapsulated by the tentorium cerebellum on the left side, pulling the tentorial incisura external and creating the externalisation of the horizontal tentorium cerebellum, taking with it the external occiput and the temporal bone.

The SCM now comes into play. Its origins – the sternal head – are at the superior part of the anterior surface of the manubrium sterni and the clavicular head at the medial third of the clavicle. While the insertion is at the lateral surface of the mastoid process of the temporal bone and the lateral half at the superior nuchal line of the occiput. The nerve supply is the spinal accessory and cervical branches of C2 and C3.

The lateral contraction of the SCM, in conjunction with the upper trapezius, causes right ipsilateral neck flexion and contralateral neck rotation. The internal opposing forces are found at the tentorium cerebellum, moving the tentorial incisura internal with the right temporal bone internalising. The right occiput is taken into internal rotation by the opposing nuchal line at the transverse and sigmoid sinuses, encapsulated by the posterior tentorium cerebellum at the occipital sulcus and the petrous portion of the temporal bone.

The left temporalis now contracts, deviating the mandible to the left, removing the canine guidance from the left mandibular/maxilla (jaw to jaw) contact. When the left temporalis muscle contracts, the left medial pterygoid also contracts – working in tandem with the left upper trapezius – and pulls the mandibular ramus to the left. The left SCM works in tandem with the ipsilateral lateral pterygoid muscle.

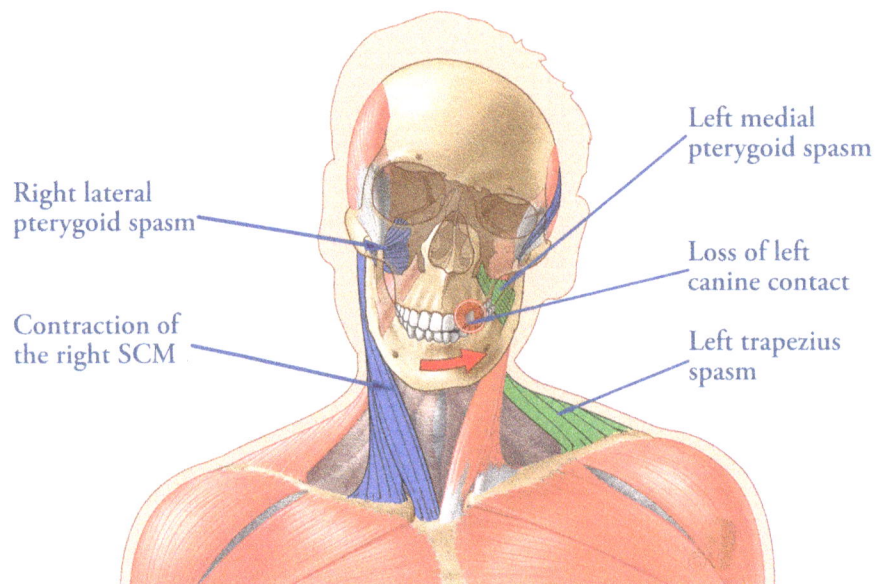

Figure 1.14 Left Mandibular Deviation: Arrow shows direction of movement of the mandible

NB When muscle testing for the lateral and medial pterygoid muscles, use the SCM – which mimics the ipsilateral lateral pterygoid muscle – and the upper trapezius muscle – which mimics the ipsilateral medial pterygoid muscle.

CRANIAL FORCES AND OPPOSING FORCES

Having described the external forces – both medial (central) and the lateral muscle groups that influence the cranium externally – we will now look at the internal cranial forces and how they come into effect, confirming Newton's Third Law.

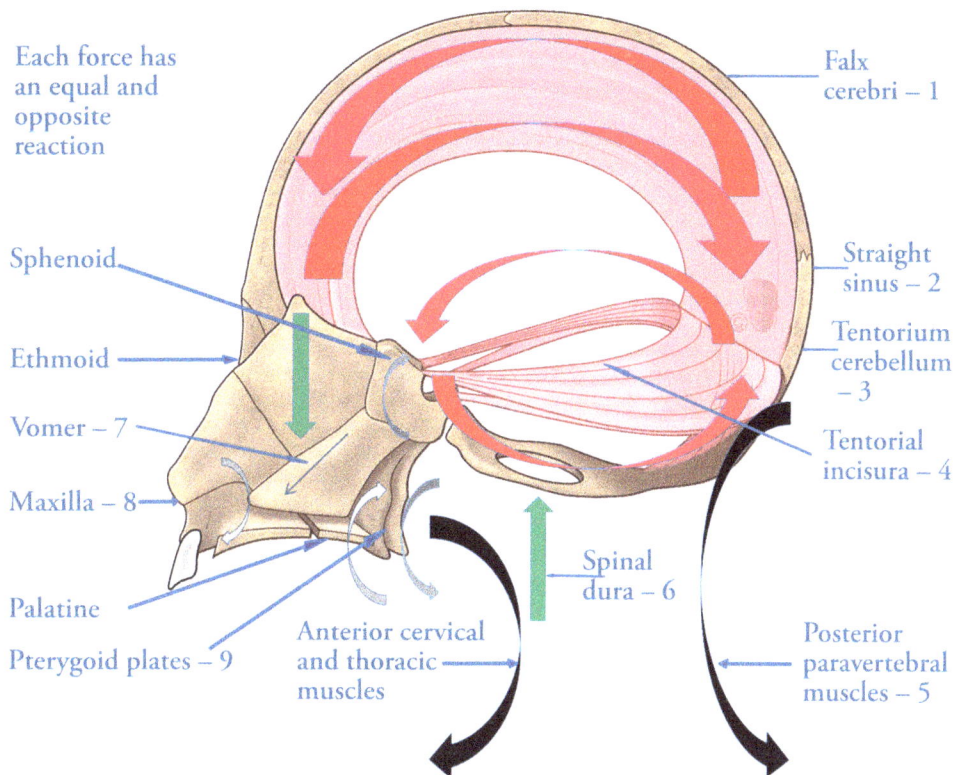

Each force has an equal and opposite reaction

Falx cerebri – 1

Sphenoid

Ethmoid

Vomer – 7

Maxilla – 8

Palatine

Pterygoid plates – 9

Straight sinus – 2

Tentorium cerebellum – 3

Tentorial incisura – 4

Spinal dura – 6

Anterior cervical and thoracic muscles

Posterior paravertebral muscles – 5

Figure 1.15 Newton's Third Law – F = ma

The intracranial RTM are placed to balance and protect the brain and cerebellum. They are also responsible for brain drainage. This would imply that the entire intracranial system, although flexible, requires a certain degree of stability to function and maintain the homeostatic balance. Trauma, or forces external to the body, will disturb, and have a profoundly negative influence on the respiration effects of that equilibrium.

a. The falx cerebri attached at the straight sinus and at the crista galli of the ethmoid bone present opposing forces within the membrane. The superior sagittal sinus and the inferior sagittal sinus must support and oppose one another in order to maintain the drainage of venous blood from the anterior and mid part of the brain. Their anchor points will become distorted and shift when the opposing forces come under tension.

b. The straight sinus at the internal occipital protuberance has to oppose the external forces and torque derived from the external muscle attachments at the external occipital protuberance. Torque at the straight sinus affects drainage to the confluence of the sinuses, destabilises the falx cerebri, the falx cerebelli and the tentorium cerebellum.

c. The tentorium cerebellum has lateral attachments at the petrous portion of the temporal bones – opposing the external actions of the temporalis muscle and the SCM at the mastoid, posterior support at the occiput – encapsulating the transverse and sigmoid sinuses – opposing the external upper trapezius and SCM at the lateral and medial parts of the nuchal line.

d. The anterior attachments of the tentorium cerebellum, to the anterior and posterior clinoid processes at the body of the sphenoid, come in the form of the two sheaths of tentorial incisura that separate at the anterior of the straight sinus and form the infratentorial compartment, encapsulating the central brain tissue – the midbrain, pons and medulla. The opposing forces to the tentorial incisura include the external central muscles into the nuchal line, the temporalis, the upper trapezius and the SCM, as well as the pterygoid plates influencing the body of the sphenoid bone.

e. The posterior paravertebral muscles oppose and counter the anterior cervical, thoracic and lumbar muscle groups. Loss of integrity in the lumbar muscle group leads to a loss of cervical, thoracic and lumbar curves, and changes in disc performance and resultant subluxations.

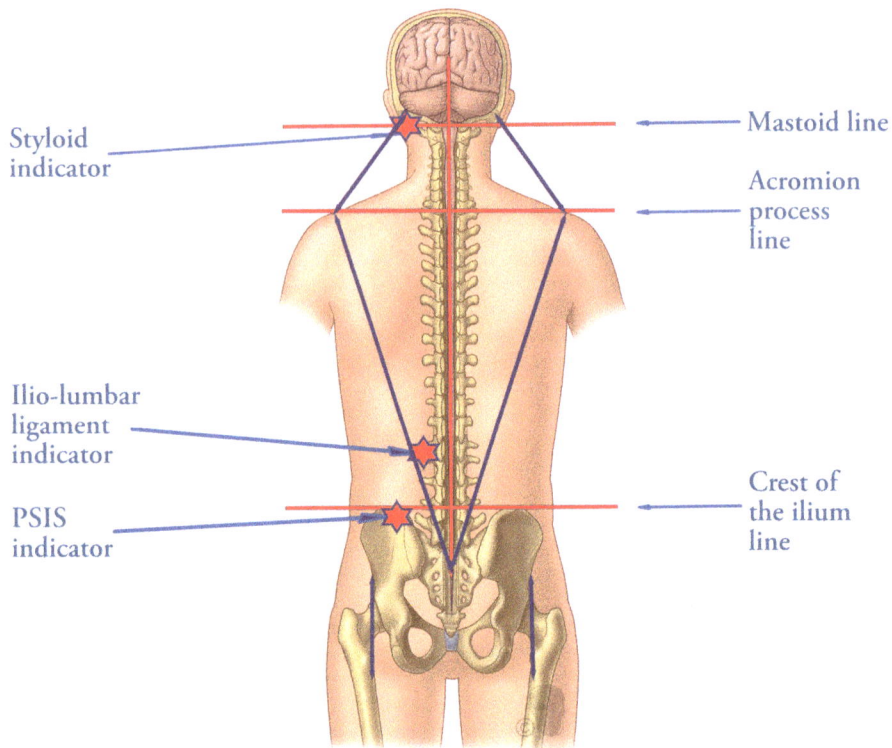

Figure 1.16 Balanced Forces in a Balanced Cranium, Spine and Pelvis

f. Spinal dura is opposed directly by the crista galli of the ethmoid bone, providing the anterior anchor for the falx cerebri and the rest of the RTM. The opposing forces include the cranial meningeal and dura and their multiple intracranial attachments, as well as the periosteal dura, with all the external muscle groups. The spinal dura is attached inferiorly to the periosteal dura of the ilia and the sacrum, completing the entire dural meningeal system. This is the reason that reciprocation exists within what started as mesenchyme on day 18 of embryological development, the benign counterclockwise torque of the cranium and its opposing benign clockwise torque of the pelvis. This is the driver of the human body's postural attitude, with all the muscles, ligaments and tendons playing the supportive role, in subservience to the fascial system – CFD.

g. The vomer is, in essence, a sheet of membrane that attaches to the ethmoid bone anteriorly and the body of the sphenoid posteriorly, anteriorly/inferiorly to the maxilla, and posteriorly/inferiorly to the palatines. The plasticity of the vomer is twofold in that the anterior part moves into an equal and opposite direction to the posterior part. This allows the falx cerebri to be driven in a motion along with the other RTM in coordination with respiration phases governed by the stomatognathic system – the motion of the maxilla and opposing motion of the palatines, pulling through the vomer, to influence the motion of the crista galli (ethmoid bone), sphenoid body (sphenobasilar synchondrosis) in one direction, while the balance of RTM and the occiput and temporal bones reciprocate. The diaphragm also brings this same motion to completion through the same respiratory phase. The maxilla and the palatines are also integral in the forces and opposing forces – activated by swallowing and mastication, influencing the vomer.

h. The pterygoid plates are responsible for the internal (medial) and external (lateral) pterygoid muscles and their dominance on mandibular activity. Where necessary, they recruit the SCM with the ipsilateral lateral pterygoid muscle, and the upper trapezius with the ipsilateral medial pterygoid muscles. The body of the sphenoid lying superior to the pterygoid plates also influences the tentorial incisura and the lesser and greater wings of the sphenoid as opposing forces to the mandible.

CFD takes into consideration Newton's Third Law as it is totally consistent with regard to balance and homeostasis in this very complex system.

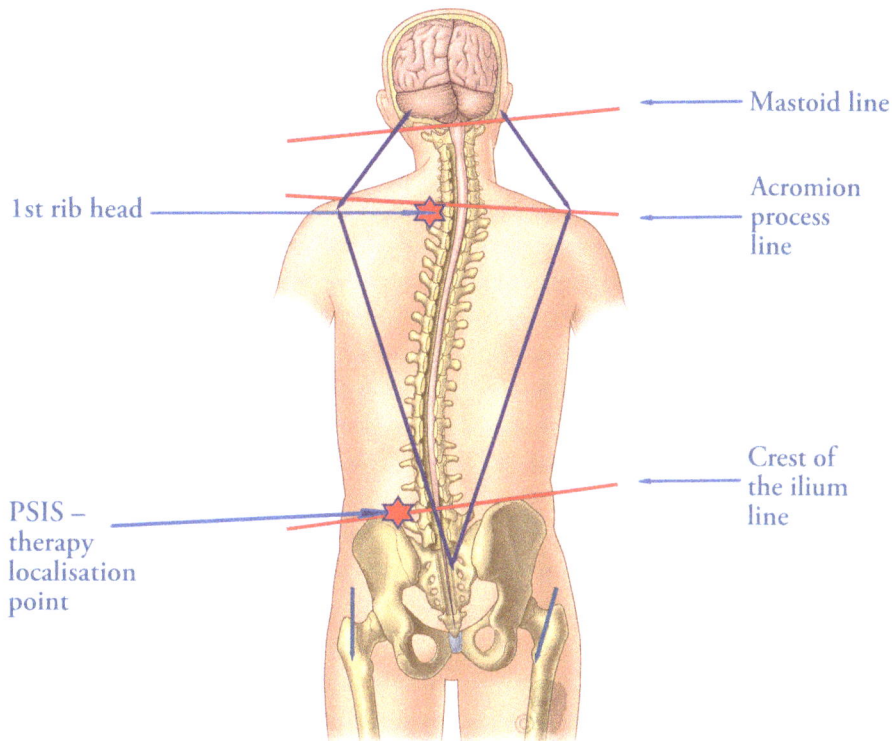

Figure 1.17 Dural Torque: Bilateral sacroiliac fixation

181

LUMBOSACRAL DISC LESION

Failure to stabilise the sacroiliac lesion, will cause more stress in an already stressed area, and while the weight-bearing problem is ignored, the lower lumbar discs become more involved as the gravitational stress starts to implicate the annulus fibrosis of the intervertebral disc, with the possibility of tearing or rupturing the outer layer of the disc.

Further damage will incur tearing and cause a disc prolapse or rupture, allowing the nucleus pulposus to break its boundary and compress the spinal nerve root or the theca.

Continued weight-bearing overload on the sacroiliac joint lesion over time, reduces its ability to function. This gradual attrition results in the lumbosacral disc lesion.

The lumbosacral disc lesion can also result from direct trauma to the body. This will present as a classic 'non-smooth' coupling in the body posture, where the two or three adjacent horizontal lines – through the mastoid, acromion and iliac crests – follow one another and an antalgia results.

As a side note, L5 reciprocates with T9 – the adrenal component. The presence of adrenal fatigue in lumbosacral disc lesion cannot be underestimated. The more the adrenal gland is used by the body under stress – pain, exhaustion and physiological imbalance – the more it needs to manufacture adrenalin. Adrenalin is made from minerals stored in muscles, ligaments and tendons, so the more minerals are needed to make adrenalin, the weaker these components become, compromising the structures they support.

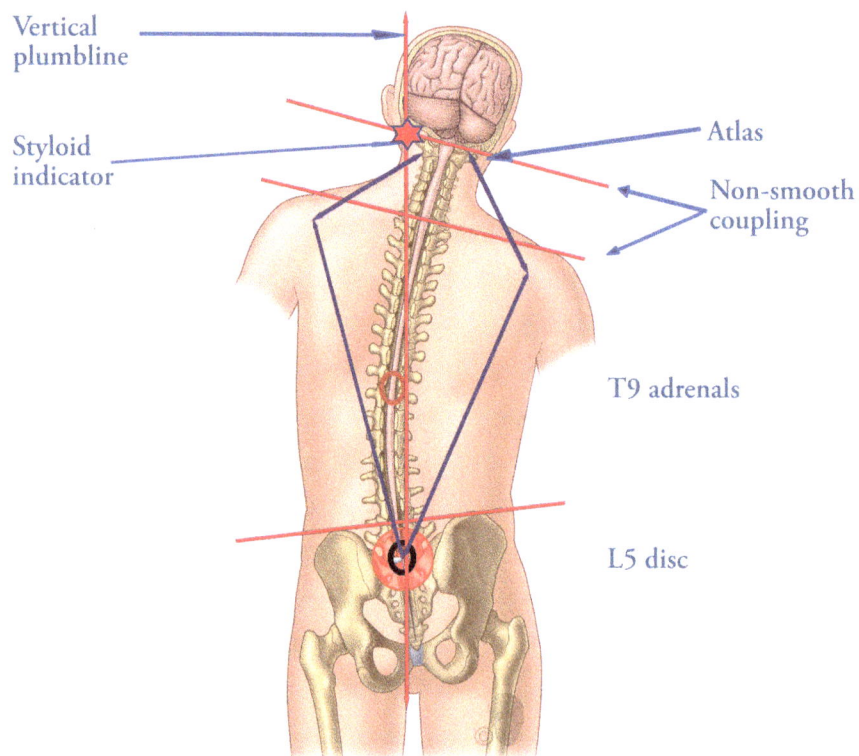

Figure 1.18 Lumbosacral Disc Lesion

LATERAL DISC BULGE

A classic lateral disc bulge occurs on the lateral aspect of the intervertebral foramen. Non-smooth coupling is present. The disc bulge is always on the same side as the sciatica. The body antalgia is in the opposite direction to the sciatica. For example: left lateral disc bulge, left leg sciatica and right antalgia; or right lateral disc bulge, right leg sciatica and left antalgia.

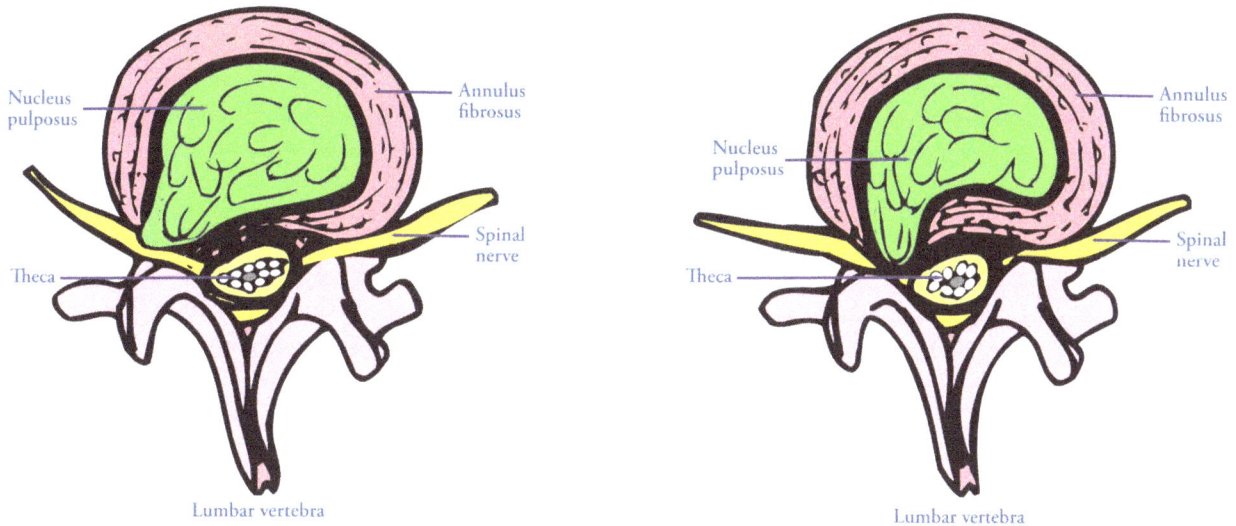

Figure 1.19 Lateral Disc Bulge (left); Medial Disc Bulge (right)

MEDIAL DISC BULGE

A medial disc bulge is where the disc bulge occurs medial to the intervertebral foramen inside the vertebral canal. Non-smooth coupling is present. The disc bulge is always on the same side as the sciatica. The body antalgia is on the same side as the sciatica. For example: right medial disc bulge, right leg sciatica and right antalgia; or left medial disc bulge, left leg sciatica and left antalgia.

This type of disc bulge should be treated with caution and conservatism, which is why pelvic blocking is the treatment of choice. No side posturing adjustment is advisable.

MUSCLES INVOLVED IN LUMBOSACRAL DISC LESION

The prime two muscles involved in this arena are the piriformis and the psoas muscles. The psoas muscle is the anterior muscle group responsible for the antalgia, while the piriformis is responsible directly for the sciatic nerve. In Figure 1.20, the left image shows lateral disc bulge to the left with left sciatica and right antalgia, while the right image shows medial disc bulge to the right with right sciatica and right antalgia.

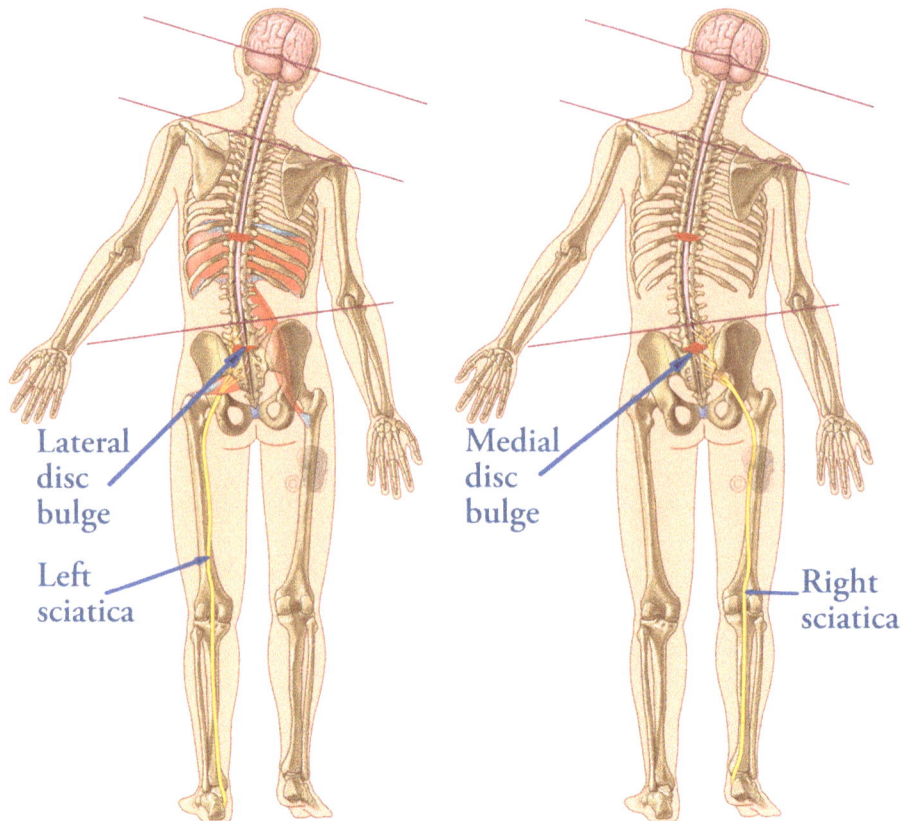

Figure 1.20 Muscle Groups in Lumbosacaeral Disc: Psoas and piriformis muscles

ANTERIOR ANTALGIA – CENTRAL DISC LESION

Anterior antalgia is produced by a central disc bulge. As Figure 1.21 shows, a central disc bulge impinges directly on the theca of the spinal cord. This can cause a vast number of potentially dangerous neurological complications and needs to be treated with the greatest care. An accurate assessment of the neurological picture needs to be performed, and 'red flags' need to be adhered to for referral purposes.

The healing of this condition may be long and arduous, and the patient needs to understand the implications and severity of the injury, which may be life-changing. MRIs and CT scans should be taken to ensure this patient is afforded the best possible outcome.

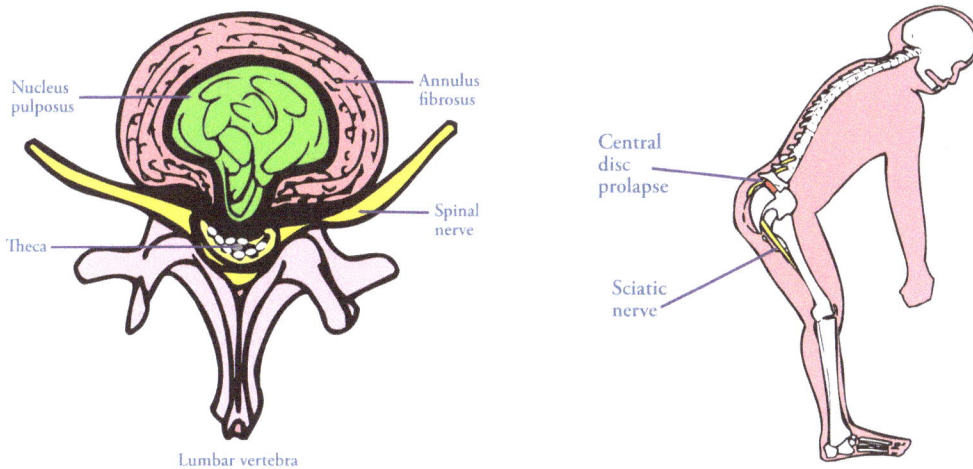

Figure 1.21 Central Disc Bulge (left); Anterior Antalgia Lumbosacral Disc Lesion

SYMMETRIC BODY MUSCULATURE

Muscles involved in a sacroiliac lesion are lateral muscle groups affected by a lateral lesion.

While they are triggered by a sacroiliac lesion, the recruitment of muscle groups takes place above, affecting the pectoral girdle and the TMJ components, and below the lesion, challenging the lower extremities.

TMJ reciprocates with sacroiliac lesion. The sacroiliac joint and the contralateral TMJ reciprocate with one another. Failure of either joint to maintain neurological integrity refers to the other joint – usually from a dental malocclusion, invoking a descending major and a weight-bearing pelvic problem.

As a side note, the insertion of the latissimus dorsi at T6 creates a potential pancreatic issue, reducing insulin and provoking hyper-glycaemia. T6 also reacts with C4 – controlling the phrenic nerve and the diaphragm – affecting respiration.

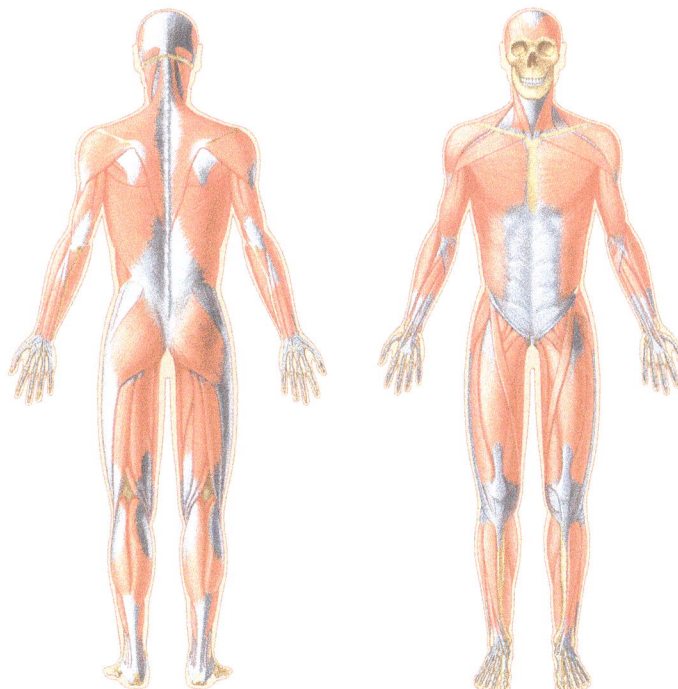

Figure 1.22 Symmetric Body Musculature

185

THE DISLOCATED BRAIN

PART IV

CRANIO VASCULAR

DYNAMICS

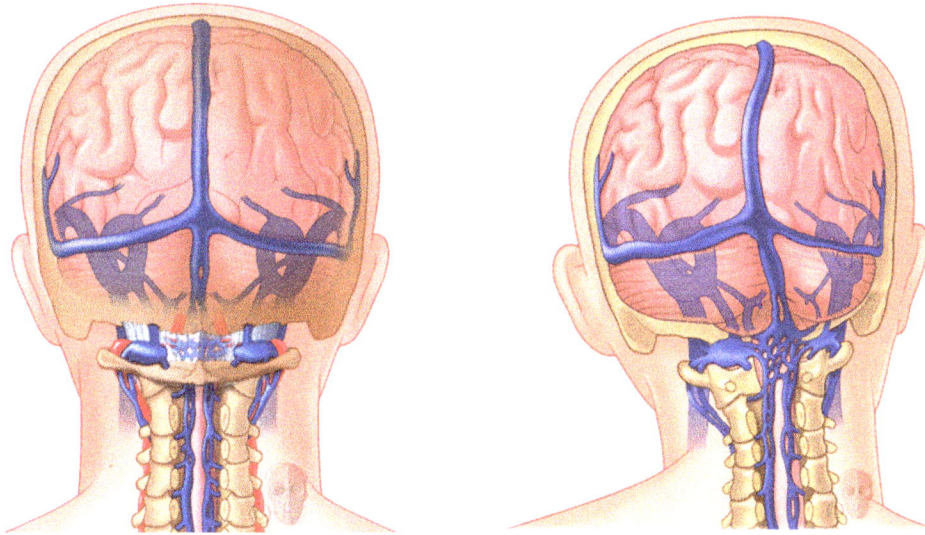

CONTENTS PART IV

ILUSTRATIONS PART IV

INTRODUCTION TO PART IV

Most people who have studied the anatomy and physiology of the cardiovascular system are aware of the intricate details involving the arterial inflow and the sinus collection of ischaemic blood that forms the basis of brain drainage. However, brain drainage is vitally dependent on the upper cervical vascular components, including the vertebral venous plexus, the atlanto-occipital membrane, the axillary plexus, and the important internal jugular vein. Injuries to the upper cervical spine from birth trauma, dental malocclusions and whiplash injuries change and congest the multitude of capillary vessels that are invested in this area, severely inhibiting the ability of the internal jugular vein to drain the venous sinus system and compromisng other drainage components. This action has massive implications for this important irrigation system. Homoeostasis requires that arterial blood in and ischaemic blood out must maintain equilised pressure within the cranial vault. When the balance of this pressure is disrupted and the brain does not drain sufficiently, intracranial pressure results. This causes a pressure build-up throughout all the potential drainage vessels and alters brain physiology. This loss of brain drainage is exacerbated by cranial dural torque to the dural membrane system, including the falx cerebri, the falx cerebellum and the diaphragma sellae. These membranes support and control the entire venous sinus system and the torqued membranes inhibit the free drainage process, creating a welling up of fluids and consequently a cytotoxic effect on any of the adjacent brain components. Over many years this results in a myriad of neurological complications which, as clinicians, we are exposed to on a daily basis. By analysing this phenomenon, it is the author's intent to tackle this complicated problem, provide strategies to help alleviate the neurological complexities, and finally, to deal with the contributing factors and the wider range of associated disorders.

CHAPTER 1

NORMAL CIRCULATION OF BLOOD

Homeostasis prevails and intracranial pressure are normal when the volumes of arterial and venous blood moving from heart to brain and back again are equalised.

Blood pressure (BP) is the pressure exerted by circulating blood upon the walls of blood vessels and generally refers to the arterial pressure in the systemic circulation. It is usually expressed in terms of systolic (maximum) pressure over diastolic (minimum) pressure and is measured in millimetres of mercury (mmHg). Normal resting systolic (diastolic) BP in an adult is approximately 120 mmHg (80 mmHg), abbreviated to '120/80 mmHg'.

BP varies, depending on situation, activity and existing disease. It is regulated by the nervous and endocrine systems. Low BP is called hypotension, and consistently high BP is called hypertension.

BP fluctuates from minute to minute and normally shows a circadian rhythm over a 24-hour period, with highest readings in early morning and evening and lowest readings at night. Without a normal fall in BP at night an increased risk of cardiovascular disease may result and there is evidence that night-time BP is a stronger predictor of cardiovascular events than daytime BP.

As adults age, systolic pressure tends to rise, while diastolic pressure tends to fall. In the elderly, systolic BP tends to be above the normal adult range, thought to be largely because of reduced flexibility of the arteries. Also, an individual's BP varies with exercise, emotional reactions, sleep, digestion and time of day.

PULSE PRESSURE

Pulse pressure is the difference between the measured systolic and diastolic pressures. The constant fluctuation of arterial pressure results from the pulsatile nature of the cardiac output, that is, the heartbeat. Pulse pressure is determined by the interaction of the stroke volume of the heart, the compliance (ability to expand) of the arterial system – largely attributable to the aorta and large elastic arteries – and the resistance to flow in the arterial tree. By expanding under pressure, the aorta absorbs some of the force of the blood surge from the heart during a heartbeat. In this way, pulse pressure is lower than it would be if the aorta were not compliant.

SYSTEMIC VENOUS PRESSURE

BP generally refers to arterial pressure in the systemic circulation. However, measurement of pressure in the venous system and the pulmonary vessels plays an important role in intensive care medicine (although requiring invasive measurement of pressure using a catheter).

Venous pressure is the vascular pressure in a vein or in the atria of the heart. It is much less than arterial pressure, with common values of 5 mmHg in the right atrium and 8 mmHg in the left atrium.

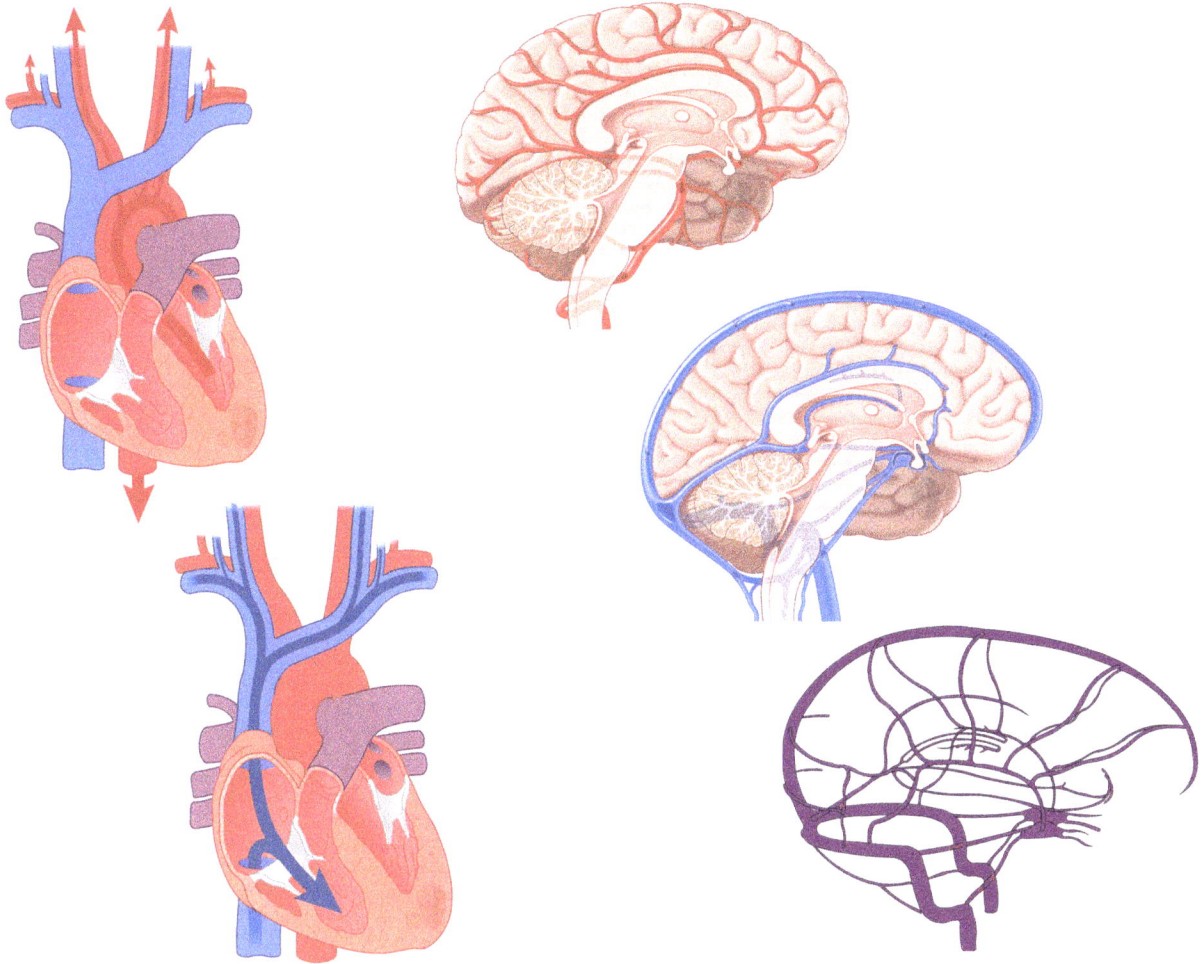

Figure 1.1 Blood Circulation

Arterial blood is pumped from the heart to the aortic arch (top left), then venous blood returns to the heart, completing the circuit (bottom left). Oxygenated blood goes into the brain (top right); deoxygenated blood is collected in the venous sinus system (middle right); spent blood leaves the brain by the dural venous sinuses (bottom right)

HYPERTENSION

Levels of arterial pressure put mechanical stress on arterial walls. Higher pressures increase heart workload and progression of unhealthy tissue growth (atheroma) that develops within the walls of arteries. The higher the pressure, the more stress that is present and the more atheroma tend to progress, with heart muscle tending to thicken, enlarge and become weaker over time.

Persistent hypertension is one of the risk factors for stroke, heart attack, heart failure and arterial aneurysm, and is the leading cause of chronic kidney failure.

HYPOTENSION

BP that is too low, hypotension, is a medical concern if it causes signs or symptoms, such as dizziness, fainting or, in extreme cases, shock.

When arterial pressure and blood flow decrease beyond a certain point, the perfusion of the brain becomes critically decreased (i.e. the blood supply is not sufficient), causing lightheadedness, dizziness, weakness or fainting.

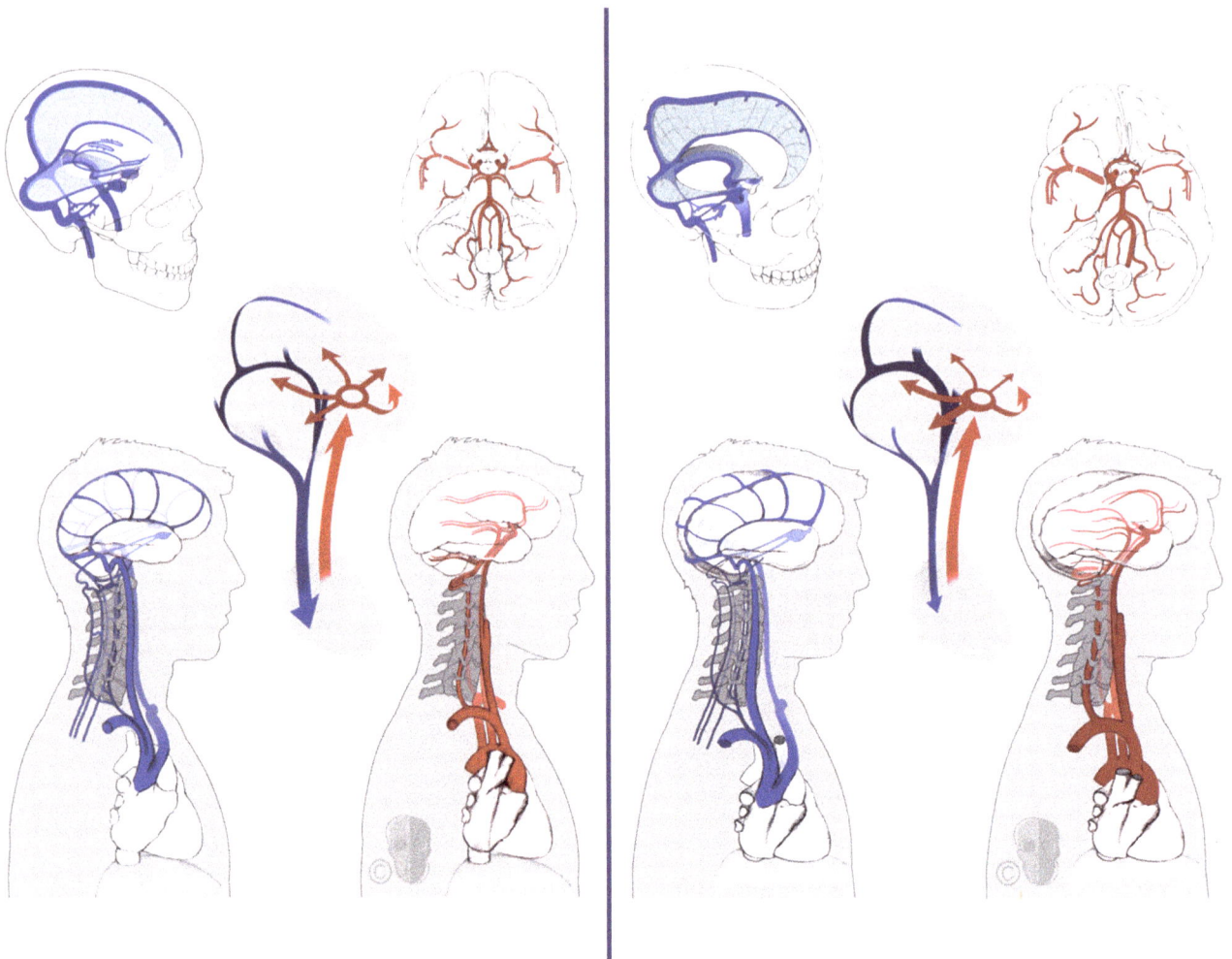

Figure 1.2 Vascular Circulation and Drainage: Normal (left); obstructive (right)

IRRIGATION SYSTEM IN NORMAL HOMEOSTASIS

The irrigation initiated by the heart sends arterial blood to the brain through the carotid arteries and the vertebral arteries into the circle of Willis. From the circle of Willis at its base, blood travels into the brain via the anterior, middle and posterior cerebral arteries, where it continues into the brain tissue. Venous blood is collected through the pacchionian bodies in the arachnoid granulation in the superior sagittal sinus, as well as other venous sinuses. It drains from the confluence of the sinuses into the transverse, sigmoid sinuses and into the internal jugular veins, the brachiocephalic veins into the heart. This represents a true homeostatic irrigation system, where blood into the cranium and blood out of the cranium is a constant volume.

However, this process is disrupted by many factors, particularly with regard to venous drainage. Given cranial and spinal trauma, this results in the volume of blood outflow becoming obstructed and restrictive, thus reducing flow back to the heart. This creates intracranial pressure and shifts the internal cranial components into a pathophysiologic dysfunction. This change in physiology has the potential to increase BP as the heart has to work harder to overcome the volume differential. This text concentrates on these changes.

THE CIRCLE OF WILLIS

The circle of Willis acts as a reservoir at the inferior aspect of the brain. It has two arterial supplies: the anterior, which is fed by the internal carotid artery; and the posterior, which is supplied by the vertebral arteries.

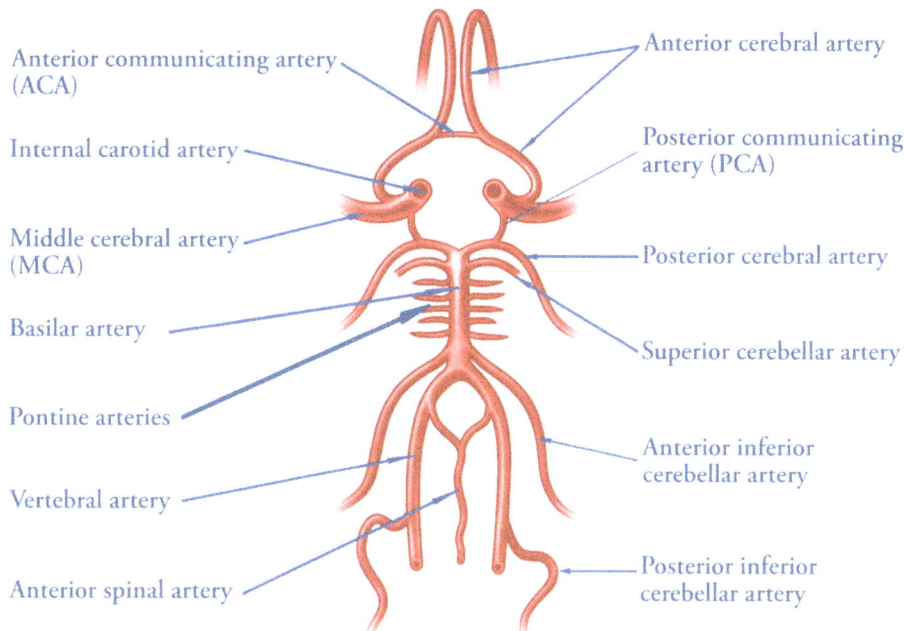

Anterior communicating artery (ACA)

Internal carotid artery

Middle cerebral artery (MCA)

Basilar artery

Pontine arteries

Vertebral artery

Anterior spinal artery

Anterior cerebral artery

Posterior communicating artery (PCA)

Posterior cerebral artery

Superior cerebellar artery

Anterior inferior cerebellar artery

Posterior inferior cerebellar artery

Figure 1.3 Circle of Willis

Anterior supply – common carotid

The common carotid artery branches off the aortic arch and bisects to form the internal carotid artery and the external carotid artery.

Internal carotid artery

The internal carotid artery divides into the middle cerebral artery (MCA) and the anterior cerebral artery (ACA).

The MCA follows the lateral sulcus/fissure, which separates the frontal and parietal lobes from the temporal lobe and divides into smaller branches called the striate arteries, supplying the basal ganglia.

The ACA passes through the interhemispheric fissure or the medial longitudinal fissure dividing the two cerebral hemispheres, and moves to the anterior part of the brain. From here the ACA divides into the pericallosal and callosomarginal arteries, at the genu of the corpus callosum, and then into the frontal lobe and the recurrent artery of Heubner, which is a large, lenticulostriate vessel which supplies the caudate nucleus, internal capsule and putamen. The two anterior cerebral arteries are connected by the anterior communicating artery that forms the anterior part of the circle of Willis. The internal carotid artery is joined to the posterior cerebral arteries by the posterior communicating artery, forming the posterior part of the circle of Willis.

The anterior cerebral arteries supply the medial, superior and lateral hemispheres. The middle cerebral arteries supply the lateral aspect of the brain, and the posterior cerebral arteries supply the occipital lobe and the inferior part of the brain.

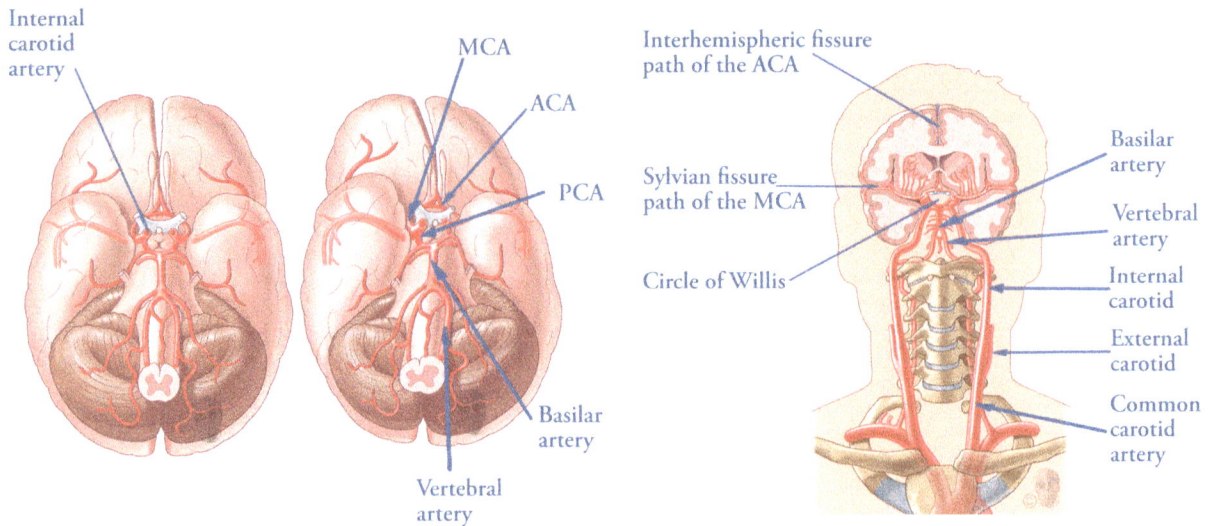

Figure 1.4 (left) Circle of Willis at Base of Brain: Inferior view– textbook symmetry (left); traumatic asymmetry (right)
Figure 1.5 (right) Internal and External Carotid Arteries

External carotid artery

The external carotid artery supplies the head and the neck through:

- Three anterior branches – the suprathyroid, the lingual and the facial
- Two posterior branches – the occipital (the posterior side of the scalp) and the posterior auricular (behind the ear)
- One medial branch – the ascending pharyngeal
- Two terminal branches – the maxillary (which goes through the infra temporal fossa) and the pterygopalatine fossa (to supply the pterygoid muscles)
- The anterior and posterior superficial arteries (which feed the anterior and posterior ear).

Posterior supply – vertebral arteries

The vertebral arteries come off the aortic arch, pass through the transverse foramen of the cervical spine and exit through the transverse foramen of the atlas, where at the base of the pons, they form the basilar artery.

Prior to this formation, the anterior spinal artery, which follows the anterior median fissure at the anterior of the spinal cord, forms the posterior inferior cerebellar artery which then feeds into the vertebral arteries. The posterior spinal artery follows the posterior spinal fissure along the posterior aspect of the spinal cord and joins the vertebral arteries as the posterior inferior cerebellar arteries.

Arteries of the brain – lateral view

Several branches come off the basilar artery, giving rise to the pontine arteries – supplying the pons, before forming the superior cerebellar artery, the anterior inferior cerebellar artery and the posterior inferior cerebellar artery – supplying the cerebellum – the brainstem, and the posterior cerebral hemispheres. The basilar artery continues to join the posterior cerebral artery (PCA) – the posterior ring of the circle of Willis – whose branches include the posteromedial choroidal artery, which supplies the midbrain, the choroid plexus of the third ventricle, the pineal gland, the medial dorsal nucleus of the thalamus, the medial geniculate body, and the posterolateral choroidal artery. This artery goes on to supply the choroid plexus of the lateral ventricle, the thalamus, the lateral geniculate bodies, the pulvinar, fornix, cerebral peduncle, pineal body, corpus callosum, tegmentum, and temporal occipital cortex.

Arteries of the brain – sagittal view

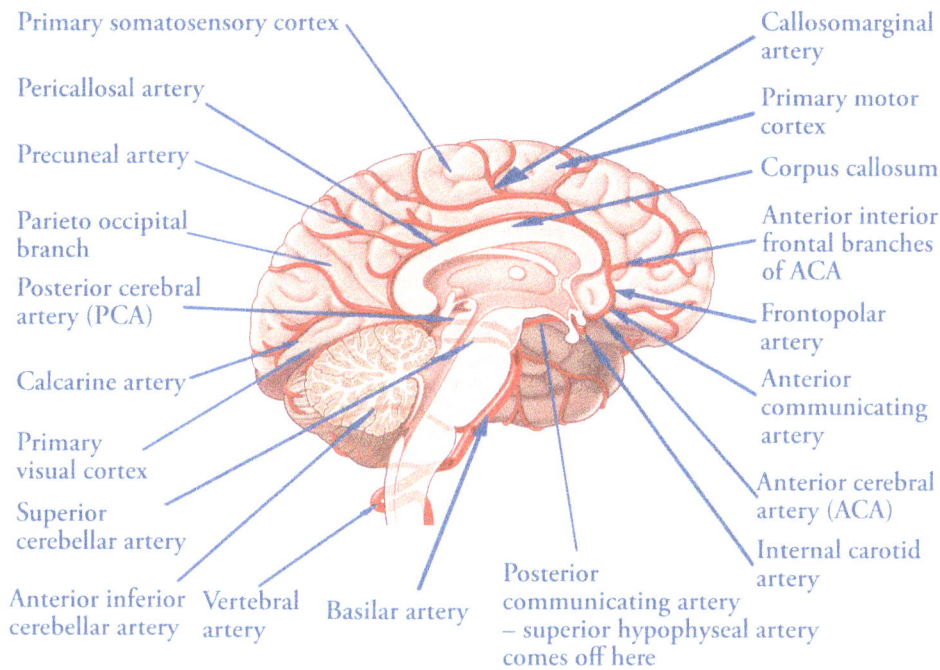

Primary somatosensory cortex

Pericallosal artery

Precuneal artery

Parieto occipital branch

Posterior cerebral artery (PCA)

Calcarine artery

Primary visual cortex

Superior cerebellar artery

Anterior inferior cerebellar artery

Vertebral artery

Basilar artery

Posterior communicating artery – superior hypophyseal artery comes off here

Callosomarginal artery

Primary motor cortex

Corpus callosum

Anterior interior frontal branches of ACA

Frontopolar artery

Anterior communicating artery

Anterior cerebral artery (ACA)

Internal carotid artery

Figure 1.6 Arteries of the Brain: Sagittal view

This sagittal view of the brain shows the PCA and all its branches at the posterior aspect of the brain (in red) feeding the occipito-parietal area, the calcarine artery supplying the lingual and cuneate gyri, and the pericallosal artery, which runs anteriorly over the splenium of the corpus callosum and anastomoses with the pericallosal branch of the ACA.

The superior hypophyseal artery comes off the posterior communicating artery or the internal carotid and supplies the primary plexus of the hypophyseal portal system – the upper part of the hypophyseal stalk, but does not supply blood to the anterior lobe directly.

The ACA, and all its branches (in white) include the anterior communicating artery, branches to the frontal areas and the callosomarginal artery covering the parieto-frontal area above the corpus callosum.

ARTERIAL FLOW TO THE BRAIN

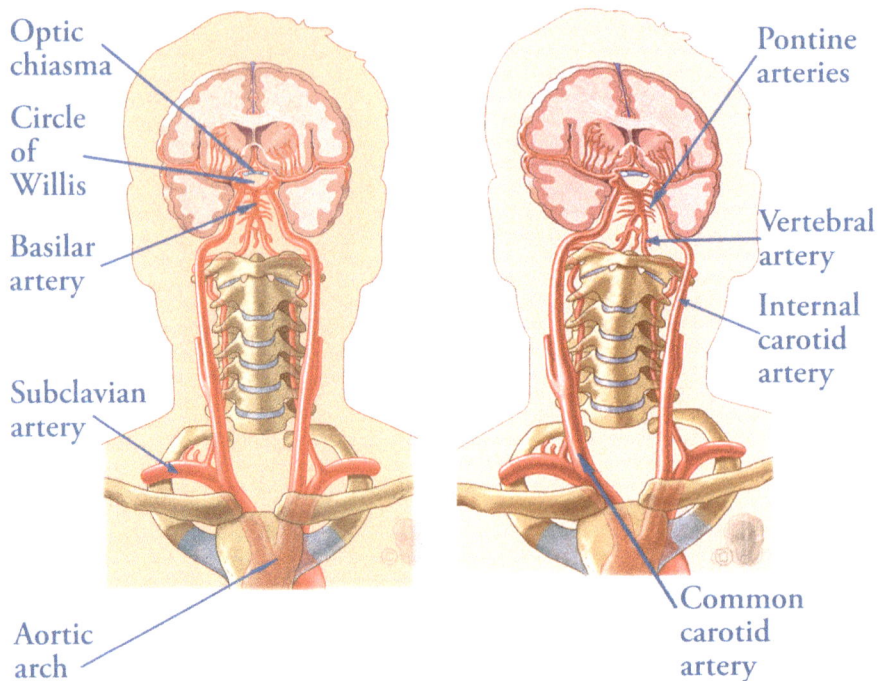

Optic chiasma
Circle of Willis
Basilar artery
Subclavian artery
Aortic arch

Pontine arteries
Vertebral artery
Internal carotid artery
Common carotid artery

Figure 1.7 Arterial Flow to the Brain: Normal (left), distorted (right)

The left vertebral artery comes off the left subclavian artery from the aortic arch, while the right vertebral artery comes off the aortic arch and then the brachiocephalic trunk. Both then thread bilaterally through the cervical transverse foramina to exit finally through the transverse foramen of the atlas, before taking a tortuous medial turn to follow the posterior arch of the atlas before taking another tortuous turn to go superiorly, penetrating the atlanto-occipital membrane and the dura mater before entering the brain through the foramen magnum. The convoluted path of the vertebral arteries in these sub-occipital areas, is critical in brain circulation and vulnerable to disruption and obstruction with upper cervical trauma.

The right common carotid artery comes off the brachiocephalic branch of the aortic arch in the superior mediastinum and bifurcates at the level of the upper border of the thyroid cartilage forming the internal and external branches of the carotid arteries. The internal carotid then travels cephalad and enters the brain through the carotid canal. The canal ascends vertically at first and then, making a bend, runs horizontally forward and medialward. The canal's internal opening is near the foramen lacerum, above which the internal carotid artery passes on its way anteriorly to the cavernous sinus. The foramen lacerum is formed by the junction of the petrous portion of the temporal bone, the lesser wing of the sphenoid bone and the basilar portion of the occiput, medial to the jugular foramen and the carotid canal. These foramina are subject to the internal rotation of the temporal bone on the right side that has the effect of closing these foramina and reducing the aperture for the vessels and nerves traversing them. The external carotid artery begins at the upper border of thyroid cartilage and curves, passing forward and upward, and then inclining backwards to the space behind the neck of the mandible, where it divides into the superficial temporal and maxillary artery within the parotid gland.

It rapidly diminishes in size as it travels up the neck, owing to the number and large size of its branches.

At its origin, this artery is closer to the skin and more medial than the internal carotid, and is situated within the carotid triangle. Cranio fascial torsion creates fascial restriction to the path of the external carotid and its branches.

CONCLUSION

A discussion of the normal avenues of arterial supply to the brain culminating in the circle of Willis.

Blood pressure evaluation

BP is the pressure exerted on the walls of blood vessels by blood circulating and usually refers to the arterial pressure in the systemic circulation, expressed in terms of the systolic (maximum) pressure over diastolic (minimum) pressure and measured in millimetres of mercury (mmHg). Normal resting systolic/diastolic BP in an adult is approximately 120 mmHg (80 mmHg), abbreviated to 120/80 mmHg.

Systemic Venous Pressure

a. Hypertension
b. Hypotension

The irrigation system in normal homeostasis allows arterial blood flowing into the brain to be at the same volume and pressure as the venous blood leaving the brain. Changes to this homeostatic model means that the venous blood return is reduced and compromised.

The circle of Willis is the complex reservoir at the base of the brain that funnels arterial blood into the brain from the main arteries.

The anterior blood supply feeding into the brain consists of the common carotid arteries, splitting into the internal and external carotids. The internal carotid artery gives rise to the ACA – both are joined together by the anterior communicating artery, forming the anterior ring of the circle of Willis – and the middle cerebral artery (MCA).

The posterior blood supply to the brain consists of the two vertebral arteries that merge to form the basilar artery. At the circle of Willis, the basilar artery bifurcates into the posterior cerebral arteries (PCA) and join with the posterior communicating artery to form the lateral and posterior ring of the circle of Willis. At the inferior aspect of the basilar artery, the anterior inferior cerebellar arteries come off, followed at the superior aspect of the basilar artery by the anterior superior cerebellar arteries. Between the two arteries are several branches of the pontine arteries, which branch off the basilar artery. The anterior and posterior spinal arteries join the vertebral arteries, before the merger into the basilar artery.

CHAPTER 2

VENOUS CIRCULATION OF THE BRAIN

VEINS OF THE CRANIUM

The venous drainage of the cranium is divided into four groups.

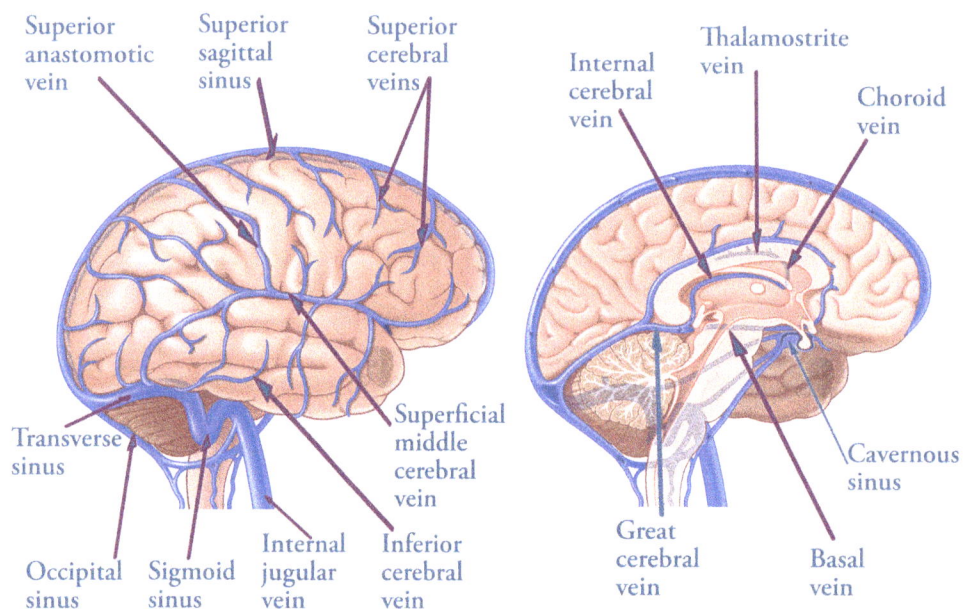

Figure 2.1 Cerebral Veins: External (left), internal (right)

I. External cerebral veins

    a. The superior cerebral veins originate in the external superior frontal, parietal and occipital lobes and the superior anastomotic vein, all drain into the superior sagittal sinus.

    b. The superior middle cerebral vein, which drains the external inferior frontal, parietal and occipital lobes and the temporal lobes, and lead into the transverse sinus.

    c. The inferior cerebral veins drain the external inferior temporal lobe and joins the superior part of the sigmoid sinus and the internal jugular vein.

II. Internal cerebral veins

These veins drain the internal cranial components of the brain and consist of:

    a. The thalamostrite vein draining the caudate nucleus, the internal capsule and the deep white matter of the posterior frontal and anterior parietal lobes.

b. The choroid vein draining the choroid plexuses of the ventricles in this area.

c. The internal cerebral vein draining the roof veins of the lateral ventricle, the veins of the posterior horn of the lateral ventricle and the thalamic veins.

d. The cavernous sinus draining the superior and inferior ophthalmic veins, superior and middle cerebral vein, the inferior cerebral veins and the sphenoparietal sinus.

e. The basal vein (of Rosenthal)which receives temporal veins and an inferior ventricular vein from the inferior horn of the lateral ventricle. These drain the deep white matter of the superior and lateral portions of the temporal lobe, the hippocampus, the dentate gyrus and the choroid plexus. The most posterior portion of the basal vein receives the lateral mesencephalic vein from the mesencephalon.

f. The great cerebral vein which receives the two basal veins, the posterior pericallosal, internal occipital, posterior mesencephalic, pre-central and superior vermian veins.

III. Superior cerebellar veins

a. The superior sagittal sinus drains into the confluence of the sinuses, where it deviates into the right transverse sinus.

b. The inferior sagittal sinus drains into the straight sinus, the confluence of the sinuses, then into the left transverse sinus.

IV. Inferior cerebellar veins

a. The confluence of the sinuses

b. The occipital sinus

c. The transverse sinuses

d. The sigmoid sinuses

e. Internal jugular vein

f. The cavernous sinuses

g. The intercavernous sinus

h. The superior petrosal sinus

i. The inferior petrosal sinus

j. The basilar plexus

k. The vertebral venous plexus

l. Sub-occipital cavernous sinus

SINUSES OF THE DURA MATER

The sinuses of the dura mater are venous channels which drain the blood from the brain into the internal jugular vein. They are devoid of valves, and are situated between the two layers of dura mater but are lined by endothelium continuous with that of the veins into which they drain.

a. Superior sagittal sinus – follows the superior border of the falx cerebri, from the glabella to the confluence of the sinuses, where it joins the right transverse sinus.

b. Inferior sagittal sinus follows the inferior border of the falx cerebri and joins the straight vein of Galen to form the straight sinus.

c. Straight sinus – situated at the junction of the falx cerebelli and the tentorium cerebellum and follows the left transverse sinus.

d. Transverse sinus – follows the border of the tentorium in both left and right directions, encapsulated by the fascia of the tentorial border from the internal occipital protuberance to the sigmoid sinuses at the junction of the temporal bones and the occiput.

e. Occipital sinus – commences at the margin of the foramen magnum by several small venous channels, one of which joins the terminal part of the transverse sinus where it communicates with the posterior internal vertebral venous plexuses and ends at the confluence of the sinuses.

f. Confluence of the sinuses – is the junction of three sinus tributaries: the superior sagittal sinus, the straight sinus and the occipital sinus, with two large transverse sinuses. The right transverse sinus usually receives the greater volume of its blood from the superior sagittal sinus, while the left transverse sinus receives its volume of blood from the straight sinus.

g. Cavernous sinus – receives the superior and inferior ophthalmic veins, some of the cerebral veins, and the sphenoparietal sinus. It has anastomoses with the transverse sinus through the superior petrosal sinus, with the pterygoid plexus through the foramen of Vesalius, foramen ovale and foramen lacerum, with the angular and facial vein through the superior ophthalmic vein. The two cavernous sinuses then anastomose with each other through the intercavernous sinuses. The cavernous sinus then drains into the inferior petrosal sinus, and then into the internal jugular vein.

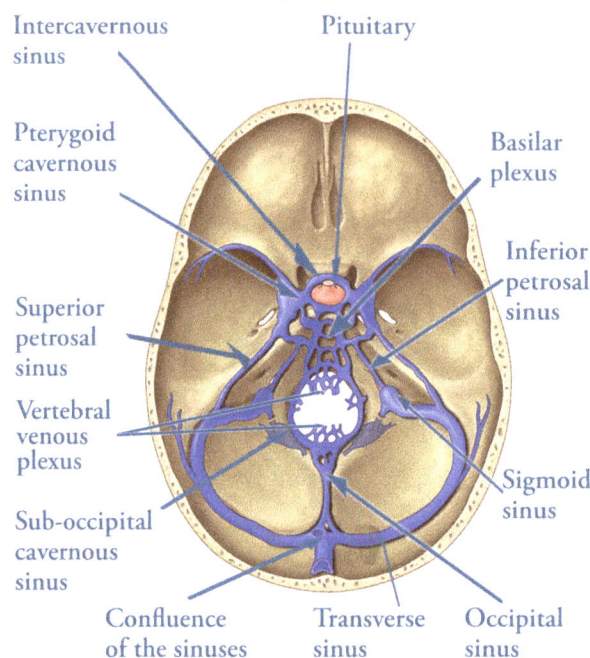

Figure 2.2 Inferior Cerebellar Veins and the Sinuses of the Dura Mater

Anatomically, the cavernous sinus lies in the space between the body of the sphenoid bone and the dura forming the medial boundary of the middle cranial fossa, over the superior orbital fissure, and inferior to the apex of the petrous portion of the temporal bone. In separate fibrous sheaths derived from the lateral wall of the sinuses lie the following nerves: the oculomotor, the trochlear, the ophthalmic and the maxillary divisions of the trigeminal nerve.

Lying medial to these nerves are the internal carotid artery and the abducens nerve.

The sphenoid sinus is one pair of four paired paranasal sinuses found in the body of the sphenoid bone under the sella turcica. The cavernous sinus surrounds the sphenoid sinus and is traversed by a number of vessels including the internal carotid artery. It is bordered laterally by the temporal lobes and the sphenoid bone and is lateral to the sella turcica. The cavernous sinus is filled with venous blood collected from the superior and inferior ophthalmic veins from the eyes and the orbits, discharging through the basilar plexus posteriorly, into the superior and inferior petrosal sinuses then the internal jugular vein. The internal carotid artery, once it leaves the cavernous sinus, turns superiorward to form the anterior communicating artery, then the ACA and the MCA of the circle of Willis. The circle of Willis lies just above the sella turcica and encircles the pituitary stalk, and so lies above the sphenoid body. Torsion to the sphenoid bone with its fascial connectors to the circle of Willis, potentially results in a torque of the circle of Willis. This warping may explain the high incidence of aneurysms in the anterior and middle cerebral arteries.

This cavernous sinus space is influenced by changes to the dura, changes to the position of the sphenoid body and the superior orbital fissure, and the petrous portion of an internally and superiorly rotated temporal bone, where cranio fascial torque becomes evident.

(This cavernous sinus space is affected by changes to the dura, changes to the position of the sphenoid body and the superior orbital fissure, and the petrous portion of an internally and superiorly rotated temporal bone when cranio fascial torque becomes evident.)

Figure 2.3 shows a coronal view of the body of the sphenoid bone surrounded laterally by the superior orbital fissures. The superior orbital fissures contain the oculomotor nerve (CN III), the trochlear nerve (CN IV), the ophthalmic division of the trigeminal nerve (CN V 1), the abducens nerve (CN VI) and the maxillary division of the trigeminal nerve (CN V 2). The internal carotid artery lies in the superior position of the superior orbital fissure. The sella turcica lies in the sphenoid body and houses the pituitary gland, suspended by the infundibulum/hypophyseal stalk, while the two sphenoidal sinuses lie just below.

The collapse of the right sphenoid body (on the right of Figure 2.3) shows congestion of all the apertures through which the aforementioned cranial nerves and internal carotid artery traverse; the collapse of the right sphenoid sinus causing congestion and pressure, while the sella turcica pulls on the infundibulum, distorting and congesting the pituitary. The anterior and posterior clinoid processes surrounding the sella turcica will become warped and alter the position of the tentorium cerebellum, the horizontal dural membrane. This sphenoid distortion can be brought about by direct trauma to the face, a shift in the occlusion and the jaw-to-jaw relationship, or trauma to the cranium, disrupting the dynamics of the reciprocal tension membranes (RTM).

Intercavernous sinus – anterior and posterior components connect the two cavernous sinuses across the midline. The anterior (usually the larger) passes anterior to the hypophyseal stalk, the posterior component posterior to it, forming with the cavernous sinus, a circular sinus around the hypophysis.

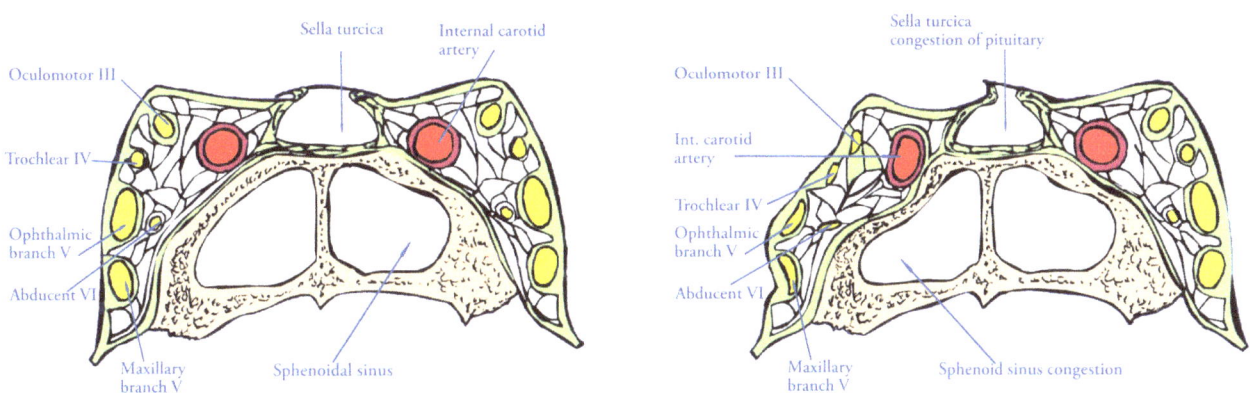

Figure 2.3 Cavernous Sinus – Sphenoid Bone (distorted on right)

h. Superior petrosal sinus – connects the cavernous sinus with the transverse sinus. It attaches to the lateral margin of the tentorium in the superior petrosal sulcus of the temporal bone and joins the transverse sinus at the junction of the sigmoid sinus. It receives cerebellar and inferior cerebral veins, and veins from the tympanic cavity.

i. Inferior petrosal sinus – is situated in the inferior petrosal sulcus formed by the junction of the petrous portion of the temporal bone with the basilar part of the occiput. It begins in the posterior inferior part of the cavernous sinus and, passing through the anterior part of the jugular foramen, ends in the superior bulb of the internal jugular vein. The inferior petrosal sinus receives the internal auditory veins, and veins from the medulla oblongata, pons, and inferior surface of the cerebellum.

j. Basilar plexus – consists of several interlacing venous channels between the layers of the dura mater over the basilar portion of the occipital bone and serves to connect the two inferior petrosal sinuses, which then communicate with the anterior vertebral venous plexus.

k. Inferior petrosal sinus lies medially with, and anterior to the meningeal branch of the ascending pharyngeal artery.

l. The transverse sinus is situated at the lateral and posterior part of the foramen with a meningeal branch of the occipital artery.

m. Between these two sinuses, are the glossopharyngeal, vagus and spinal accessory cranial nerves.

The junction of the inferior petrosal sinus with the internal jugular vein is located at the lateral aspect of the nerves.

All these veins are supported by both the sphenoid and temporal bones, so are influenced by the dural meningeal tissue that embraces their osseous partners. The presence of cranio fascial torque therefore has a bearing on their overall performance, particularly with the obstruction of nerves and fluid retention of vascular vessels.

Baroreceptors and chemoreceptors

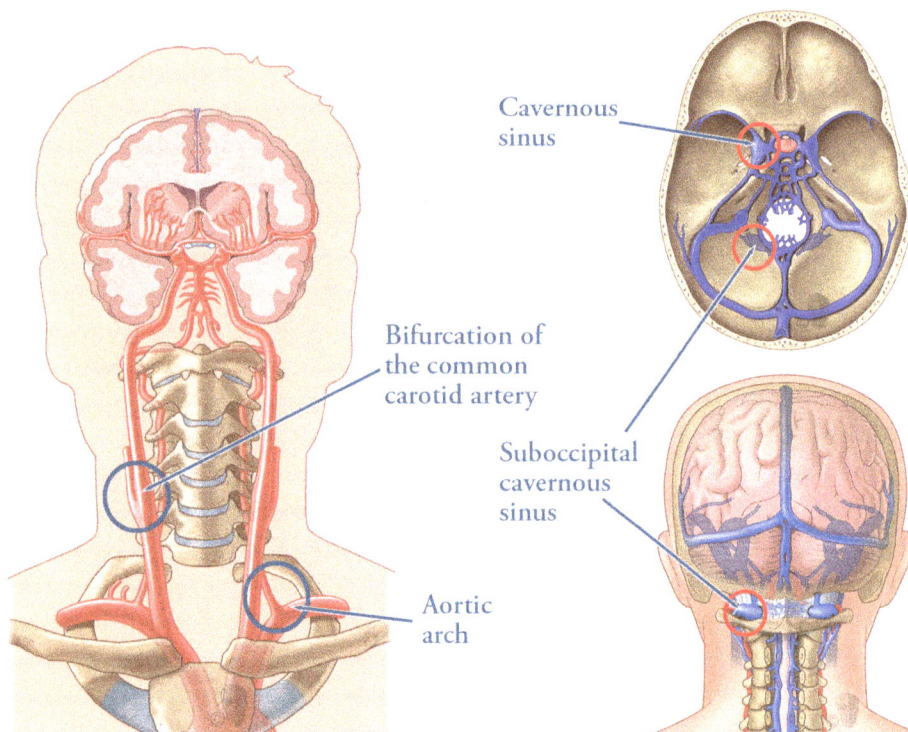

Figure 2.4 Baroreceptors and Chemoreceptors

These receptors are found in certain parts of the body to measure the O_2, CO_2 and pH values and to autoregulate the body towards homeostasis where required.

Baroreceptors are mechanoreceptors that are found in the aortic arch and in the aorta that help regulate BP through a stretch reflex.

Chemoreceptors measure the O_2, CO_2 and pH changes, and when there is a change in the chemical composition, either an increase in carbon dioxide (hypercapnia) or a decrease in blood levels of oxygen (hypoxia). That information is sent to the central nervous system to stimulate responses to restore homeostasis.

Baroreceptors are found in the aortic arch and at the bifurcation of the internal carotid artery – the carotid sinus. The reflex from the aortic arch stimulates the glossopharyngeal nerve (CN XI) and increases the BP, while the stimulus sent from the carotid sinus stimulates the vagus nerve (CN X) and increases or decreases the BP as required.

The vasomotor centre is found in the medulla oblongata of the brainstem and regulates BP through the vagus and glossopharyngeal nerves.

The suboccipital cavernous sinus and the cavernous sinus both contain baroreceptors and chemoreceptors sensitive to BP changes and O_2, CO_2 and pH concentrations.

The cavernous sinus is a part of the neurovascular myogenic autoregulatory reflex mechanism known as cerebral autoregulation. If BP decreases, autoregulation responds with a reduction in cerebral vascular resistance in an attempt to prevent cerebral hypoperfusion – decrease in brain vascularisation.

The cavernous sinus is a blood-filled sinus that receives venous blood from the ophthalmic veins that has been cooled by conduction, convection, radiation and evaporation in the eyes and orbits. This outgoing venous blood passing through the cavernous sinus, cools the arterial blood from the internal carotid and maintains the brain two or three degrees cooler than the rest of the body. This phenomenon is also specific to the suboccipital cavernous sinus which is cooled by the scalp and neck and cools the incoming vertebral arteries.

The pterygoid plexus

The pterygoid plexus lies between the temporalis muscle and the lateral pterygoid muscle and partly between the medial and lateral pterygoid muscles. This is a large plexus that communicates with the anterior facial vein and then through the cavernous sinus by branches through the foramen Vesalii, foramen ovale and foramen lacerum. The pterygoid plexus becomes the maxillary vein and the superficial temporal vein, which later combine to become the retromandibular vein (lying between the ramus of the mandible and the sternocleidomastoid muscle) and together with the posterior auricular vein forms the external jugular vein leading to the subclavian vein and to the heart.

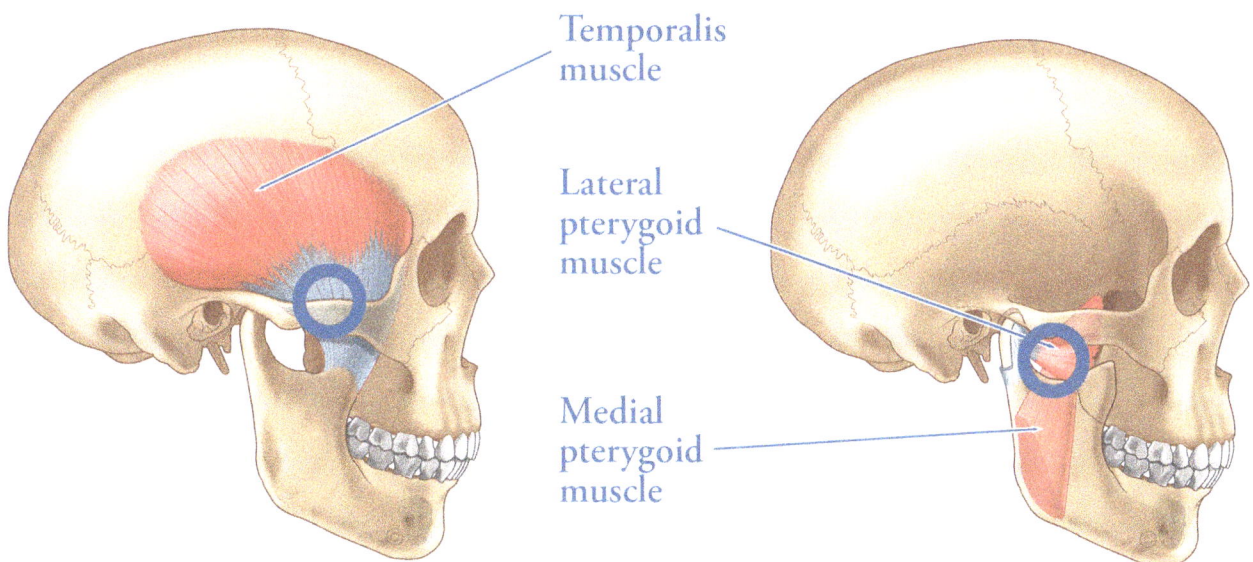

Temporalis muscle

Lateral pterygoid muscle

Medial pterygoid muscle

Figure 2.5 Pterygoid Plexus

Some sheaths

Spinal nerves – dural sheath

As the spinal nerve roots leave the foramen, the dura that covers the spinal cord continues to cover the nerve roots. This dural sheath blends with the outer covering (the epineurium) of the spinal nerve, which continues to the end organ.

CNS and PNS – myelin sheath

Layers of Schwann cell membrane (peripheral nervous system) or oligodendrocytes (central nervous system) wrapping the nerve fibres, providing electrical insulation and increasing the velocity of impulse transmission.

Vascular components – carotid sheath

A portion of the cervical fascia enclosing the carotid artery, internal jugular vein, vagus nerve and sympathetic nerves supplying the head.

Venous sinuses – dural sheath

The dura mater is made up of the endosteal layer – the outermost covering – and the meningeal layer, which are fused to each other except where they form folds enclosing the cranial venous sinuses between them.

Cranial nerves – endosteum and periosteum

The endosteal layer covers the internal surface of the cranial bones and continues with the periosteal layer on the outside surface of the cranial bones. These two layers are continuous and pass through the sutures as a continuous membrane by fibrous and vascular processes. Embryologically they surround the early cranial plates and form the fontanelles.

The periosteal lining of the ocular orbit through the superior orbital fissure provides, for example, sheaths for the cranial nerves which fuse with the epineureum of the nerve.

CRANIAL VESSELS – PIA MATER SHEATHS

Pia mater provides perivascular sheaths for vessels entering or leaving the brain.

Diploic veins

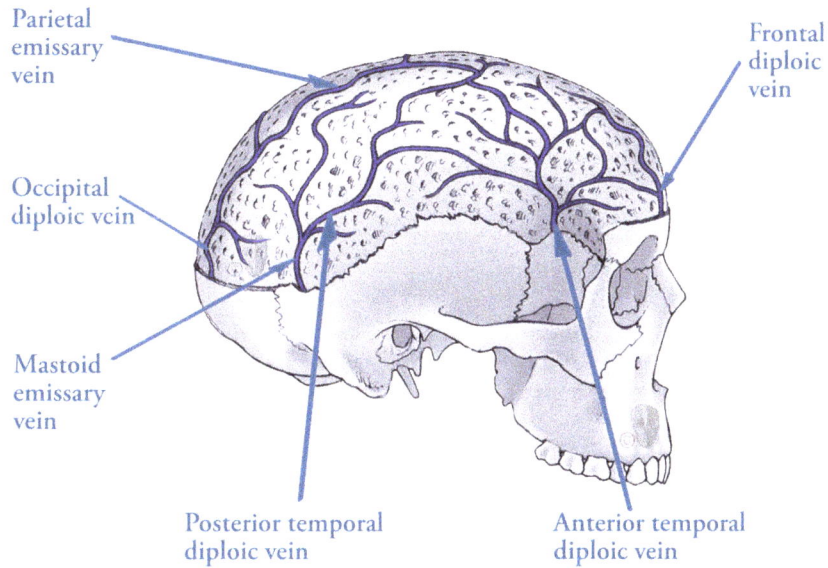

Figure 2.6 Diploic Veins

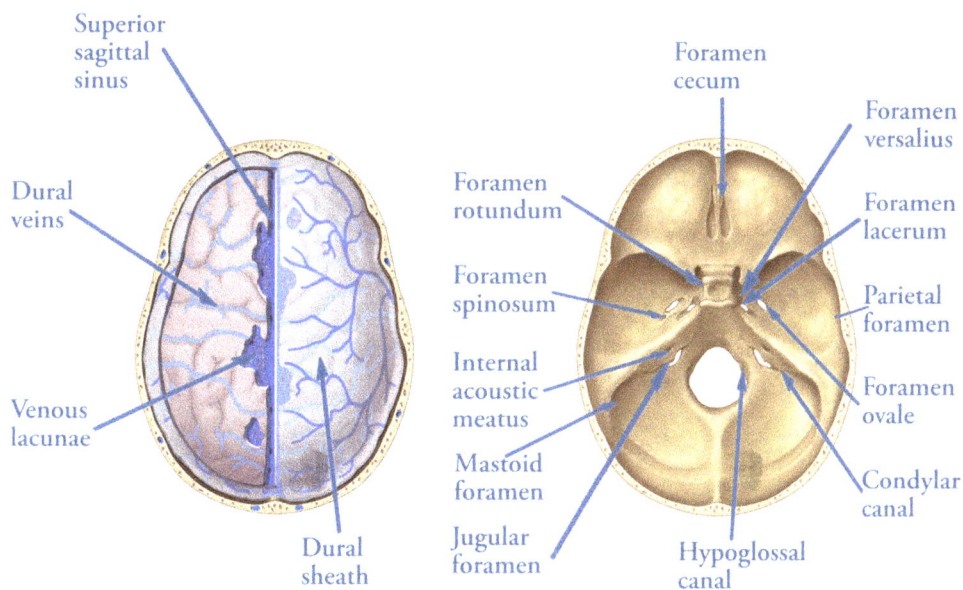

Figure 2.7 Diploic Veins (left); Emmisary Foramena (right)

The diploic veins occupy channels in the diploe of the cranial bones. They are large and exhibit at irregular intervals pouch-like dilations; their walls are thin, and formed of endothelium resting upon a layer of elastic tissue.

So long as the cranial bones are separated from one another, these veins are confined to particular bones, but when the sutures are obliterated, they unite with each other and increase in size. They communicate with the meningeal veins and the sinuses of the dura mater, and with the veins of the pericranium.

They consist of:

• Frontal – anastomoses with the supraorbital vein and the superior sagittal sinus

- Anterior temporal – confined chiefly to the frontal bone, anastomoses with the sphenoparietal sinus and the deep temporal veins through the aperture of the greater wing of sphenoid
- Posterior temporal – which is in the parietal bone and ends in the transverse sinus, through an aperture at the mastoid angle of the parietal bone or through the mastoid foramen
- Occipital – the largest of the four, which is confined to the occipital bone and opens externally in the occipital vein, or internally into the transverse sinus or the confluence of the sinuses.

Emissary veins

The emissary veins pass through the various foramena and openings in the cranial wall and establish anastomoses between the sinuses of the dura inside the skull, and veins on the exterior of the skull.

They connect the veins outside the cranium to the venous sinuses inside the cranium. The emissary veins connect the extracranial venous system with the intracranial venous sinuses. They drain from the scalp, through the skull, into the larger meningeal veins and dural venous sinuses.

Emissary veins have an important role in selective cooling of the head. They also serve as routes where infections are carried into the cranial cavity from the extracranial veins to the intracranial veins. Because the emissary veins are valveless, they are an important part in selective brain cooling through bi-directional flow of cooler blood from the evaporating surface of the head.

In general, blood flow is from external to internal but the flow can be altered by increased intracranial pressure. There are also emissary veins passing through the foramen ovale, jugular foramen, foramen lacerum and hypoglossal canal.

A type of emissary vein goes through the sphenoidal emissary foramen, inferior to the zygomatic arch with the cavernous sinus on the inside of the skull.

This is an important route for the spread of infection, because cranial nerve VI and the internal carotid pass through the cavernous sinus, with cranial nerves III, IV, VI, and V2 passing alongside the lateral wall of the sinus.

Subsequent infection or inflammation in the cavernous sinus can result in damage to any of the cranial nerves that pass through it or the meninges – resulting in meningitis.

Furthermore, rupturing the emissary veins will result in a subdural haematoma that will compress the brain.

Emissary foramena

The emissary veins pass through the various foramina and openings in the cranial wall and establish anastomoses between the sinuses of the dura inside the skull, and veins on the exterior of the skull.

a. Mastoid emissary vein – runs through the mastoid foramen, connecting the transverse sinus with the occipital vein.
b. Parietal emissary vein – passes through the parietal foramen to connect the superior sagittal sinus with the veins of the scalp.
c. Hypoglossal emissary vein– traverses the hypoglossal canal and joins the transverse sinus with the vertebral vein and the deep veins of the neck.
d. Condyloid emissary vein– passes through the condyloid canal and connects the transverse sinus with the deep veins of the neck.
e. Foramen ovale emissary vein– connects the cavernous sinus with the pterygoid plexus through the foramen ovale.
f. Foramen lacerum emissary vein– connects the cavernous sinus with the pterygoid plexus through the foramen lacerum.
g. Foramen of Vesalius vein– also connects the cavernous sinus with the pterygoid plexus through the foramen of Vesalius.

h. Internal carotid plexus vein– traverses the carotid canal between the cavernous plexus and the internal jugular vein.

i. Foramen cecum vein – connects the superior sagittal sinus with the veins of the nasal cavity.

CONCLUSION

This chapter discusses the venous and venous sinus systems, their anatomy, and how the format for brain drainage takes place.

Cerebral veins

External cerebral veins

Internal cerebral veins

Cerebellar veins

Superior cerebellar veins

Inferior cerebellar veins

Sinuses of the dura mater

Anterior/superior group draining through the right transverse sinus

- Superior sagittal sinus
- Confluence of the sinuses
- Right transverse sinus
- Right sigmoid sinus
- Right internal jugular vein

Anterior/inferior group draining through the left transverse sinus

- Inferior sagittal sinus
- Straight sinus
- Occipital sinus
- Confluence of the sinuses
- Left transverse sinus
- Left sigmoid sinus
- Left internal jugular vein

Relationship of the jugular foramen components

Diploic veins

The diploic veins occupy channels in the diploe of the cranial bones:

- Frontal
- Anterior temporal
- Posterior temporal
- Occipital

Emissary veins

a. Mastoid emissary vein

b. Parietal emissary

c. Hypoglossal emissary

d. Condyloid emissary
e. Foramen ovale emissary
f. Foramen lacerum emissary
g. Foramen of Vesalius
h. Internal carotid plexus
i. Foramen cecum

CHAPTER 3

THE VENOUS SINUS SYSTEM

The venous sinus system is made up of continuous connective fascia – dural meningeal tissue. The dural membranes totally support and encapsulate the entire venous sinus system. After passage through the ventricles, cerebrospinal fluid (CSF) leaves the forth ventricle and enters the subarachnoid spaces. The meningeal layers, the pia mater and arachnoid mater form the subarachnoid space, and these are formed from neural crest cells made of mesenchyme. The subarachnoid spaces form the cisterna magna, cisterna basalis and cisterna pontis providing a CSF bed for the pons, the medulla oblongata (including the nuclei of the third through to the twelfth cranial nerves) and the cerebellum. From the cisterns of the subarachnoid space, CSF is absorbed through the pacchionian bodies into the superior sagittal sinus. The venous sinus system drains blood from two areas. The posterior superior group and the anterior inferior group both service the areas of the brain and cavities of the cranium.

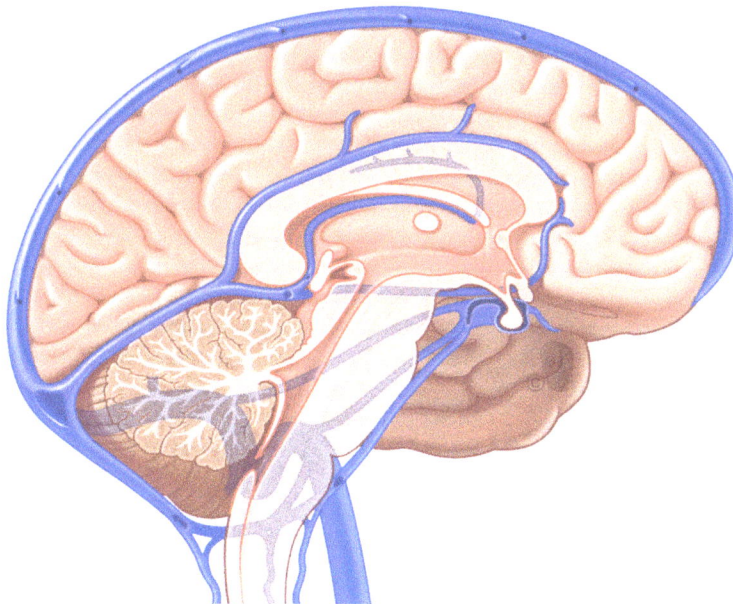

Figure 3.1 Venous Sinus System: All these vessels are encapsulated in dura

According to Upledger and Vredevoogd (1983), there exists an arachnoid granulation at the junction between the straight sinus and the great cerebral vein of Galen, in which they described the following:

> This body (arachnoid granulation at the junction) contains a sinusoidal plexus of blood vessels which become engorged and act as a ball-valve mechanism. This mechanism may control the outflow from the great cerebral vein. This in turn, by increasing back pressure, effects the secretion of the CSF by the choroid plexuses of the lateral ventricles. The drainage of these regions of the brain is from the internal cerebral vessels which empty into the great cerebral vein.

The superior petrosal sinus drains the anterior inferior group – the cavernous sinus and the circular sinus. The transverse sinus leads from the confluence of the sinuses and drains the posterior superior group of sinuses – the superior and inferior sagittal sinuses. These two major drainage areas converge at the transverse sinus, which then leads into the internal jugular vein.

THE VENTRICLES

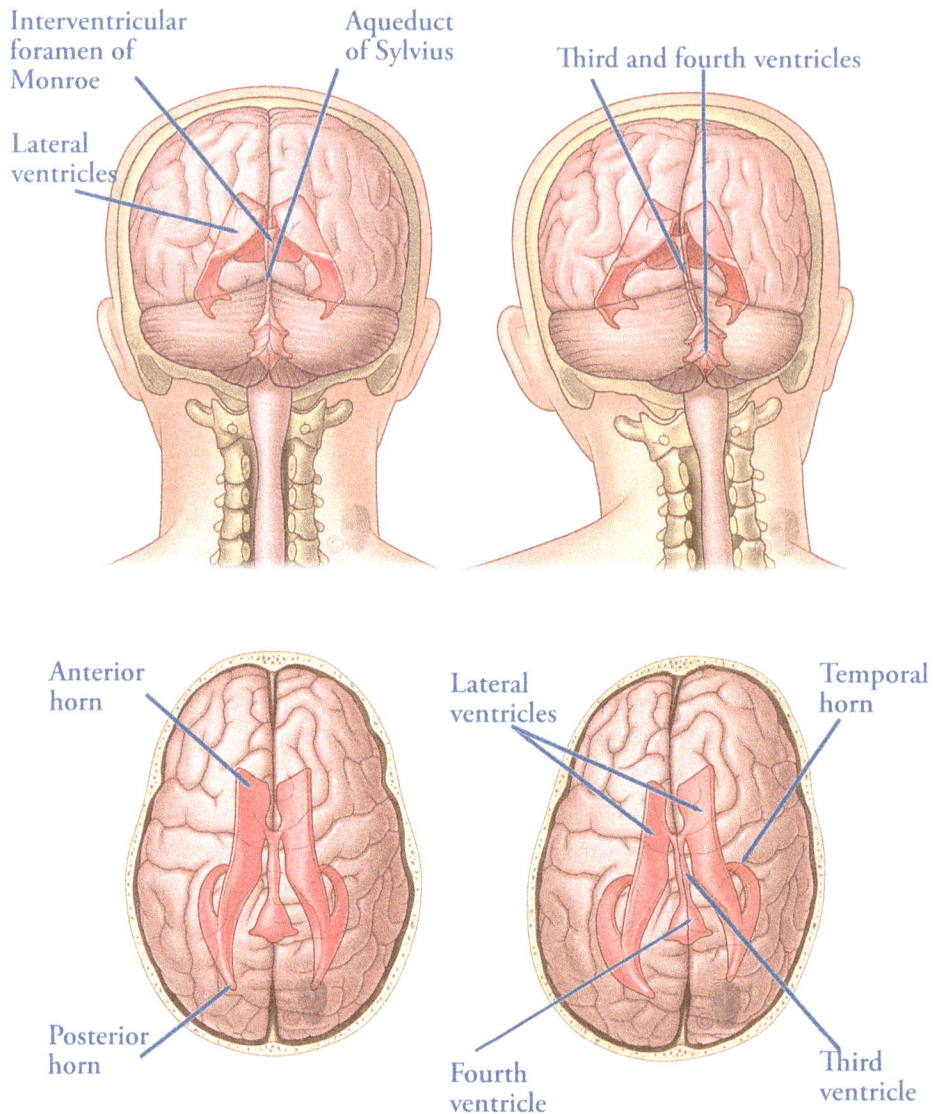

Figure 3.2 Posterior (top) and Lateral (bottom) Views of the Ventricles:
Textbook symmetry (left), traumatic asymmetry (right)

The brain vesicles, the prosencephalon, the mesencephalon and the rhomencephalon basically form the fore brain, the midbrain and the hind brain. Within those structures are formed the ventricular system; the two lateral, and the third and fourth ventricles.

The ventricles produce CSF. The two lateral ventricles feed into the third ventricle through the interventricular foramen of Monro, and from the third to the forth ventricle by the aqueduct of Sylvius. From the forth ventricle, CSF flows laterally through the two apertures of Luschka and medially through the aperture of Magendie. Within the lining of each of the ventricles are areas known as choroid plexuses, which are derived as double layers of pia mater richly invested into tuft-like processes called the tela choroidea, which emerge from the linings of each of the four ventricles. The ventricles receive their vascular supply via the circle of Willis. The two lateral ventricles are fed by the internal carotid artery, the third ventricle by the basilar artery, and the fourth ventricle by the posterior inferior cerebellar arteries. These arteries are developed from embryonic mesenchyme of the third and fourth pharyngeal/branchial arches during the 4th and 5th weeks of embryogenesis

Once it leaves the dominant system CSF flows helically in a caudal direction around the spinal cord to the sacrum (the sacral bulb – dural arachnoid sac) and then in a cephalic direction into the cisterna and perivascular spaces of the brain. CSF is finally absorbed through the subarachnoid space by the arachnoid granulation into the superior sagittal sinus and then through the venous sinus system to the internal jugular vein, and finally the heart.

CONFLUENCE OF THE SINUSES

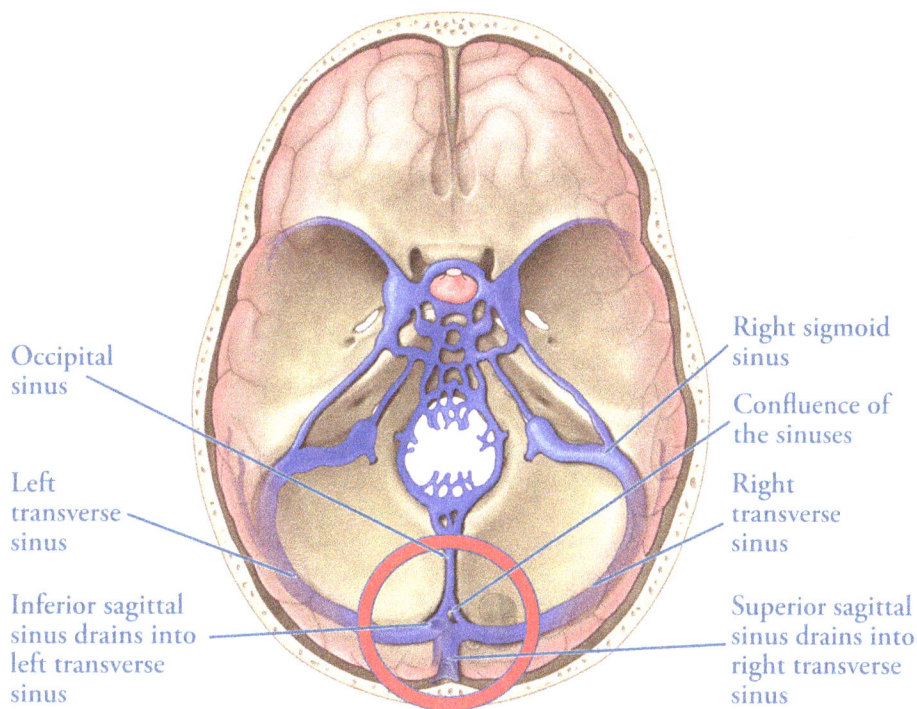

Occipital sinus

Left transverse sinus

Inferior sagittal sinus drains into left transverse sinus

Right sigmoid sinus

Confluence of the sinuses

Right transverse sinus

Superior sagittal sinus drains into right transverse sinus

Figure 3.3 Confluence of the Sinuses
Note the separate pathways of the superior and inferior sagittal sinuses

The confluences of any major communicating pathways are always designed to allow for maximum through flow of the specific entity that is required to move. The expectation is always to anticipate that free passage to exist, and when that passage is altered, the transport system is compromised and chaos ensues. The confluence of the sinuses is the junction point where the various venous sinuses drain.

Early anatomy illustrators and writers depict the "confluence of the sinuses" as the point where the superior sagittal sinus joins the right transverse sinus, the right sigmoid sinus and the right internal jugular vein, while the straight sinus and the occipital sinus join the left transverse sinus, the left sigmoid sinus and the left internal jugular vein. The author has noted that in more recent times these four vessels all converge at the "confluence of the sinuses" making the flow of venous blood an arbitrary selection depending on intracranial pressure and gradient (probably recently drawn from fMRI studies that show a venous congestion at that point, where the three major sinuses converge, in a congested brain).

However, illustrations by early anatomists – (probably more accurately informed by their knowledge of human dissection) – show a distinct flow of right-sided drainage and left-sided drainage. In addition some anatomical differences manifest occasional anastomotic joining of small sections of the straight sinus and the superior sagittal sinus, but with minor influence on the volume of either sinus. This underlines the theory that a benign asymmetric dural torque would facilitate a haemodynamic effect on cranial drainage by producing a helical motion of vascular blood. This flow moves in a counterclockwise movement out of the transverse sigmoid sinuses into both the internal jugular veins before arriving at the left and right brachiocephalic veins and into a right field superior vena cava to the heart. Indeed the vascular dimensions are larger on the right side of this drainage system, confirming the greater volume of blood flow through the superior sagittal sinus than that through the straight sinus.

THE VENOUS SINUS SYSTEM

Production and flow of CSF is essential to brain flotation, support and protection, as well as metabolic waste removal. The primary drainage route for the brain is the accessory drainage system through the foramen magnum emptying into the spinal canal of the cervical spine. Each vertebra in the spinal column contains its own vertebral venous plexus also referred to collectively as the axillary plexus, and basically acts as a supplementary reservoir for the brain. A giraffe, when feeding from the succulent leaves at the top of a tree, then bends forward to drink, a distance of possibly twenty or so feet, relies on the ballast tank at the end of its proboscis to allow blood to freely flow backwards and forwards to create a cranial balance. The human similarly relies on the axillary plexus to do the same.

The basilar plexus drains into the anterior vertebral venous plexus at the anterior rim of the foramen magnum. The sigmoid plexus drains partially into the lateral vertebral venous plexus, while the sub-occipital cavernous sinuses drain into the posterior vertebral venous plexus – all at the base of the foramen magnum.

The atlanto-occipital junction comes under immense restrictive pressure when the atlas and foramen magnum lose their juxtaposition, and the torsion of the cranial and spinal dura at that junction cause a restrictive flow between the brain and spinal cord. The membrane which encapsulates the peripheral vertebral venous plexus around that junction – the atlanto-occipital membrane – torsionstwists and warps under influence of the cranio fascial distortion and compromises the valveless flow of these vessels as well as the vertebral arteries – a major congestion area at the base of the brain.

THE VERTEBRAL VENOUS PLEXUS

The VVP is the accessory drainage inside the spinal canal. None of these veins have valves to prevent the backflow of venous blood as elsewhere in the body – blood can flow in either direction according to prevailing pressure gradients. The primary respiratory mechanism facilitates CSF flow, as well as the cerebral perfusion pressure (CPP), which is the difference between the arterial pressure in the anterior and posterior blood supply going into the brain and the venous blood in the superior sagittal sinus known as the SSVP (superior sagittal venous pressure). Venous blood, which is generally cooler than arterial blood, is warmed by the passage of the vertebral and carotid arteries passing in close proximity to the venous drainage (at the atlanto-occipital membrane). Brain cooling is also facilitated by the emissary veins that link to veins in the face and scalp to the dural sinuses, and cooling is performed by radiation, convection and conduction. Production and flow of CSF is essential to brain flotation, support and protection, as well as metabolic waste removal.

The primary drainage route for the brain is the accessory drainage system through the foramen magnum emptying into the spinal canal of the cervical spine, and the occipital marginal sinus system, which drains into the vertebral venous plexus.

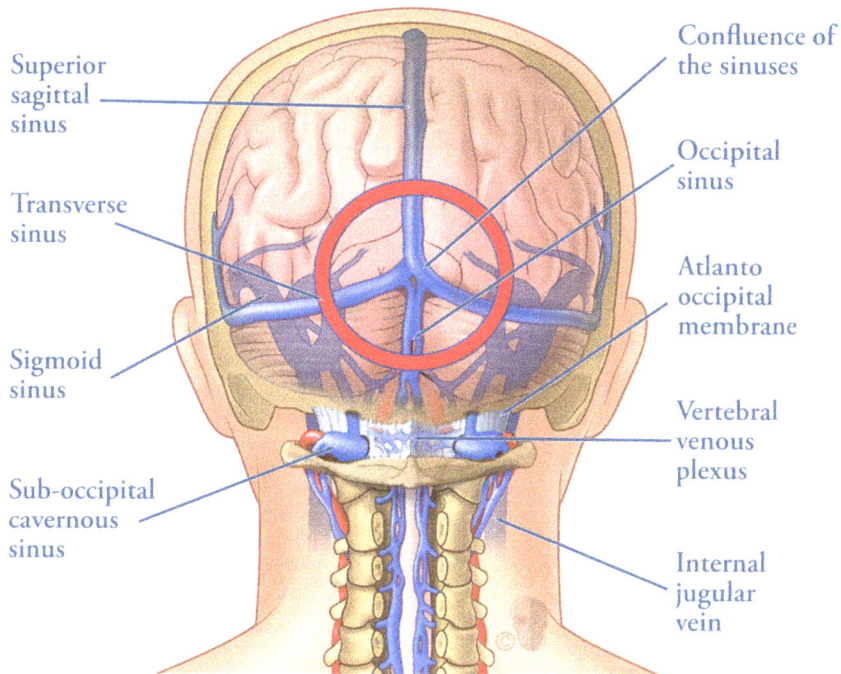

Figure 3.4 Vertebral Venous Plexus
Note the separate pathways of the superior and inferior sagittal sinuses

RECIPROCAL TENSION MEMBRANES

The meningeal dura also form what are called the RTM, the four membranes which act as sagittal, vertical and horizontal partitions providing structural stability within the cranial vault.

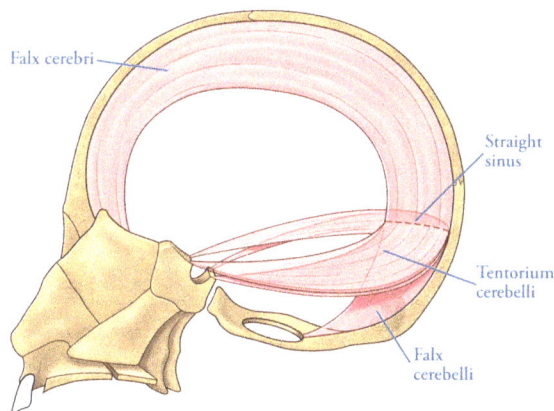

Figure 3.5 Reciprocal Tension Membranes

The Anterior Pole

The falx cerebri separates the two cerebral hemispheres, the left and right brain and anchors anteriorly at the crista galli of the ethmoid bone, forming the 'anterior pole' of the RTM. It is sickle-shaped and acts as a sagittal dynamic vector anchoring posteriorly at the internal occipital protuberance forming the straight sinus, becoming continuous with the falx cerebelli – the vertical dynamic vector separating the left and right cerebellar hemispheres.

The falx cerebri and the falx cerebelli as a vertical membrane anchored at the crista galli of the ethmoid, the superior sagittal suture, the straight sinus at the internal occipital protuberance and internal occipital crest.

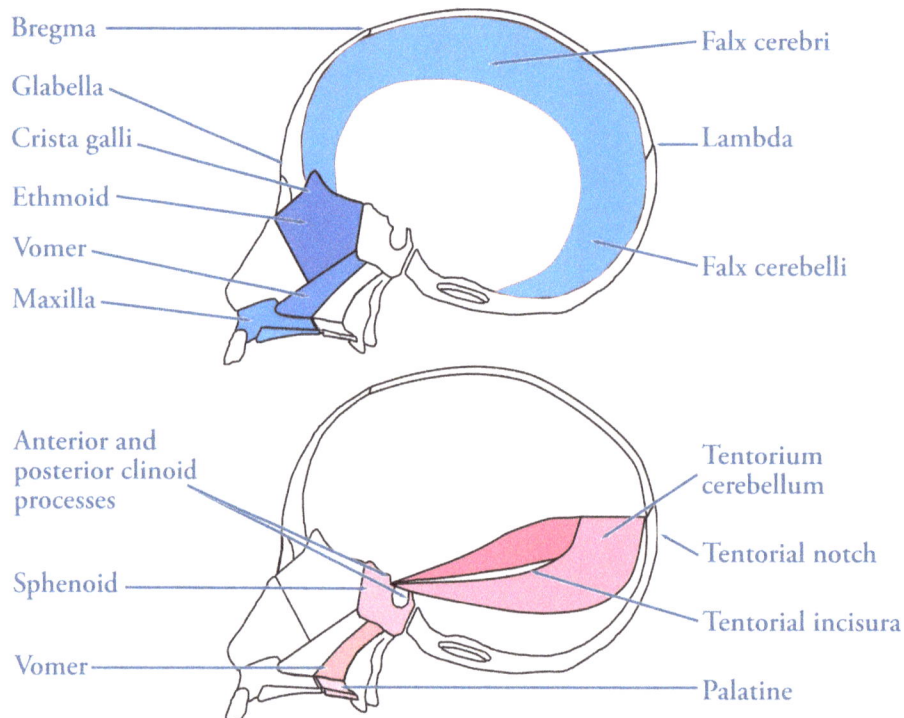

Figure 3.6 Anterior Pole (top), Posterior Pole (bottom)

The Posterior Pole

The junction of the straight sinus, with the great vein of Galen feeding in at the anterior end, and the confluence of the sinuses at the posterior, forms a cross or cruciate structure with the horizontal dynamic vector – the tentorium cerebelli, which anchors at the anterior and posterior clinoid processes of the sella turcica of the sphenoid body. The inferior aspect of the horizontal tentorium forms an oval opening called the 'tentorial incisura', which is occupied by, among other structures, the midbrain and the anterior part of the superior vermis, the cerebellum.

The tentorium cerebelli anchors into the occipital bone at the transverse sinuses and into the temporal bone at the petrous portion that contains the superior petrosal sinus.

The underside of the tentorium which is derived from the falx cerebelli, anchors at the posterior clinoid processes of the sphenoid bone, while the superior layer of the tentorium derived from the falx cerebri anchors at the anterior clinoid processes at the sphenoid bone – the sphenoid bone is the 'posterior pole' of the RTM. Between the anterior and the posterior clinoids of the sphenoid bone is anchored the diaphragma sellae which is a dural membrane which supports the hypophyseal stalk, the pituitary, and is thought to influence anterior and posterior pituitary function. The RTM are an extension of the periosteal and endosteal dural meningeal tissue – the external and internal cranial fascia.

At the apex of the petrous portion and beneath the cavernous sinus is a recess, which is created by an anterolateral evagination of the lower section of the tentorial membrane called the 'trigeminal cave'. The trigeminal cave (also known as Meckel's cave or cavum trigeminale) is an arachnoidal pouch containing CSF. It forms a dural encapsulation with the roots and sensory ganglia of the trigeminal ganglion. Cranio fascial torsion will distort the trigeminal cave and compress the trigeminal ganglion, on the right internal temporal bone. Adjacent structures include the tentorial incisura, the jugular foramen and the carotid canal.

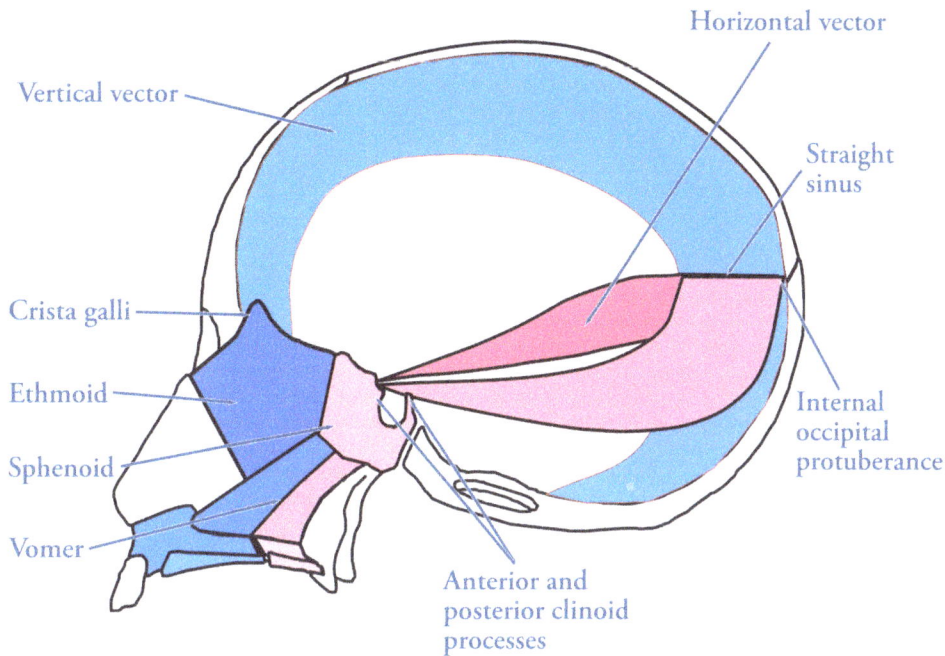

Figure 3.7 Anterior and Posterior Pole: Textbook balance with vertical and horizontal vectors

ACTIVATION OF MEMBRANES BY FLEXION AND EXTENSION

Inhalation and exhalation phases of respiration cause the RTM to flex and extend in the various phases of respiration. The primary respiratory mechanism activated by diaphragmatic function, causes the occiput to move into external rotation on the inhalation phase while the sacrum moves into the flexed position, with the sacral apex coming forward, tightening the spinal cord and reducing its length as the balance of the reciprocal membranes are pulled into the cranium. Flexion of the occiput drives the temporal bones into external rotation, activating the petrous portions, elevating the greater wings of the sphenoid and bringing the frontal bones into external rotation. The parietal bones also flex, activating the superior sagittal sinus, the pacchionian bodies and the arachnoid granulations to assist venous drainage into the superior sagittal sinus, the confluence of the sinuses, then into the transverse and sigmoid sinuses into the internal jugular vein. The entire membrane system flexes activating venous sinus drainage. This entire process is reversed on the exhalation phase, resulting in the balance of the membranes being pulled out of the cranium, as the spinal cord lengthens and the sacral apex moves posterior into extension.

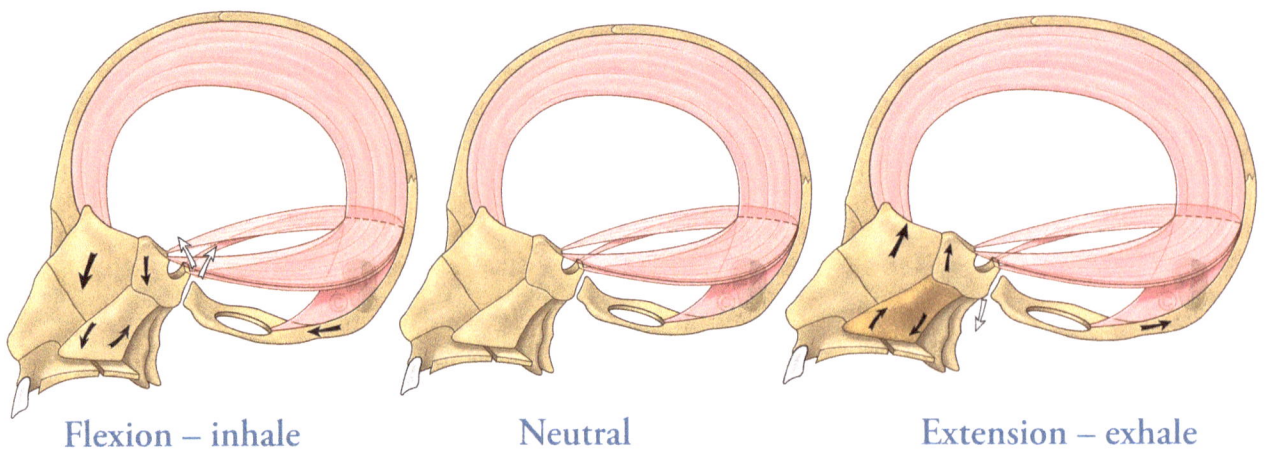

| Flexion – inhale | Neutral | Extension – exhale |

Figure 3.8 Cranial Motion with Respiratory Phases

At the junction of the ethmoid (anchor of the anterior pole) and the sphenoid body (anchor of the posterior pole) the two bones have a sutural intersection allowing them to flex and extend with one another, as well as being able to rotate laterally on their common axis (not unlike placing the knuckles of opposing clenched fists together at the index and middle fingers where flexion and extension and lateral rotation can be achieved). This junction has a common bone – the vomer – which connects the inferior body of the ethmoid at the anterior margin, the sephnoid body at its superior margin, the anterior pterygoid plates of the sephnoid bone at the posterior margin and the maxillae and palatines at its inferior margin. The vomer, made of membrane, works by pulling the various bones that it attaches to rather than pushing them, and acts like a tarpaulin so is very thin, and undergoes a degree of torsion in its activity. The superior and inferior borders are made of cartilage which allows for a firm attachment and anchor point at the ethmoid/sphenoid and the maxillae/palatine borders, while in between, the major part of the vomer is made up of membrane.

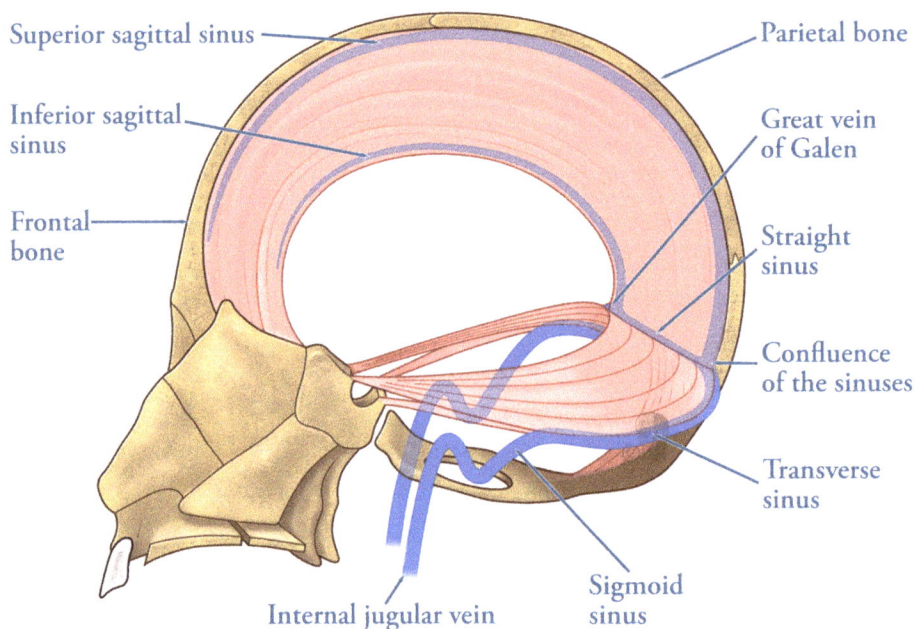

Figure 3.9 Sinuses Encapsulated in Dural Membrane

It is important to mention at this juncture the sphenobasilar mechanism, and why in reading cranial texts there is some confusion about its importance. In the neonate, the sphenobasilar junction is an important synchondrosis, as it lies at that point of the skull where an enormous amount of growth and development are taking place.

As mentioned earlier, a complex collection of dura, endosteum and periosteum converge at that point. These and the spinal dural attachments at the foramen magnum and the atlas are all dynamics that require movement, compensation and adaption to allow particularly the brainstem, pons and cerebellum to develop, along with the association, projection and radiation fibres. Around the end of puberty, the sphenobasilar synchondrosis starts to fuse forming one bone – the sphenoid with the occiput, which fuses between the ages of 18 to 25 years. Therefore in the adult skull, there is no joint at the sphenobasilar junction, so cranial motion, initiated from the anterior and posterior poles, relies totally on the falx cerebri, (and the falx cerebelli) and the tentorium cerebelli. These should be regarded as two dynamic membranes, vertical and horizontal, controlling the RTM, without interference from a sphenobasilar synchondrosis. As the sphenoid/occiput go into flexion, the sphenoid body moves superiorwardpulling the posterior part of the vomer superior and consequently pulls the palatines superior, taking the palatines into internal rotation. Conversely, the ethmoid bone is pulled inferior by the anterior part of the vomer, tightening the falx cerebri (and the falx cerebelli), while the dynamic of the anterior vomer allows the maxillae to relax and go into external rotation. The maxillae and the palatines are paired bones, joined at the intermaxillary and interpalatine sutures. The two maxillae and the two palatines are separated by the cruciate suture. This entire process is reversed on the exhalation phase, reversing the dynamics of the vomer and its importance in the integrity of the anterior and posterior poles.

The ethmoid plate, a continuation of the crista galli, is also an extension of the vomer, so the vertical anchorage of the falx cerebri is substantial, and why occlusal activity of the maxillae and palatines – the upper jaw – with the mandible – the lower – have such an influence on the RTM. For example, a monolateral bite (chewing on the same side continually) will change the palate, the vomer, the ethmoid, the falx cerebri, the superior sagittal sinus drainage and so on. This is why occlusion plays such a major role in cranial bio-physiology.

THE CAVERNOUS AND INTERCAVERNOUS SINUSES

The anterior and inferior sinuses involve the cavernous and intercavernous sinuses and their drainage into the basilar, superior and inferior petrosal sinuses, is an integral part of brain cooling. Most of this drainage involves the sphenoid body, the pterygoid plates (part of the anterior sphenoid body) and the basilar part of the occiput. Changes in the cranio fascial dynamic distort all these areas, particularly those driven by the tentorium cerebelli, and drainage can be inhibited, causing congestion at the pituitary.

VENOUS DRAINAGE

The anterior superior drainage through the superior sagittal and inferior sagittal sinuses, along with the diploic veins, is activated through the falx cerebri as the main vertical membrane that services this drainage process. Changes to the tentorium cerebelli at the sphenoid change the dynamics at the falx cerebri and the falx cerebelli, and therefore affect the anterior and posterior poles and the efficiency of the drainage process, causing congestion in the cerebrum and central cranial organs. This involves the cingulated gyrus, the corpus callosum, the fornix, the caudate nucleus and the hippocampus. This sort of distortion is seldom a singular event and can persist for years, laying, the foundation for extreme congestion later in life.

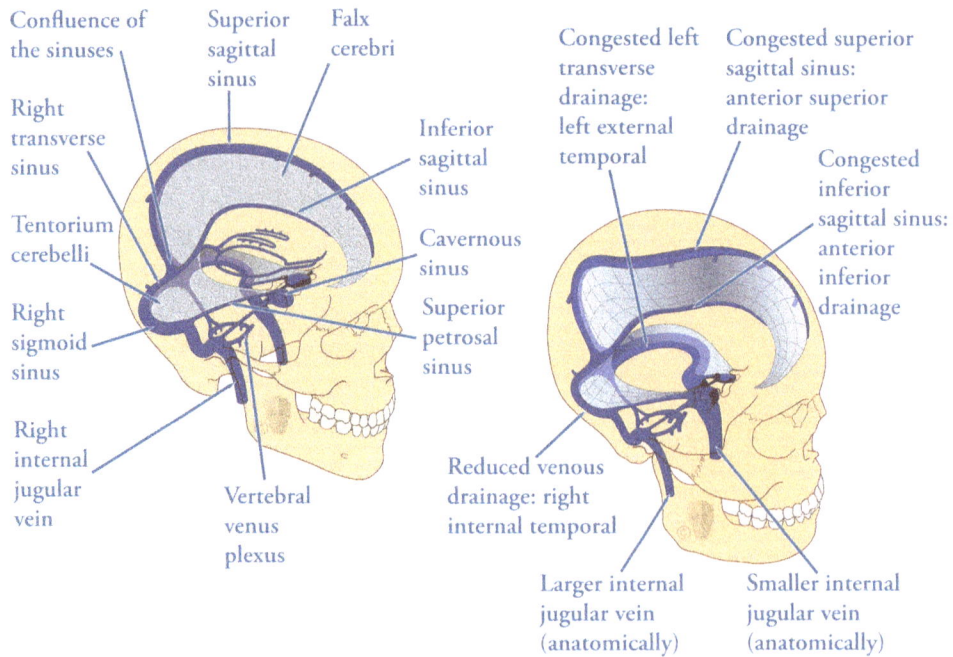

Labels (left figure):
Confluence of the sinuses
Superior sagittal sinus
Falx cerebri
Right transverse sinus
Inferior sagittal sinus
Tentorium cerebelli
Cavernous sinus
Right sigmoid sinus
Superior petrosal sinus
Right internal jugular vein
Vertebral venus plexus

Labels (right figure):
Congested left transverse drainage: left external temporal
Congested superior sagittal sinus: anterior superior drainage
Congested inferior sagittal sinus: anterior inferior drainage
Reduced venous drainage: right internal temporal
Larger internal jugular vein (anatomically)
Smaller internal jugular vein (anatomically)

Figure 3.10 Complete Venous Sinus Drainage: Textbook symmetry (left), corrupted (right) Counterclockwise traumatic torque of the brain

SUPERIOR AND INFERIOR DRAINAGE

When the dural membranes are under the influence of cranio fascial distortion and accumulated trauma takes its toll, drainage issues become paramount.

The superior and inferior pathways become more congested, not only as detailed above, but also the final drainage of vessels including the straight sinus, the occipital sinus and the confluences of the sinuses. The right drainage process is significantly reduced at the right transverse, sigmoid sinuses and the right internal jugular vein, as the right temporal and occipital bones move more into internal rotation, closing the right jugular foramen. The left transverse, sigmoid sinuses and the left internal jugular vein become more congested by the overload of the left drainage process, and so together the drainage pathways become equally compromised.

THE DURAL MEMBRANE SUPPORT SYSTEM

The anterior and posterior poles of the RTM, which are responsible for cranial drainage, are further frustrated, not only by the cranio fascial torque, but also the accumulation of other life-changing factors. As a person ages, one has to consider relevant details of chemical interjection – pharmaceuticals, diet, vaccinations and antibiotics – that contain elements that cross the blood brain barrier, the retention of cytotoxic oedema, the congestion of ventricular sustainability and, of course, drainage efficiency. All these matters will be discussed in later chapters.

CONCLUSION

This chapter defines and discusses the venous sinus system, and its intricate involvement with cranial, and more specifically, brain drainage.

Venous sinus system

The venous sinus system is made up of continuous connective fascia – dural meningeal tissue. The dural membranes totally support and encapsulate the entire venous sinus system. After its passage through the ventricles, CSF leaves the forth ventricle and enters the subarachnoid spaces.

Ventricles

The brain vesicles, the prosencephalon, the mesencephalon and the rhomencephalon basically form the fore brain, the midbrain and the hind brain. Within those structures are formed the ventricular system; the two lateral, and the third and fourth ventricles.

Confluence of the sinuses

The confluence of the sinuses is the junction point where the various venous sinuses drain. It is the point where the superior sagittal sinus joins the right transverse sinus, the right sigmoid sinus and the right internal jugular vein, while the straight sinus and the occipital sinus join the left transverse sinus, the left sigmoid sinus and the left internal jugular vein.

Vertebral venous plexus

The VVP is the accessory drainage inside the spinal canal. None of these veins have valves to prevent the backflow of venous blood as elsewhere in the body – blood can flow in either direction according to prevailing pressure gradients. The primary respiratory mechanism facilitates CSF flow, as well as the CPP, which is the difference between the arterial pressure in the anterior and posterior blood supply going into the brain and the venous blood in the superior sagittal sinus known as the SSVP (superior sagittal venous pressure).

Reciprocal tension membranes

The meningeal dura also forms the four RTM, which act as sagittal, vertical and horizontal partitions promoting equilibrium within the cranial vault.

Anterior pole – the falx cerebri and the falx cerebelli anchors at the crista galli of the ethmoid, the superior sagittal suture to the straight sinus at the internal occipital protuberance.

Posterior pole – the tentorium cerebelli anchor at the anterior and posterior clinoid processes of the sphenoid, the petrous portion of the temporal bone to the straight sinus and finally to the internal occipital protuberance.

Activation of membranes by flexion and extension

Inhalation and exhalation phases of respiration cause the RTM to flex and extend in the various phases of respiration. The primary respiratory mechanism is activated by diaphragmatic function.

At the junction of the ethmoid (anchor of the anterior pole) and the sphenoid body (anchor of the posterior pole) the two bones have a sutural intersection. This allows them to flex and extend with one another, as well as being able to laterally rotate with each other on their common axis (not unlike placing the knuckles of opposing clenched fists together at the index and middle fingers where flexion and extension and lateral rotation can be achieved).

Cavernous and intercavernous sinuses

The anterior and inferior sinuses involve the cavernous and intercavernous sinuses, and their drainage into the basilar, superior and inferior petrosal sinuses, which is an integral part of brain cooling.

Venous drainage

The anterior superior drainage through the superior and inferior sagittal sinuses, along with the diploic veins, is activated through the falx cerebri as the main vertical membrane that services this drainage process. Changes to the tentorium cerebelli at the sphenoid alter the dynamics at the falx cerebri and the falx cerebelli, therefore affecting the anterior and posterior poles and the efficiency of the drainage process, causing congestion in the cerebrum and central cranial organs.

Superior and inferior drainage

When the dural membranes are under the influence of cranio fascial distortion and accumulated trauma takes its toll, drainage issues become paramount.

Dural membrane support system

The anterior and posterior poles of the RTM, which are responsible for cranial drainage, are further frustrated, not only by the cranio fascial torque, but by the accumulation of other life-changing factors.

CHAPTER 4

CONGESTION OF THE UPPER CERVICAL SPINE

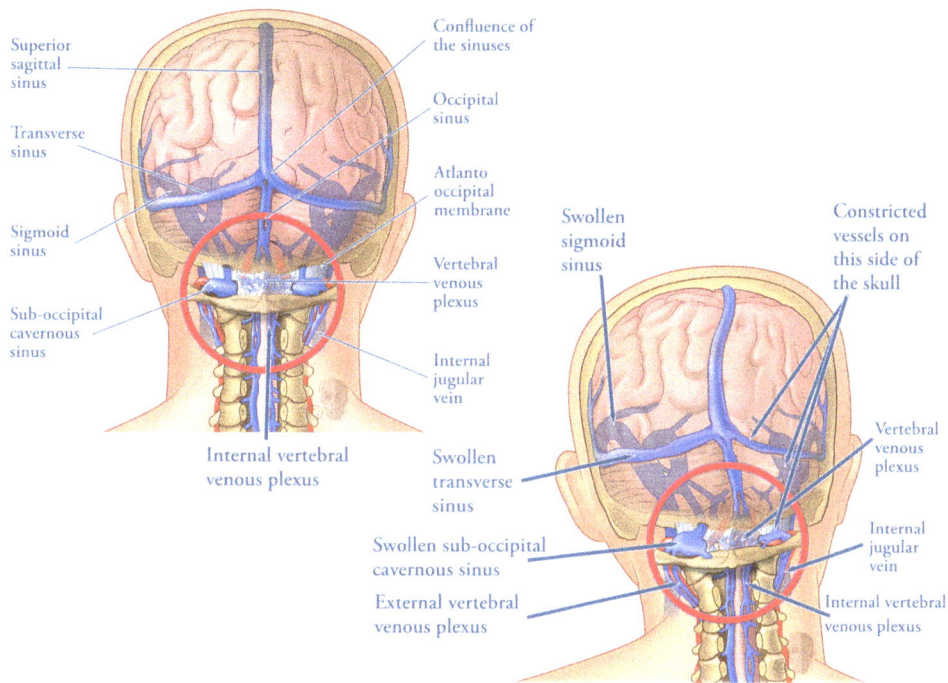

Figure 4.1 Complex Accessory Drainage Plexus (left); Distorted Pathway (right)
Note the separate pathways of the superior and inferior sagittal sinuses

Damage to the fragile junction of the brain and spine at the atlas occipital junction causes most disruption to the drainage mechanism of the brain. With so many vessels, both arterial and venous, as well as the spinal cord and the brainstem traversing the foramen magnum, this area has warranted scrutiny by many anatomists and physiologists over the years to try and alleviate the congestion in this complex area.

The main drainage vessels include: the vertebral venous plexus which lines the ring of the foramen magnum, draining into the axillary plexus which drains down into the spine; the transverse and sigmoid sinuses which drain into the internal jugular veins; and the sub-occipital cavernous sinuses which also drain into the axillary plexus. The arterial distribution in this delicate junction includes the two vertebral arteries and the common carotid arteries, which provide the inflow to the brain of arterial blood.

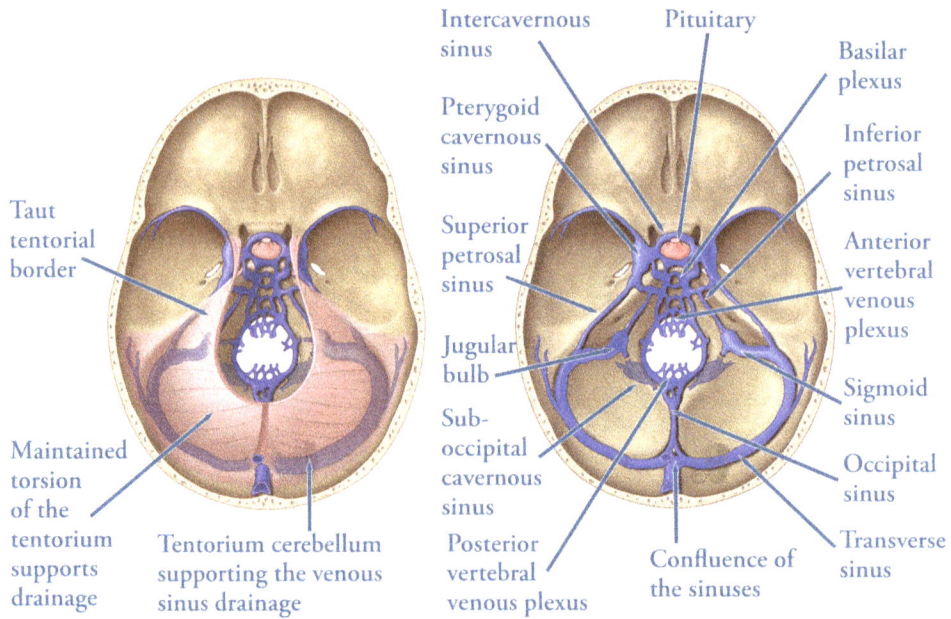

Figure 4.2 Brain Irrigation; Venous Return Drainage (right)

The four main concerns of obstruction in this area are outlined as follows:

a. Birth trauma
b. Whiplash injuries
c. Dental malocclusion
d. Chiari malformation

BIRTH TRAUMA

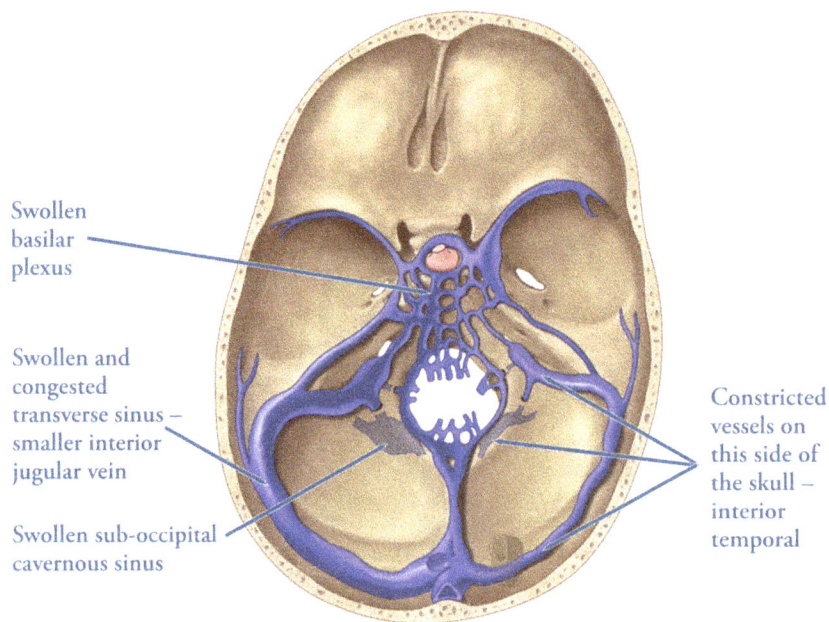

Figure 4.3 Loss of drainage ability

One of the main factors possibly causing birth trauma is the higher frequency and clinical acceptance of induced births.

For various reasons, whether due to the pressure on obstetric departments, the number of available midwives, medical concern over late births or wishes of the parents, birth induction has become more common.

Arguably an induced birth by its very nature, is forced on mother and baby, potentially resulting in a 'train smash'. It increases the likelihood of the baby becoming stuck and unable to make the passage of birth on its own with the help of the mother. The foetal head goes directly into the pelvic ring without any normal gentle contractions, and the maternal muscles contract and tear at the sudden onset of the unwanted intrusion. The introduction of assisted delivery comes into play, with the tearing of the birth canal – possibly both anteriorly and posteriorly – or an episiotomy being performed which, if not repaired properly has the effect of permanent damage to the mother, both in elimination functions and intercourse for the rest of her life, unless reconstructive surgery is performed. Damage to the upper cervical vertebrae and the neonate cranium from the use of forceps, ventouse or emergency caesarean section, becomes a contentious issue. The result of this damage causes drainage issues with the VVP, emissary veins, the axillary plexus and the internal jugular veins. This blockage effect causes backup pressure through the venous system, back into the cranium causing intracranial pressure.

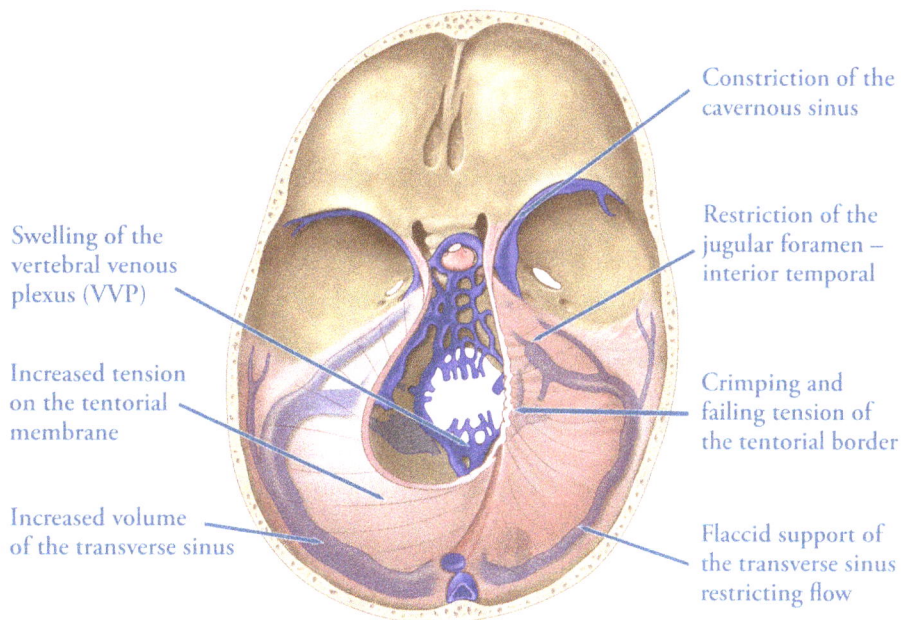

Constriction of the cavernous sinus

Restriction of the jugular foramen – interior temporal

Swelling of the vertebral venous plexus (VVP)

Increased tension on the tentorial membrane

Crimping and failing tension of the tentorial border

Increased volume of the transverse sinus

Flaccid support of the transverse sinus restricting flow

Figure 4.4 Irrigation Congestion

Forceps Delivery

In short, the mother, through anaesthesia, is not able to feel or push. One must question whether the epidural crosses the placental barrier and what affects it has on the baby. The child is distressed and the tissues are tearing, so a forceps delivery could be considered. Forceps are placed bilaterally over the temporal, parietal and sphenoidal area. Traction is applied in line with the axis of the pelvis, and delivery is effected by the head anteriorly and rotationally. The pressure of the forceps blades over the pterion area causes sutural jamming at the fronto-parietal-temporo area (coronal and squamosal) and the greater wing of the sphenoid, locking the sphenobasilar mechanism, and the body of the sphenoid – sella turcica, optic chiasma, superior orbital fissure, diaphragma sellae and tentorial attachments – the 'posterior pole'. It may also result in considerable maternal laceration, urethral rupture, and bladder and bowel damage. Foetal damage may also involve facial bruising and nerve damage, intercranial haemorrhage, and a loss in cranio fascial dynamics (CFD).

Ventouse Delivery

The alternative to forceps delivery is the application of a suction cap to the foetal scalp with extraction by traction. The suction cap is placed posterior to the bregma on the superior sagittal suture and traction applied with contractions and a rotation of the head, as it is pulled onto the pelvic floor. Laceration of the scalp and haematoma may be the result of ventouse extraction. Causing vacuum pressure on the superior sagittal suture may affect the superior sagittal sinus, the arachnoid granulation, and the pacchionian bodies, effecting CSF drainage. This results in changes of intercranial pressure and loss of homeostasis.

Caesarean Section

Finally, if both these methods do not achieve the objective, an emergency caesarean is performed. The child is removed from the uterus by a direct incision though the abdominal wall and uterus. Once the infant's head has been located in the birth canal, it has to be freed and then pulled cephalad, turned and removed from the abdominal cavity.

All three of these methods can cause irreparable damage to the infant skull, changing the internal dynamics of the fascia, changing the production, circulation and absorption of CSF. The internal cranial bones – the temporal, the ethmoid (anterior pole) and sphenoidal bones (posterior pole) – become distorted in their formation resulting in cranial nerve damage. Reciprocal tension membranes torque, reducing sensory communication in the limbic system, transcranial communication with the corpus callosum and possible damage to the amygdala and hippocampus.

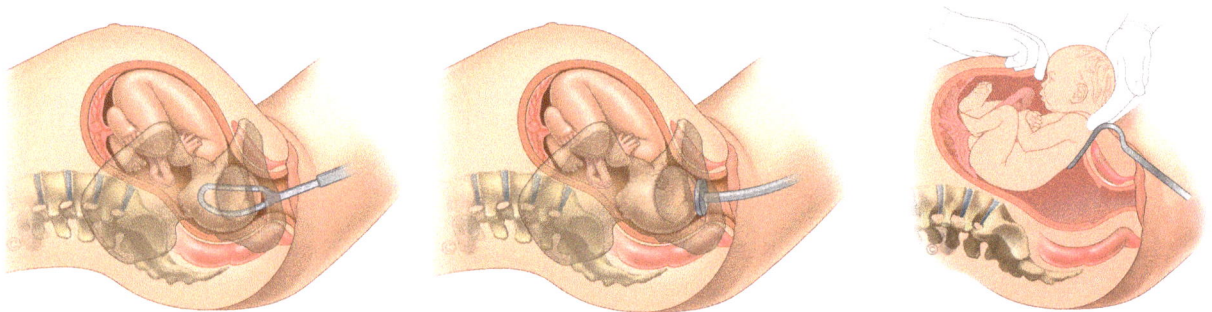

Figure 4.5 (left) Forceps Trauma: Compressing the parietal, temporal and sphenoid;
(centre) Ventouse Trauma: Pressure on the superior sagittal sinus, bregma and lambda;
(right) Caesarean Trauma: Vaginal delivery not possible – emergency or elective

Conclusion of Birth Trauma

In a normal uninterrupted birth process where mother and baby are allowed to go to full term, skull moulding allows the cranio fascial dynamic to respond and reflex back to a normal position, allowing the RTM, the ventricular system, the venous sinus system and the entire dural meningeal system, to respond to the compression of the birth process. Induction means that a collision between the baby's skull and the internal maternal pelvis might cause obvious catastrophic damage. Foetal and maternal distress is complicated by the fact that the pelvic floor resists the passage of the infant skull. Internal fascia dynamics change and become distorted, sensory input is dulled by anaesthetic epidurals. Once the foetal head has made its presentation there is an inability for the cranio fascial dynamic to spring back into the position that the body requires for homeostasis function. The anterior and posterior poles become permanently distorted and the neurological implications are huge and persist for life. Chiropractic and dental treatment remain impervious to change unless 'brain balancing' occurs, to reinstate the CFD . Obstetricians may have limited options when faced with a difficult/problematic birth.

FACIAL CHANGES AND THE INFANT SKULL

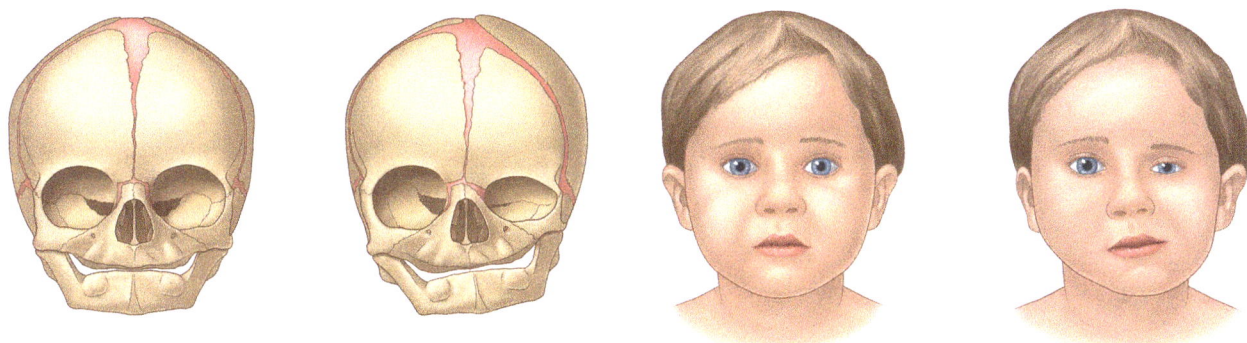

Figure 4.6 Infant Skull and Cranio Fascial Distortion

By examining Figure 4.6 distortions in the facial expression of the child are immediately obvious. The eye on the right is large, involved and engaging, while its counterpart has moved posteriorly, is smaller and not part of the intellectual composition. Similarly, the left ear is flared, there is a clear left deviation of the mandible – changing the occlusion, a high cheek on the left and the flat expansive cheek on the right.

The vaginal compression of the baby's body down the birth canal, helps kick-start the natural maturation of the infant reflexes, allowing proper neural development to take place. The very act of giving birth through the vagina stimulates the production of oxytocin – the hormone known to play a primary role throughout the whole birthing process, as it floods the mother's brain with powerful maternal signals. Breastfeeding is often easier with a natural birth, possibly because of the better psychological bonding between mother and child after a natural delivery.

Vaginal deliveries also activate another hormone – prolactin – a gonadotrophic hormone secreted by the anterior lobe of the pituitary, which decreases the levels of oestrogen, increases the levels of progesterone, promotes lactation by stimulating the alveoli of the mammary glands and contributes to surfactant synthesis to increase healthy lung function after birth. The sheer physical pressure on the baby being expelled through the birth canal improves lung function by expelling extravenous fluids from the baby's lungs in preparation for initial breaths of oxygen.

As the foetal head accomplishes the expulsion phase and exits through the pelvis, there is a spring back effect on the frontal, parietal and occiput bones. The compression of the occiput and frontal bones underneath the parietals means that the falx cerebri and the falx cerebelli become compressed towards one another and the tentorium becomes horizontally extended. The endosteal and meningeal fascia become taut, pulling with them the periosteal external dura and the dural membranes (the pia, the arachnoid and the dura mater) of the spinal meningeal system. With the entire fascial system under torsion, skull moulding takes place, and the internal dynamics of the fascia spring back in an almost elastic type dynamic – like a cork coming out of a champagne bottle – which activates the dominant system, the venous sinus system, the RTM, the cranial floor, the ethmoid, ('anterior pole'), the sphenoid, ('posterior pole'), the temporals, the occiput, the spinal dura, diaphragm, pelvic floor and the entire fascial system.

WHIPLASH TRAUMA

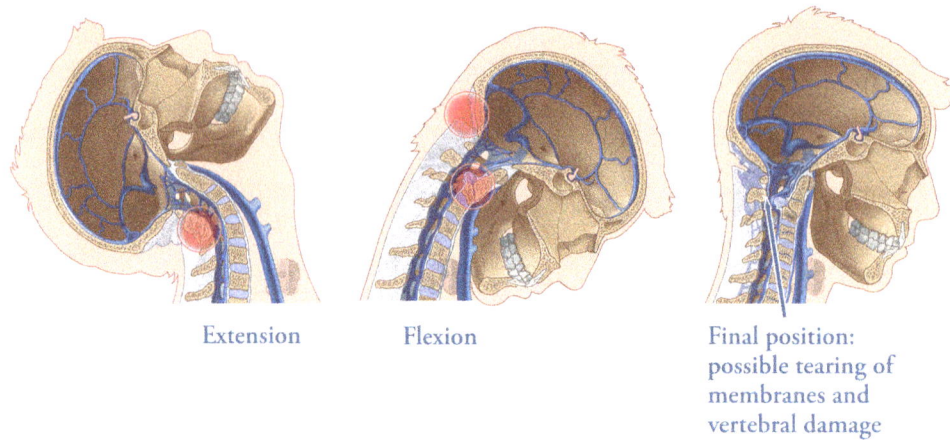

Extension   Flexion   Final position: possible tearing of membranes and vertebral damage

Figure 4.7 Whiplash Injury

Whiplash injury is the violent acceleration/deceleration of the head and the spine, with inevitable lifelong consequences. Whiplash is not only a type of trauma received in a vehicle accident or the severe trauma seen in contact sports, but may even be caused by an over-exuberant father throwing an infant up into the air and catching it. This subtle damage usually occurs when the infant is not weight-bearing. It lacks maturity in development of the spinal and cervical muscles, so the head and neck become flexed and extended in a nanosecond, normal muscular recovery being completeletly prevented by the immaturity of its reflexes.

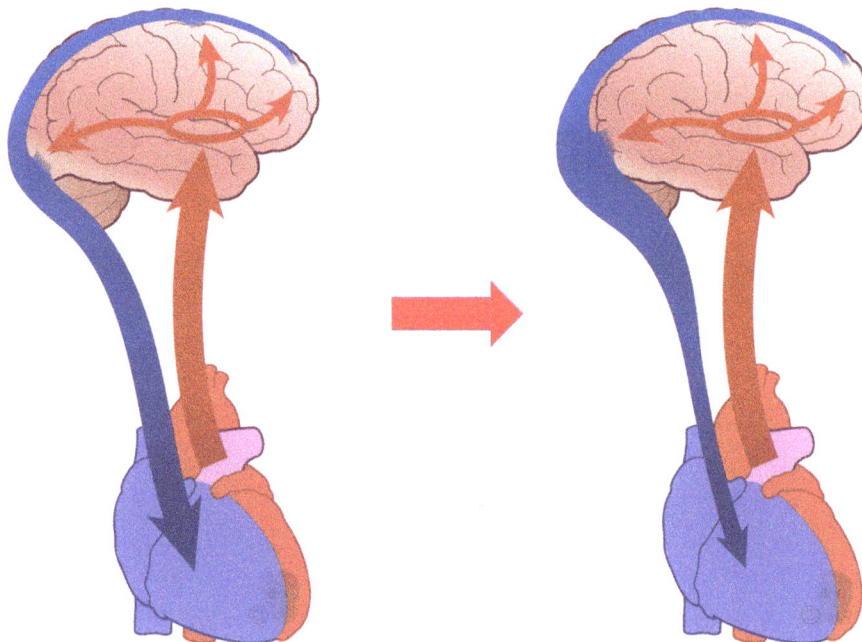

Figure 4.8 Whiplash Reduces Brain Drainage

The consequences in all these types of injuries, extreme or subtle, can have a severe effect on:

- The brain first being forced posteriorly (acceleration), crashing into the occiput, and then anteriorly (deceleration), by collision with the frontal bone, contusing the brain tissue, often severely enough to cause haematomas
- The dural meningeal tissues – which become stretched, can often tear away from their insertion and anchor points, disturbing their equilibrium and the dynamics that hold the brain in position. More importantly the central (midline) components – the cerebral cortex, the corpus callosum, the fornix, the hippocampus, the amygdala, the thalamus, the caudate nucleus, the cingulate gyrus, the pons and the cerebellum – may also be compromised
- The venous sinus system – brain swelling and fascial disturbance from the trauma will disrupt brain drainage and create obstruction to the venous flow out of the brain – oedema retention, the spinal column – stretching the pre and post zygapophyseal joints, the anterior and posterior common ligaments, the spinal dura, spinal nerve roots, the inter-vertebral foramina, the spinal canal and the composition of the inter-vertebral discs and their position, changing the lordosis into a kyphosis. The atlanto-occipital membrane – obstructing the vertebral arteries, the vertebral venous plexus, the internal jugular vein (through the jugular foramen), the brainstem and the cranial and spinal dura. The sacrum and sacroiliac joints – the adverse reciprocal movement of the occiput and atlas, have a profound effect on the L5-S1 junction, and change the pelvic balancing ability at the sacroiliac joints, changing pelvic and spinal equilibrium.

DENTAL MALOCCLUSION

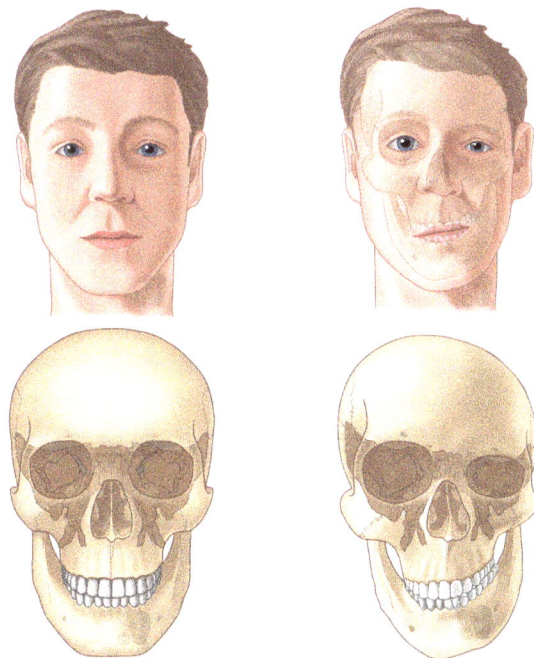

Figure 4.9 Dental Malocclusion: Facial distortion
Left eye closes down as a result of the depression of the left greater wing of the sphenoid, which pulls the right occiput and temporal bone internally and closes the right jugular foramen – possibly caused by a lack of posterior dental support

Each tooth in its alveolus, both upper and lower jaws, is connected and dedicated to a visceral organ, a muscle group and thereby its corresponding neurological supply. In a normal homeostatic occlusion, the teeth come together and occlude at the bucal cusps simultaneously, symmetrically and with the same force evenly on each cusp of the tooth. This is a smooth, non-frictional encounter of symphonic acoustic precision. This occlusion resets the brain between 2,000 and 2,500 times a day when one swallows and masticates, putting the mandibular condyle within the mandibular (glenoid) fossa in a superior anterior position, which enables the condyle to articulate on the articular disc at its superior pole. This resting effect includes all the cusps of each tooth and their relationship on each organ, their nerve supply and their corresponding muscle groups through the trigeminal ganglion – there are three sensory nuclei and one motor nucleus of the trigeminal nerve found in the brainstem; the sensory nuclei comprise the mesencephalic nucleus, the nucleus of the descending tract, and the principal sensory nucleus, but none is exclusive to the trigeminal nerve, all of them receive sensory inputs from other cranial nerves.

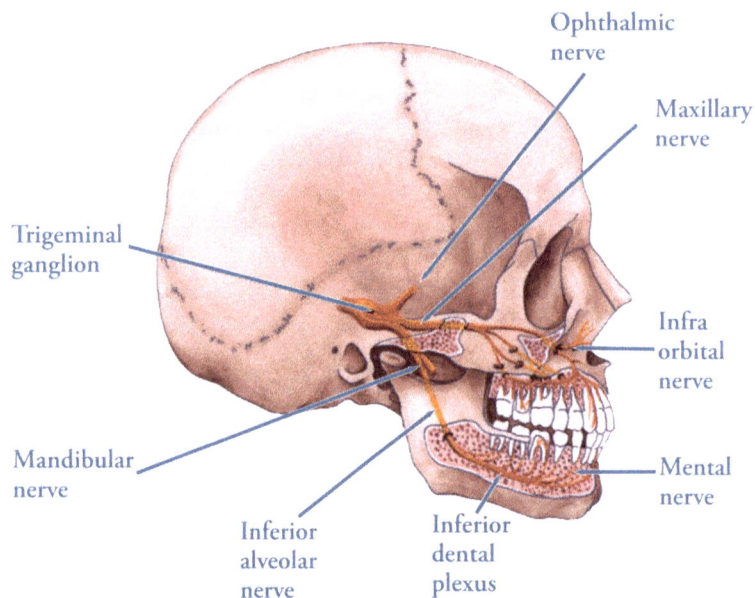

Figure 4.10 Trigeminal Nerve Distribution

The retrodiscal tissue – these tissues are highly vascularised, well innervated, loose connective tissue – posterior to the condyle that registers the condylar position within the temporomandibular joint (TMJ), and has neurological ties through the mandibular branch to the trigeminal ganglion, which lies just superior to the TMJ. When this occlusion establishes this juxtaposition, the mandibular, maxillary and ophthalmic branches of the trigeminal nerve are uninterrupted in their neurological pathways.

The sphenoid bone is the central bone in the cranium (posterior pole), articulating with the occiput posteriorly, and the maxillae and palatines with the ethmoid (anterior pole) anteriorly. It provides the orbit for the eye and at the superior orbital fissure supplies the cranial nerves to the eye.

The position of the pterygoid muscles is symmetric and balanced. The medial and lateral pterygoid muscles, are attached to the medial and lateral pterygoid plates respectively. Their action within the normal occlusion, allows the symmetric movement of the condyles to sit within the juxtaposition of their respective TMJs. This means that the muscles of mastication – the temporalis, the masseters and the buccinators – all establish an even and symmetric occlusion during mastication.

CRANIO FASCIAL DISTORTION FROM TRAUMA

When cranio fascial distortion takes place, the sphenoid bone moves out of its juxtaposition, the right greater wing of the sphenoid is elevated and rotated anteriorly, pulling the right temporal bone and occiput into internal rotation, while the left greater wing becomes depressed and rotates posteriorly taking the left temporal bone and occiput into external rotation. The pterygoid plates move and rotate with the sphenoid body, changing the muscle tonus and dynamic of the medial and lateral pterygoid muscles influencing the mandibular condyles within the mandibular fossa.

When, after dental malocclusion occurs, the maxillary and mandibular components are thrown out of synchronisation as well as the trigeminal ganglion.

The trigeminal ganglion activates the mesencephalic nucleus in the cortex, which then fires the spinal nucleus of the cervical spine moving the upper three cervical vertebrae, especially to the atlas, to try and re-establish a balance to the malocclusion. Dental malocclusions cause atlas subluxations.

Compression of the retrodiscal tissue causes temporomandibular joint dysfunction (TMJD), and with continual percussion of this area, affects the internal auditory meatus (the vestibulocochlear and acoustic VIII cranial nerves – balance and hearing), the tympanic membrane (causing tinnitus) and the auditory ossicles (the incus, malleus and stapes) causing distortion of hearing. TMJD is a dysfunctional, life-changing experience, which can then be exacerbated into trigeminal neuralgia, tic douloureux and Bell's palsy, all of which are devastating to the patient.

In conclusion, the action of the posterior position of the mandibular condyle in this malocclusion pulls the head forward, changing the cervical lordosis into a kyphosis, subluxating the atlas and possibly C2 and C3 (spinal dural attachments); distorts the atlanto occipital membrane and affects the vertebral venous drainage, the axillary plexus drainage, and the internal jugular vein drainage, restricting venous drainage from the brain, and arterial flow into the brain through the vertebral arteries.

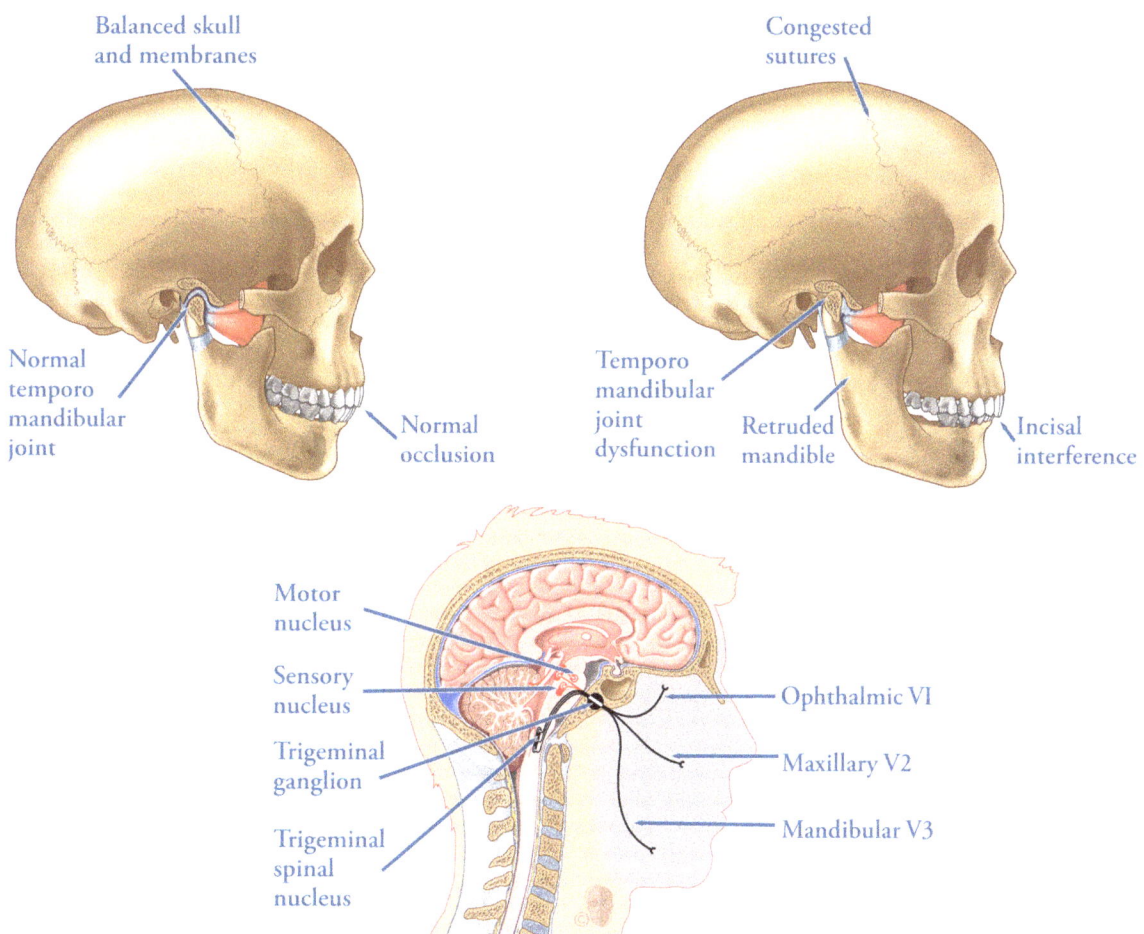

Figure 4.11 Trigeminal Balance: Normal occlusion (top left); malocclusion (top right); malocclusal effect on the trigeminal nerves (bottom)

CHIARI MALFORMATION

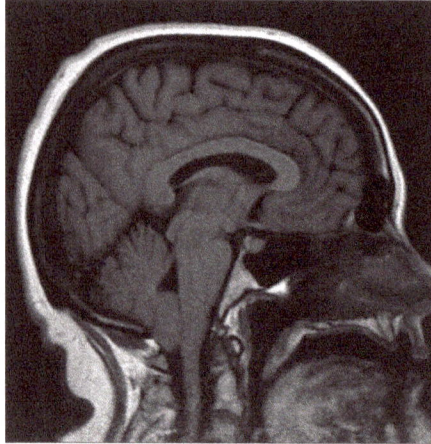

Figure 4.12 Chiari Malformation

This is a serious neurological disorder where the bottom part of the brain, the cerebellum, descends out of the skull and crowds the spinal cord, putting pressure on both the brain and spine and causing many symptoms. The brainstem sinks slightly into the foramen magnum, compresses the occipital marginal sinus system, the three cisterns, the vertebral arteries and the posterior and anterior spinal arteries, compressing the VVP of the accessory drainage system, causing localised venous congestion, hypertension & neurogenic claudication.

Mayo Clinic classifies the three main types of Chiari malformation as:

- Type I – occurs when the occiput is too small or deformed, the cerebellar tonsils are displaced, exerting pressure onto the upper spinal cord
- Type II – nearly always associated with a form of spina bifida (myelomeningocele), pushing the cerebellum into the upper spinal canal interfering with CSF flow
- Type III – occurs when the cerebellum or the brainstem extends through the foramen magnum and is diagnosed at birth or by an ultrasound during pregnancy.

The reason for the descent of the cerebellum and more specifically the cerebellar tonsils, is 'pressure conus', where the intracranial pressure becomes significant enough to push the cerebellum inferior to the only aperture in the cranium – the foramen magnum – to relieve pressure. The waterbed effect of the cisterna magna, the cisterna basalis and the cisterna pontis are severely diminished, as this fluid is pushed superiorward, back into the ventricular system, causing more cephalad pressure, and into the brain, exacerbating the effect of pressure on the conus. The brainstem sinks slightly into the foramen magnum, compresses the occipital marginal sinus system, the three cisterns, the vertebral arteries and the posterior and anterior spinal arteries, compressing the VVP of the accessory drainage system, causing localised venous congestion, hypertension and neurogenic claudication.

TONSILAR ECTOPIA

The term tonsillar 'ectopia' is used to characterize any condition in which the cerebellar tonsils are found to be below the basion-opisthion line (B-OL), regardless of symptom presence. Other authors have suggested that the range of normal tonsil position ends at 2 mm below the B-OL.

The threshold for diagnosis is variable: most authors have suggested that to be considered pathologic the cerebellar tonsils must be 5 mm or more below an imaginary line that runs from the basion (the most anterior point of the foramen magnum) to the opisthion (the posterior point of the foramen magnum).

Symptoms that are most often associated with Chiari type I malformation are occipital headache, neck pain, upper extremity numbness and paraesthesia and weakness. In a few cases there can also be lower extremity weakness and signs of cerebellar dysfunction. The criterion for diagnosis of a Chiari type I malformation is most frequently given as magnetic resonance imaging (MRI) evidence of low cerebellar tonsils relative to the foramen magnum.

SYRINX – SYRINGOMYELIA

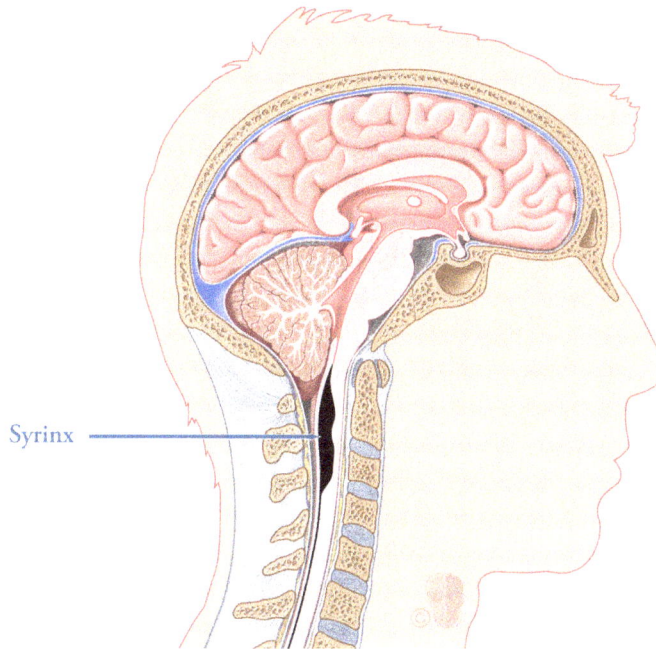

Syrinx

Figure 4.13 Spinal Cord Syrinx

A syrinx in the spinal cord is a rare condition called syringomyelia.

A syrinx is a cyst filled with CSF that forms within the cord. Syrinxes develop anywhere along the spinal cord, however, they often start in the neck and grow downward, affecting the entire cord, as explained in the Merck Manuals.

As the cyst grows and lengthens, it destroys a portion of the spinal cord from the inside out. It also damages nerve fibres that conduct information from the brain to the body's extremities. Syrinxes may be congenital or develop because of a tumour or injury.

Syringomyelia causes progressive stiffness, pain and weakness in the back, arms, shoulders and legs and loss of ability to feel pain and cold.

CONCLUSION

Congestion of the Upper Cervical Spine

The fragile junction of the brain and spine, at the atlas occipital junction is the area in the body that causes most disruption to the drainage mechanism of the brain. The four main concerns of obstruction in this area are outlined as follows:

> e. Birth trauma
> f. Whiplash injuries
> g. Dental malocclusion
> h. Chiari malformation

Birth Trauma

One of the potential causes of birth trauma is the clinical practice of inducing births, an intervention that has become more frequent in recent years with the increased volume of maternity cases. The result of this damage causes drainage issues with the VVP, emissary veins, the and the internal jugular veins. This blockage effect causes backup pressure through the venous system and back into the cranium causing intracranial pressure.

Forceps delivery

Forceps are placed bilaterally over the temporal, parietal and sphenoidal area. Traction is applied in line with the axis of the pelvis, and delivery is effected by the head anteriorally and rotationally.

Ventouse delivery

The alternative to forceps delivery is the application of a suction cap to the foetal scalp with extraction by traction. The suction cap is placed posterior to the bregma on the superior sagittal suture and traction applied with contractions and a rotation of the head, as it is pulled onto the pelvic floor.

Caesarean section

Finally, if both these methods do not achieve the objective, an emergency caesarean is performed. The child is removed from the uterus by a direct incision though the abdominal wall and uterus. Once the infant's head has been located in the birth canal, it has to be freed and then pulled cephalad, turned and removed from the abdominal cavity.

Conclusion of birth trauma

Once the foetal head has made its presentation there is an inability for the cranio fascial dynamic to spring back into the position that is required by the body for homeostasis function. The anterior and posterior poles become permanently distorted and the neurological implications are enormous and persist for life. Chiropractic and dental treatment remains impervious to change unless 'brain balancing' occurs to reinstate the CFD .

Whiplash Trauma

Whiplash injury is the acceleration/deceleration of the head and the spine resulting in an injury with massive lifelong consequences. Whiplash is not only the trauma received in a vehicle accident or the severe trauma seen in contact sports but could be initiated by an over exuberant father throwing an infant up into the air and catching it.

The consequences in all these types of injuries, severe or subtle, can have a severe effect on:the brain first being forced posteriorly (acceleration), crashing into the occiput, and then anteriorly (deceleration) by collision with the frontal bone, contusing the brain tissue, often severely enough to cause haematomas. the dural meningeal tissues – which become stretched and can often tear away from their insertion and anchor points, disturbing their equilibrium and the dynamics that hold the brain in position, more importantly the central (midline) components – the cerebral cortex, the corpus callosum, the fornix, the hippocampus, the amygdala, the thalamus, the caudate nucleus, the cingulate gyrus, the pons and the cerebellum. The venous sinus system – brain swelling and fascial disturbance from the trauma will disrupt drainage from the brain and create obstruction to the venous flow out of the brain – oedema retention. The spinal column – stretching the pre and post zygapophyseal joints, the anterior and posterior common ligaments, the spinal dura, spinal nerve roots, the inter-vertebral foramina, the spinal canal and the composition of the inter-vertebral discs and their position, changing the lordosis into a kyphosis. The atlanto-occipital membrane – obstructing the vertebral arteries, the vertebral venous plexus, the internal jugular vein (through the jugular foramen), the brainstem and the cranial and spinal dura.

The sacrum and sacroiliac joints – the adverse reciprocal movement of the occiput and atlas have a profound effect on the L5-S1 junction and change the pelvic balancing ability at the sacroiliac joints, changing pelvic and spinal equilibrium.

Dental Malocclusion

Each tooth in its alveolus, both upper and lower jaws, is connected and dedicated to a visceral organ, a muscle group and thereby its corresponding neurological supply. In a normal homeostatic occlusion, the teeth come together and occlude at the bucal cusps simultaneously, symmetrically and with the same force evenly on each cusp of the tooth.

The malocclusion also changes the position of the inter-cusp relationship of the tooth within the alveolus, and the smooth inter-cusp relationship changes into an abrasive percussion alarming the mandibular and maxillary branches of the trigeminal nerve and activating the trigeminal ganglion.

Cranio fascial Distortion from Trauma

When cranio fascial distortion takes place, the sphenoid bone moves out of its juxtaposition, the right greater wing of the sphenoid is elevated and rotated anteriorly, pulling the right temporal bone and occiput into internal rotation, while the left greater wing becomes depressed and rotates posteriorly taking the left temporal bone and occiput into external rotation. The pterygoid plates move and rotate with the sphenoid body, changing the muscle tonus and dynamic of the medial and lateral pterygoid mucles influencing the mandibular condyles within the mandibular fossa.

Chiari Malformation

The result of Chiari malformation changes the physiology at the junction of the foramen magnum and the atlas creating arterial and venous congestion and stasis affecting brainstem, pons and cerebellum. Failure of the venous return to drain venous blood from the brain gives rise to ventricular reabsorption of CSF, stretching and changing the ventricular boundaries, and then encroachment onto central cranial organs affecting their ability to perform neurologically. The stasis of fluid not being able to drain, leaves cytotoxic fluid (unable to assimilate due to its synthetic makeup), accessible to myelin covering and degeneration of insulating tissue occurs.

Tonsilar Ectopia

Compression of the brainstem will affect both blood and CSF flow and a build-up of CSF in the ventricles, while upright, but a reduction when recumbent continually changing the CSF pressure gradient, causing the cerebellum to be constantly pushed into the posterior fossa and pulled down through the foramen magnum.

Syrinx – Syringomyelia

A syrinx in the spinal cord is a rare condition called syringomyelia.

A syrinx is a cyst filled with CSF that forms within the cord.

CHAPTER 5

CRITICAL ASPECTS OF CRANIAL DRAINAGE

Cranial drainage is the most important aspect of brain homeostasis that is often ignored by most authorities in neurology, Brain drainage is crucial to an irrigation system that ensures that the amount of blood entering the brain equals that leaving it. For obvious reasons, a build-up of fluid in the cranium leads to an inevitable increase in intracranial pressure. This adversely affects the internal cranial organ systems and their sophisticated ability to communicate with each other and compromises effective systemic function.

THE VENTRICULAR SYSTEM

The ventricular system includes the two lateral ventricles, feeding into the third ventricle through the inter-ventricular foramen of Monro, and the Aqeduct of Sylvius draining from the third ventricle into the fourth ventricle. From the fourth ventricle CSF drains out through the two lateral apertures of Lushka and the single medial aperture of Magendie, as well as the central canal into the spinal cord.

The ventricular system involves primarily, the individual choroid plexuses in each ventricle supplying CSF in the correct amount thus allowing the hydro-dynamic of the ventricles to function at optimum levels. This system also depends on the amount of CSF coming into the lateral ventricles and generated by the choroid plexuses to equal the same volume leaving the fourth ventricle thus establishing homeostasis. If this does not happen, the ventricles engorge changing their shape and impacting on the cranial organs that surround it.

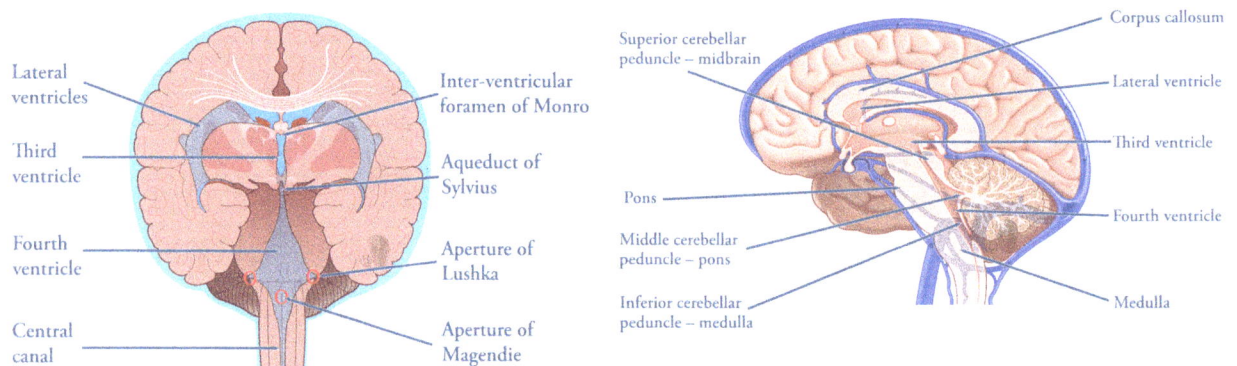

Figure 5.1 The Ventricular System and its Boundaries: The cerebellar pdeuncles connect the cerebellum to the midbrain, pons and medulla

Supporting organs of the dominant system

The roof of the lateral ventricles is the corpus callosum (which also supports the supracallosal gyrus and the cingulate gyrus). The floor of the lateral ventricles is supported by the fornix, separated by the septum pellucidum, and the lateral aspect of the lateral ventricles is supported by the caudate nucleus, the body and tail, all part of this crescent shaped cranial organ. All these particular cranial systems communicate with each other through a network of communicating fibres – commissural fibres, association fibres and projection fibres. Engorgement of the lateral ventricles inhibits the CSF flow through the inter-ventricular foramen of Monro, and disrupts the communicating ability of the other fibres. They can be stretched or compressed, but they do not relay the information as required.

The third ventricle is surrounded by the thalamus and the hypothalamus, both acting as 'junction boxes' between the spinal cord and the cerebral cortex. Engorgement in the third ventricle reduces flow of the aqueduct of Sylvius, and must have an impact on the communicating ability of these systems, as well as the adjacent fibre network of the internal capsule and the nuclei of the putamen and globus pallidus – part of the basal ganglia.

The fourth ventricle is supported and is surrounded by the cerebral peduncles, the communicators from the cerebellum to the midbrain, pons and medulla. The posterior wall of the fourth ventricle is supported by the pons. Engorgement of the fourth ventricle has an impact on the drainage of the apertures of Lushka, Magendie and the central canal, as well as affecting the surrounding systems and influencing their communicating ability.

The critical function of ventricular drainage is also reduced by cranio fascial torque – trauma. The membrane system that ultimately supports the dominant system distorts the framework of the ventricles and has an impact on their ability to drain.

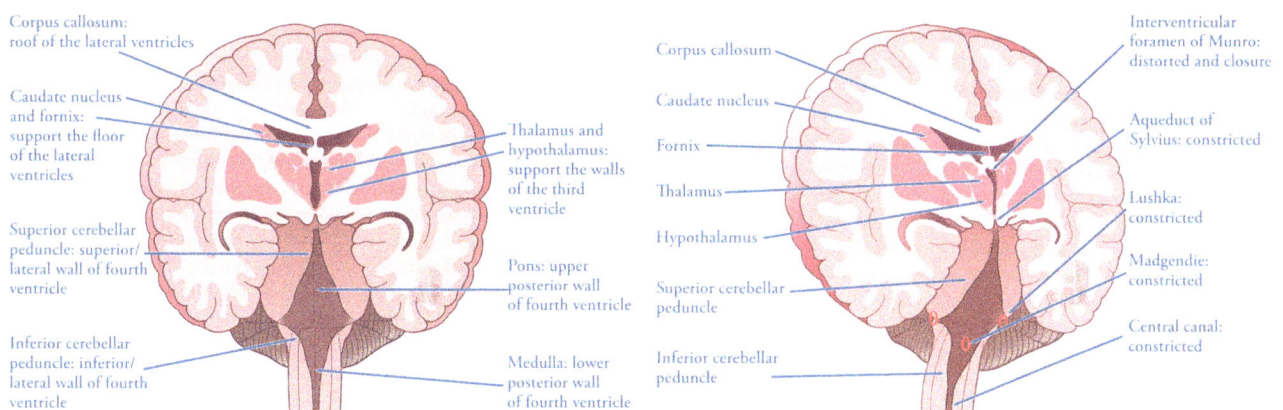

Figure 5.2 Brain Component Support for the Ventricles; (right) Distorted: CSF Reduced flow and fluid retention

THE TENTORIAL INCISURA

Probably the most critical membrane in the cranium because it influences so many parts of the brain systems, and is often ignored in the referred damage it can cause to the disruption of vital communication fibres, the arterial and venous circulation and its impact on the central brain organs.

The tentorium incisura is the bilateral crest shaped membrane, as an extension of the tentorium cerebellum, coming off the anterior aspect of the straight sinus, with its medial borders forming the 'tentorial notch', a large opening which surrounds the cerebral peduncles, the midbrain, the pons and the brainstem and anchoring into the anterior and posterior clinoid processes of the sphenoid body. The lateral borders attach to the petrous portion of the temporal bones and anchors with the medial portion at the sphenoid body.

The tentorial incisura is divided into three spaces – the anterior, the middle and the posterior spaces.

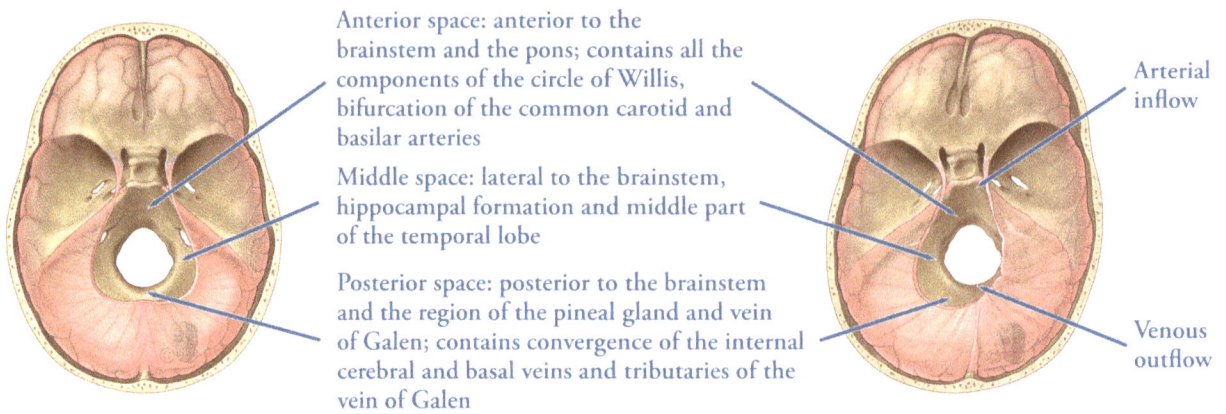

Anterior space: anterior to the brainstem and the pons; contains all the components of the circle of Willis, bifurcation of the common carotid and basilar arteries

Middle space: lateral to the brainstem, hippocampal formation and middle part of the temporal lobe

Posterior space: posterior to the brainstem and the region of the pineal gland and vein of Galen; contains convergence of the internal cerebral and basal veins and tributaries of the vein of Galen

Arterial inflow

Venous outflow

Figure 5.3 Sectors and influence of the tentorial incisura

From a vascular standpoint, the arterial vessels are found in the anterior space and the venous vessels are found in the posterior space. These are complex relationships, since the anterior space contains all of the components of the circle of Willis and the bifurcation of the common carotid and basilar arteries. The middle space incorporates the PCA and the superior cerebellar artery which pass around the brainstem; the posterior space contains the convergence of the internal cerebral and basal veins and many of their tributaries to the vein of Galen. The 'tentorial incisura' is intimately related to the depths of the cerebrum and cerebellum, the first six pairs of cranial nerves, and the upper brainstem and the pons.

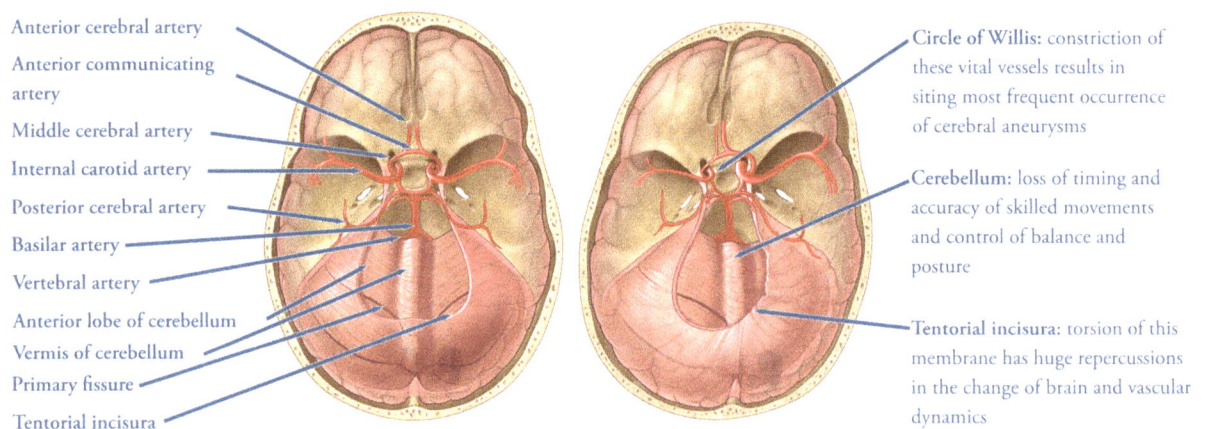

Anterior cerebral artery

Anterior communicating artery

Middle cerebral artery

Internal carotid artery

Posterior cerebral artery

Basilar artery

Vertebral artery

Anterior lobe of cerebellum

Vermis of cerebellum

Primary fissure

Tentorial incisura

Circle of Willis: constriction of these vital vessels results in siting most frequent occurrence of cerebral aneurysms

Cerebellum: loss of timing and accuracy of skilled movements and control of balance and posture

Tentorial incisura: torsion of this membrane has huge repercussions in the change of brain and vascular dynamics

Figure 5.4 Cerebellum and Circle of Willis with Torsion of the Tentorial Incisura

When the cranium is subjected to trauma and cranio fascial torque takes place, the anterior space will experience a constriction of the circle of Willis, where these vital vessels distort to produce the most frequent occurrence of cerebral aneurysm and interfere with normal circulation. Equally the posterior space warps the straight sinus, the venous tributaries to the great vein of Galen and reduces the venous distribution of the internal cerebral and basal veins – outgoing drainage.

The torsion of the tentorium incisura will also pull the brainstem, pons, medulla and the cerebral peduncles out of their juxtaposition, as well as the dominant system and all the aforementioned surrounding internal cranial components that maintain homeostasis. Changes to neural communication fibres, so vital to brain system processing, lose their ability to transmit effectively. Could this be the precursor to brain changes that see a reduction in neurological capability, the failure of the auto-immune system and conditions such as PTSD, poor allergic responses and the myriad of neurological disturbances recognised today?

CRANIAL FLOOR APERTURES AND VITAL LINKS

These are some of the points of reference visible on the inferior aspect of the infant cranium. The most important point to take into consideration is the cranial plate configuration of the infant skull. The formation of the occiput, which includes four components – the basilar part, attaching to the body of the sphenoid, the two condylar parts lying adjacent to the two temporal bones and the occipital squama which articulate with the parietals superiorly and the squamosal part of the temporal bones laterally and inferiorly. The temporal bone is made up of three components – the tympanic part, housing the glenoid fossa, the tympanic membrane and the external auditory meatus, the petrous portion which houses the internal acoustic meatus, the petrous ridge and affords the opening for the jugular foramen and the carotid canal, and the squama which articulates with the parietal bones and the occiput.

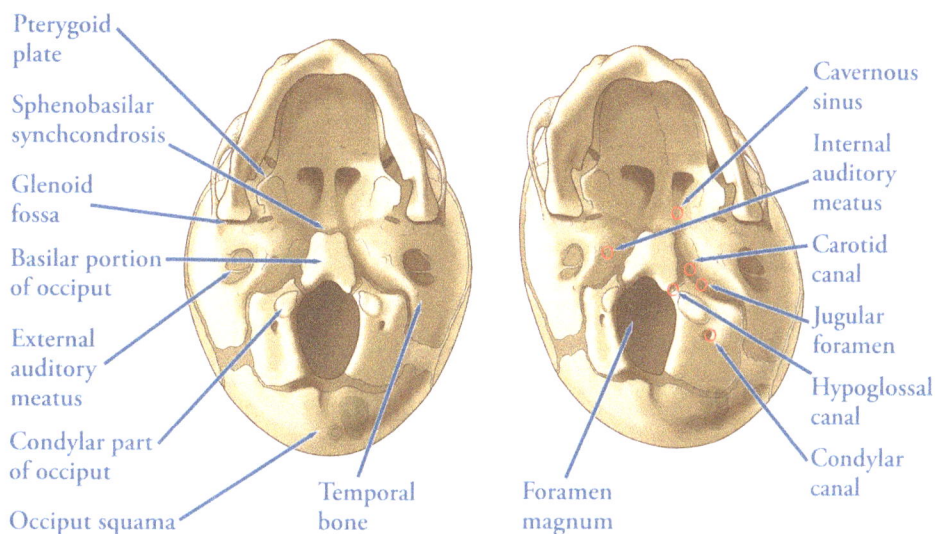

Figure 5.5 Inferior Infant Skull: Cranial floor apertures, (left) counterclockwise torque

The multiple small bones that make up this area are important, as they are encapsulated by the endosteal and periosteal dura acting as a sleeve around these bones. It ensures that the reinforcement of dura (endosteal and periosteal) is exaggerated and complex to give the area strength and flexibility in the early development of the skull. The dural sleeve also leaves the foramen magnum and becomes continuous with the spinal dura attaching firmly at C1, C2 and C3. This entire area requires enormous resilience, as it is responsible for massive movement of the heavy skull on the upper cervical spine, where the brainstem, major arteries and the spinal cord all converge. The base of the skull also supports the jugular foramen (vagus nerve, spinal accessory nerve and the internal jugular vein), the carotid canal (internal carotid artery), the vertebral venous plexus (brain drainage), the sub-occipital cavernous sinus, the occipital sinus, the occipital emissary vein (inferior condylar canal), the hypoglossal canal and the foramen magnum.

The tentorium cerebellum, at its posterior borders encapsulates the transverse sinus, the sigmoid sinus, at the occipital squama, before becoming the internal jugular vein. The increased volume and, the larger vessels on the right side, drive the brain into a counterclockwise motion and therefore this area requires more versatility and strength to facilitate this activity – hence the multiple dural attachments and the heavy investment of these membranes at the cranial base.

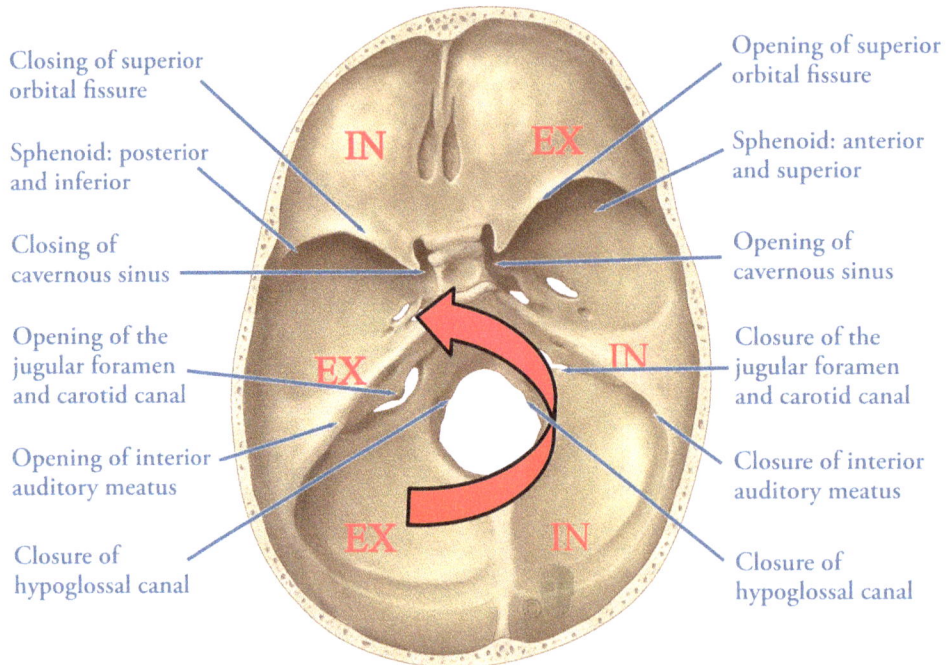

Closing of superior orbital fissure

Sphenoid: posterior and inferior

Closing of cavernous sinus

Opening of the jugular foramen and carotid canal

Opening of interior auditory meatus

Closure of hypoglossal canal

Opening of superior orbital fissure

Sphenoid: anterior and superior

Opening of cavernous sinus

Closure of the jugular foramen and carotid canal

Closure of interior auditory meatus

Closure of hypoglossal canal

Figure 5.6 Important cranial floor apertures: Counterclockwise torque

With the counterclockwise motion, comes a cranio fascial distortion, which changes aperture size as the dural membrane goes through flexion (external rotation) on the left, and extension (internal rotation) on the right, following this haemodynamic motion. Once maturity and ossification of the cranial bones, occurs, the apertures – lined with dural membrane – of the adult skull become established and these important factors need to be recognised.

The sphenoid bone is central to all these considerations, as it is the lynch pin to cranial activity. The right sphenoid greater wings move anterior and superior, while the left sphenoid greater wings move posterior and inferior. This changes the superior orbital fissure, the right side becomes more enlarged, affording a bigger orbit for the right eye – hence the protruded eye and a larger pathway for all the vessels passing through it. The left side is reduced making the orbit smaller and impacting the eye, and compressing all the vessels passing through it. The left oculomotor nerve (medial rectus muscle) is inhibited hence the lack of convergence with the left eye.

The cavernous sinus is compressed on the left, reducing flow of the internal carotid and the other components, while the right side is open and the vessels have freer movement.

The body of the sphenoid presents the sella turcica – housing the pituitary and the dural attachments of the diaphragma sellae – at the anterior and posterior clinoid processes. These processes are also the anchor points for the tentorium cerebellum, but more importantly, the tentorial incisura.

This is a crucial area in whiplash type trauma, whether to the skull or the upper cervical spine. Lateral whiplash injuries are the most severe and the most common, as the lateral forces drive the 'tentorial incisura' into a lateral rotational torque, distorting the three incisural spaces in a twisting, throttling manner. This leads to the greater wings of the sphenoid, the anterior insertion points of the tentorium cerebellum at the clinoid processes moving in one direction, while the posterior margins of the tentorium cerebellum at the occiput and transverse sinuses, move in the other direction twisting the 'straight sinus' and tributaries feeding the great vein of Galen. This helical action involves constriction of the pons (the posterior border of the pons makes up the anterior wall of the fourth ventricle), the brainstem, the hippocampal and amygdala formation and the medial portion of the temporal lobe, the six pairs of cranial nerves and the arterial inflow and venous outflow of vessels lying in the invested tissue of the 'tentorial incisura'.

When the sphenoid rotates as described, there is an anterior pull on the right tentorial incisura, taking the tentorium cerebellum into internal rotation and reducing the apertures of the jugular foramen, the carotid canal, the hypoglossal canal and the internal acoustic meatus. This affects arterial blood flow into the cranium (internal carotid artery) and drainage out of the cranium (internal jugular vein), the vagus, acoustic, facial, spinal accessory and trigeminal nerves. The torque on the diaphragma sellae also twists the hypophysial stalk of the pituitary.

Conversely, the left sphenoid body moves posteriorly, taking the left tentorial incisura and tentorium cerebellum in external rotation, opening those same apertures to increase the viability of all the incumbent vessels. This same movement will also pull the central brain components away from the mid-line, as discussed earlier. As already discussed, the posterior rotation of the sphenoid on the left, pulls the left glenoid fossa of the temporal bone posterior, as well as the left pterygoid plate, which deviates the mandible to the left on opening and creates a malocclusion with the lower jaw. This in turn irritates the maxillary and mandibular branches of the trigeminal nerve ultimately resulting in TMJ dysfunction.

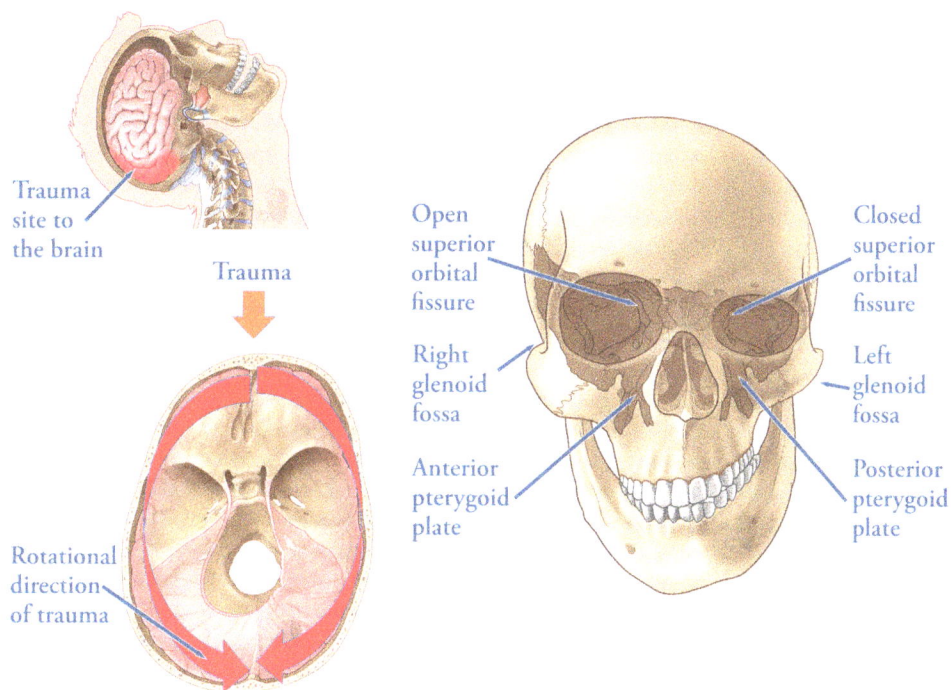

Figure 5.7 (left) Brain Trauma After Whiplash of the Spine: Magnified distortion of tentorial incisura; (right) Sphenoid Collapse

DRAINAGE AND THE HAEMODYNAMIC EFFECTS

The haemodynamic effects of drainage were covered in Part 1, Chapter 3. The main function of the haemodynamic force arises as a result of larger drainage vessels and a larger drainage capacity found in the anterior–superior drainage of the brain: the superior sagittal sinus draining into the right transverse sinus, the right sigmoid sinus and the right internal jugular vein. This is the right drainage system separated at the confluence of the sinuses.

The anterior–inferior drainage includes the inferior sagittal sinus, draining into the straight sinus and at the separation at the confluence of the sinuses, which drains into the left transverse sinus, the left sigmoid sinus and the left internal jugular vein. This system has smaller vessels and less drainage capacity. The volume/pressure differential between the left and right internal jugular veins has the propensity to drive the brain in a counterclockwise direction (more pressure and volume on the right).

The cardiovascular rhythm drives this drainage rate at between 68 and 72 cycles per minute, thereby enhancing the arterial flow into the brain and the venous drainage out, maintaining the brain irrigation system at homeostatic levels. The significance of this balance is paramount to normal brain function within the meningeal dura.

Trauma to the brain or to the brainstem changes these parameters. It increases the arterial supply, but decreases the venous drainage and the propensity for the brain to work in a rhythmic pulsating manner. As a result, drainage, perfusion, medulla oblongata autoregulation, stroke and infarction are among some of the issues that arise.

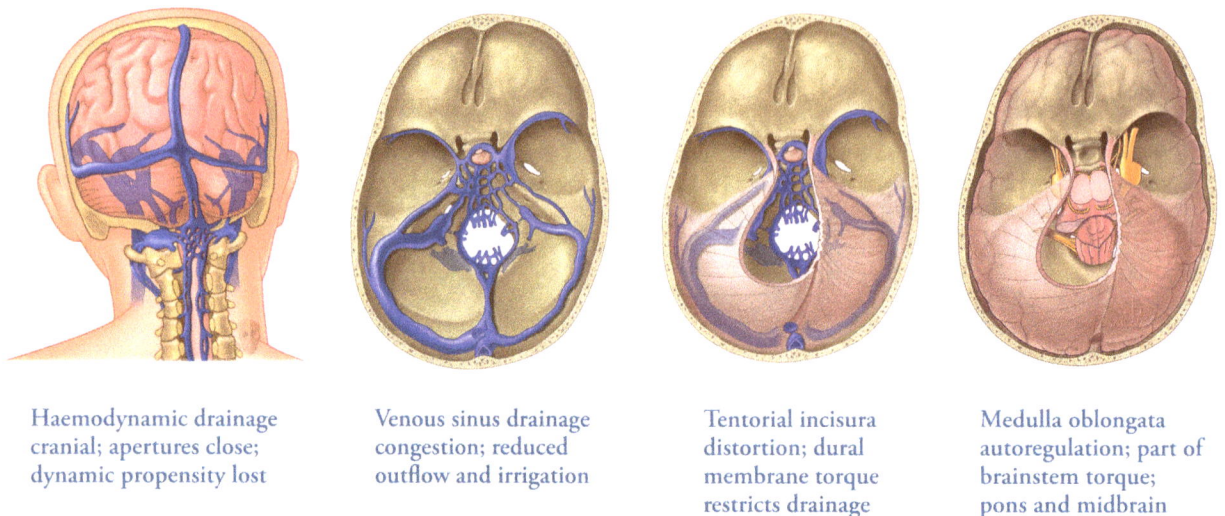

Haemodynamic drainage cranial; apertures close; dynamic propensity lost

Venous sinus drainage congestion; reduced outflow and irrigation

Tentorial incisura distortion; dural membrane torque restricts drainage

Medulla oblongata autoregulation; part of brainstem torque; pons and midbrain

Figure 5.8 Some issues that may arise from loss of haemodynamic propensity and cardiovascular rhythmic pulses

CONCLUSION

The drainage potential of the brain – and the arterial inflow – is a subject that is not addressed to the optimum, possibly because the apertures of vascular circulation are many and not considered worthy of further study(as part of the 'big' picture)and possibly because they cannot be measured or accurately assessed. In considering the importance of vascular flow and the effects of the overall irrigation system, it is imperative that the facts be looked at on an individual basis and each system evaluated on its merit. The complete drainage complex must be considered with specific reference to the function of the 'dural membranes', rather than the cranial bones that are attached to them. – this attitude reverts to the embryological development and the timetable that shows the fascial system precedes the introduction of the cranial plates, and therefore by nature takes precedence.

The ventricular system

The two lateral ventricles flowing into the interventricular foramen of Monro then into the third ventricle, with its flow into the fourth ventricle, the aqueduct of Sylvius, all these make up the dominant system.

The fourth ventricle drains CSF from the lateral appertures of Lushka, the medial aperture of Magendie and the central canal into the spinal cord. The choroid plexuses generate CSF in the lateral, third and fourth ventricles, while the blood-CSF barrier involving the choroid plexus epithelium is present in the third ventricle and the two lateral ventricles – a very important factor.

The entire dominant system is also supported and surrounded by central brain components, namely:

a. The corpus callosum – roof of the lateral ventricles
b. The fornix – the floor of the lateral ventricles
c. The caudate nucleus – the lateral walls of the lateral ventricles
d. The thalamus and hypothalamus – the walls of the third ventricle
e. The pons – the posterior wall of the fourth ventricle
f. The cerebral peduncles – the walls of the superior and inferior parts of the fourth ventricles

When the dominant system is distorted by cranio fascial torque, all these organs, apertures and the neurological fibres must be influenced and their transmission of information compromised. The apertures will also be reduced, affecting their circulatory ability to move CSF. This could lead to engorgement of the ventricular framework, altering the shape of the ventricles and all their surrounding components.

The tentorial incisura

This is possibly the most influential membrane in the cranium, with the anterior bifurcation of the tentorium cerebellum, creating the 'tentorial notch' at the straight sinus, the two crescent shaped folds anchor at the anterior and posterior clinoid processes of the sphenoid body. When cranio fascial torque takes place, the right tentorial incisura is pulled anterior, as the dural membrane goes into internal rotation, and the left tentorial incisura is pulled posterior as the left dural membrane goes into external rotation. This torque changes;

a. The sella turcica – the diaphragma sellae – the pituitary
b. The pterygoid plates – influence mandibular deviation
c. The superior orbital fissure – ocular nerve control
d. The cavernous sinus – internal carotid artery
e. The petrous portions of the temporal bone – drainage from the superior petrosal sinuses
f. The jugular foramen – internal jugular vein, vagus and spinal accessory nerves
g. The carotid canal – internal carotid artery
h. The hypoglossal canal – hypoglossal nerve
i. The foramen magnum – brainstem, VVP. Vertebral arteries
j. Anterior tentorial incisura space – the circle of Willis and the bifurcation of the common carotid and basilar arteries
k. Middle tentorial incisura space – the PCA and the superior cerebellar artery which pass around the brainstem
l. Posterior tentorial incisura space – the straight sinus, the venous tributaries to the great vein of Galen and reduces the venous distribution of the internal cerebral and basal veins
m. The torsion of the tentorium incisura will also pull the brainstem, pons, medulla and the cerebral peduncles out of their juxtaposition, as well as the dominant system and all the surrounding internal cranial components that maintain homeostasis.

The cranial floor apertures

With the counterclockwise motion, comes a cranio fascial distortion, which changes aperture size as the dural membrane goes through flexion (external rotation) on the left, and extension (internal rotation) on the right, following this haemo-dynamic motion. Once maturity and ossification of the cranial bones occurs, the apertures – lined with dural membrane – of the adult skull become established and these important factors need to be taken into consideration.

CHAPTER 6

DISTRIBUTION OF CONGENITAL

CEREBRAL ANEURYSMS

An aneurysm is a balloon-like bulge or weakening of an arterial wall. As the bulge grows it becomes thinner and weaker. It can become so thin that the BP within it can cause it to burst or leak. Most aneurysms develop from a weakness or abnormal artery wall. Aneurysms usually occur on larger blood vessels where an artery branches. Approximately 85% of aneurysms form in the anterior circulation of the brain, while the remaining 15% form in the back posterior circulation of the brain. Continued restriction to arterial flow in vulnerable parts of the circle of Willis as a result of cranio fascial torsion can lead to the formation of an aneurysm and if not reduced can lead to rupturing of the aneurysm.

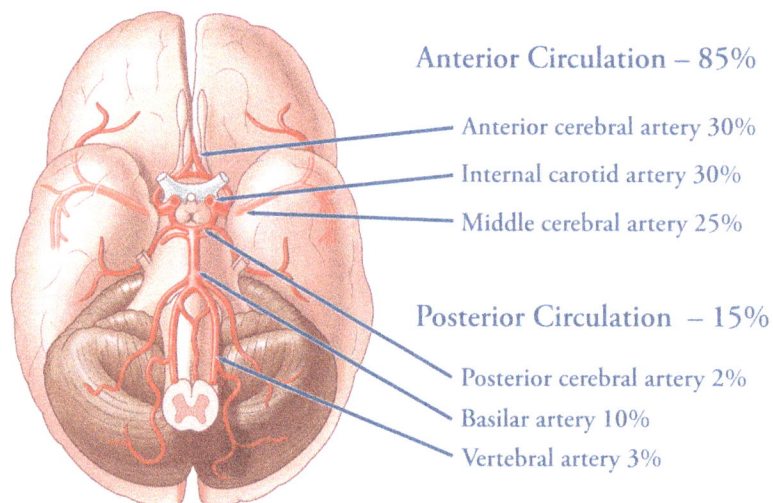

Anterior Circulation – 85%

Anterior cerebral artery 30%

Internal carotid artery 30%

Middle cerebral artery 25%

Posterior Circulation – 15%

Posterior cerebral artery 2%

Basilar artery 10%

Vertebral artery 3%

Figure 6.1 Distribution of Congenital Cerebral Aneurysms

Stroke is a sudden interruption of the blood supply to the brain. Most strokes are caused by an abrupt blockage of an artery (ischaemic stroke). Other types of stroke are caused by bleeding into brain tissue when a blood vessel bursts (haemorrhagic stroke). The effects of a stroke depend on the severity and which area of the brain is injured. Strokes may cause sudden weakness, loss of sensation, or difficulty speaking, seeing, or walking. Since different parts of the brain control different areas and functions, it is usually the area immediately surrounding the stroke that is affected. Haemorrhagic strokes have a much higher death rate than ischaemic strokes.

Ischaemic strokes occurring in the anterior circulation are the most common of all ischaemic strokes, accounting for approximately 70% of all cases. They are caused most commonly by occlusion of one of the major intracranial arteries. The most common causes of arterial occlusion involving the major cerebral arteries are: (1) emboli, most commonly arising from: atherosclerotic arterial narrowing at the bifurcation of the common carotid artery; cardiac sources; or atheroma in the aortic arch, and (2) a combination of atherosclerotic stenosis and superimposed thrombosis.

The anterior circulation of the brain describes the areas of the brain supplied by the right and left internal carotid arteries and their branches. The internal carotid arteries supply the majority of both cerebral hemispheres, except the occipital and medial temporal lobes, which are supplied from the posterior circulation.

The ACA supplies the whole of the medial surfaces of the frontal and parietal lobes, the anterior four-fifths of the corpus callosum, the frontobasal cerebral cortex, the anterior diencephalon, and the deep structures.

The MCA is the largest of the intracerebral vessels and through its pial branches supplies almost the entire convex surface of the brain, including the lateral frontal, parietal, and temporal lobes; insula; claustrum; and extreme capsule. The lenticulostriate branches of the MCA supply the basal ganglia, including the caput nuclei caudati, the putamen, the lateral parts of the internal and external capsules, and sometimes the extreme capsule.

Embolic stroke – caused when a clot breaks off from the artery wall which becomes an embolus, which can travel farther down the bloodstream to block a smaller artery. Emboli usually come from the heart, where different diseases cause clot formation.

Haemorrhagic stroke – (less common – 17% of cases) is caused by rupture or leaking of an artery either within or around the brain. It can occur when a weakened blood vessel ruptures, releasing blood into the space surrounding the brain – a subarachnoid haemorrhage (SAH). It can be caused by a ruptured aneurysm, arteriovenous malformation (AVM), or head trauma.

ARTERIAL LESIONS

Primary consideration and aetiology for arterial lesions must include birth trauma, whiplash injuries to the cervical spine and dental malocclusions. No matter what the intensities of these injuries at inception, the long-term effects of arterial flow into the brain through the anterior (vertebral arteries) and the posterior (carotid arteries) supply may manifest into serious obstructions and flow later in life, when other issues such as aneurysms, emboli, infarctions and traumas are added to the list. Cranio fascial torsion may be a major contributor to aetiology of stroke because of the the way arterial circulation is retarded from birth trauma. In addition, cervical trauma then causes venous congestion through the sub-occipital stasis of the vertebral venous plexus thus resulting in the restriction of the internal jugular vein.

As the brain's vascular system attempts to complete the balanced exchange of arterial and venous blood, this cervical trauma can cause ischaemia in specific areas when the dynamic of hypertension becomes evident.

This slowing down of vascular circulation then gives rise to the eventual occurrence of aneurysms, emboli, infarctions and trauma – the latent pathophysiology of brain circulation.

The most significant event occurring during week 3 of embryonic development is gastrulation, the process that establishes all three germ layers in the embryo beginning with the primative streak at day sixteen. The formation of mesenchyme (day 18) the loosely organised embryonic connective tissue that provides the inductive stimulus and determines the path of differentiation from which the germ layers, ectoderm, mesoderm and endoderm develop by the end of week 3. The entire cardiovascular system – the heart, blood vessels and blood cells – originate from the mesodermal germ layer. The distortion of cranial fascia, which embraces all the cranial vessels, should be the primary consideration.

REGIONS SUPPLIED BY THE THREE CEREBRAL ARTERIES

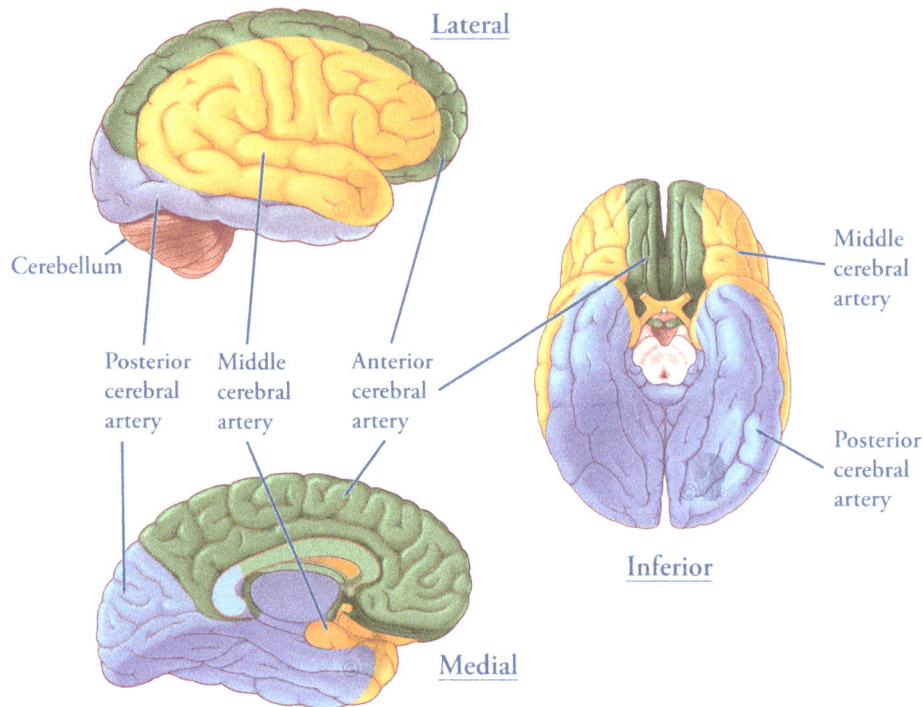

Figure 6.2 Lateral, Medial and Inferior Cerebral Cortexes

The three main arteries (ACA, MCA – anterior circulation – and the PCA – posterior circulation) give rise to numerous branches that travel to the subarachnoid space over the surface of the brain and into the sulci. Small penetrating branches arise from these vessels to supply the superficial portions of the brain, including the cortex and the underlying white matter. The deep structures of the brain, such as the basal ganglia, the thalamus and the internal capsule, are supplied by small penetrating branches that arise from the initial segments of the main cerebral arteries near the circle of Willis at the base of the brain.

Anterior cerebral artery

The ACA leaves the circle of Willis and moves anterior through the interhemispheric fissure as it sweeps back over the corpus callosum as the pericallosal artery to the primary somatosensory cortex, and the callosomarginal artery to the primary motor cortex. The ACA thus supplies most of the cortex on the anterior medial surface of the brain from the frontal to the parietal lobes, usually including the medial sensorimotor cortex.

Middle Cerebral Artery

The MCA leaves the ACA at the circle of Willis and travels laterally giving off several branches of lenticulostriate arteries which penetrate into the anterior perforated substance to supply large regions of the basal ganglia (caudate nucleus, putamen and the globus pallidus) and the internal capsule before entering into the Sylvian fissure where it eventually bifurcates into the superior division and the inferior division. The 'superior division' supplies the cortex above the Sylvian fissure, including the lateral frontal lobe and the perirolandic cortex. The 'inferior division' supplies the cortex below the Sylvian fissure, including the lateral temporal lobe and a portion of the parietal lobe.

In hypertension, the lenticulostriate arteries are particularly prone to narrowing, which can lead to lacunar infarction, as well as to rupture causing intracerebral haemorrhage.

Posterior cerebral artery

The PCA comes off the basilar artery at the posterior aspect of the circle of Willis and predominantly supplies the supratentorial structures, the upper part of the midbrain, branches over the inferior and medial temporal lobes and over the medial occipital cortex. The main cortical branches include the posterior pericallosal, the parieto-occipital, the calcarine and the posterior temporal branches.

The proximal part of the PCA, from which many perforating arteries arise, has peduncular (supplying the tectum, cerebral peduncles of the midbrain, multiple branches to the thalamus and hypothalamus, subthalamus and midline and nuclei of the thalamus) and ambient branches (supplying the geniculate bodies, the lateral geniculate nucleus is a relay center in the thalamus for the visual pathway). It receives a major sensory input from the retina. The medial geniculate nucleus or medial geniculate body is part of the auditory thalamus and represents the thalamic relay between the inferior colliculus and the auditory cortex.

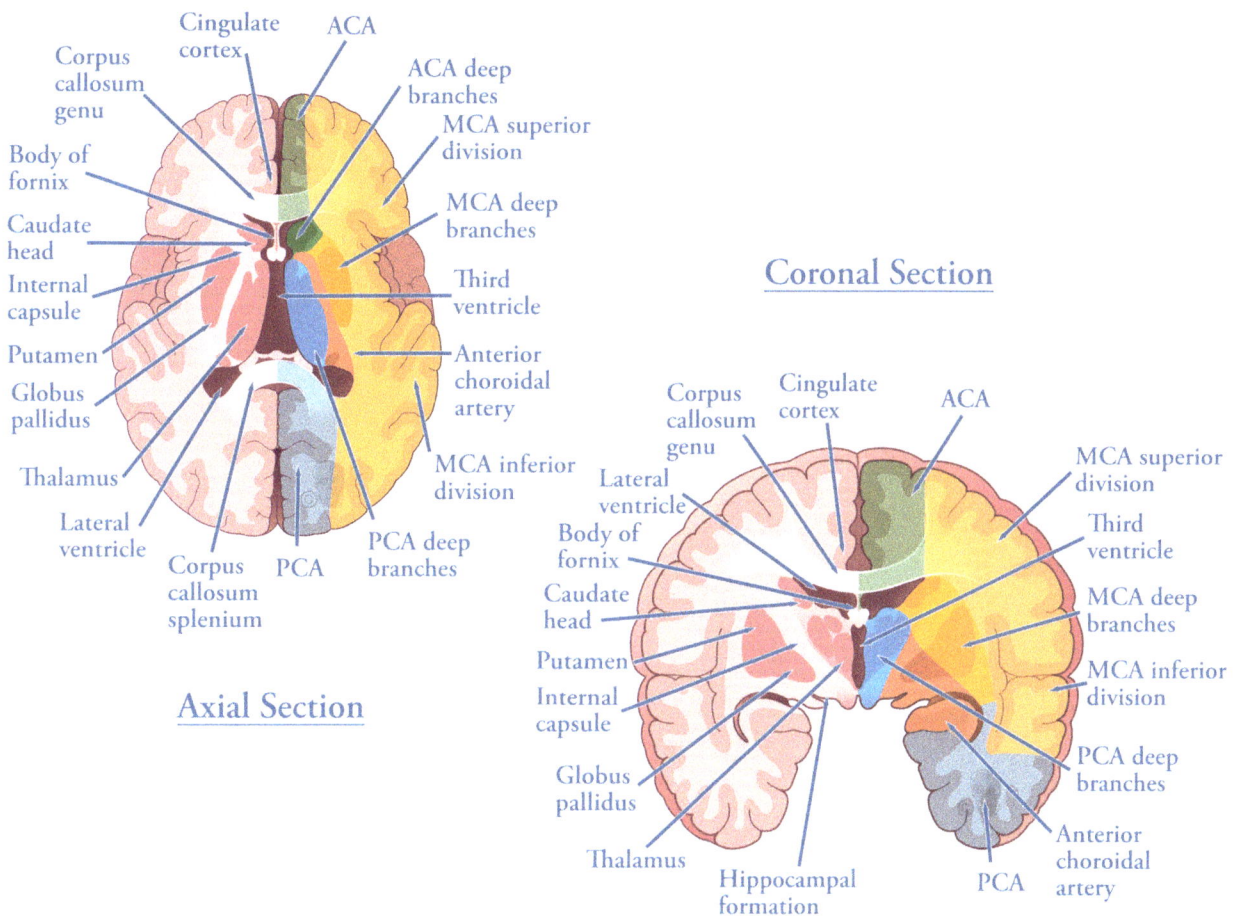

Figure 6.3 Superficial and Deep Blood Supply to the Cerebral Hemispheres: Axial and coronal sections

WATERSHED ZONES FOR THE MAIN CEREBRAL ARTERIES

When a cerebral artery is occluded, ischaemia and infarction occur in the territory supplied by that vessel but has little effect on other areas. However, when the blood supply from two adjacent cerebral arteries is compromised, the regions between the two vessels are most susceptible to infarction and ischaemia. These regions are known as the 'watershed zones' and can produce proximal arm and leg weakness and because the regions of the homunculus involved can influence the trunk and proximal limbs, while the dominant hemisphere watershed can cause transcortical aphasia syndromes.

Bilateral watershed infarcts in both the ACA-MCA and MCA-PCA watershed zones can cause severe drops in systemic BP, with a sudden occlusion of the internal carotid artery or stenosis of the internal carotid, as both are fed by the common carotid artery.

ACA-MCA watershed infarcts – carotid obstruction.

MCA-PCA watershed infarcts affecting the occipital lobe can cause disturbances to higher order visual processing.

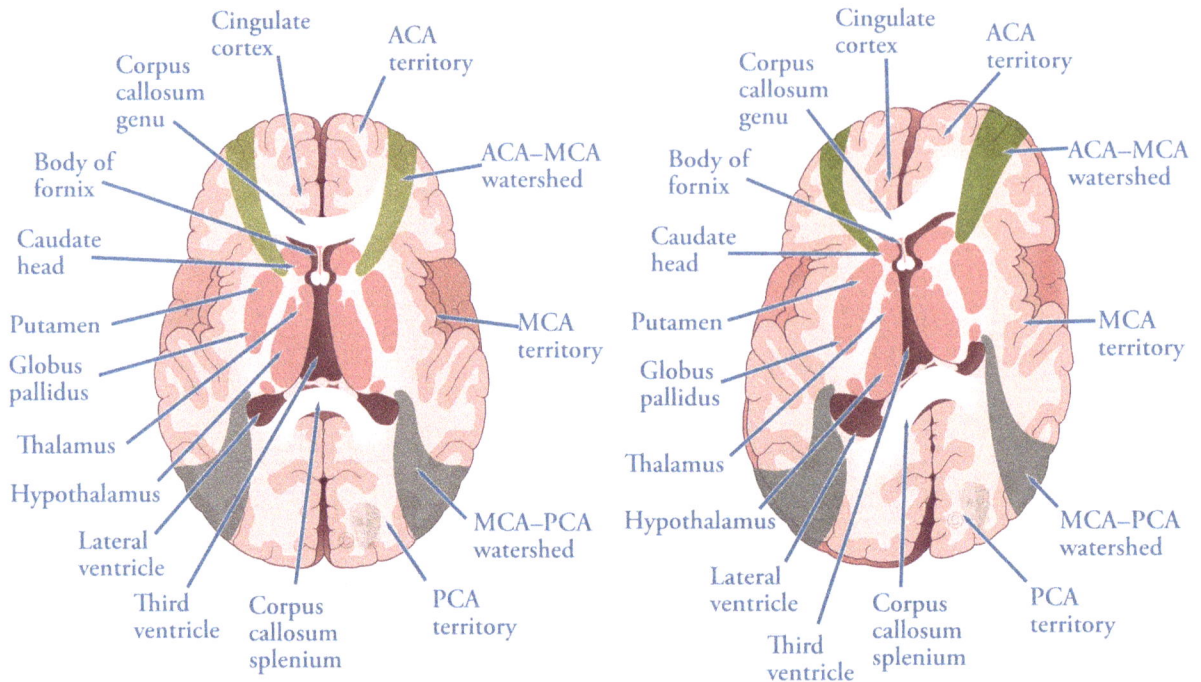

Figure 6.4 Watershed Zones for the Major Cerebral Arteries: Axial views of the diencephalon, torqued on right

FASCIAL TORSIONAL EFFECTS ON THE WATERSHED

Cranio fascial torsion will only increase potential damage and risk to the central cranial components including the three main arterial supplies and their overlap in the watershed zones. Most evident in these are the two lateral, and the third and fourth ventricles, where torsion, obstructed flow through the interventricular foramen of Monro, the aqueduct of Sylvius and the apertures of Luschka and Magendie may inhibit drainage potential in the ventricular system leading to increasing intracranial pressure and brain congestion.

OCCLUSION OF ANTERIOR AND MIDDLE CEREBRAL ARTERIES

Occlusion of the main stem of the ACA or the MCA or their superficial branches is most often caused by an embolus from the heart or proximal vessels, especially from the cervical segment of the internal carotid artery.

Occlusion of the deep penetrating branches is most often caused by lipohyalinosis resulting from hypertension. Occasionally, atherosclerosis narrows the lumina of the major intracranial arteries, leading to thrombosis and occlusion. Intracranial atherosclerosis, in the absence of severe extracranial disease, usually involves the proximal main stem of the MCA.

The extent of infarction following occlusion of the anterior or MCA and their branches is extremely variable and depends on the location and rapidity of the occlusive process; the variable anatomical features of the circle of Willis; previous occlusive lesions; and systemic circulatory, haematologic and serologic factors.

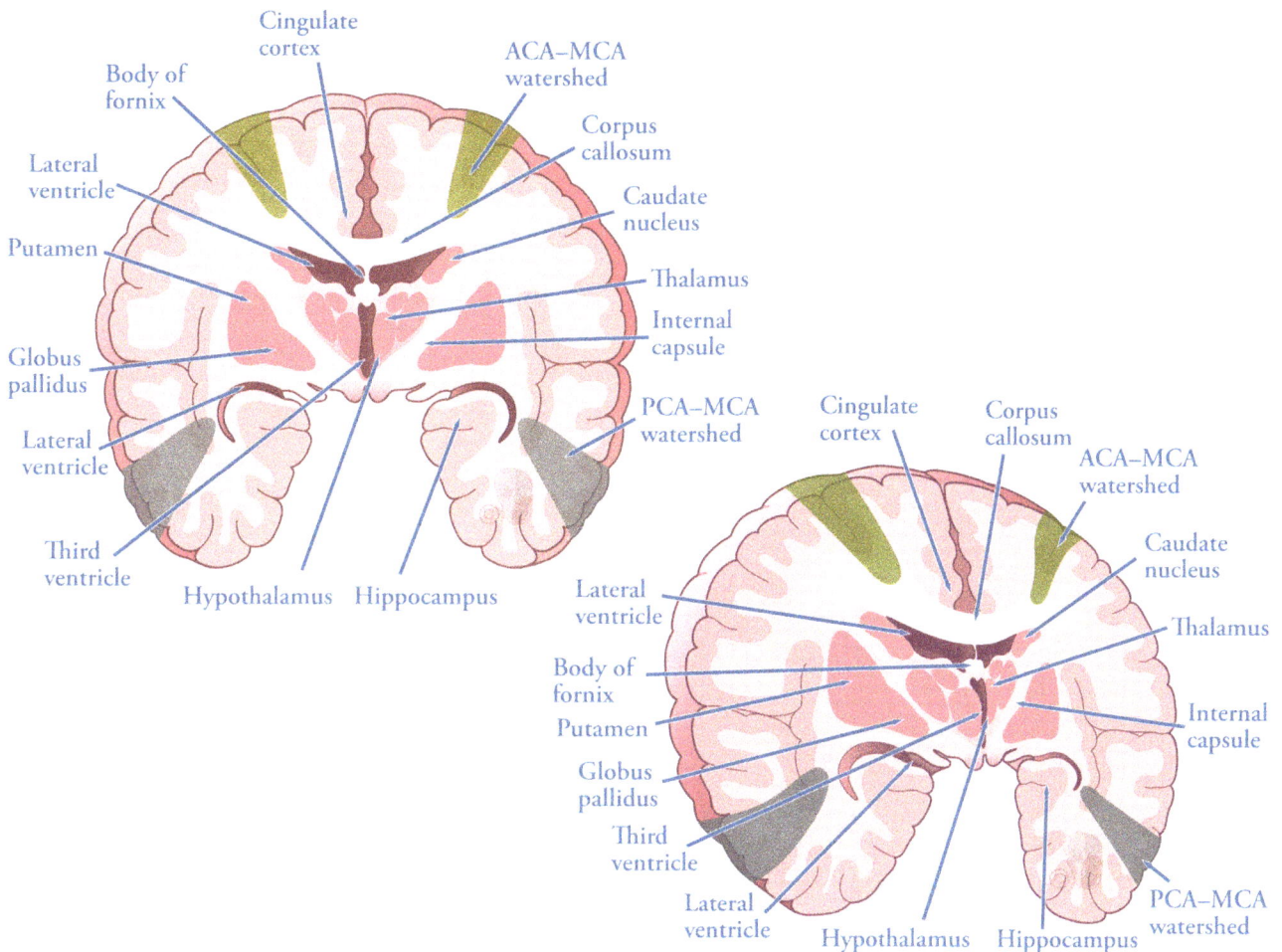

Figure 6.5 Watershed Zones for the Major Cerebral Arteries: Coronal views of the diencephalon, torqued on right

ANTERIOR CEREBRAL ARTERY – ENTIRE TERRITORY 30%

Blockage of the right ACA at its source can affect its entire distribution and can produce the following clinical manifestations:

- Incontinence
- Contralateral hemiplegia – left leg weakness of the upper motor neuron type and left leg cortical-type sensory loss
- Abulia, a pathological inability to make decisions. Damage to the nerve circuits of the frontal lobes of the brain that impact the dopaminergic system, is thought to be the cause of abulia

- Transcortical motor aphasia, or motor and sensory aphasia – affecting the production, or comprehension of speech and the ability to read or write
- Left hemineglect can also be seen – left limb dyspraxia; and larger infarcts may cause left hemiplegia – paralysis of the left side of the body.

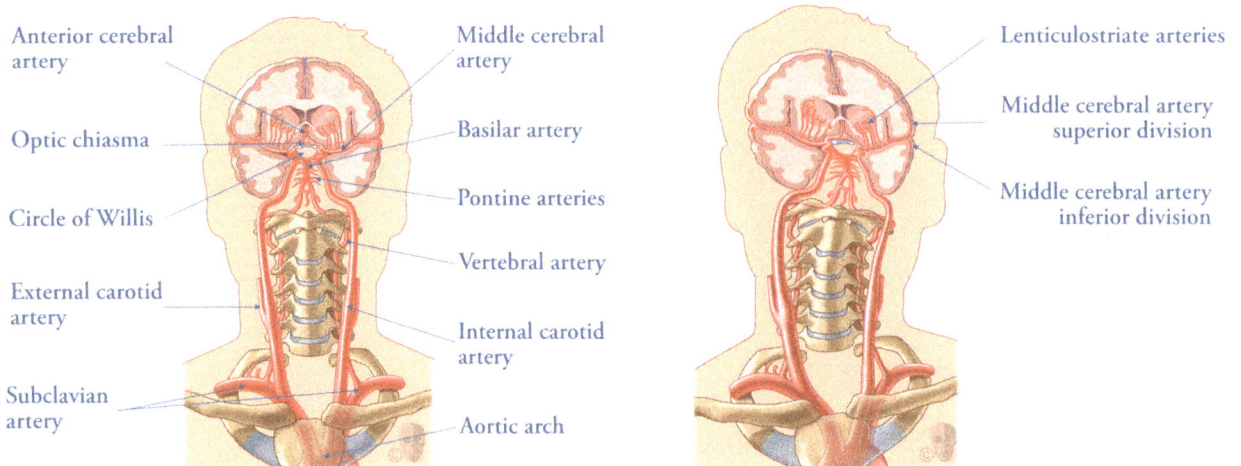

Figure 6.6 Anterior View of the Arterial Supply to the Brain

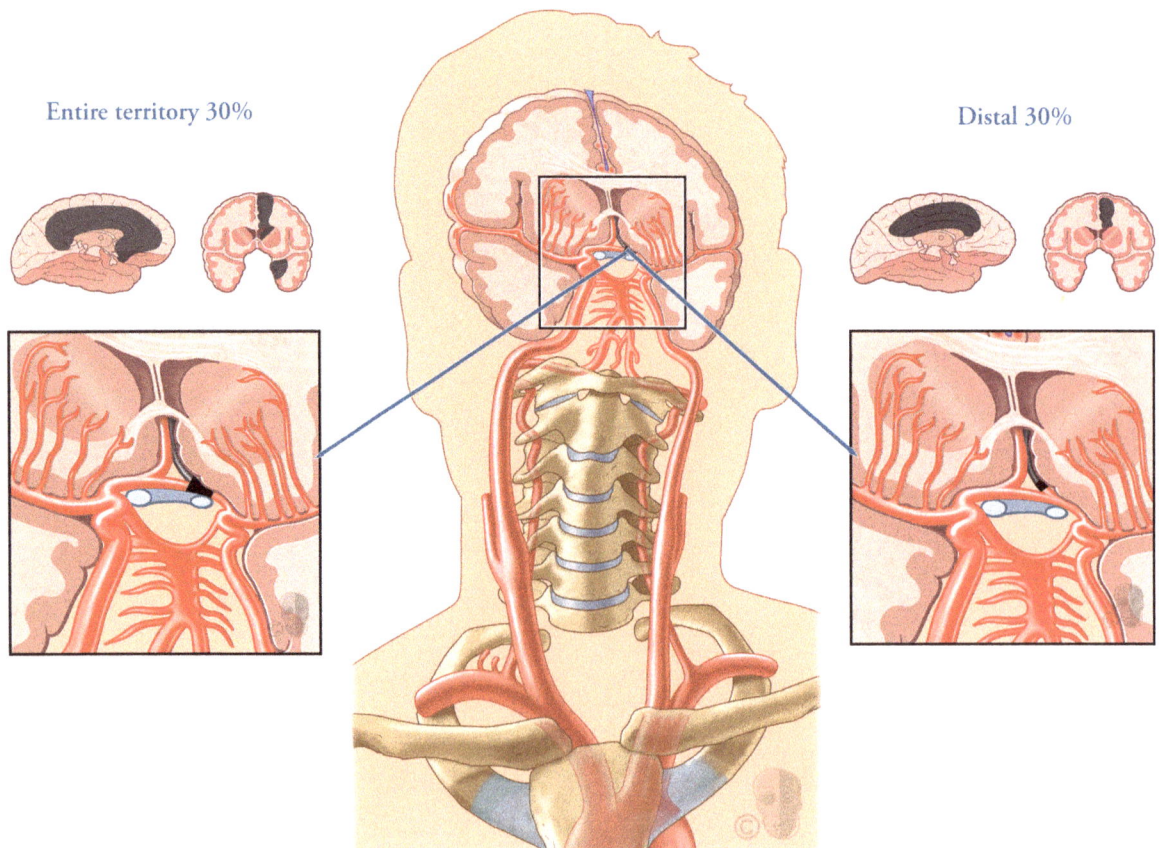

Figure 6.7 Anterior Cerebral Artery: Entire territory (30%) and distal (30%)

252

ANTERIOR CEREBRAL ARTERY – DISTAL 30%

Blockage towards the distal circulation of the ACA can cause the following clinical manifestations:

- Contralateral weakness of the hip, leg, foot and shoulder
- Sensory loss in the foot
- Left limb dyspraxia (makes it harder to understand spatial relationships)
- Transcortical motor aphasia (TMA), or motor and sensory aphasia (TSA) –

  - TMA is characterised by halting speech output, with good comprehension and repetition. Patients with TMA have impaired writing skills, difficulty speaking and difficulty maintaining a clear thought process. Furthermore, TMA is caused by lesions in cortical motor areas of the brain as well as in the anterior portion of the basal ganglia, and can be seen in patients with expressive aphasia
  - TSA is a kind of aphasia that involves damage to specific areas of the temporal lobe of the brain, resulting in symptoms such as poor auditory comprehension, relatively intact repetition, and fluent speech with semantic paraphasia present. TSA is a fluent aphasia similar to Wernicke's aphasia, with the exception of a strong tendency to repeat words and phrases. The person may repeat questions rather than answer them.

MIDDLE CEREBRAL ARTERY – ENTIRE TERRITORY 20%

Blockage of the entire proximal MCA involves the medial and lateral lenticulostriate arteries as well as a superior and inferior division. These clinical manifestations can cause:

- Contralateral gaze palsy – there is usually a right gaze preference, usually at the onset, caused by damage to the right hemisphere cortical areas important for driving the eyes to the left
- Hemiplegia
- Hemisensory loss
- Spatial neglect
- Hemianopsia
- May lead to coma, secondary to oedema
- Global aphasia (if on the left side)

  - This is the most severe form of aphasia and applies to patients who can produce few recognisable words and understand little or no spoken language. Persons with global aphasia can neither read nor write. Global aphasia may often be seen immediately after the patient has suffered a stroke and may rapidly improve if the damage has not been too extensive. However, with greater brain damage, severe and lasting disability may result.

MIDDLE CEREBRAL ARTERY – DEEP 20%

Blockage to the more distal part of the MCA, involving the lenticulostriate arteries can produce the following clinical manifestations:

- Contralateral gaze palsy
- Hemiplegia
- Hemisensory loss – left pure hemiparesis of the upper motor neuron type. Larger infarcts may produce 'cortical' deficits as well – such as left hemineglect

- Hemineglect, also known as unilateral neglect, hemispatial neglect or spatial neglect, is a common and disabling condition following brain damage in which patients fail to be aware of items to one side of the visual field. Neglect is most prominent and long-lasting after damage to the right hemisphere of the human brain, particularly following a stroke. Such individuals with right-sided brain damage often fail to be aware of objects to their left, demonstrating neglect of leftward items
- Transcortical motor and/or sensory aphasia (if on the left side).

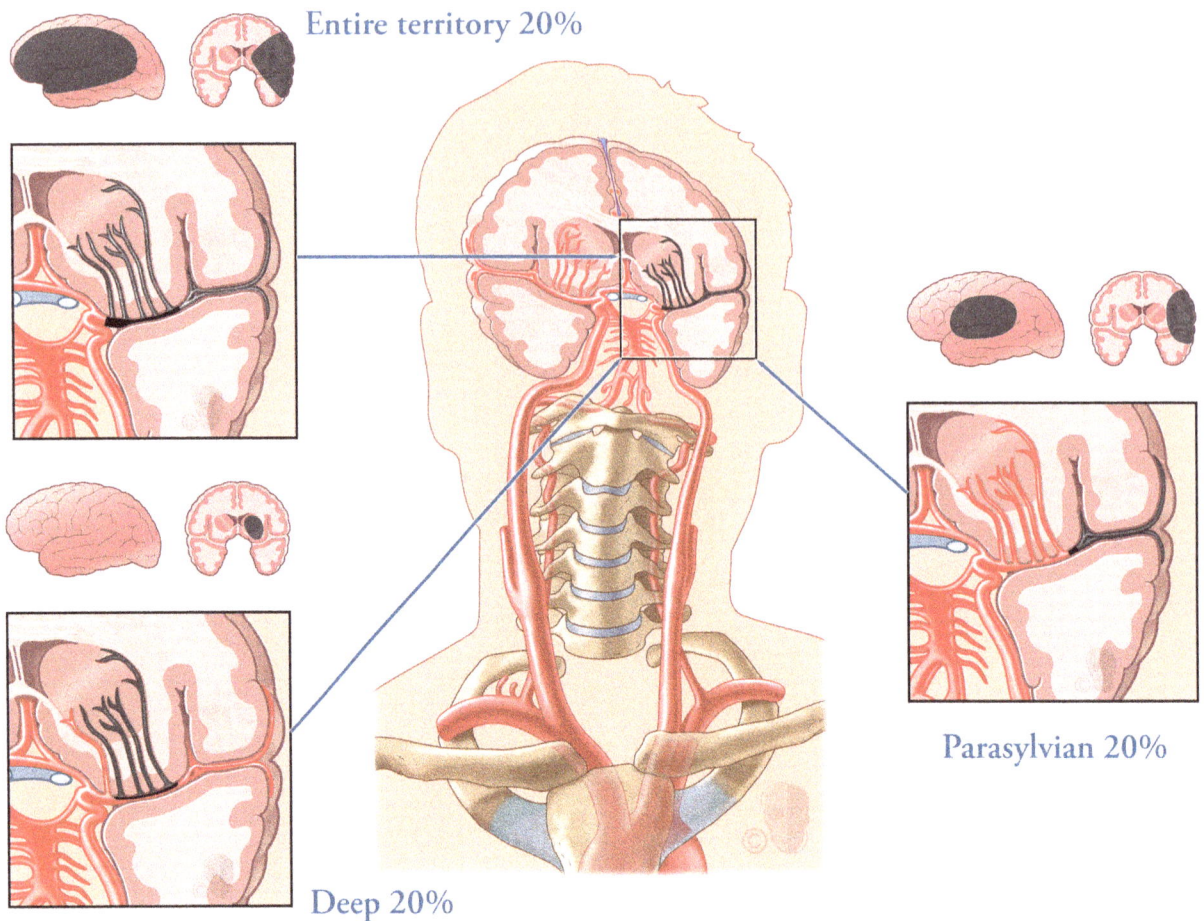

Figure 6.8 Middle Cerebral Artery: Entire territory (20%), deep (20%) and parasylvian (20%)

MIDDLE CEREBRAL ARTERY – PARASYLVIAN 20%

Blockage to the MCA after the lenticulostriate arteries terminate, prior to the bifurcation of the superior and inferior divisions, can produce the following clinical manifestations:

- Contralateral weakness and sensory loss of the face and hands
- Conduction aphasia, apraxia
- Gerstmann's syndrome (if on the left side)
  - Gerstmann's syndrome is a neuropsychological disorder that is characterised by a constellation of symptoms suggesting the presence of a lesion in a particular area of the brain. Destruction to the inferior parietal lobule of the dominant hemisphere results in Gerstmann's syndrome.
- Constructional dyspraxia (if on the right side)

- Constructional apraxia is characterized by an inability or difficulty to build, assemble, or draw objects. Apraxia is a neurological disorder in which people are unable to perform tasks or movements even though they understand the task, are willing to complete it, and have the physical ability to perform the movements. Constructional dyspraxia may be caused by lesions in the parietal lobe, following stroke, or it may serve as an indicator for Alzheimer's disease.

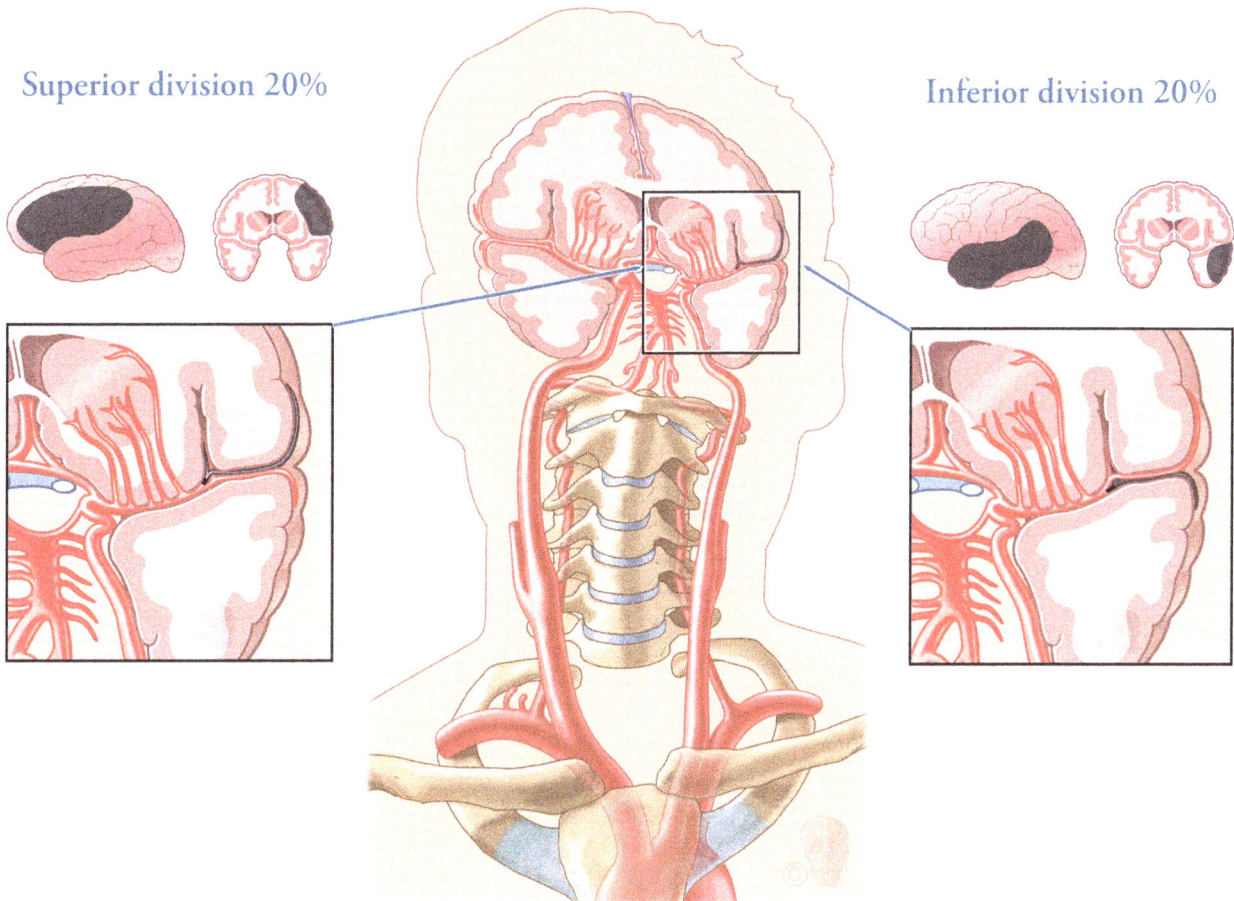

Superior division 20%   Inferior division 20%

Figure 6.9 Middle Cerebral Artery: Superior division (20%) and inferior division (20%)

MIDDLE CEREBRAL ARTERY – SUPERIOR DIVISION 20%

Blockage to the superior division of the MCA can produce the following clinical manifestations:

- Contralateral hemiplegia
- Hemisensory loss
- Gaze palsy
- Spatial neglect
- Broca's aphasia (if on the left side)
  - Speech output can be severely reduced with short utterances of a few words in this sort of aphasia, with limited access to vocabulary, while in Broca's aphasia the formation of sounds is often clumsy and laboured. These people may be limited in writing but will read well and understand speech.

MIDDLE CEREBRAL ARTERY – INFERIOR DIVISION 20%

Blockage to the inferior division of the MCA can produce the following clinical manifestations:

- Constructional dyspraxia (if on the right side)
- Contralateral hemianopsia or upper quadrant anopsia

  - Hemianopsia is a decreased vision or blindness (anopsia) in half the visual field, usually on one side of the vertical midline. The most common causes of this damage are stroke, brain tumour, and trauma.

- Wernicke's aphasia (if on the left side)

  - In this form of aphasia the ability to grasp the meaning of spoken words is chiefly impaired, while the ease of producing connected speech is not much affected. Therefore Wernicke's aphasia is referred to as a 'fluent aphasia.' However, speech is far from normal. Sentences do not hang together and irrelevant words intrude – sometimes to the point of jargon in severe cases. Reading and writing are often severely impaired.
  - Wernicke-Korsakoff syndrome in alcoholics particularly is associated with atrophy/infarction of specific regions of the brain, especially the mamillary bodies. Other regions include the anterior region of the thalamus (accounting for amnesic symptoms), the medial dorsal thalamus, the basal forebrain, the median and dorsal raphe nuclei, and the cerebellum.

POSTERIOR CEREBRAL ARTERY

PCA supply the occipital lobes, the thalami, splenium of the corpus callosum and medial and inferior temporal lobes. Symptoms associated with PCA strokes are diplopia, visual field defects, dysphagia, vertigo, alteration in consciousness, memory impairment. Blockage to the PCA can produce the following clinical manifestations:

- Contralateral homonymous hemianopsia (occipital infarction), hemisensory loss (due to thalamic infarction) and hemibody pain

  - Homonymous hemianopia is characterised by visual field loss in either or both eyes, and on either the left or right side of the vertical midline. It occurs because the right half of the brain has visual pathways for the left hemifield of both eyes, and the left half of the brain has visual pathways for the right hemifield of both eyes. When one of these pathways is damaged, the corresponding visual field is lost.

- Extension to the splenium of the corpus callosum can cause alexia without agraphia, disconnection of visual information in right visual cortex from left temporal speech areas
- Larger infarcts including the thalamus and internal capsule, may cause aphasia, left hemisensory loss and left hemiparesis.

CONCLUSION

The distribution of cerebral aneurysms. Most aneurysms develop from a weakness or abnormal artery wall. Aneurysms usually occur on larger blood vessels where an artery branches. Approximately 85% of aneurysms form in the anterior circulation of the brain, while 15% form in the posterior circulation of the brain.

Embolic stroke – is caused when a clot breaks off from the artery wall then becoming an embolus, which can travel further down the bloodstream to block a smaller artery. Emboli usually come from the heart, where different diseases cause clot formation.

Haemorrhagic stroke – (less common – 17% of cases) is caused by rupture or leaking of an artery either within or around the brain.

Arterial lesions – primary consideration and aetiology for arterial lesions must include birth trauma, whiplash injuries to the cervical spine and dental malocclusions. No matter what the intensities of these injuries at inception, the long-term effects of compromised arterial flow into the brain through the anterior (carotid arteries) and the posterior (vertebral arteries) supply may manifest into serious obstructions and flow later in life. These are exacerbated when the later diagnosis of aneurysms, emboli, infarctions and traumas is added to the list.

Regions supplied by the three main arteries

The three main arteries (ACA, MCA – anterior circulation – and the PCA – posterior circulation) give rise to numerous branches that travel to the subarachnoid space over the surface of the brain and into the sulci.

When blood supplies from two adjacent cerebral arteries are compromised, the regions between the two vessels are most susceptible to infarction and ischaemia. These regions are known as the 'watershed zones':

ACA-MCA watershed infarcts – carotid obstruction.

MCA-PCA watershed infarcts affecting the occipital lobe can cause disturbances to higher order visual processing.

Anterior cerebellar artery – entire territory 30%

Blockage of the right ACA at its source can affect its entire vascular distribution and can produce the following clinical manifestations: incontinence;, contralateral hemiplegia – left leg weakness of the upper motor neuron type and left leg cortical-type sensory loss.

Anterior cerebral artery – distal 30%

Blockage towards the distal circulation of the ACA can cause the following clinical manifestations: contralateral weakness of the hip, leg, foot and shoulder; sensory loss in the foot; left limb dyspraxia (makes it harder to understand spatial relationships); transcortical motor aphasia, or motor and sensory aphasia.

Middle cerebral artery – entire territory 20%

Blockage of the entire proximal MCA involves the medial and lateral lenticulostriate arteries as well as a superior and inferior division. These clinical manifestations can cause: contralateral gaze palsy – there is usually a right gaze preference, usually at the onset, caused by damage to the right hemisphere cortical areas important for driving the eyes to the left; hemiplegia; hemisensory loss; spatial neglect and hemianopsia; may lead to coma, secondary to oedema; global aphasia (if on the left side).

Middle cerebral artery – deep 20%

Blockage to the more distal part of the MCA, involving the lenticulostriate arteries can produce the following clinical manifestations: contralateral hemiplegia and hemisensory loss – left pure hemiparesis of the upper motor neuron type; larger infarcts may produce 'cortical' deficits as well – such as left hemineglect.

Middle cerebral artery – parasylvian 20%

Blockage to the MCA after the lenticulostriate arteries terminate, prior to the bifurcation of the superior and inferior divisions, can produce the following clinical manifestations: contralateral weakness and sensory loss of the face and hands; conduction aphasia; apraxia; and Gerstmann's syndrome (if on the left side).

Middle cerebral artery – superior division 20%

Blockage to the superior division of the MCA can produce the following clinical manifestations: contralateral hemiplegia; hemisensory loss; gaze palsy and spatial neglect; Broca's aphasia (if on the left side).

Middle cerebral artery – inferior division 20%

Blockage to the inferior division of the MCA can produce the following clinical manifestations: constructional dyspraxia (if on the right side); contralateral hemianopsia or upper quadrant anopsia.

Posterior cerebral artery

Blockage to the PCA can produce left homonymous hemianopia – a visual field loss in either or both eyes, and on either the left or right side of the vertical midline. It occurs because the right half of the brain has visual pathways for the left hemifield of both eyes, and the left half of the brain has visual pathways for the right hemifield of both eyes.

CHAPTER 7

THE CISTERNS OF THE BRAIN

The cisterns are large compartments made of meningeal tissue, specifically, the subarachnoid space that is filled with CSF and supports the brain rather like an insulating pad between the surface of the brain and the internal surface of the skull.

These three large cisterns – the cisterna pontis, the cisterna basalis and the cisterna magna – form a waterbed at the base of the brain supporting the brainstem and all the surrounding neurological tissue and drainage vessels.

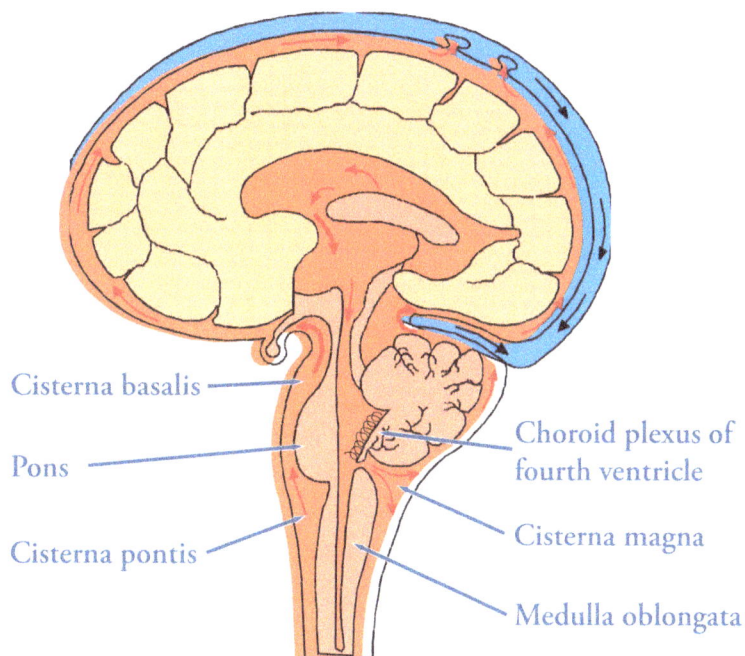

Figure 7.1 The Three Principal Subarachnoid Cisternae

Pressure build-up in the cisterns may cause compression on the parts of the brain or brainstem that they come into contact with, and this could result in physiological changes to those areas.

Pressure on the cisterna pontis, one of the first areas to be subjected to pressure, lies against the substantia nigra, and is currently being reviewed as a possible root cause of Parkinson's disease. Cerebellar dysfunction must be a primary concern in all CSF pressure changes, not only from a cisternal standpoint, but also from the fourth ventricle.

Pressure around the cisterna magna (cerebromedullary cistern) could compress the cerebellum, the lower cranial nerves (cranial nerves IX – the glossopharyngeal, X-the vagus and XI – the spinal accessory, all exit the internal jugular foramen) and brainstem, resulting in displacement of the tentorium cerebellum and distortion of the confluence of the sinuses, the transverse sinuses, sigmoid sinuses and the venous drainage process of the brain.

THE FOURTH VENTRICLE

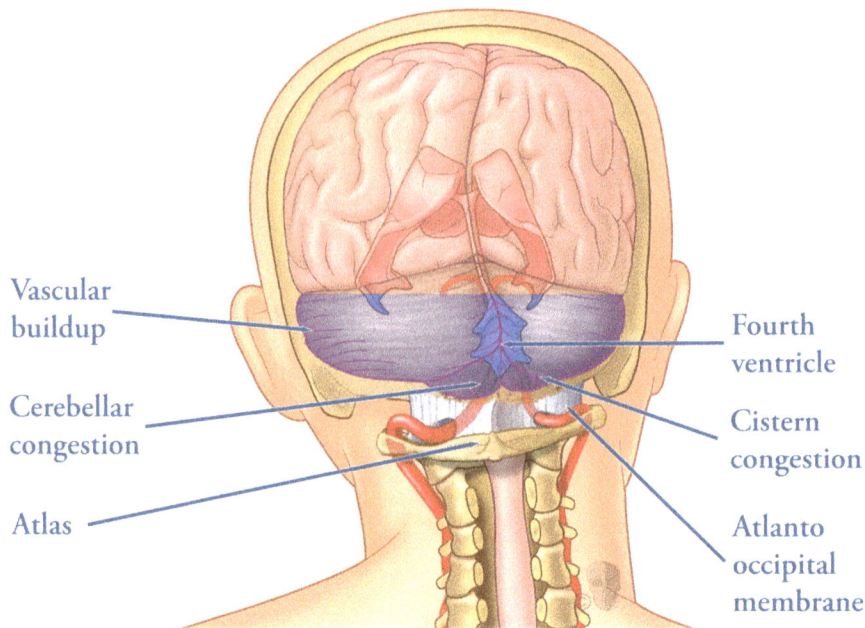

Figure 7.2 Congestion of the Fourth Ventricle

The fourth ventricle is connected to the third ventricle by the narrow cerebral aqueduct of Sylvius. The fourth ventricle is a diamond-shaped cavity located posterior to the pons and upper medulla oblongata and anterior inferior to the cerebellum. The superior cerebellar peduncles and the anterior and posterior medullary vela form the roof of the fourth ventricle. The apex (or fastigium) is the extension of the ventricle up into the cerebellum. The floor of the fourth ventricle is named the rhomboid fossa. Within the floor is the facial colliculus, sulcus limitans, and the obex, which represents the caudal tip of the fourth ventricle. The obex is also a marker for the level of the foramen magnum of the skull and therefore is a marker for the imaginary dividing line between the medulla and spinal cord. The lateral recess is an extension of the ventricle on the dorsal inferior cerebellar peduncle.

Inferiorly, it extends into the central canal of medulla. The fourth ventricle communicates with the subarachnoid space through the lateral foramen of Luschka, located near the flocculus of the cerebellum, and through the median foramen of Magendie, located in the roof of the ventricle. Most of the CSF outflow passes through the medial foramen. The cerebral aqueduct contains no choroid plexus. The tela choroidea of the fourth ventricle, which is supplied by branches of the posterior inferior cerebellar arteries, is located in the posterior medullary velum which forms the infero-posterior part of the fourth ventricle. Somewhat semi-lunar in shape, its convex edge is contiguous with the white substance of the cerebellum, while its thin concave margin is apparently free. In reality, however, it is contiguous with the epithelium of the ventricle, which is prolonged downward from the posterior medullary velum to the taeniae – a coiled band like anatomic structure. The main function of the fourth ventricle is to protect the human brain from trauma (via a cushioning effect) and to help form the central canal, which runs the length of the spinal cord.

When vascular build occurs and after filling the cisterns, the CSF will start to fill the fourth ventricle, increasing the pressure on the flocculonodular lobe found on the front part of the cerebellum, and forms part of the rear wall of the fourth ventricle (responsible for a stooped posture, rigidity, gait abnormalities and loss of balance)need to separate symptoms from anatomical description, (while the pons and upper part of the medulla line the anterior wall.)

THE THIRD VENTRICLE

The third ventricle is bound by the thalamus and hypothalamus on both the left and right sides. The lamina terminalis forms the anterior wall. The floor is formed by hypothalamic structures, including all the thalamic nuclei. The roof is formed by the ependyma, lining the undersurface of the tela choroidea of the third ventricle, and the blood brain barrier.

The importance of these subcortical nuclei for normal brain function and behaviour is emphasised by the numerous and diverse neurological conditions associated with basal ganglia dysfunction. These conditions include: disorders of behaviour control, such as Tourette's syndrome, hemiballismus, and obsessive-compulsive disorder, dystonia, addiction, and movement disorders. Parkinson's disease (involving the degeneration of the dopamine-producing cells, in the substantia nigra pars compacta), and Huntington's disease primarily involving damage to the striatum being the two most well known. The caudate nucleus is highly innervated by dopamine neurons that originate from the substantia nigra, located in the midbrain, containing cell projections to the caudate and putamen and utilise the neurotransmitter dopamine.

The caudate nucleus and the putamen send their axonal signals back to the globus pallidus, the output component of the basal ganglia. The globus pallidus, in turn, forwards the signals to the ventral anterior nucleus of the thalamus. The thalamus then relays signals to the motor and premotor cortex of the cerebrum, where the motor cortex provides the executive commands for movement, while the premotor cortex provides the programs to write and store in memory, where they need to be retrieved.

The basal ganglia, because of its extensive anatomy, becomes subject to craniofacial torsion and ventricular congestion, and transmission of processed neurological information will be reduced and retarded.

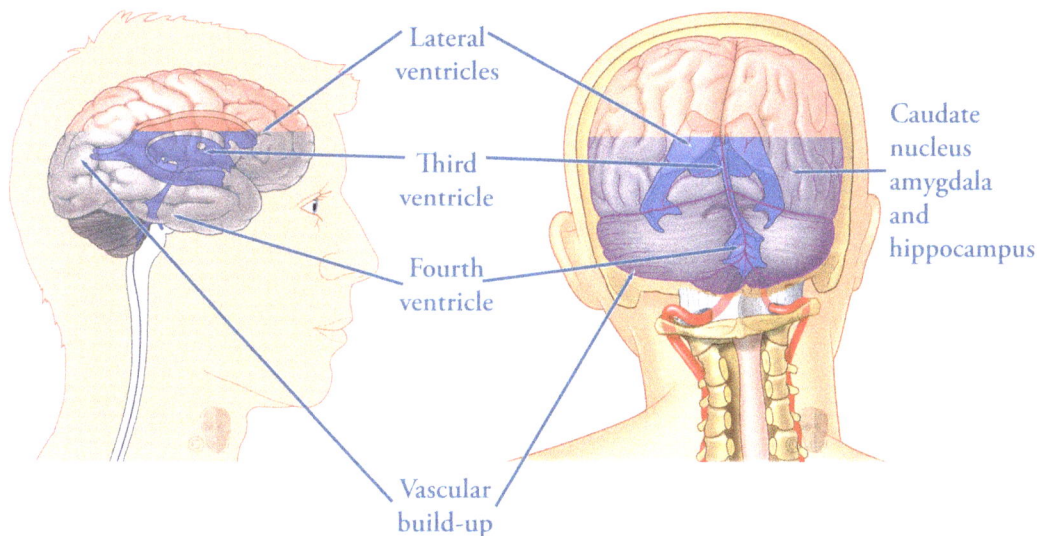

Figure 7.3 Congestion and Engorgement of the Ventricular System

The motor symptoms of the disease result from the death of cells in the substantia nigra. This causes a lack of dopamine in these areas. The reason for this cell death is poorly understood, but involves the build-up of proteins into Lewy bodies in the neurons. Lewy bodies are abnormal clumps of protein that have been found in the brains of people with Lewy body dementia, Alzheimer's disease and Parkinson's disease.

Torsion of the midline and vertical falx cerebri changes the third ventricle boundaries and, with ventricular congestion and retention of CSF, these borderline tissues also change position and format. The position of the adjacent tissues and nerve fibres, both projection and radiation fibres, will also affect their efficiency and transmission.

Several studies have found evidence of ventricular enlargement to be associated with major depression, particularly enlargement of the third ventricle. These observations are interpreted as indicating a loss of neural tissue in brain regions adjacent to the enlarged ventricle, leading to suggestions that cytokines and related mediators of neurodegeneration may play a role in giving rise to the disease.

THE LATERAL VENTRICLES

Each lateral ventricle resembles a C-shaped structure that begins at an inferior horn in the temporal lobe, travels through a body in the parietal lobe and frontal lobe, and ultimately terminates at the interventricular foramina where each lateral ventricle connects to the single, central third ventricle. Along the path, a posterior horn extends backwards into the occipital lobe, and an anterior horn extends farther into the frontal lobe. The lateral ventricles have three horns or cornu, the anterior, the posterior and the inferior.

The anterior horns of the lateral ventricle wrap around the caudate nucleus, while the posterior lateral horns form the floor of the corpus callosum. The inferior horn traverses the temporal lobe, forming a curve around the posterior end of the thalamus. Its roof is formed by the upper surface of the reflected portion of the corpus callosum, the rostrum. It is bound medially by the front part of the septum pellucidum, and laterally by the head of the caudate nucleus. Its apex reaches the posterior surface of the genu of the corpus callosum.

Its floor and medial border present the following parts: the hippocampus, the fimbria hippocampi, the collateral eminence, and the choroid plexus.

The C-shaped caudate nucleus lies just below the lateral ventricles, and below the caudate nucleus lies the C-shaped fornix, under which lies the C-shaped hippocampus. Above the lateral ventricles lies the C-shaped corpus callosum, and above that the C-shaped cingulated gyrus, upon which lies the inferior sagittal sinus.

When cranio fascial distortion takes place, the midline dynamic of the falx cerebri becomes distorted, possibly displacing all of the above central cranial organs and systems and changing their function and vitality.

The volume of the lateral ventricles is known to increase with age. They are also enlarged in a number of neurological conditions and are, on average, larger in patients with schizophrenia, bipolar disorder and Alzheimer's disease.

A severe asymmetry, or an asymmetry with midline shift or diffuse enlargement may indicate brain injury early in life, particularly in cases of a longer right occipital horn.

MULTIPLE SCLEROSIS

Multiple sclerosis is a chronic illness involving the central nervous system. The immune system attacks myelin, which is the protective layer around nerve fibres. This causes inflammation and scar tissue, or lesions which can make it difficult for the brain to send and receive signals to and from the rest of the body.

DEMENTIA

Dementia involves damage of nerve cells in the brain, which can occur in several areas of the brain. Dementia affects people differently, depending on the area of the brain affected.

Dementias are often grouped by what they have in common, such as the part of the brain that's affected or whether they worsen over time (progressive dementias). Some dementias, such as those caused by a reaction to medications or vitamin deficiencies, might improve with treatment.

Progressive Dementias

Types of dementias that progress and are not reversible include:

Alzheimer's Disease

In people age 65 and older, Alzheimer's disease is the most common cause of dementia. Although the cause of Alzheimer's disease is not known, plaques and tangles are often found in the brains of people with Alzheimer's. Plaques are clumps of a protein called beta-amyloid, and tangles are fibrous tangles made up of tau protein. Certain genetic factors might make it more likely that people will develop Alzheimer's.

A low level of insulin in the brain is linked to brain cell degeneration, while good levels of insulin are essential for their survival and function. After reviewing all the evidence showing a connection between Alzheimer's and type 2 diabetes, pathologists from Brown Medical School and Rhode Island Hospital demonstrated that insulin levels are reduced in the frontal cortex, hippocampus and the hypothalamus, all areas affected by Alzheimer's, whereas the cerebellum, which is not affected by Alzheimer's, did not show the same low insulin levels.

Vascular Dementia

This second most common type of dementia occurs as a result of damage to the vessels that supply blood to the brain. Blood vessel problems can be caused by stroke or other blood vessel conditions.

Frontotemporal Dementia

This is a group of diseases characterized by the breakdown (degeneration) of nerve cells in the frontal and temporal lobes of the brain, the areas generally associated with personality, behaviour and language. As with other dementias, the cause is not known.

Mixed Dementia

Autopsy studies of the brains of people 80 and older who had dementia indicate that many had a combination of Alzheimer's disease, vascular dementia and Lewy body dementia. Studies are ongoing to determine how having mixed dementia affects symptoms and treatments.

OTHER DISORDERS LINKED TO DEMENTIA

Huntington's Disease

Caused by a genetic mutation, this disease causes certain nerve cells in the brain and spinal cord to waste away. Signs and symptoms, including a severe decline in thinking (cognitive) skills usually appear around age 30 or 40.

Traumatic Brain Injury

This condition is caused by repetitive head trauma, such as that experienced by boxers, football players or soldiers. Depending on the part of the brain that's injured, this condition can cause dementia signs and symptoms, such as depression, a short temper, memory loss, uncoordinated movement and impaired speech, as well as slow movement, tremors and rigidity (Parkinsonism). Symptoms might not appear until years after the trauma.

Creutzfeldt-Jakob Disease

This rare brain disorder usually occurs in people without known risk factors. This condition might be due to an abnormal form of a protein – prions. Creutzfeldt-Jakob disease can be inherited or caused by exposure to diseased brain or nervous system tissue. Signs and symptoms of this fatal condition usually appear around age 60.

Parkinson's Disease

Many people with Parkinson's disease eventually develop dementia symptoms (Parkinson's disease dementia).

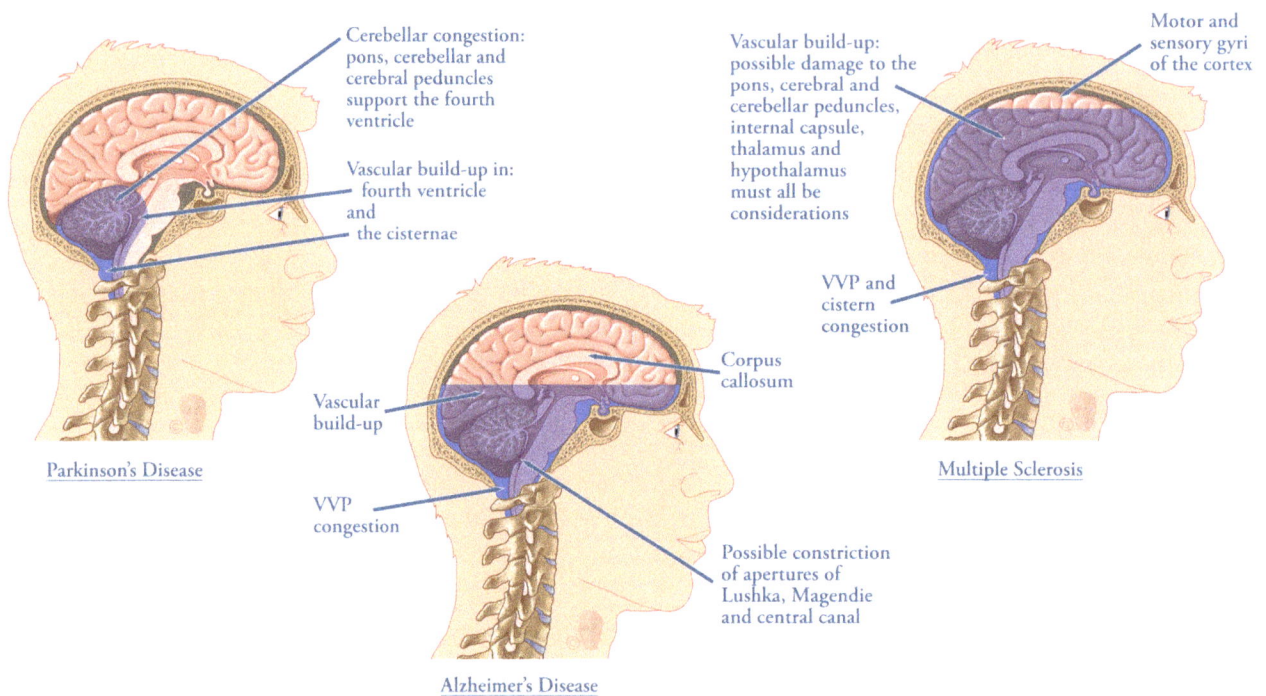

Figure 7.4 Parkinson's Disease; Alzheimer's Disease; Multiple Sclerosis

INTERSTITIAL OEDEMA

Cerebral oedema of the brain is caused by the accumulation of fluid in the brain substance. It may result from head injury, stroke, infection, hypoxia, brain tumours, obstructive hydrocephalus, and lead to encephalopathy; it may also be caused by disturbances in fluid and electrolyte balance that accompany haemodialysis and diabetic ketoacidosis. The most common type is vasogenic oedema, which may result from increased capillary pressure or from increased capillary permeability caused by trauma to the capillary walls. Cellular oedema may occur in ischaemia or hypoxia of the brain. Because the brain is enclosed in the solid vault of the skull, oedema compresses the blood vessels, decreasing the blood flow and causing ischaemia and hypoxia, which, in turn, result in further oedema. Unless measures are taken to reverse the oedema, destruction of brain tissue and death will result.

Interstitial oedema creates two problems for the brain:

It can cause cytotoxic oedema due to the accumulation of metabolic waste products. Cytotoxic oedema has also been implicated as a possible causative factor in demyelination, similar to the effects of ketoacidosis. Ketoacidosis is seen in diabetes and is the result of burning fats and proteins instead of carbohydrates, (Fats are the protective coverings of the nerves, and proteins form the cellular membrane) which can cause more erosion of delicate tissues such as nerves, resulting in diabetic neuropathy.

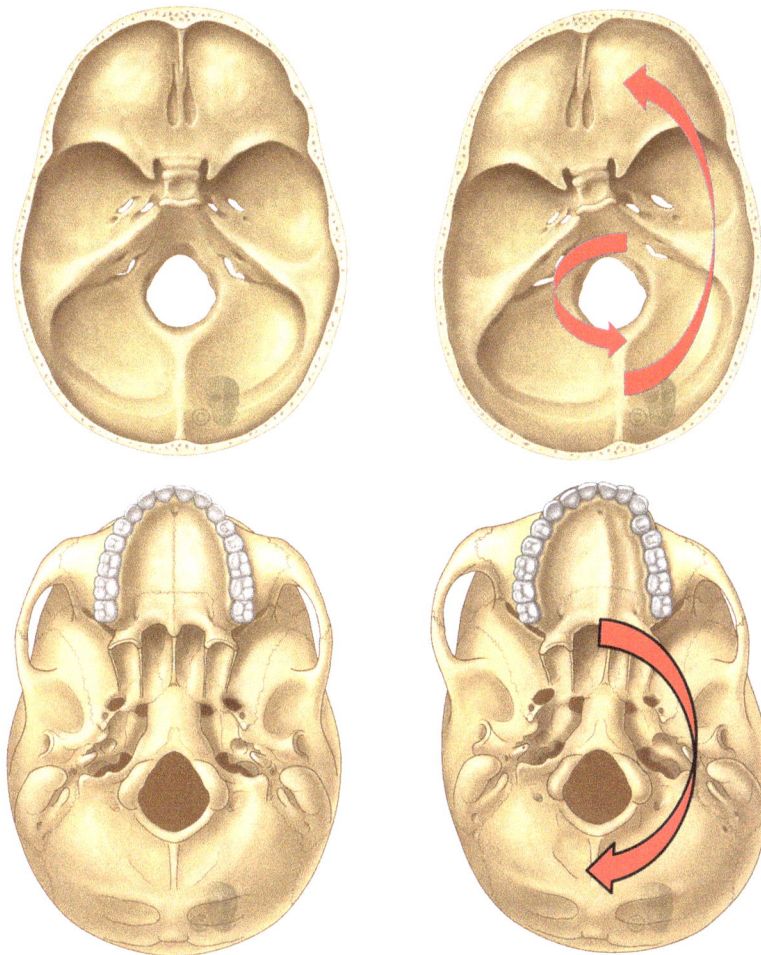

Figure 7.5 Counterclockwise Torque

This can result in a cascade of neurodegenerative events, with a sluggish and stagnant blood flow keeping by products and toxins in circulation longer than necessary. This toxic exposure of healthy tissues leads to further nerve damage and chemical destruction – lysis of myelin.

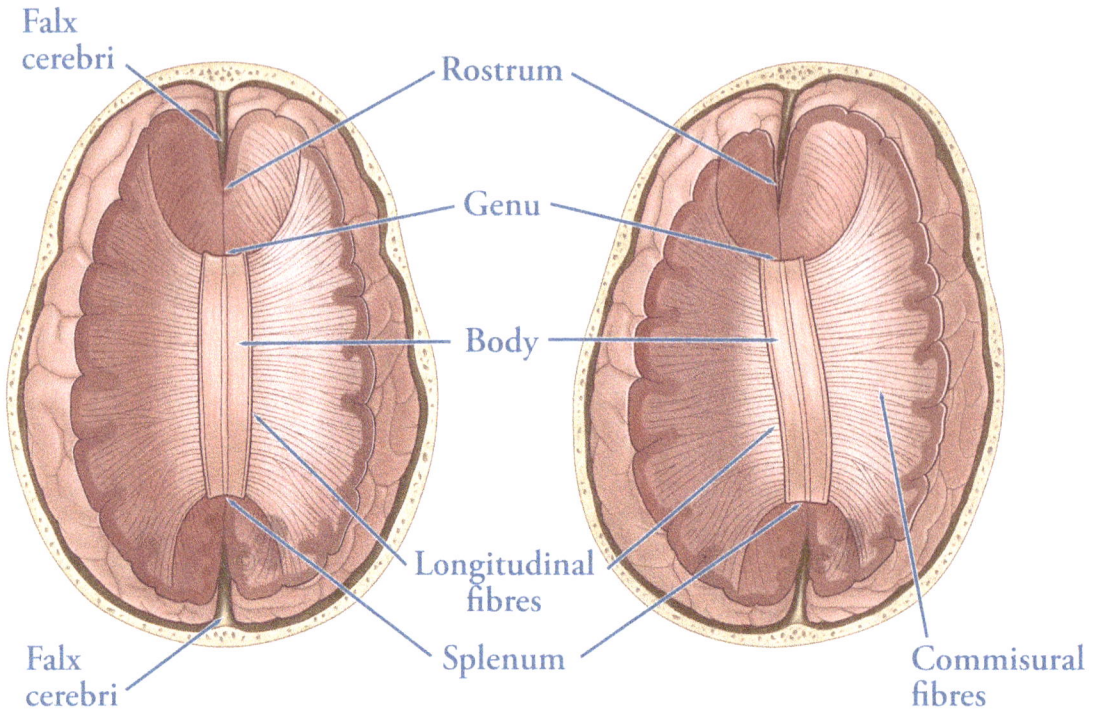

Figure 7.6 Corpus Callosum: Torsion of the falx cerebri

The second problem caused by interstitial brain oedema is that it can cause damage to myelin by simply overstretching it, as it does to the periventricular areas including the myelinated pathways of the corpus callosum. The corpus callosum forms the roof of the lateral ventricles, while the hippocampus forms part of the posterior lower floor. This hypersensitivity and neurodegeneration are frequently found in the corpus callosae of patients with Alzheimer's disease, multiple sclerosis and Parkinson's disease.

Interstitial oedema occurs in obstructive hydrocephalus due to a rupture of the CSF-brain barrier. This results in trans-ependymal flow of CSF, causing CSF to penetrate the brain and spread to the extracellular spaces and the white matter. Interstitial cerebral oedema differs from vasogenic oedema as CSF contains almost no protein.

CHAPTER 8

CLINICAL ASSESSMENT OF CFD

Since its inception, CFD has demonstrated amazing and dramatic changes to patient symptoms and outcomes. Since 2004 this protocol has been used on over 50,000 patients and has produced substantial changes to the parameters that were tested.

Quite apart from the clinical effects of the protocol and having detailed the internal problems arising from cranial torsion and examples of conditions having benefited from treatment, the author has for the last decade looked for clinically accepted ways of measuring these results (to demonstrate the effectiveness of the procedures). Although cranial applied science has been little understood in its application, the overall way in which the brain functions has in my opinion been misunderstood, in effect, that the brain essentially works around a central axis.

CFD has a radical appreciation of the developing brain guided by the hierarchical process of foetal development. At day one, conception occurs, with the egg and sperm cell uniting in the zygote, then at day sixteen we see development of the primitive streak, the future brain and spinal cord and the nervous system that controls every function for that body throughout life. Day eighteen sees the formation of mesenchyme, the future fascia or clingfilm that wraps, encapsulates, supports and protects every part of the body and system. Day twenty-three produces the four pairs of mixed cranial nerves, from the pharyngeal arches that evolve from the three primary brain vesicles at the end of week 3 beginning of week 4 and finally the formation of the five secondary brain vesicles that make up the central brain component, the ventricular system – the dominant system.

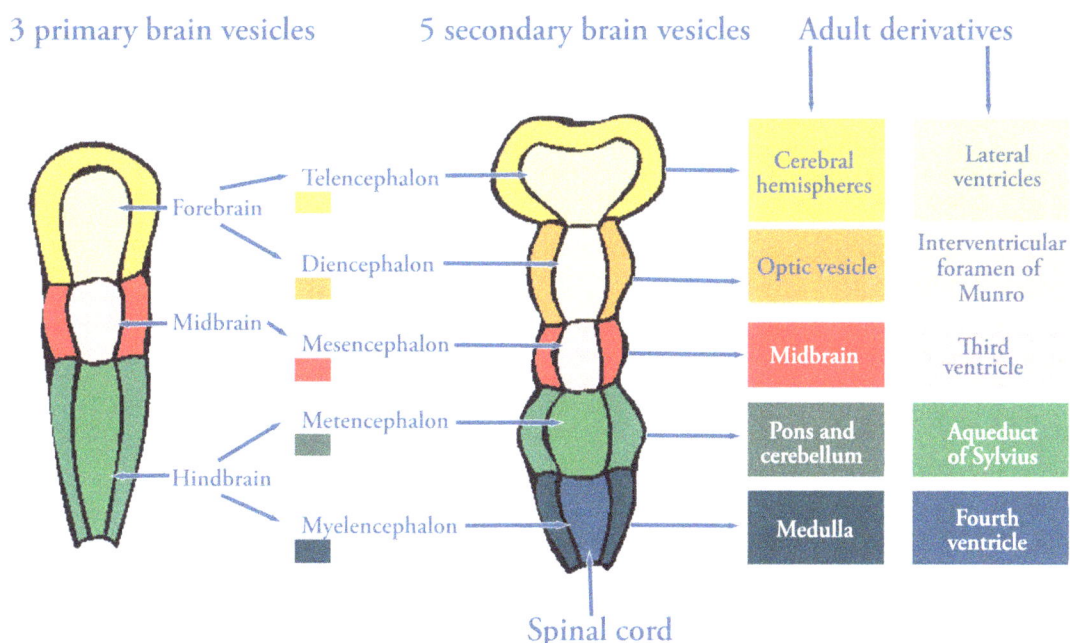

Figure 8.1 Central Canal at Five Weeks: The ventricular system becomes the central core support of the brain

The ventricular system is made up of the two lateral ventricles, joined to the third ventricle by the interventricular foramen of Monro, then the fourth ventricle joined to the third by the aqueduct of Sylvius, which has four outlets. The two lateral apertures of Luska, the medial aperture of Magendie and the central canal that exits into the spinal cord.

The ventricular system generates cerebro spinal fluid which bathes the brain and spinal cord, and acts as a protection against neural injury, creates buoyancy allowing the brain to float, thereby reducing the weight of the brain on the base of the brain with the help of the cisterns also filled with cerebro spinal fluid and retains chemical stability to allow the brain to function normally, by retaining a low extracellular level of potassium for synaptic transmission.

The entire ventricular system supports the brain and is surrounded by and influences all the immediate brain components. The corpus callosum provides the roof of the lateral ventricles and supports both the supracallosal gyri and the cingulate gyrus – the 'processing and retrieval centres'. The base of the lateral ventricles is supported by the caudate nucleus and the fornix, while the third ventricles support the thalamus and the hypothalamus which wrap around it – the 'junction boxes'. The fourth ventricle is surrounded by the cerebellum, cerebellar peduncles at the posterior and the pons and the cerebral peduncles to the anterior – the 'junction boxes transmitting information from cortex to spine and vice versa'. The fourth ventricle is an extension of the spinal cord. The cisterns support this entire structure, followed by the occiput and the spinal column supporting the spinal cord.

Any change in the status of the ventricular system, the surrounding central brain components and the spinal cord will change the homeostasis of the entire central core of the brain. This is introduced by trauma. Trauma comes in any form that potentially changes the delicate balance of the CSF. Its consistency, buoyancy and volume will change the defined border of the ventricles implicating all the central core brain components. That will potentially change the neural pathways, the conduits and the neural connectors to other parts of the brain and spinal cord and can potentially create brain chaos, compromisng retrieval, processing and dissemination capabilities.

CFD has based all its concepts and protocols around the central axis of the ventricular system as well as the potential damage that trauma brings to the entire central nervous system, the autonomic nervous system and the peripheral nervous system.

Quantifying these potentially critical areas of performance has been challenging and initially unrewarding. This is equivalent to the 'hair in the mouth' scenario, where a 'hair in the mouth' causes an enormous sensory activity in a reactive mouth which, once removed, everything changes and the mouth returns to normal. When measuring that hair, it is infinitesimal in its dimensions but can cause annoyance. The same applies to changes in neurological transmission, the torsion is apparently insignificant but the consequences are substantial. Trauma is an ongoing recurrence throughout life, with trauma upon trauma being inflicted on the brain. If this trauma is not reduced or neutralised, then the significance/long term effects become profound.

THERMAL IMAGING AND THE HOWAT SWEEP

We can assess CFD treatment by employing thermal imaging. Thermal imaging cameras showed the build-up of vascular retention and congestion in the skull. Unfortunately, areas covered by hair do not give accurate evidence of vascular congestion over the top of the calvarium, as the heat is diffused and absorbed, thus readings are corrupted The movement of blood from the face and cranium to the neck and shoulders was substantial, as shown in Figure 8.2. A solution was perhaps to shave the patients beforehand, which would not be taken kindly – even for the sake of science.

The other problem with thermal imaging was the inability to measure the change in heat dispersal and accumulation. This method was then aborted.

After thermal imaging showed the build-up of vascular congestion, the Howat Sweep was performed. Immediately after the sweep, thermal images were taken of the face and neck at intervals of 5 minutes, 10 minutes and 15 minutes. The images show how the vascular build-up had drained from the original congested area and appeared to be more diffuse over the face and neck. This demonstrates, initially, the efficacy of the Howat Sweep, but a more analytical approach is needed to substantiate these findings.

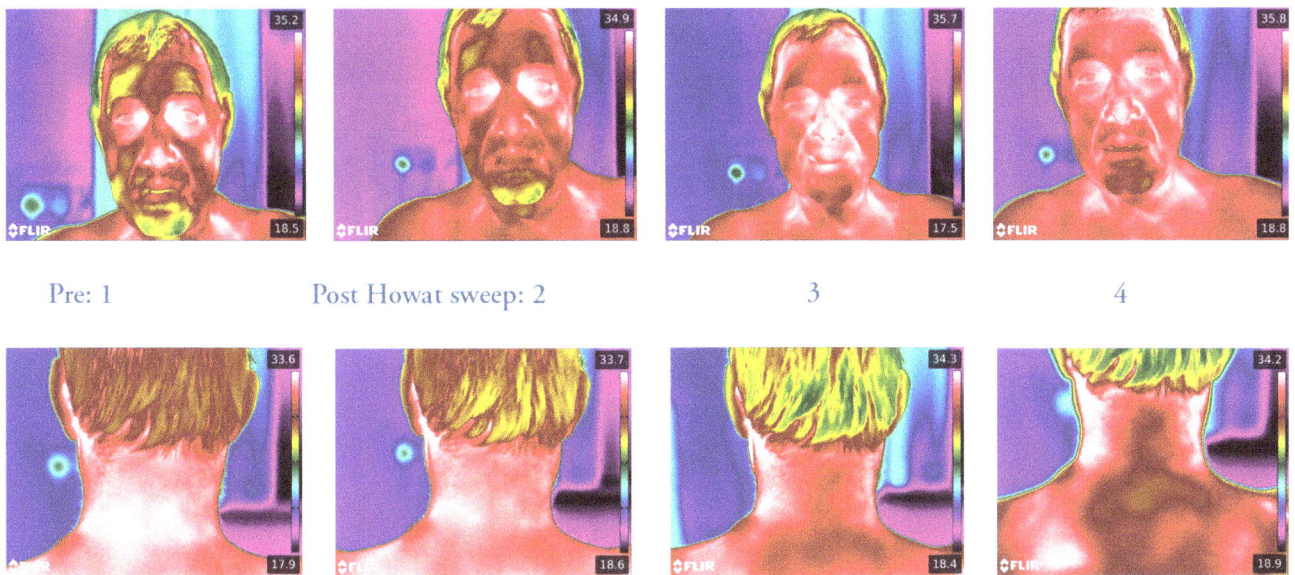

Pre: 1   Post Howat sweep: 2   3   4

Figure 8.2 Thermal Imaging

Transcranial Dopler Ultrasound (TCD)

CFD looks at the brain as an 'irrigation system' with blood flow into the brain being equal to volume of blood flowing out. This would be homeostasis. Transcranial dopler ultrasound measures the arterial blood flow of the basal cerebral arteries into the brain through windows created by the sutural fontanelles, which are then compared to common carotid arterial flow. There should be consistency in volumes and BP, changes in cerebral vasoactivity (changes in CO_2) and cognitive and motor activation. TCD is also used in the clinical diagnosis of a number of cerebrovascular disorders.

The principle idea in CFD, was to compare the arterial inflow to the circle of Willis and to compare it to the venous outflow through the internal jugular veins, the vertebral venous plexus and the sub-occipital cavernous sinus – not usually undertaken by TCD. The data was difficult to collect, was variable and inconsistent. This method, too, was abandoned.

Transcranial Doppler (TCD) and transcranial colour Doppler (TCCD) are types of Doppler ultrasonography that measure the velocity of blood flow through the brain's blood vessels by measuring the echoes of ultrasound waves moving trans-cranially (through the cranium). These modes of medical imaging provide a spectral analysis of the acoustic signals they receive and can therefore be classified as methods of active acoustocerebrography. They are used as tests to help diagnose emboli, stenosis, vasospasm from a subarachnoid haemorrhage (bleeding from a ruptured aneurysm).

The volume of typical blood flow can be measured through specific cranial 'windows' with the transcranial Doppler, specifically, the ACA, the MCA, the PCA and the internal carotid artery (ICA).

Pupillometry (PLR)

A few years ago, Reflex created an app used on a handheld device, which for access and simplicity, was easy and effective in reading pupillary light reflex (PLR).

This shows the pupillary light reflex response with the Reflex app. When the light is shone in the eye, the first response is light on the retina, transmitted by the optic nerve through the optic chiasma, by way of the optic tract to the midbrain, to the pretectal nucleus in the lateral geniculate nucleus, then to the Edinger-Westphal nucleus, where the oculomotor nerve, with parasympathetic fibres, takes over, taking the stimulus to the ciliary ganglion, and through the short ciliary nerve fibres and to the pupillary constriction muscles.

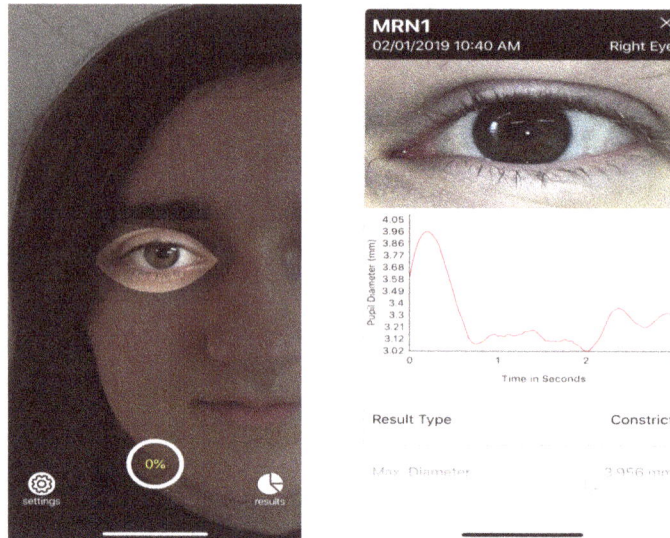

Figure 8.3 Handheld Device for Measuring PLR from Reflex

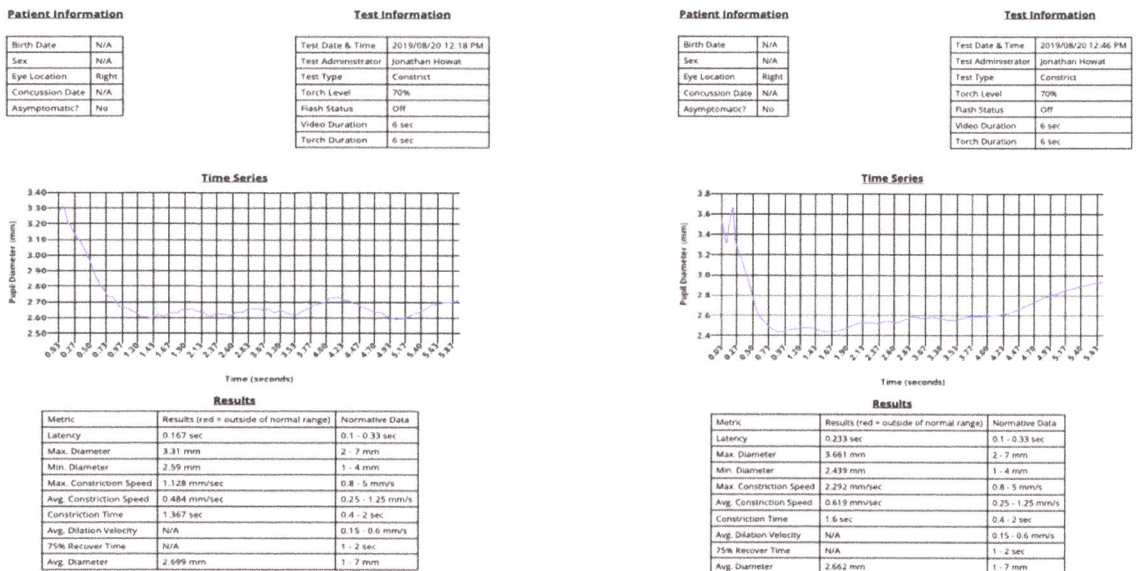

Figure 8.4 Reading from Stroke Victim: (left) Pre reading, (right) post reading

These are the measurements Reflex takes, which are then downloaded onto either an Excel spreadsheet or by way of an email address onto a laptop.

a. Latency – time taken for the pupil to respond to a light stimulus, measured in seconds. From retina CN II to pretectal nucleus to EW nucleus, to red nucleus to constriction

b. Maximum diameter – maximum diameter of the pupil observed by Reflex measured in millimetres (mm)

c. Maximum constriction velocity observed by Reflex over the constriction period measured in mm/sec

d. Average constriction velocity – the average velocity observed by Reflex over the total constriction period measured in mm/sec

e. Minimum diameter – the minimum diameter observed by Reflex measured in mm

f. Dilation velocity – the average velocity observed by Reflex over the total dilation period measured in mm/sec

g. 75% recovery time – time taken for the pupil to reach 75% of its initial diameter value measured in secs.

h. Average diameter – average of all diameter measurements taken in a time series measured in mm.

The diameter of the pupil is controlled by smooth muscle within the iris. The pupillary size, shape and reactivity to light are regulated by the autonomic nervous system. The parasympathetics will constrict the pupil using the pupillary constrictors by way of the neurotransmitter norepinephrine (Phase 1).

Once the light source terminates, there is a recalibration of the pupil, where the parasympathetics are reduced, and the sympathetics come into play, dilating the pupil by way of the sympathetic neurotransmitter acetylcholine to the pupillary dilators – the radial muscles within the iris (Phase 2).

Once the parasympathetics cease being reactive, the sympathetics will come into play, returning the pupil to the accommodation state (Phase 3).

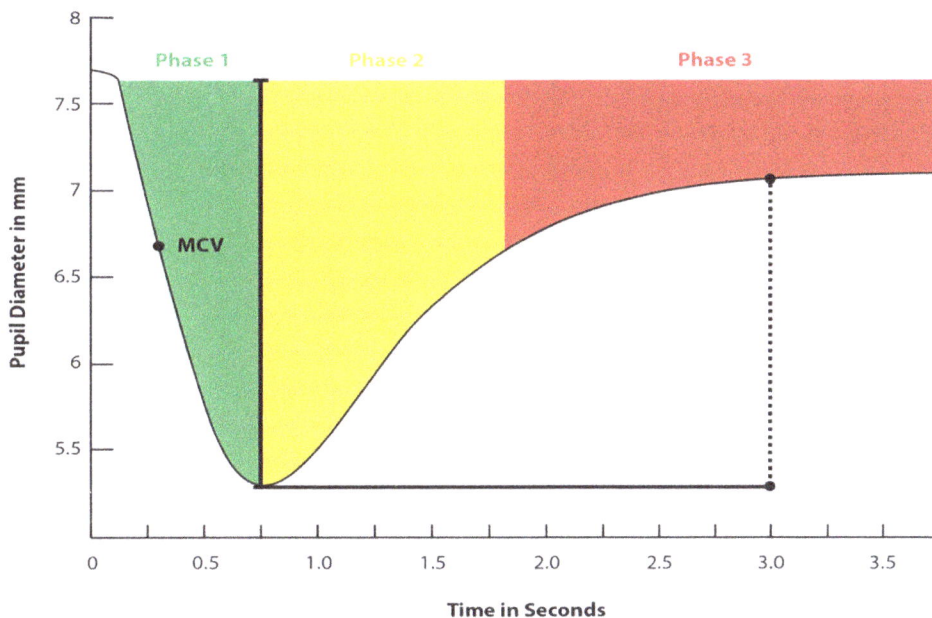

Figure 8.5 Pupillary Eye Reflex Chart: Phase 1 – parasympathetic; phase 2 – sympathetic and parasympathetic; phase 3 – sympathetic

The Autonomic Nervous System (ANS) consists of the Sympathetic Nervous System (SNS) and the Parasympathetic Nervous System (PNS) and is regulated by the Hypothalamus. The ANS receives monitoring input from the Limbic System (cingulate gyrus, hippocampus, amygdala) and is regulated by the Hypothalamus, just above the brain-stem. Brain trauma and whiplash injuries may torque the brainstem and medulla, along with the ventricular system, potentially changing the neurological pathways and conduits conveying vital nerve communications. The first of these distortions occur with the peripheral and adjacent central core brain organs, the thalamus and the hypothalamus and thereby has influence on ANS activity. The parasympathetic pathway stimulates the constrictor muscles of the iris constricting the pupils, where the neurotransmitter is acetylcholine, while the sympathetic pathway stimulates the dilator muscles of the iris, dilating the pupils – where the stimulating neurotransmitters are epinephrine and norepinephrine.

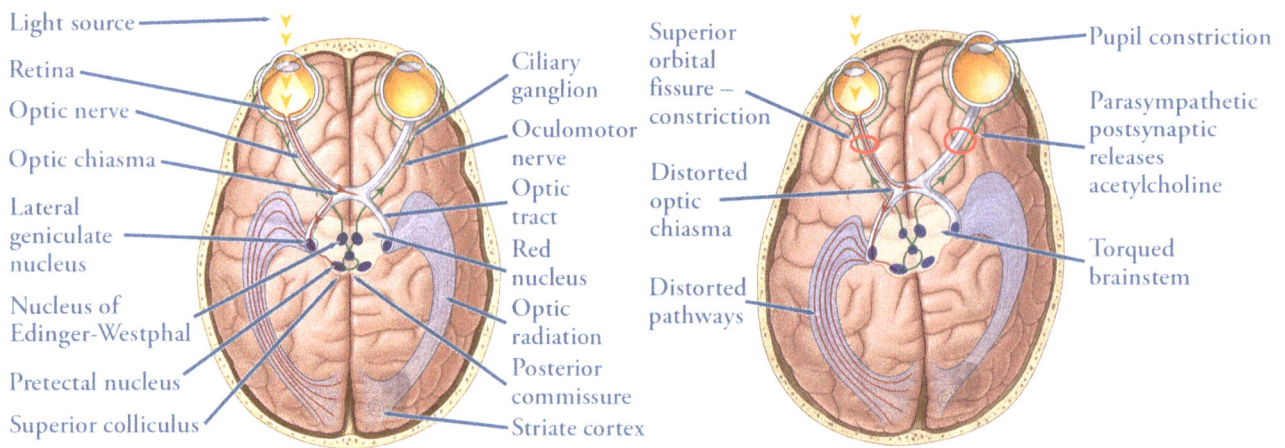

Light source
Retina
Optic nerve
Optic chiasma
Lateral geniculate nucleus
Nucleus of Edinger-Westphal
Pretectal nucleus
Superior colliculus

Ciliary ganglion
Oculomotor nerve
Optic tract
Red nucleus
Optic radiation
Posterior commissure
Striate cortex

Superior orbital fissure – constriction
Distorted optic chiasma
Distorted pathways

Pupil constriction
Parasympathetic postsynaptic releases acetylcholine
Torqued brainstem

Figure 8.6 PLR Pathway: (left) normal; (right) distorted

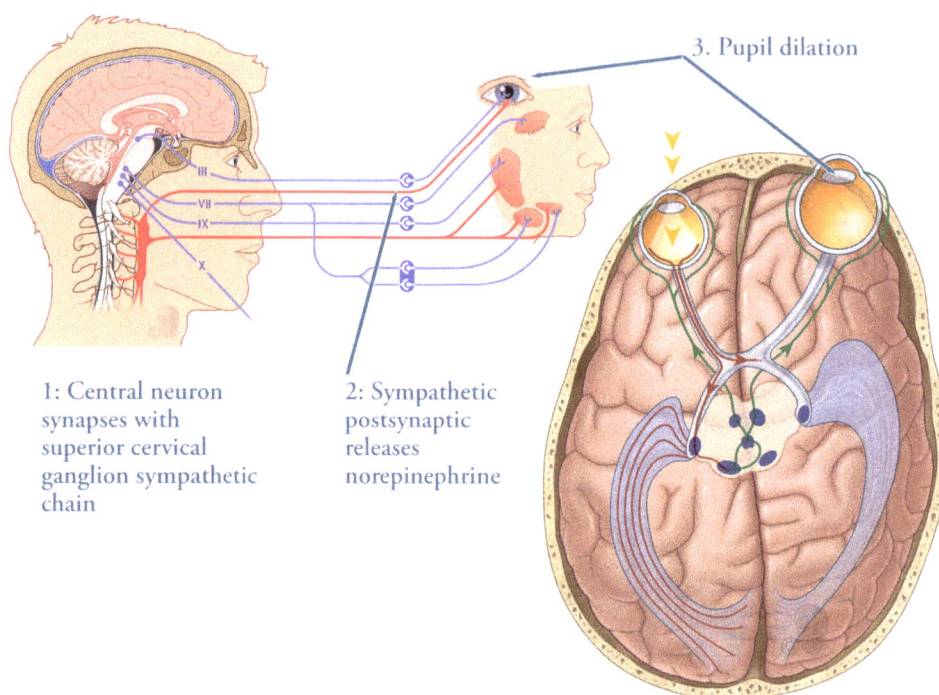

3. Pupil dilation

1: Central neuron synapses with superior cervical ganglion sympathetic chain

2: Sympathetic postsynaptic releases norepinephrine

Figure 8.7 Distorted PLR

For the last six months the Neuroptics NPI-200 has been used to measure the PLR, and while still in its infancy is providing useful and promising information. (The advantage of this handheld unit, is there are no variables in the light intensity in the room, as the device uses an infrared camera,)

The principle advantage of this device is its infrared camera which is unaffected by variables in surrounding light intensity. Infrared light intensity is a constant vital when measuring light reflexes This handheld device has been used almost exclusively in critical care facilities in hospitals, more specifically for head injury patients, to monitor and measure on almost an hourly basis how the patient is progressing. The Neurological Pupillary Index (NPI) is an algorithm of several readings taken as one value, which works in an inverse relationship to intracranial pressure (ICP). If the NPI stays above a given figure between 5 and

3, the ICP is much lower. When the NPI goes down (below 3) the ICP goes up and allows physicians to investigate why the ICP has elevated – possibly a sub-dural haematoma or some other injury requiring surgical intervention. This measurement has been consistent for a sample of about 400 patients, and is finding itself becoming more and more reliable.

The use of this device to measure changes in cranial function is a new deviation from the original concept of measuring NPI, but the device also indicates that the Howat 8-Step Protocol modifies brain function. The speed of 'constriction velocity' and 'pupil size' has already been flagged as a 'change' in brain activity.

The PLR monitors the latency – the retina reaction time from the light source, the optic nerve transmission to the pretectal nucleus in the lateral geniculate body, the transmission to the nucleus of Edinger-Westphal, then, the transmission via the oculomotor nerve to the ciliary ganglion and finally to the iris for parasympathetic reaction with acetylcholine to constrict the pupil.

Apart from the torque at the midbrain, affecting the geniculate body, the pretectal and Edinger-Westphal nuclei, the optic and oculomotor nerves have to go through the optic chiasma and finally through the superior orbital fissure in the sphenoid, both of which are subjected to cranial torque. There is also the activation of both the parasympathetic and sympathetic nervous systems depending on the intensity of the light source – either 'bright' or 'dim', releasing acetylcholine or norepinephrine.

In effect there are many issues to be aware of in measuring the PLR. This is an exciting modality, which we will be testing for some time to come.

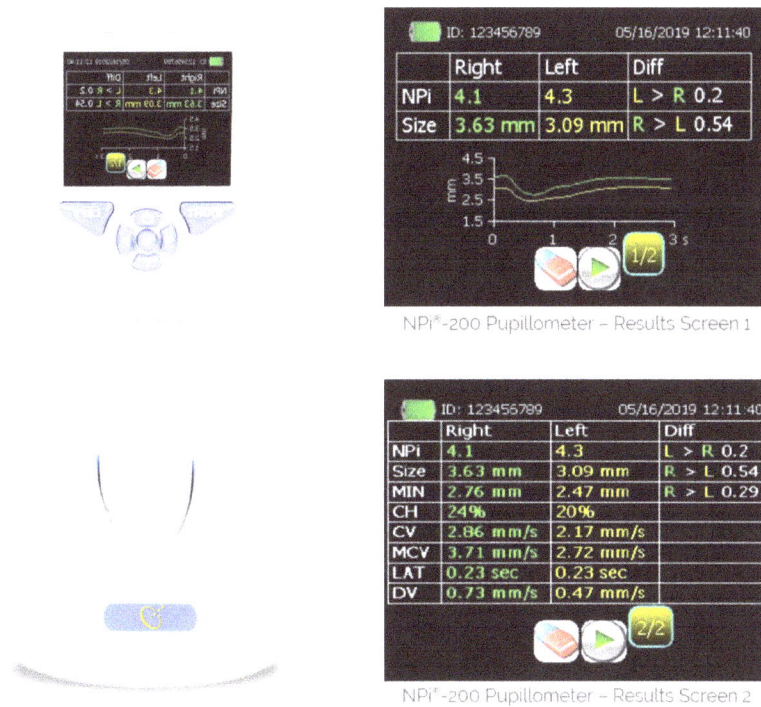

Figure 8.8 NPi®-200 Pupillometer

Variable heart rate elite HRV

Heart rate variability (HRV) is an accurate, non-invasive measure of the autonomic nervous system (ANS) – which responds to everything: how you exercise, recover, eat, sleep and perceive stress.

Unlike basic heart rate (HR) that counts the number of heartbeats per minute, HRV looks much closer at the exact changes in time between successive heartbeats (also called inter-beat intervals, RR intervals, NN intervals, etc.).

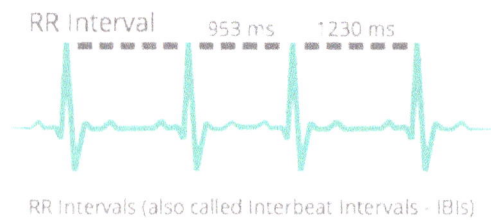

RR Interval   953 ms   '230 ms

RR Intervals (also called Interbeat Intervals - IBIs)

Figure 8.9 Heart Rate Variability Graph

By trending short HRV readings on a daily basis, our adaptive algorithms learn what our "normal" Autonomic Nervous System patterns look like, help us gain insights into our nervous system, stress and recovery activity, and then automatically guide us in improving those patterns over time

The sympathetic nervous system controls the body's "fight or flight" reactions in response to internal or external stressors. It stimulates blood glucose (to fuel the muscles), pupil dilation (to detect threats), slows digestion/peristalsis (to focus energy on the present danger), and increases heart rate (to ensure adequate blood circulation to run or fight). The SNS is ideally activated to overcome short term stress situations such as running from a tiger or fighting an intruder. But this same response also occurs when exercising, performing challenging mental tasks, getting into an argument, or even launching a kickstarter.

The parasympathetic nervous system controls the body's "rest and digest" responses and is associated with recovery. Parasympathetic activation conserves energy, constricts pupils, aids digestion, and slows heart rate. The PSNS is meant to help build for the long term and is needed to grow faster, stronger, and healthier.

The SNS and PSNS control the same organs with opposite effects. Both branches are always working and both are needed to maintain homeostasis (balance or equilibrium) in the body. With every single heartbeat, the nervous system is saying "slow down – speed up" based on feedback from all the senses and emotions. A healthy nervous system has a balanced but strong push and pull between the sympathetic and parasympathetic branches. Heart rate variability is an accurate, non-invasive measure of the ANS and the balance between the SNS and PSNS branches.

WHY DOES THIS MATTER?

The Sympathetic Nervous System's physiological response to stress focuses on short term survival in lieu of long-term health. This acute response can become chronic (constant, long term) in the presence of stress from modern daily life such as work, relationships, financial, environmental, dietary, physical and lifestyle choices. Chronically accumulated stress from multiple sources can all contribute to drastically reduced health and performance over the long term.

A significant amount of research published over the past 50 years correlates HRV to:

- Disease risk and progression (diabetes, cardiovascular disease, respiratory diseases, gastrointestinal diseases, autoimmune conditions, etc.)
- Morbidity and mortality
- Biological aging and health
- Mental health, mood, depression, anxiety, PTSD
- Physical performance (HRV is heavily used in elite endurance and team sports to guide training and recovery)
- Injury prevention
- Guided rehabilitation

- Mental cognition

CFD protocols have a direct impact on the traumatised brain, ultimately reducing the torque to central brain components, the thalamus and hypothalamus, the pons and related cerebral peduncles and the cerebellar peduncles, the primary neural pathways. These pathways have an impact on the limbic system, including the sympathetic and parasympathetic nervous systems and their ability to counter stress.

Studies with this heart rate monitor will be used to evaluate any changes to the HRV using the Howat 8-Step Protocol.

The Autonomic Nervous System (ANS) controls the unconscious bodily processes and influences the functions of internal organs.

Some internal processes regulated by the ANS:

- Heart rate
- Blood pressure
- Body temperature
- Electrolyte balance
- Digestion
- Respiratory rate
- Pupillary response
- Urination
- Sexual arousal

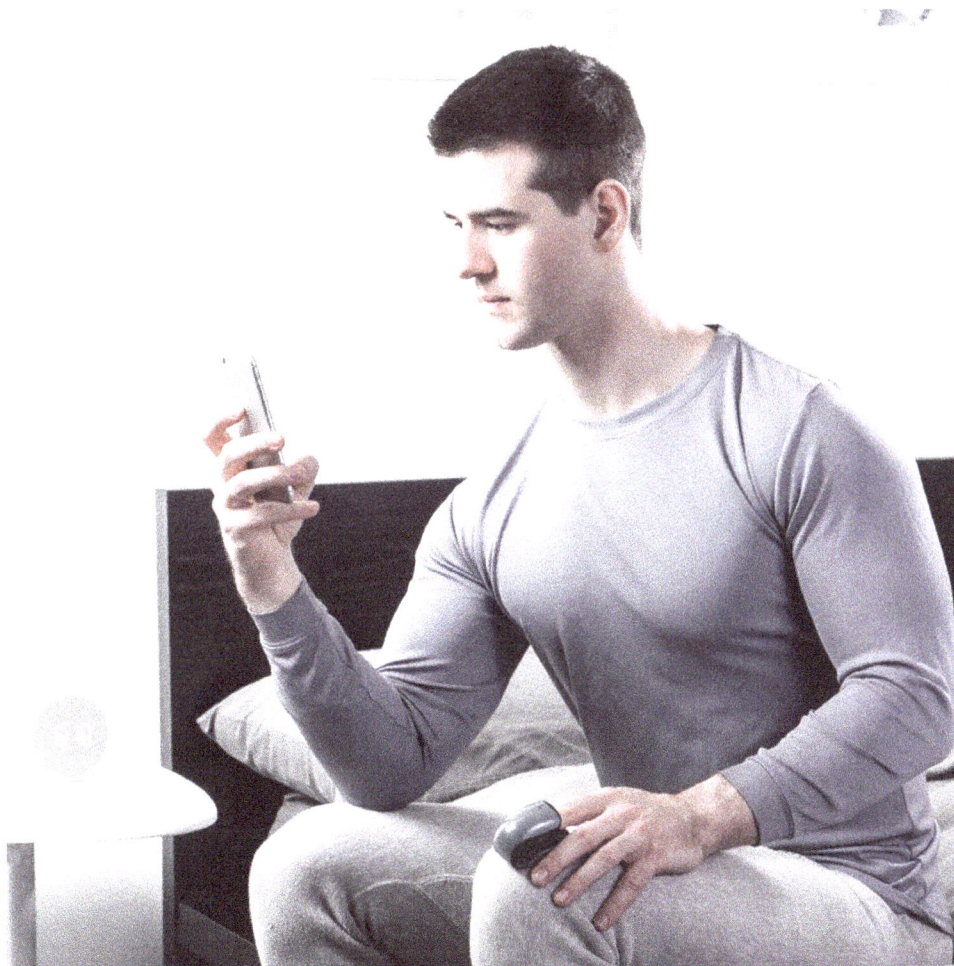

Figure 8.10 Using the Elite HRV App and CorSense® (© elitehrv.com)

THE DISLOCATED BRAIN

PART V

CRANIO DENTAL

DYNAMICS

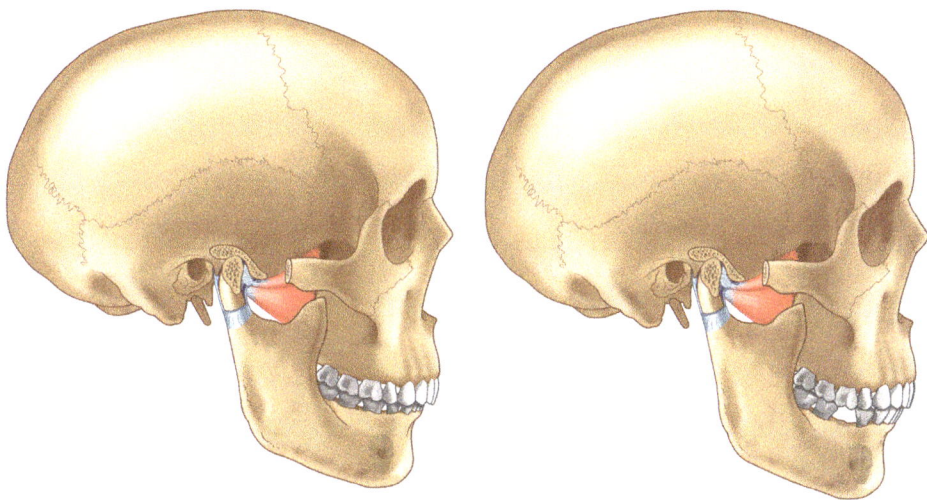

CONTENTS PART V

ILLUSTRATIONS PART V

CHAPTER 7

INTRODUCTION TO PART V

In recent years the chiropractor's understanding of descending stomatognathic problems has led to the use of 'brain-balancing' techniques to try and neutralise the descending cranial major, provided these changes are of a fascial nature. To a large degree this negates the necessity of dental intervention, both orthopaedically and orthodontically, which for most patients is of great benefit. However, if the cause of the descending major is directly rooted in a dental issue, such as missing dentition, loss of vertical, incisal interference and so on, then functional dentistry will be required to remove the descending major before attempting to correct the fascial drag – disruption to normal fascial function.

Fixed orthopaedic and orthodontic appliances introduce vectors into the skull, which are reinforced for 24 hours of the day for the duration of the treatment. These vectors are manmade and although assessed/ selected using modern technology/diagnostic methods, the author questions whether any (functional) orthodontist/orthopaedist can introduce the finely tuned fixed appliance to provide the vectors required in the skull to the degree the body or brain need.

The mutual understanding between functional dentistry and cranio-fascial rebalancing is an essential component in trying to resolve a descending stomatognathic problem. The assessment by these professionals of the patient's needs is vital to making this happen. There are dental issues that can only be resolved by a dentist, but they are fundamental to changing the status quo of toxic vectors that are the basis of the descending major. Once that has been achieved, then removing the torque and allowing the cranium to unwind with a non-registered lower plate appliance will allow a recalibration of the cranium and the RTMs to take place. However, if the aetiology of the descending major is not a dental issue then appliances could be inappropriate and cranio-fascial rebalancing may be all that is needed to neutralise the descending major. The reason for a relapse of an inappropriate orthodontic or orthopaedic intervention is the action of vectors and dynamics within the mouth, tongue and masticatory muscles that will combine to try and reinstate the original stomatognathic system, because the 'forced' change to the system has been unsuitable and misplaced.

CHAPTER 1

PROPRIOCEPTION

The central nervous system coordinates information from receptors located in the muscles, joints and tendons. These are sensory receptors called proprioceptors and are responsible for the kinaesthetic sense and perception of movement in the individual.

In normal temporomandibular joint (TMJ) function proprioceptors are found in the periodontal ligaments, muscles of mastication and the retrodiscal tissue, and those sensory receptors feed back to the central nervous system (CNS) the state of the periodontal tissue and tooth position, muscle tension and the length of the muscle spindle, and the state of the retrodiscal tissue. Two types of receptors make up this information – the muscle spindle and the Golgi tendon organ apparatus. The muscle spindle monitors the length of the muscle and consists of a connective tissue sheath that contains several intrafusal muscle fibres located deep in the muscle tissue and is formed by several thin striated fibres. The muscle spindle contains sensory and motor fibres.

The Golgi tendon organ is found in the musculotendinous junction and is a simpler receptor than the muscle spindle. It discharges sensory impulses with both the stretch or contracture of a muscle and records the degree of stretch a tendon is experiencing. The muscle spindle emphasis is on the muscle length and facilitates or contracts the muscle, whereas the Golgi tendon organ has an inhibitory effect at the muscle origin. Therefore, stretching a muscle receptor – either a Golgi tendon organ or a muscle spindle – sends sensory impulses to the CNS. When a muscle contracts, the response of the two receptors is different. The tendon organ reacts while the muscle spindle will relax or shorten. The stretch reflex is initiated by stretch of the muscle spindle, whereby the muscle contracts, thus enabling the muscle to maintain a constant length. Inhibitory impulses are transmitted to the motor neurons of the antagonistic muscles allowing the reflex to be more effective.

In the mandible the stretch reflex is referred to as a jaw jerk reflex. When the jaw closing muscles are stretched the muscle spindle mechanism sends information to the brainstem causing a reflex contraction of those muscles. With the teeth together in occlusion the proprioceptive mechanisms of the periodontal membrane stimulate the jaw opening muscles to prevent excessive contraction of the jaw closing muscles thus providing a homeostatic occlusion.

In malocclusions caused by bruxing, or loss of dentition, or loss of posterior support, or incisal interference or loss of vertical support, the muscles would attempt to shorten themselves through the stretch reflex mechanism resulting in muscle fatigue and muscle soreness. A constant force on the TMJ and periodontal membrane proprioceptive mechanisms will cause the nerve endings to reversibly deteriorate to a level where they cannot contribute to the reflex control of the jaw muscles thereby promoting temporomandibular joint dysfunction (TMJD).

Trigeminal Nerve – Mandibular Branch – Neuroanatomy

Proprioceptive sensory stimuli from the Golgi tendon organ, the muscle spindles, the periodontal ligament and the retrodiscal tissue are conducted through the mandibular division of the trigeminal nerve to the trigeminal ganglion and to the mesencephalic nucleus in the brainstem. Then a monosynaptic arc to the masticatory (motor) nucleus creates a jaw jerk reflex into the muscles of mastication – the temporalis, masseter, lateral and medial pterygoid muscle – for coordination and control of chewing movements and the bite.

Sensation from the meninges of the anterior and middle cranial fossae is carried by the meningeal branch of the mandibular division. Two major meningeal trunks that travel with the middle meningeal artery converge into a single nerve that exits through the skull via the foramen spinosum and joins the main trunk of the mandibular nerve prior to returning to the cranial cavity through the foramen ovale.

The sensory nucleus of the trigeminal nerve is the largest of the cranial nerve nuclei. It extends caudally into the spinal cord as far as the second cervical segment. The nucleus of the spinal tract of the trigeminal nerve extends from the chief sensory nucleus in the pons caudally into the spinal cord where it emerges with the dorsal grey matter of the spinal cord. Its function is perception of pain and temperature.

DENTAL OCCLUSAL CLASSIFICATION

The dental classification is a hereditary type of jaw to jaw position, as defined by the relationship between the upper and lower teeth. The jaw to jaw position and relationship is defined as the shape and size of the two maxillae, the height of the palate at the apex junction of the two bones, the lateral width of the maxillae at the base and its contact with the mandible, and the position achieved by the anterior protrusion of the maxillae.

How the mandible fits with the maxillae under these circumstances determines the final classification.

CLASS I – NORMOGNATHIC

Dental classification is based on the relationship between the canines and first premolars. In centric occlusion there are three relationships that can exist between the first molars. In a normal relationship the maxillary first molar is slightly posterior to the mandibular first molar. The mesiobuccal cusp of the maxillary first molar is directly in line with the buccal groove of the mandibular first molar. Such a relationship is called a Class I occlusion relationship.

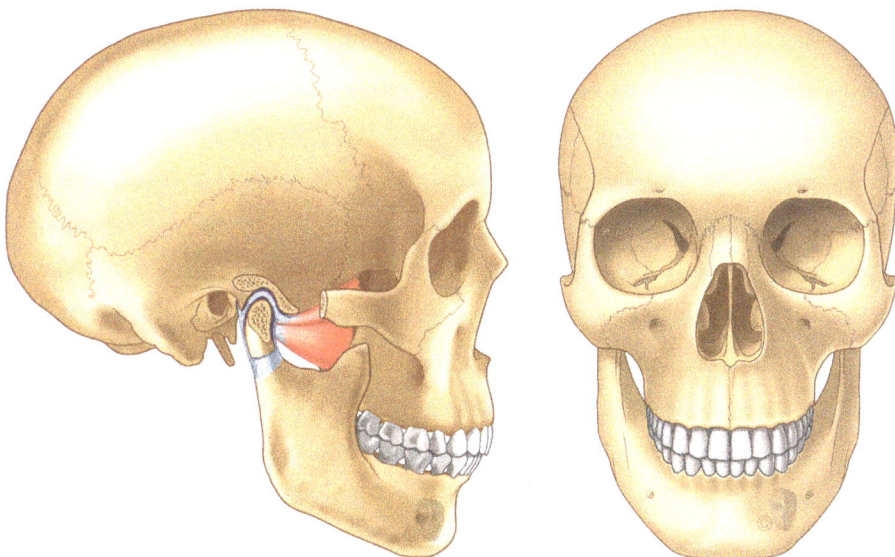

Figure 1.1 Class I – Normognathic

CLASS II DIVISION 1 – RETROGNATHIC

A Class II distocclusion exists when the maxillary first molar is anterior to the mandibular first molar. In this relationship, the buccal groove of the mandibular first molar is posterior to the mesiobuccal cusp of the maxillary first molar. There are two divisions:

Division 1 occurs when the permanent first molars are in Class II and the permanent maxillary central incisors are in a slightly protruded position. This is brought about by an inferior vertical strain where the sphenoid is depressed creating an internal rotation of the frontal bone.

CLASS II DIVISION 2 – RETROGNATHIC

Division 2 occurs when the permanent first molars are in a Class II relationship and the permanent maxillary central incisors are retruded and inclined lingually. This results in hyperflexion of the sphenobasilar synchondrosis.

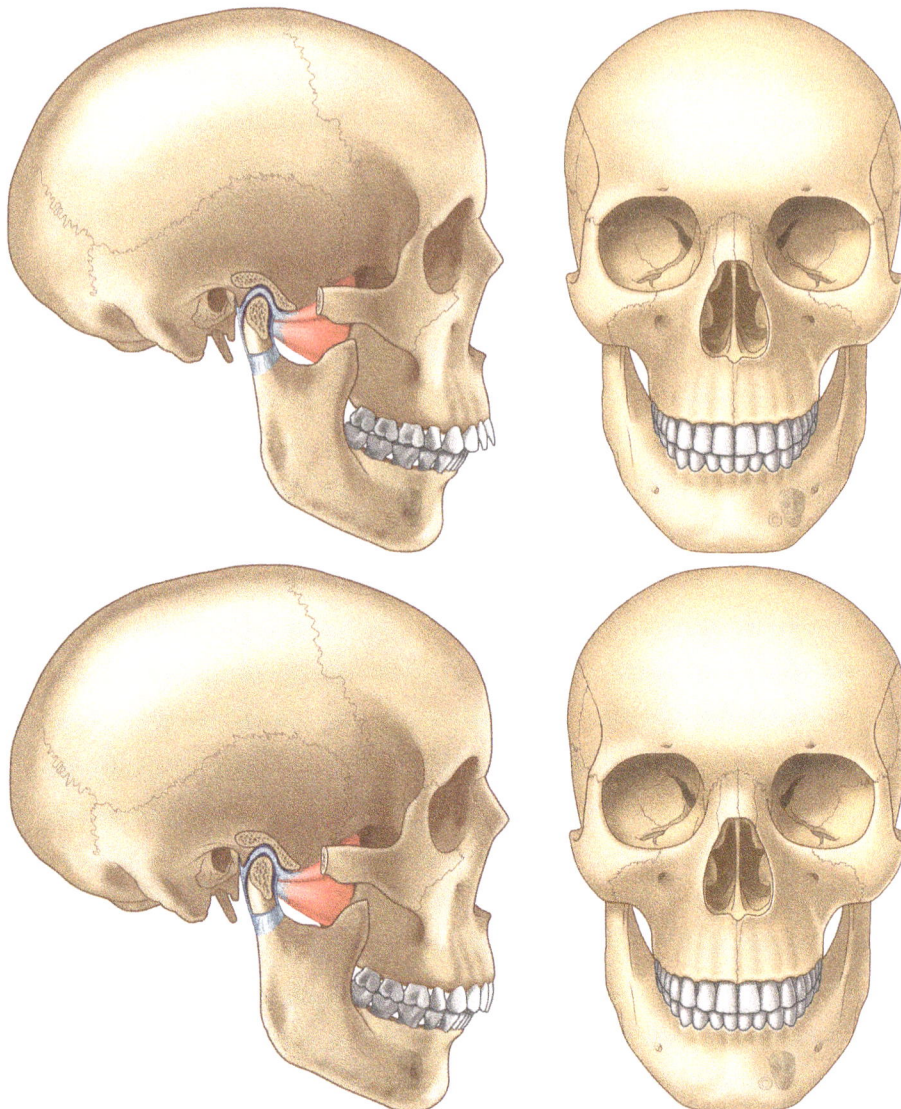

Figure 1.2 Class II – Retrognathic: (top) Division 1, (bottom) Divison 2

CLASS III – PROGNATHIC

A Class III mesi-occlusion exists when the buccal groove of the mandibular first molar is more anterior than normal to the mesiobuccal cusp of the maxillary first molar. This results in a superior vertical strain elevation of the sphenoid and external rotation of the frontal bone. When the jaws are completely closed together there are two possible relationships: either there is a relationship of the upper jaw to the lower jaw centric relation or a relationship of the upper teeth to the lower teeth centric occlusion.

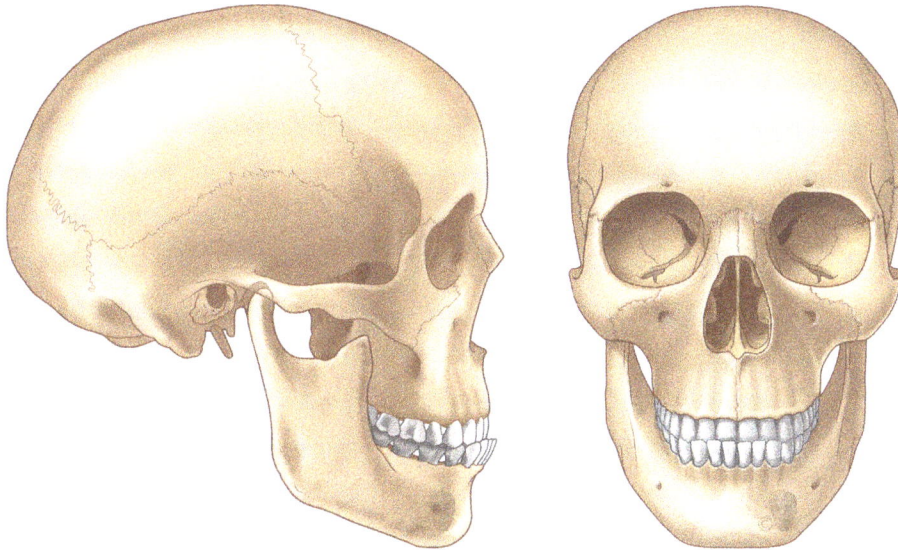

Figure 1.3 Class III – Prognathic: Protruding mandible

CENTRIC OCCLUSION AND RELATION

When you think of centric occlusion/centric relation, think of the condylar head in the fossa and its relative position. CO, or habitual position, is the position of the condylar head in the fossa when the teeth come together. This is often dictated by habit and the teeth that give you the "feel right" feeling when you bite down. In this position, the condylar head can be ANYWHERE within the fossa. CR is when the condylar head is in its most ANTERIOR and SUPERIOR position and in this position most often the teeth do not come together normally. If you put yourself in CR and close, you will feel the bite is off. So, the teeth and habit dictate CO position while condylar head/fossa dictates CR position.

> Centric Relation (CR) is not an occlusion at all. It has nothing to do with teeth because it is the only 'centric' that is reproducible with or without teeth present. Centric relation is a jaw relationship: it describes a conceptual relationship between the maxilla and mandible. All attempts to lay down rigid definitions of CR are plagued by the fundamental difficulty that there is no sure or easy way of proving that the locating criteria have been achieved. Centric relation has been described in three different ways: anatomically, conceptionally, and geometrically. (*British Dental Journal*)

Centric occlusion also refers to a position when the jaws are closed, but this position is determined by the way the teeth fit together. It is a jaw position that affords the greatest interdigitation of the teeth. It is dependent on the position that allows the most inter-cuspation. It is related to tooth occlusion and not determined by muscle or bone. It is a habitual way that the teeth come together. With the jaws closed the occlusal surfaces of the maxillary teeth touch the occlusal surfaces of the mandibular teeth. The lingual cusps of the maxillary premolars and molars rest in the deepest part of the occlusal sulci of the mandibular premolars and molars, and the buccal cusps of the mandibular premolars and molars rest in the deepest part of the sulci of the maxillary premolars and molars.

CONCLUSION

Proprioception – The central nervous system coordinates information from receptors located in the muscles, joints and tendons. These are sensory receptors called proprioceptors and are responsible for the kinaesthetic sense and perception of movement in the individual.

This chapter address the classification of the various occlusions:

- Class I – normognathic
- Class II – retrognathic
  - Division 1
  - Division 2
- Class III – prognathic
- Centric relation (CR) – the position of the condyle, which is the most viable position within the TMJ, regardless of the interdigitation of the teeth
- Centric occlusion (CO) – the position of the condyle in the TMJ when the teeth are interdigitated.

CHAPTER 2

DESCENDING – MAJOR STRESS

The following characteristics are known as major stresses. The most important aspect of testing for cranio fascial dynamic torsion is to assess if the patient is an ascending or descending major. The ascending/descending major test was first put together by Dr Jean Pierre Meersseman from Como in Italy. He was able to differentiate whether a problem had its aetiology in the stomatognathic area or whether in fact the stomatognathic area was not involved. The stomatognathic area deals with the jaws and the TMJs and the highly invested trigeminal nerve complex. The stomatognathic area can potentially influence the cranial primary respiratory mechanism in either a positive or negative way, or plainly put, the stomatognathic area, the teeth and the TMJs directly influence fascial drag – if the primary aetiology is a stomatognathic problem. If fascial drag is NOT part of the stomatognathics then the problem is an ascending problem, which means it is primarily weight bearing, a bilateral sacroiliac fixation, a sacroiliac strain, an inferior or superior sacral involvement, a lumbar sacral lesion or problems with the hips, knees, ankles and feet.

STOMATOGNATHIC SYSTEM

The combination of organs, structures, and nerves involved in speech and reception, mastication, and deglutition of food. This system is composed of the teeth, the jaws, the masticatory muscles, the tongue, the lips, the surrounding tissues, and the nerves that control these structures.

The following components make up the stomatognathic system:

- Jaws – premaxilla, both the maxillae and mandible, palatines and the soft palate
- Teeth – both the alveolus and periodontium and the dentate ligaments
- Palate – the maxillae and the palatines
- Tongue, the lips and the soft palate
- Muscles include the internal (medial) and external (lateral) pterygoids masseters, buccinators and the temporalis muscles
- Sphenoid, vomer and ethmoid.

All the nerves that facilitate these functions – namely, the trigeminal, facial, glossopharyngeal and vagus nerves – are all the mixed cranial nerves.

DESCENDING – MAJOR STRESS

These are considered to be major stress configurations that will possibly require some dental intervention, once the cranio fascial torsion has been removed. Once cranio fascial torque has been removed, further assessment is required to establish whether the outstanding malocclusion requires dental intervention, in the form of re-establishing tooth height to counter a vertical height deficit with overlays on the teeth, implants to rectify the loss of dentition to establish posterior support, or in the case of a Class II upper arch, the need to expand the arch with orthopaedics and orthodontics, to try and regain a proper occlusion. The importance of cranial work alongside this dental work cannot be overstated, as the new position of the upper and lower jaw relationship will be defined by the stress vectors allowed within the cranial dynamics. This part of treatment, if neglected, will possibly cause a relapse of the orthodontics and orthopaedics as time goes on, as these vectors are part of the innate protection of the autoimmune system.

INCISAL INTERFERENCE

Caused by the conflict of the lower incisors coming into contact with the inferior aspect of the upper incisors, retruding the mandible and pushing the mandibular condyle against the retrodiscal tissue of the TMJ.

OVERCLOSED

Caused by the loss of dentition, a loss of vertical or wearing down of teeth through bruxing.

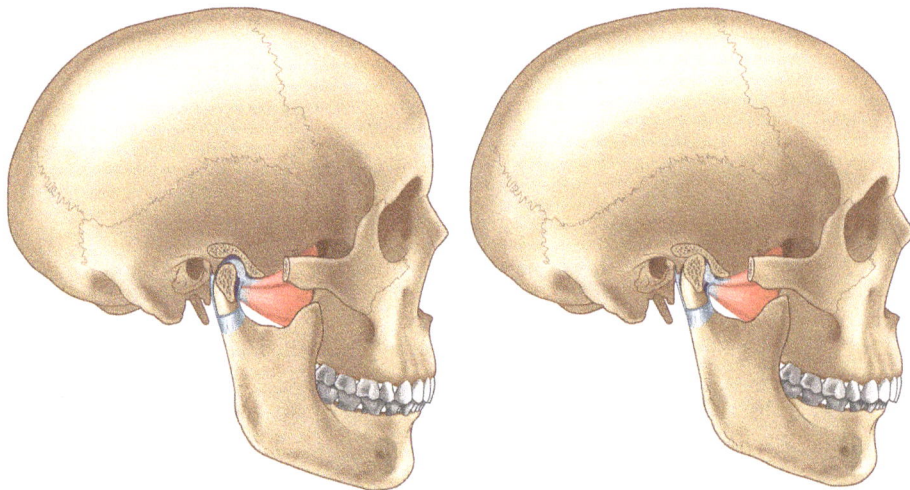

Figure 2.1 (left) Incisal Interference: Mandibular condyle crushes retrodiscal tissue in the TMJ; (right) Overclosed: Incisal interference causes TMJ compression by the mandibular condyle

LOSS OF DENTITION

Caused by dental decay, gingivitis or trauma. The loss of dentition as shown, will cause the teeth on either side of the lost tooth to collapse towards one another, reducing the vertical dimension, and forcing the condyle superior into the glenoid/mandibular fossa.

LOSS OF POSTERIOR DENTAL SUPPORT

Caused by changes in the occlusion with dynamic stress on the posterior teeth.

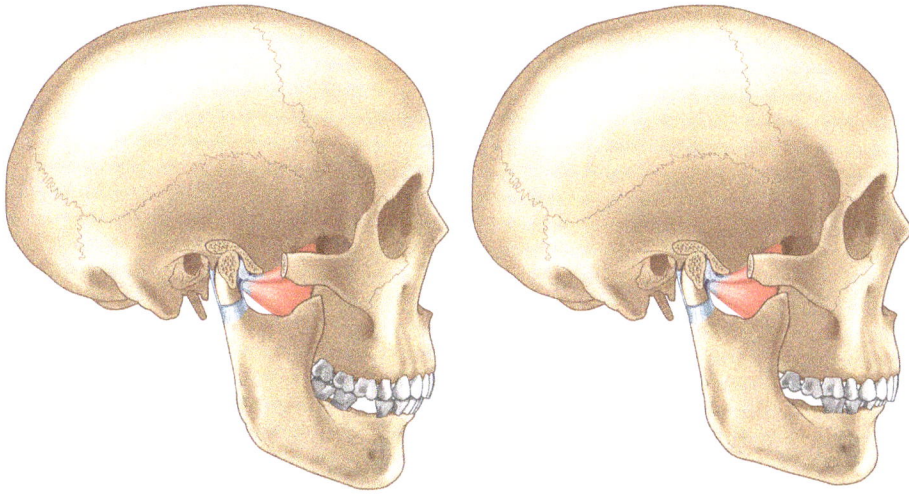

Figure 2.2 (left) Loss of Dentition – Loss of Vertical, (right) Loss of Posterior Dental Support: Mandibular condyle crushes retrodiscal tissue in the TMJ

BILATERAL CROSSBITE

Caused by abnormal muscular forces on the mandible, changes in the TMJ and cranio fascial torque.

EDGE TO EDGE

Usually by orthodontics trying to take a Class III into a Class I to bring the mandible as far forward as possible to change the aesthetics.

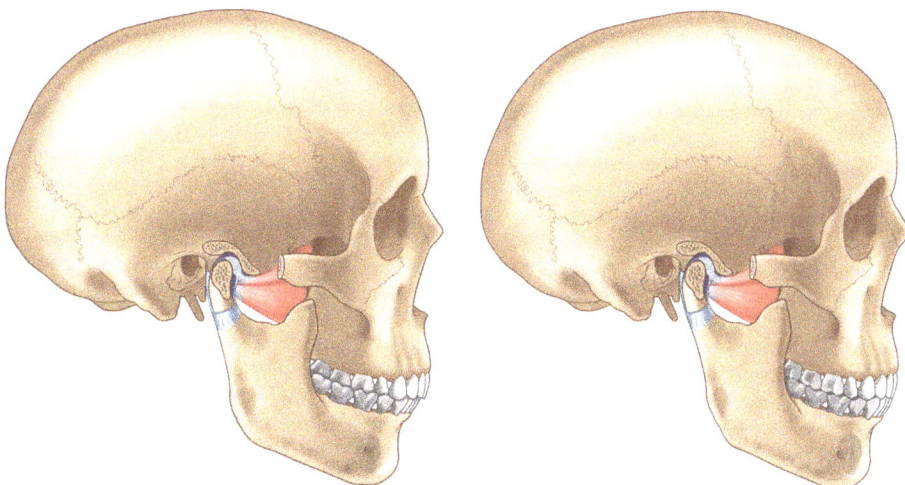

Figure 2.3 (left) Crossbite: Noxious stimulae change the dynamics in the brain; (right) Edge to Edge: Noxious stimulae create abnormal dynamics in the brain

NEUROLOGIC TOOTH

In some instances there is no evidence during occlusal evaluation why a tooth will show positive therapy localisation. There are two possibilities:

- Pathology of the tooth or periodontal tissues
- Disturbance in the receptors in the periodontal ligaments.

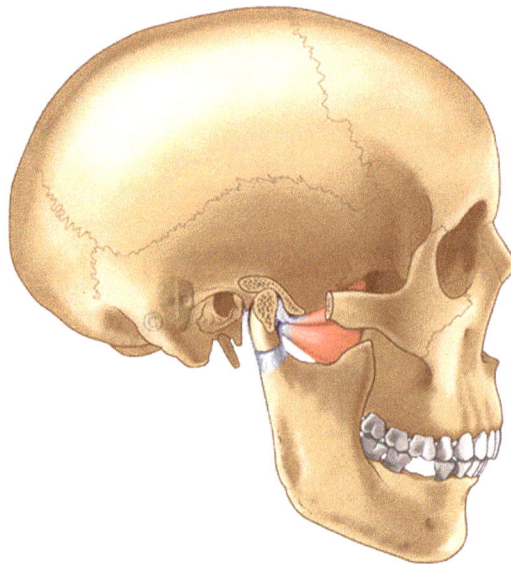

Figure 2.4 Neurologic Tooth: Periodontal disease, gingivitis, tooth decay

DESCENDING – MINOR STRESSES

These minor stresses can be changed by chiropractic and cranial care as they are dynamics that are controlled by neuro-muscular activity. Muscular fatigue and spasms, trauma, both cranially and upper cervically, change through the spinal nucleus of the trigeminal nerve complex.

Premature Contact

Caused by muscular derangement, putting one tooth into occlusion before the others.

Jaw Derangement – TMJD

Caused by one temporal bone going into extension, while the opposite goes into internal rotation, changing the TMJ position.

Bruxing, Clenching

Caused by cranial distortion and cranial stress, usually at the sphenoid bone at both the greater wings and the pterygoid plates.

Crossbite

Caused by cranial stress and cranio fascial torsion, pulling the mandible to one side.

Monolateral Mastication

A habitual problem caused initially by bruxing and cranial stress, and then by ease of chewing on one side.

ASCENDING STRESS – NOT STOMATOGNATHIC IN ORIGIN

Ascending stresses, by their nature, are not stomatognathically driven, and fall under the classification of factors that are foremost in the chiropractic compendium. These are factors that change spinal, pelvic and cranial function, but are NOT major considerations as primary causes to body malfunction.

1. Feet and foot lock – Bjorner

2. Ilio – Sacral – Coccygeal – Logan (1925)

3. Occiput – Atlas – Axis – BJ Palmer (1924)

4. Sacro Occipital Technique – MB Dejarnette (1924)

CONCLUSION

Descending majors refer to any disruption in the stomatognathic system caused by malocclusions, cranio fascial torque and neuro-muscular deviations that change the stomatognathic system.

Ascending majors are the effects that do not compromise the stomatognathic system.

CHAPTER 3

TEMPOROMANDIBULAR JOINT DYSFUNCTION

The complexity of TMJD is outlined below and gives the reader some idea as to the far-reaching effects and symptoms experienced by our patients. It also outlines how incorrect diagnosis of sole symptomatology, particularly by medical practitioners, may drive inappropriate treatment protocols, often with negative consequences.

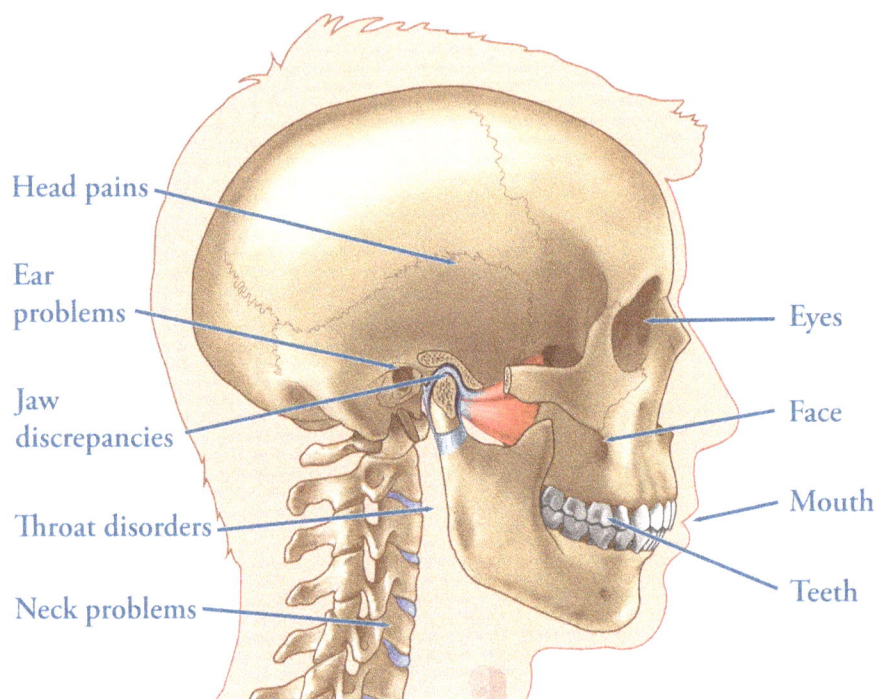

Head pains

Ear problems

Jaw discrepancies

Throat disorders

Neck problems

Eyes

Face

Mouth

Teeth

Figure 3.1 Temporomandibular Joint Dysfunction

Eyes

This is caused primarily by the sphenoid bone when distorted by cranio fascial distortion. The superior orbital fissure becomes distorted and compresses all the nerve and arterial vessels that pass through the fissure, including the optic nerve, through the optic foramen, the oculomotor nerve, trochlear nerve and the abducens nerve, which all control the eye. As the greater and lesser wings of the sphenoid become distorted, (the backdrop of the socket) the pressure pushes the eye forward and compresses it, restricting all the arterial and venous vessels .

Symptoms
- Pain behind the eyes
- Bloodshot appearance
- Bulging eyes

- Hypersensitive to sunlight
- Visual disturbances

Jaw

Derangement of the mandible will result in changing the occlusion between the mandible and maxillae, changing the occlusal surfaces, retruding the mandible into the TMJ, and compressing the retrodiscal tissue by the posterior movement of the mandibular condyle creating an abnormal temporomandibular relationship.

Symptoms

- Clicking popping jaw joints
- Grating sounds and tinnitus
- Pain in the cheek muscles
- Uncontrollable tongue and jaw movements

Head Pain

This is an intracranial pressure problem, caused by cranio fascial torsion and distortion changing the dynamics of the reciprocal tension membranes (RTM) and the points to which they are anchored in the cranium. The anterior pole torsions affect the falx cerebri, the ethmoid, vomer and maxillae anteriorly and then at the internal occipital protuberance posteriorly, and at the glabella, bregma and lambda superiorly.

The posterior pole at the sphenoid body distorts, changing the dynamic of the tentorium cerebellum at the sphenoid, the petrous portion of the temporal bone and the sigmoid and transverse sinuses at the occiput. The effects of this reciprocal tension membrane torsion change the venous sinus drainage of the cranium and creates intracranial pressure.

The falx cerebelli also distorts at the anchor points of the occipital sinus and the confluence of the sinuses.

These sites of the intracranial attachments and torsion points will generate more stasis of venous blood that is retained by blockage or obstruction and create the head pain.

Symptoms

- Headaches
- Migraine-type headaches
- Sinus congestion
- Temporal pains
- Sub-occipital pain

Face

Changes to the occlusion will affect the maxillary and ophthalmic branches of the trigeminal nerve and the facial nerve, both mixed cranial nerves with their specific nuclei at the pons and which emanate through the superior orbital fissure of the sphenoid and the internal auditory meatus of the temporal bone, respectively. Both pathways will be changed by the malocclusion with devastating effects.

Symptoms

- Tic douloureux
- Bell's palsy
- Facial neuralgia

Throat

The action of a retrusive mandible, jamming the condylar head into the retrodiscal tissue, results in all the anterior cervical musculature compressing the throat, the oesophagus, the pharynx, the larynx, the tonsils, the thyroid and para-thyroid glands. This situation opens the door to numerous changes in all these organs resulting in compression of the airways and the passage to the stomach, congestion of lymphatic drainage, irritation of the tonsils and, possibly the most important, a resultant malfunction of the thyroid and para-thyroid glands, possibly resulting over the long term in underactive thyroids and a goitre.

Symptoms
- Laryngitis
- Swallowing difficulties
- Sore throats with no infections
- Voice irregularities or changes
- Frequent coughing or constant clearing of the throat
- Constant feeling of foreign object stuck in the throat
- Thyroid function irregularities

Teeth

Poor occlusion and irregular interdigitation of the teeth arising from a poor mandibular condylar position in the TMJ, will cause a clenching and bruxing of the teeth line from cranial congestion, and the muscles of mastication try, through these noxious strain dynamics, to find an equilibrium position to try and release their tension.

Symptoms
- Clenching, grinding and bruxing, especially at night
- Loosing and soreness of the back teeth
- Long-term abscesses and bleeding gums from the alveolus

Ears

With the constant and persistent compression of the retrodiscal tissue by the condylar head in the TMJ, the internal and external meatus come under consistent bombardment of noxious dynamics. The resultant changes to the ossicles' position and structure, mostly change the perfection of the tympanic membrane sound transmission into the medial geniculate nucleus – the auditory relay nucleus of the thalamus. This gives rise to hearing malfunction, deafness, tinnitus and distorted transmission. The ossicles become damaged and confused in their ability to work as a functional component creating a wax build-up in the ears to protect and nurse these vital components – removal of such will render permanent damage to these bones. The vestibular mechanism in the mastoid bodies – the housing of the TMJs – is also relentlessly challenged by the action of the posterior condyle onto the retrodiscal tissue, changing the equilibrium dynamics producing, at worst, the likes of Meniere's disease.

Symptoms
- Tinnitus, buzzing or ringing in the ears
- Decrease in hearing at either end of the hearing spectrum
- Earache, ear pain inside the ear but no infection
- Itchy clogged ears, with a build-up of wax, laid down to protect the ossicles of the ear. **NB** This ear should not be syringed as the wax is protection
- Vertigo, loss of equilibrium, dizziness and Meniere's disease

Neck

The retrusive mandible – up and back – into the mandibular/glenoid fossa changes the vertical balance of the spinal curves, mostly seen in the loss of cervical lordosis, changing it into a cervical kyphosis, at the levels of C4 and C5. The trigeminal spinal nucleus at the levels of C1, C2 and C3, are already compromised by the malocclusion – the maxillary and mandibular branches of the trigeminal ganglion and their anchoring dural attachments at C1, C2 and C3, so the 'free' C4 and C5 are the next in line to become compromised in the kyphotic dynamics. The resultant changes, as seen on an fMRI, show stretching of the dural sheath, compression of the spinal cord and interference of normal nerve transmission – the perfect example of subluxation.

These subluxations at the upper cervical spine, unless changed by the position of the mandible, will result in lack of cranial drainage – from the controlling position of the atlanto-occipital membrane – impeding the flow of the vertebral arteries into the brain. They will also restrict external flow from the brain by the vertebral venous plexus – blood and cerebrospinal fluid (CSF) stasis. The long-term effects on the C4 and C5 complex will eventually produce degenerative joint disease (DJD) at these levels, without any further trauma.

Symptoms
- Loss of cervical mobility and stiffness
- Neck pain and torticollis
- Tired sore muscles
- Shoulder aches and lower backache
- Arm and finger pain and/or numbness
- Vascular equilibrium, intracranial pressure

Mouth

The muscles of mastication are designed to open uniformly, smoothly and simultaneously, when all the muscle groups work in unison. Changing the mandible/maxillary relationship, by retrusion of the mandibular condyles in the mandibular/glenoid fossa, changes the temporalis, masseters and buccinators muscles, and the internal (medial) and external (lateral) pterygoid muscles, creating abnormal muscle tensions and dynamics. The motor nucleus of CN IV receives cortical fibres for voluntary control of the muscles of mastication. These fibres are mostly crossed. It also receives input from the mesencephalic and sensory nuclei. The axons emerge anterior to the sensory root from the lateral surface of the pons. This motor root joins the semilunar ganglion together with the sensory root. Fibres control the mucous membranes, the lateral side of the face and proprioception in the muscles of mastication. All are run by the trigeminal ganglion and are all changed by TMJD.

Symptoms
- Limited opening of the mouth
- Inability to open evenly and smoothly
- Jaw deviates to one side on opening
- Jaw locks shut or open
- Irregular bite
- Involuntary biting of tongue, cheeks and lips
- General mouth discomfort
- Excessive salivation or dry mouth

CONCLUSION

TMJD has far-reaching effects on: eyes; jaw; head pain; face; throat; teeth; ears; neck; mouth.

CHAPTER 4

MALOCCLUSIONS: CAUSES AND EFFECTS

INCISAL INTERFERENCE

Incisal interference describes the contact of the mesial surface with the lower incisor to the distal inner surface of the upper incisor. This contact will be prior to any posterior molar contact and the consequences of incisal interference upon swallowing/chewing are that the upper incisors force the mandible into a posterior retruded position as the maxillae incisor closes over the mandibular incisor. Incisal interference is responsible for retrodiscal tissue damage and articular disc damage. As the mandible moves posterior and retrudes into the mandibular fossa the head flexes forward, the cervical spine loses its lordosis and becomes kyphotic particularly in the region of C3/C4 and C5. Over a period of time this will account for early DJD of the mid-cervical spine. Disruption of the cervical spine leads to overcompensation within the thoracics and into the lumbar spine changing spinal skeletal stability.

Causes

- Retruded incisors
- Loss of dentition
- Deviated mandible

Effects

- Retruded mandible
- Compression of the TMJ
- Loss of vertical support, dental damage
- Hearing distortions, tinnitus, vertigo, balance
- Throat, larynx, pharynx, thyroid, dysfunctions

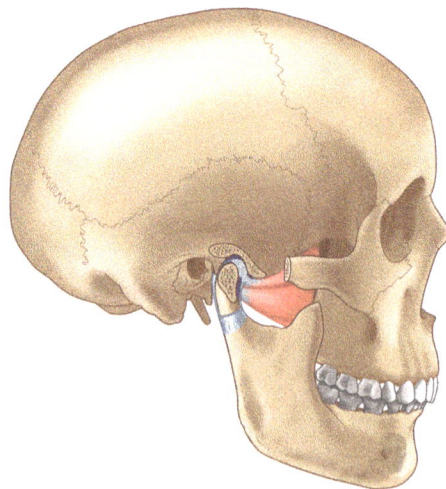

Figure 4.1 Incisal Interferences: Mandibular condyle crushes retrodiscal tissue in the TMJ

OVERCLOSED

The overclosed occlusion is brought about by a lack of vertical height, a collapse of the posterior molars and loss of dentition creating an overclosed situation where the upper incisors almost cover the lower incisors. This again may gradually lead to incisal interference, retruding the mandible and creating disruption in the TMJ.

Causes

- Loss of posterior dentition – usually 6s, 7s and 8s
- Incisal/canine interference
- Retruded mandible

Effects

- Compression of the TMJ
- Loss of vertical height
- Compression of the TMJ

LOSS OF DENTITION, LOSS OF VERTICAL HEIGHT

Causes
- Loss of dentition
- Retrusive mandible

Effects
- Loss of vertical height
- Compression of the TMJ
- Overclosure/Incisal interference
- Crossbite

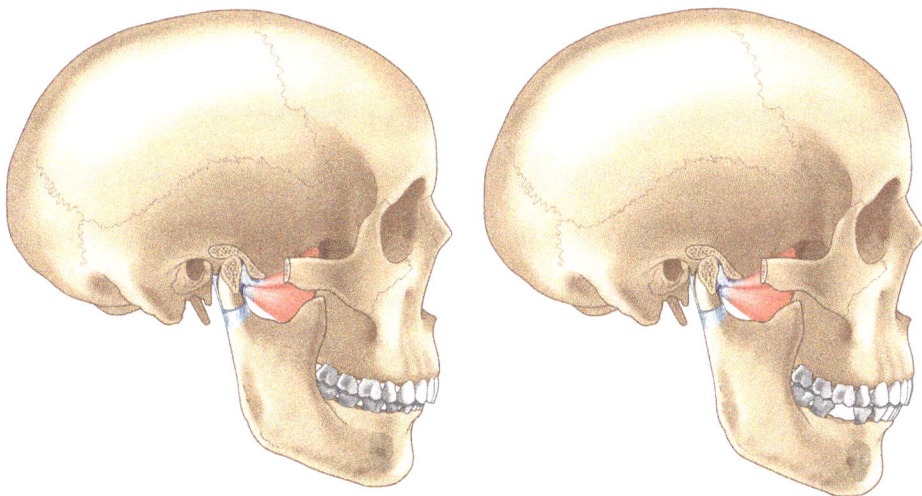

Figure 4.2 (left) Overclosed: Incisal interference causes TMJ compression by the mandibular condyle; (right) Loss of Dentition, Loss of Vertical Height: Mandibular condyle crushes retrodiscal tissue in the TMJ

LOSS OF POSTERIOR SUPPORT/LOSS OF DENTITION

A loss of dentition in either the upper or lower jaw can and will eventually cause problems with the vertical height if the dentition is not restored. As illustrated, the reason for this is that if a lower molar is removed, lost or not bridged and replaced (implant) then the molars on the other side of the gap will gradually tend to collapse towards one another and collapse medially. This will eventually lead to a loss of contact and ultimately a loss of vertical height. The unopposed teeth will gradually super-erupt causing all sorts of distorted patterns on that side of the mouth.

Causes

- Maxillae becomes over-closed
- Incisal interference
- Crossbite

Effects

- Retrusion of the mandible
- Compression of the TMJ

CROSSBITE

In a normal bite the buccal cusps on the maxillae overlap the buccal cusps of the mandible. In a crossbite however one maxilla is in internal rotation and the other is in external rotation. The buccal cusps of the internally rotated maxilla are overlapped by the buccal cusps of the mandible on that side, while on the other side the buccal cusps of the externally rotated maxilla overlap the corresponding buccal cusps of the mandible. The crossbite can occur anywhere within the upper arch and needs to be addressed as soon as it is evident. With one maxilla internally rotated and the other externally rotated this distorted pattern affects the sphenoid maxillae relationship and in turn the sphenobasilar relationship, creating a torquing effect at the base of the cranium and ultimately affecting the tentorium cerebelli and the diaphragma sellae. Distortion of the RTM can also affect the spinal dural meningeal system and influence the skeletal structures.

Causes

- Changes in the upper and lower jaw relationship, either from early TMJD, incorrect orthodontics or trauma
- Deviating mandible, where the maxillary dentition is overlapped by the mandibular dentition. This can be either a unilateral or a bilateral overlap

Effects

- Incisal interference – mandibular retrusion – TMJD

- Edge to edge contacts – noxious vectors into the skull

- Mandibular deviation – TMJD – Retrodiscal tissue inflammation

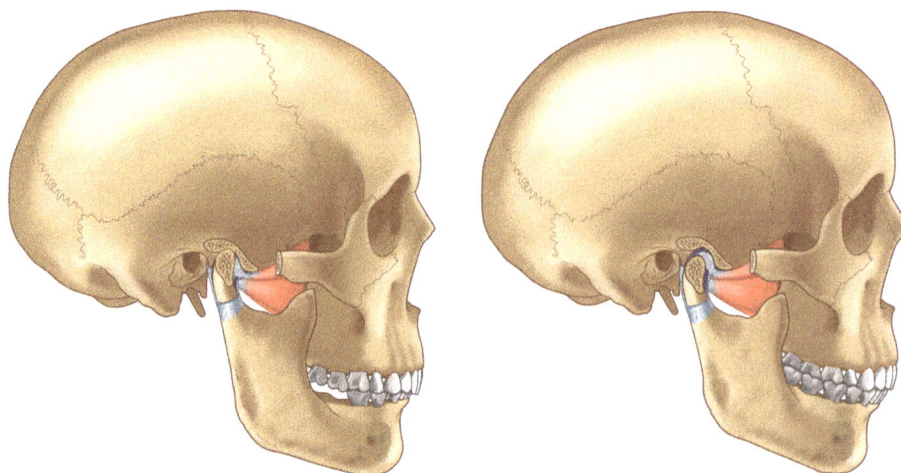

Figure 4.3 (left) Loss of Posterior Support/Loss of Dentition: Mandibular condyle crushes retrodiscal tissue in the TMJ; (right) Crossbite: Noxious stimulae from the crossbite changes the dynamics in the brain

EDGE TO EDGE

Edge to edge contact refers to the inferior surfaces of the upper incisors in contact with the superior surface of the lower incisors. Provided that the edge to edge incisal contact and the posterior molars contact simultaneously the occlusion will be normal. However, if the incisal edge to edge contact is made prior to any posterior molar contact this will create enormous problems through the premaxillae into the naso-frontal sinuses and into the frontal part of the cranium.

Causes	*Effects*
Protruded mandible	Poor condylar positioning in the mandibular fossa, retrodiscal irritation and misalignment of the articular disc
Orthodontics – changing Class III to Class I	Trigeminal ganglion irritation and consequent neurological damage and pain
Trauma – changing position of the mandibular condyle within the mandibular fossa	
Loss of posterior support – loss of inter-cuspidal integration	

NEUROLOGIC TOOTH

In some instances there is no evidence during occlusal evaluation as to why a tooth will show positive therapy localisation.

There are two possibilities:

* Pathology of the tooth or periodontal tissues
* Disturbance in the receptors in the periodontal ligaments.

The objective of evaluation and treatment is to return the tooth and its periodontal ligament receptors to normal function. Each of the four quadrants is therapy-localised separately. The quadrant containing the neurologic tooth will then be isolated and each tooth in that quadrant is therapy-localised separately to establish which tooth is corrupt.

To find the offending tooth, and to determine the receptor dysfunction, the tooth can be challenged in all directions, rotational and through the axial lines of the tooth in the alveolus.

To establish the offending position, the muscle weakness becomes evident, and that weakness shows the direction that creates the malfunction. The strong reactive muscle shows the direction of correction to which the tooth needs to be taken to resolve the dysfunction. This pressure on the tooth following the line of drive to correct the tooth is maintained through three respiratory phases.

Once the correction has been made, the quadrant and the offending tooth are re-challenged again, to confirm that the correction has been made satisfactorily.

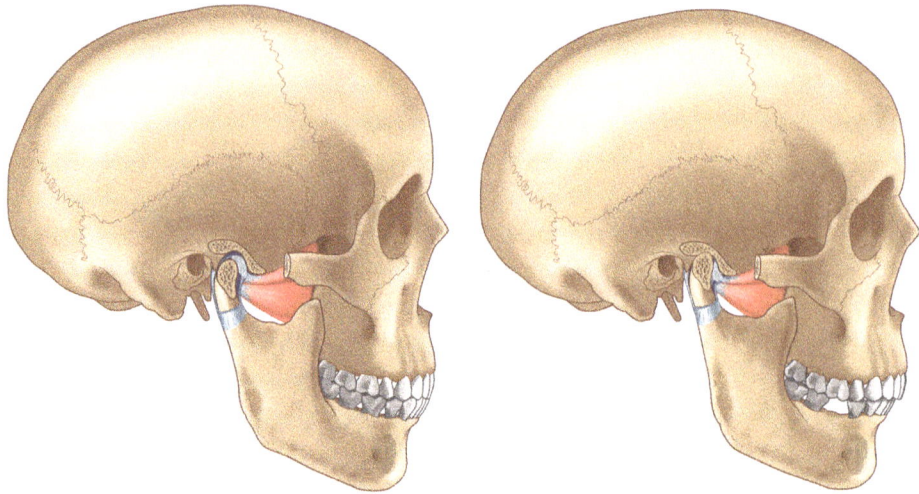

Figure 4.4 (left) Edge to Edge: Noxious stimulae create abnormal dynamics in the brain; (right) Neurologic Tooth: Periodontal disease, gingivitis, tooth decay

CONCLUSION

Malocclusions that occur, their causes and effects.

- Incisal interference
- Overclosed
- Loss of dentition, loss of posterior support
- Crossbite, unilateral and bilateral
- Edge to edge
- Neurologic tooth

CHAPTER 5

CRANIAL MUSCLES

MUSCLES OF MASTICATION

The muscles of the skull that control the mandible, and mastication, have a great influence on position of the occlusion, and are therefore critical in cranial balance. Apart from the buccinator muscle, all the muscles of mastication are controlled by the motor part of the mandibular branch of the trigeminal nerve.

The temporalis muscle is innovated by a nerve supply from the deep temporal branches of the anterior trunk of the mandibular nerve.

The nerve supply for the masseter muscle is the masseteric nerve from the anterior trunk of the mandibular division of the trigeminal nerve.

The nerve supply for the internal pterygoid muscle is the medial pterygoid nerve of the mandibular division of the trigeminal nerve.

The nerve supply for the external pterygoid muscle is the lateral pterygoid nerve of the anterior trunk of the mandibular division of the trigeminal nerve.

The nerve supply for the buccinator muscle is the buccal branches of the facial nerve.

To assess and correct cranial fascial dynamics one has to use indicators to fully evaluate the problem.

TEMPORALIS MUSCLE

The temporalis muscle is broken down into the anterior, medial and posterior portions. The temporalis muscle covers the entire sutural system of the lateral part of the skull. Because of its wide origin the fascial attachments cover the frontal, parietal, occipital, temporal and sphenoid bones. All the fibres of the temporalis muscle insert into the coronoid process of the mandible and sometimes into the distal part of the third molar. The action of the temporalis muscle when functioning symmetrically is to pull the coronoid process and elevate the mandible closing the jaw. The temporalis muscle is innervated by the mandibular branch of the trigeminal nerve or fifth cranial nerve.

ANTERIOR TEMPORALIS

When the anterior temporalis goes into the spasm it pulls the mandible into an anterior horizontal direction. The distal cusps of the posterior molars on the lower jaw will pull forward and contact the mesial cusps of the molars in the upper jaw. This sort of action can cause a premature contact.

303

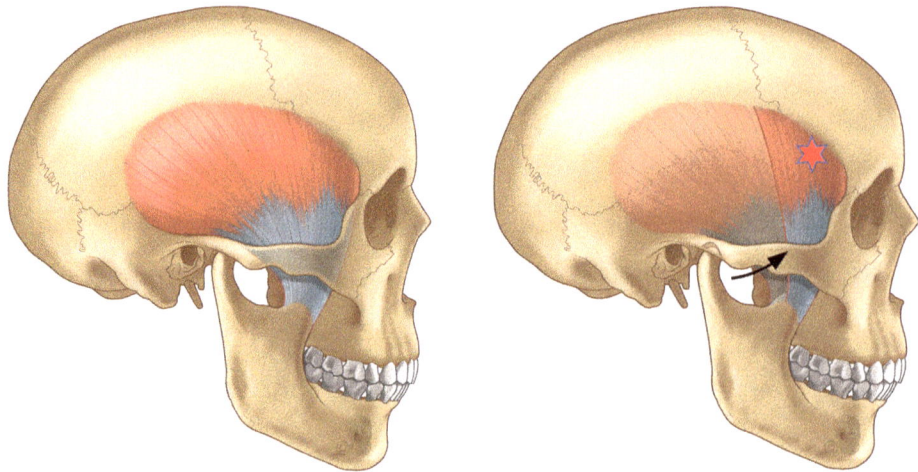

Figure 5.1 (left) Temporalis Muscle; (right) Anterior Temporalis: Arrow shows direction of movement of the mandible

BILATERAL ANTERIOR TEMPORALIS SPASM

The effect of bilateral anterior muscle spasm is to pull the mandible forward, in effect decompressing the TMJ.

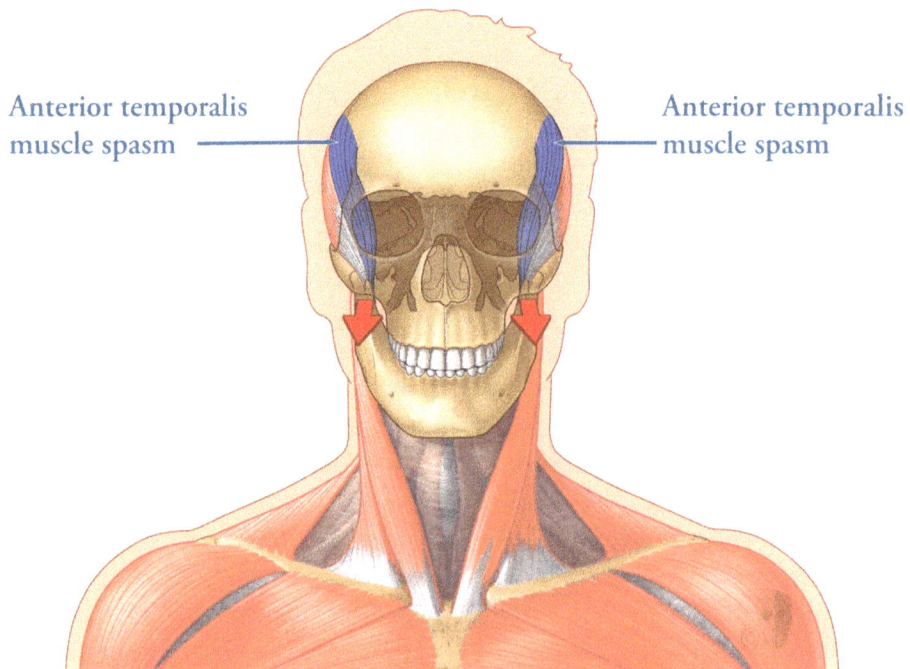

Anterior temporalis muscle spasm

Anterior temporalis muscle spasm

Figure 5.2 Bilateral Anterior Temporalis Muscle Spasm: Arrow shows direction of movement of the mandible

MEDIAL TEMPORALIS

This will cause a vertical and retruded movement of the mandibular condyle in towards the mandibular fossa of the temporal bone. This sort of spasm will produce a diminished vertical dimension (vertical height), the distance between the superior surface of the condyle and the inferior surface of the mandibular fossa. This loss of vertical will cause inflammation and irritation to the retrodiscal tissue and the posterior part of the articular disc. This action also compresses the premolars; the 4s and the 5s, can bring the maxillae into an over-closed position, restricting the incisors and the canines.

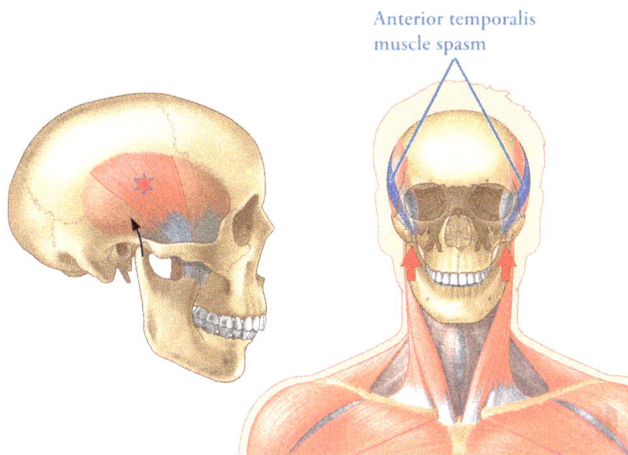

Figure 5.3 (left) Medial Temporalis;
(right) Bilateral Medial Temporalis Muscle Spasm:
Arrows show direction of movement of the mandible

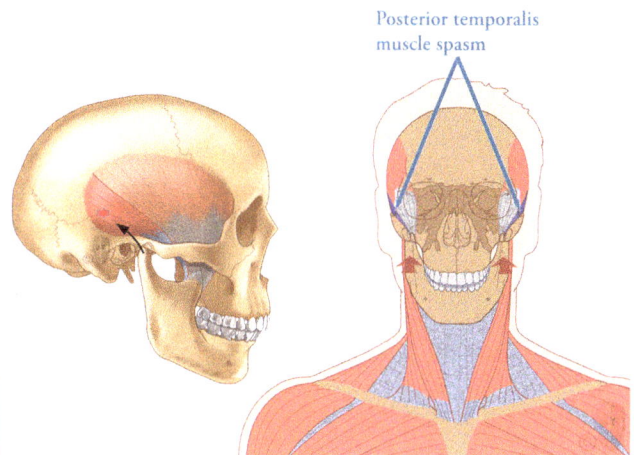

Figure 5.4 (left) Posterior Temporalis;
(right) Bilateral Posterior Temporalis Muscle Spasm:

POSTERIOR TEMPORALIS

The posterior temporalis spasm pulls the mandible into a horizontal posterior position with the mesial cusps of the posterior lower teeth driving the mesial cusps of the posterior upper teeth into a posterior direction (distal direction). Damage incurred by the posterior temporal spasm occurs to the retrodiscal tissue and the vestibular mechanism of the temporal bone. The long-term effects of this action are that it causes fibrillation of the ossicles of the ears resulting in tinnitus and possible changes in hearing and balance.

RIGHT POSTERIOR/LEFT ANTERIOR TEMPORALIS MUSCLE SPASM

The effect of a right posterior/left anterior temporalis muscle spasm is that the mandible will deviate to the right taking the mid-lines out of alignment, possibly causing a crossbite, interfering with the left incisors and canines, compressing the right temporomandibular fossa and decompressing the left temporomandibular fossa.

LEFT POSTERIOR/RIGHT ANTERIOR TEMPORALIS MUSCLE SPASM

The effect of a left posterior/right anterior temporalis muscle spasm is that the mandible will deviate to the left taking the mid-lines out of alignment, possibly causing a crossbite, interfering with the right incisors and canines, compressing the left temporomandibular fossa and decompressing the right temporomandibular fossa.

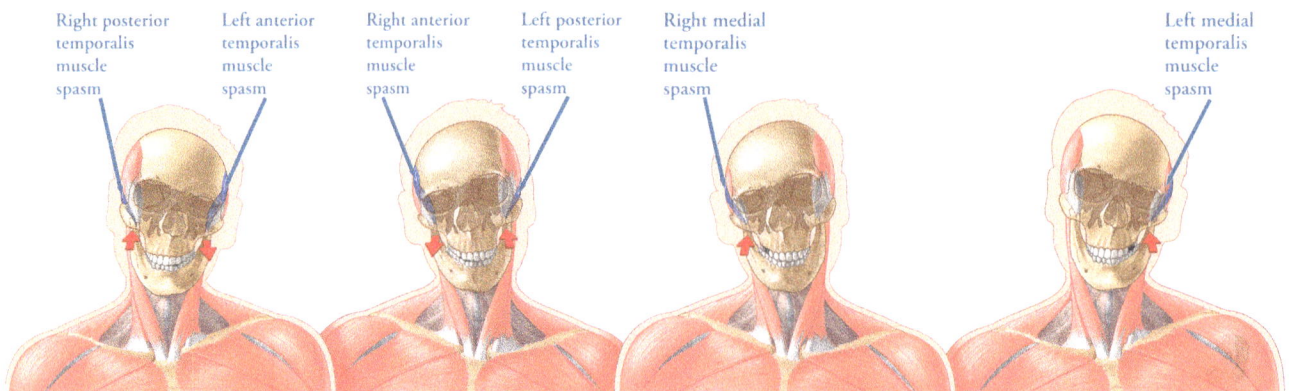

Figure 5.5 (far left) Right Posterior/Left Anterior Temporalis Muscle Spasm; (centre left) Left Posterior/ Right Anterior Temporalis Muscle Spasm; (centre right) Right Medial Temporalis Spasm; (far right) Left Medial Temporalis Spasm (arrows show direction of movement of the mandible)

RIGHT MEDIAL TEMPORALIS SPASM

Right medial temporalis spasm results in a loss of vertical dimension on the right side – the distance between the mandibular condyle and the roof of the mandibular/glenoid fossa. The loss of vertical occurs at the premaxillars – the 4s and 5s. This causes over-closure of the occlusion, incisor interference, and canine interference.

LEFT MEDIAL TEMPORALIS SPASM

Left medial temporalis spasm results in a loss of vertical dimension on the left – the distance between the mandibular condyle and the roof of the mandibular/glenoid fossa. The loss of vertical height occurs at the premaxillars – the 4s and 5s. This causes over-closure of the occlusion, incisor interference, and canine interference.

LATERAL/EXTERNAL PTERYGOID MUSCLE

This muscle has two separate origins. The smaller superior origin arises from the area known as the infratemporal crest of the greater wing of the sphenoid bone. The larger inferior origin arises from the lateral side of the lateral pterygoid plate. Some of the fibres of the superior head penetrate the capsule of the TMJ and insert into the anterior border of the disc of the joint. The remainder of the fibres from that origin and the fibres of the inferior head insert into the neck of the condyle. The action of the muscle is twofold.

The inferior head pulls the condyle forward while the disc is also brought forward. The function of the lateral pterygoid when both inferior heads function together is to protrude the mandible. If only one lateral pterygoid is contracted there will be lateral excursion to the opposite side of the contracted muscle. The superior head functions to guide posterior movement of the disc and condyle as it goes back into its centric position. The overall action of the lateral pterygoid is to open the jaw, protruding the mandible and moving the mandible from side to side. The innervation of the lateral pterygoid muscle is from the mandibular division of the trigeminal nerve (CN V.3)

MEDIAL/INTERNAL PTERYGOID MUSCLE

The medial or internal pterygoid muscle has two origins, the larger and major origin is from the medial side of the lateral pterygoid plate and the pterygoid fossae; the smaller origin lies just anterior to that area and comes from the maxillary tuberosity just behind the third molar. The insertion point is into the angle of the mandible on the medial side just opposite the masseter insertion on the lateral side. The function of this muscle is to elevate the mandible and close the mouth. The nerve innervation is from the trigeminal nerve (5th cranial nerve).

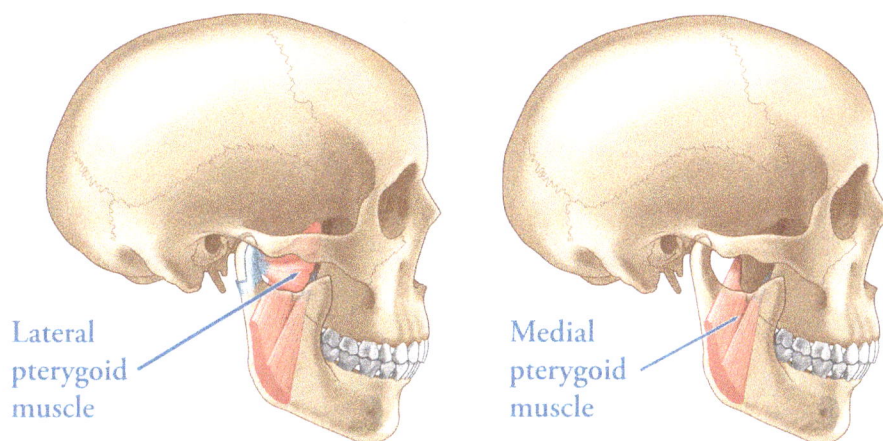

Lateral
pterygoid
muscle

Medial
pterygoid
muscle

Figure 5.6 (left) Lateral/External Pterygoid; (right) Medial/Internal Pterygoid

CANINE GUIDANCE

Canine guidance relates to the superior surface of the lower canines making contact with their opposite canine on the inferior/labial surface. This is an emphatic contact, and not a contact that influences the mandible being put into a retrusive position – as in incisal interference. This contact ensures that the canines control their respective muscles – no contact means the muscles are corrupted in their function.

The canines control the ipsilateral trapezius muscle (medial pterygoid component) and the contralateral sternocleidomastoid (SCM) muscle (lateral pterygoid component). The medial and lateral pterygoid muscles couple with the trapezius and SCM in their action, and can be muscle tested using the trapezius and SCM, respectively.

Canine control is achieved by the contact of the upper and lower canines making contact with the enamel part of each canine tooth. This contact is literally like an electrical terminal, where the contact ensures an electrical circuit is established through the tooth, through the periodontal ligament in the alveolus, to the mandibular and maxillary nerves of the trigeminal nerve and being registered by the trigeminal ganglion.

This neurological circuitry applies to all the teeth in both jaws – the incisors, the canines, the pre-maxillary and the molars. This would indicate a balanced occlusion, without any deficit to the trigeminal ganglion. This is the objective in establishing a physiological occlusion.

The embryological development of the canine shows the canine as a locking and guiding tooth in creating the balanced jaw to jaw relationship. The canine is the first tooth in the maxillary bone next to the medial and lateral incisors which develops from the premaxilla bone. At maturity it acts in isolation to the other teeth in the dental configuration and controls the upper and lower jaw relationship.

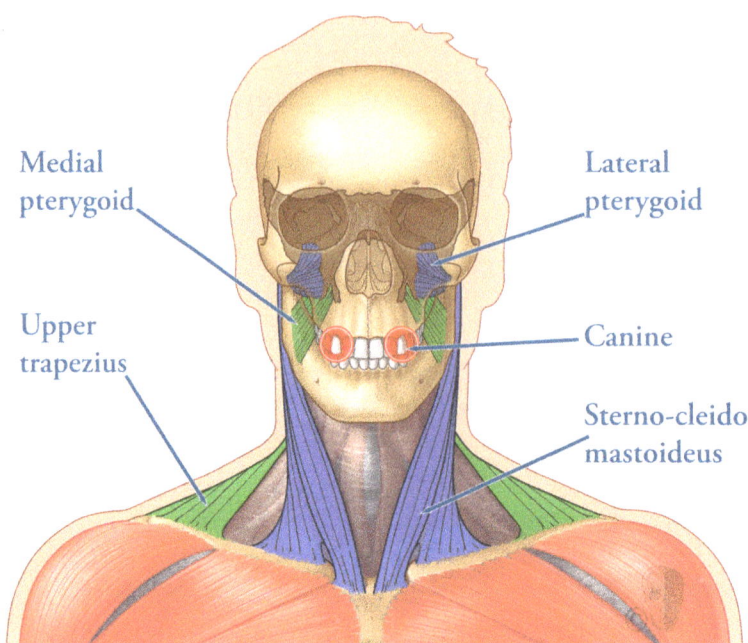

Figure 5.7 Canine Guidance

LOSS OF BILATERAL CANINE CONTROL

The canines control the ipsilateral upper trapezius muscle (medial/internal pterygoid), and the contralateral SCM (lateral/external pterygoid). The upper canines control the lower canines, by holding the lower canines in place, preventing them from moving the mandible too far forward on either side. This canine guidance action means there is bilateral control on both the upper trapezius and SCM muscles, keeping the mandibular condyles within their juxtaposition within the glenoid fossae.

RIGHT MANDIBULAR DEVIATION

If the right upper canine loses its guidance from the lower right canine and is not checked, the right upper trapezius muscle will contract, pulling the head over to the right. This, in turn, contracts the ipsilateral medial pterygoid muscle pulling the mandible to the right.

The contralateral SCM (left) pulls the head to the right, while its muscle partner, the left lateral pterygoid muscle pulls the mandible forward and right achieving right mandibular deviation, compressing the right TMJ with a possible crossbite ensuing.

LEFT MANDIBULAR DEVIATION

If the left upper canine loses its guidance from the lower left canine and is not checked, the left upper trapezius muscle will contract, pulling the head over to the left. This, in turn, contracts the ipsilateral medial pterygoid muscle pulling the mandible to the left.

The contralateral SCM (right) pulls the head to the left, while its muscle partner, the right lateral pterygoid muscle pulls the mandible forward and left achieving left mandibular deviation, compressing the left TMJ with a possible crossbite ensuing.

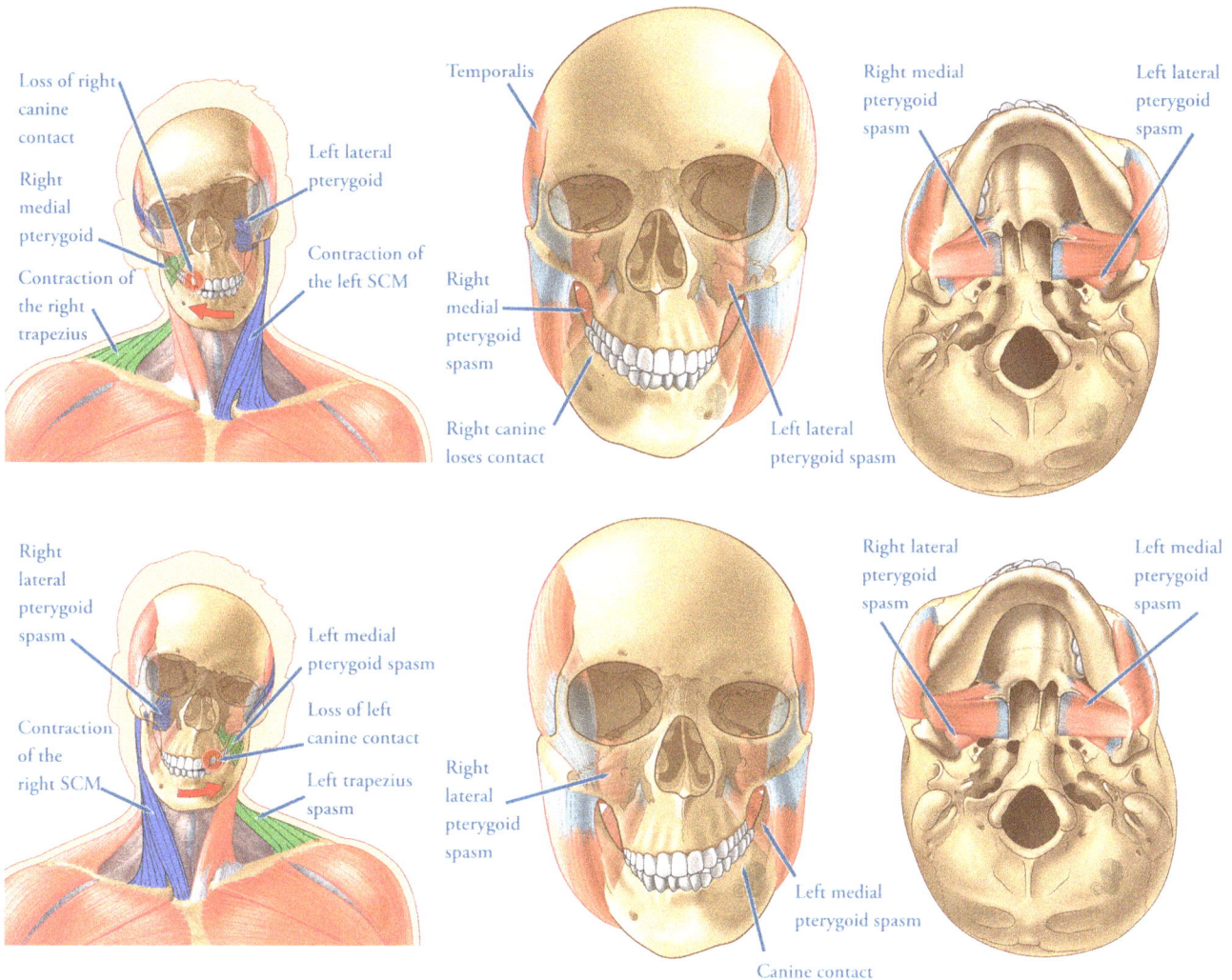

Figure 5.8 (top) Right Mandibular Deviation; (bottom) Left Mandibular Deviation:
Arrows show direction of movement of the mandible

MALOCCLUSIONS – DISTURBANCES OF THE STOMATOGNATHICS

A malocclusion occurs when the maxillary and mandibular teeth come together asymmetrically, out of synchrony and with uneven pressure. The malocclusion changes the maxillary/mandibular relationship and will create stomatognathic dysfunction either at the tooth edge, or within the TMJ, reducing dental stability and increasing neurological dysfunction. The malocclusion will create irritability through the mandibular and maxillary branches of the trigeminal nerve. This in turn will be counterbalanced and compensated, by increasing muscle loading on one or several of the mastication muscles (masseter, buccinator, lateral and medial pterygoid and temporalis) all of which are controlled and innervated by the mandibular/motor branch of the trigeminal nerve.

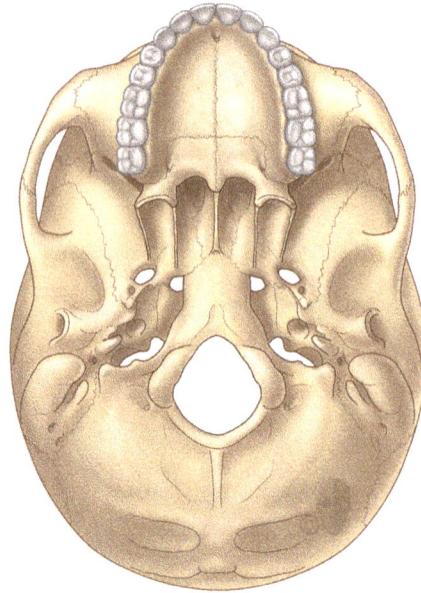

Figure 5.9 Normal Occlusion Inferior View

BALANCED MAXILLAE AND MANDIBLE

The balanced maxillae should occlude with the mandible at the junction of the central cusps of the three molars and the two premolars, then at the buccal surfaces of the canines, the lateral incisors, and the medial incisors. The latter three teeth should make contact with their opposing numbers in a way that the contact is made without influence on retrusive mandibular function that might cause compression of the retrodiscal tissue. This contact should be simultaneous, symmetric and with even pressure to ensure that all contacts maintain a cranial vector of equilibrium.

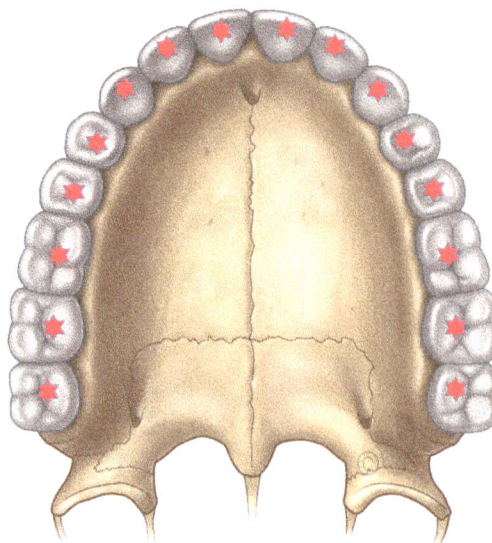

Figure 5.10 Balanced Maxillae: Contact points where mandibular teeth occlude with the maxillae

MAXILLARY DISTORTION

Collapse of the left maxilla into internal rotation, means that the dentition in the upper left quadrant does not occlude with the opposing mandible in an inter-cuspidal relationship. The medial and lateral incisors teeth on the left maxilla are involved in incisal interference, while the canine has no contact. As the arch has become more internal on the left, the teeth have jostled for the ever decreasing space resulting in the irregular alignment of the premolars, followed by the molars, reducing the curve of the left maxilla more and more, moving them out of direct contact with their opposing number in the mandible. The new contact points in this scenario are only the cusps during mastication, which will bring forceful dynamics and pressure through different various fragile cusp edges, rather than through the whole solid tooth body. Over a period of time this continual abrasive bombardment on the fragile cusp edges sends reverberations through the tooth body and root, shaking and loosening the strong root foundation of the tooth, until they ultimately loosen in the alveolus. This loosening now creates a break in the tooth seal at the alveolar/tooth body border. This is now new territory – the neurologic tooth.

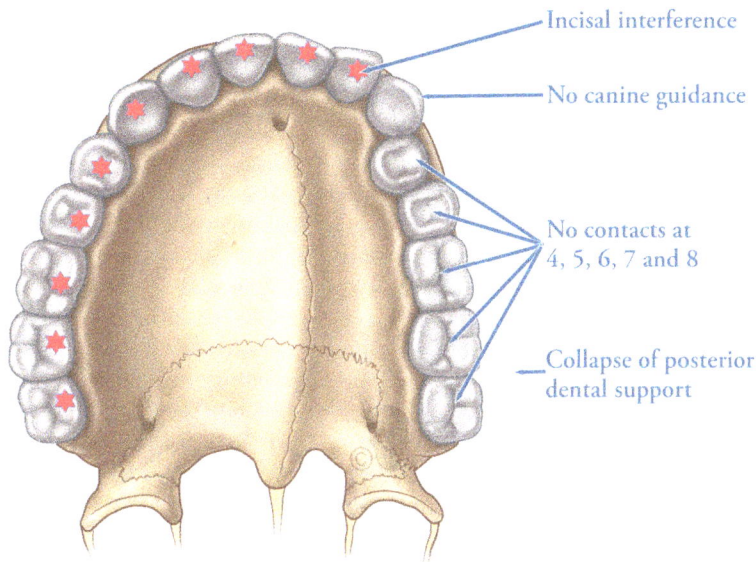

Figure 5.11 Maxillary Occlusal Distortion: Contact points where mandibular teeth malocclude with the maxillae

This broken seal means the junction is now exposed to oxygen. Oxidation provides an environment for foreign matter such as bacteria and fungi to grow, the start of gingival issues around the tooth, later gingivitis, infection, pus, abscess formation, pain and bleeding, antibiotics, mouth washes, sore throats, tonsillitis and laryngitis. This becomes a site of full blown infection, which can bubble on for years and years. Treatment includes the hygienist, multiple scouring around the edge of the alveolar/tooth root junction; X-rays on most visits to see whether an abscess has developed; and antibiotics to quell infection. When the abscess is finally located there is likely to be bone infection, regression of gums, bigger spaces between tooth and gums – more infection, more pain and bleeding. Resolution is now in the order of a root canal treatment. This means every passage, tunnel or venial has to be blocked off to prevent the presence of oxygen.

When done correctly, and all oxygen presence has been removed by the blockage of these pathways, the tooth has now become inert – rather like a dead tooth or a foreign body. This is a very controversial subject, as many believe that root canal treatment may result in a concentrated focal infection site, with too strong a negative effect on overall body health, or that it causes disease. Others feel that the presence of that tooth represents a 'gap filler' that maintains the integrity of the occlusal surface, the gums and the bone until the process recurs.

The subject of implants is equally contentious. If teeth are lost as a result of compromised stasis at the tooth/gingival junction because of poor hygiene, large gaps between the teeth and the presence of oxygen for oxidation purposes, then what sort of artificial material will survive those rigours after the patient's own tissue and bone have failed? The new type of implant has to be inert and impervious to the presence of oxygen. Currently titanium has become the latest material to face exclusion, as it forms titanium oxide in the presence of oxygen, and thus becomes a potential bed for infection. Zirconia however, is the dioxide form of the metallic element Zirconium, similar in properties to a natural diamond, and therefore reputed to be biocompatible.

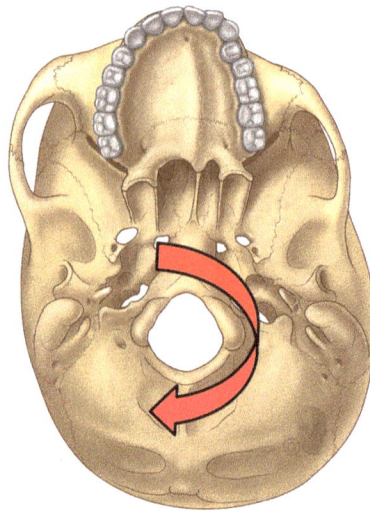

Figure 5.12 Counterclockwise Torque

The superior and inferior views of the cranium show the presence and importance of the sphenoid bone. The insertion of the petrous portion of the temporal bone into the junction of the body and lesser wing of the sphenoid, and the basilar part and condylar area of the occiput in the neonate, bring together a swathe of fascia which reinforces the cartilage in the neonate to become bone later. The jugular foramen and the carotid canal – bearing the glossopharyngeal, vagus and spinal accessory cranial nerves, the internal jugular vein and the internal carotid artery respectively – will become compressed and restrictive at these apertures, and because of the cranial torque, the dural coverings around these vessels will be further constricted cutting off the venous and arterial flow, and diminishing nerve conduction. In close proximity to these apertures is the foramen magnum and the hypoglossal canal, both of which come under the influence of this torqued dural membrane.

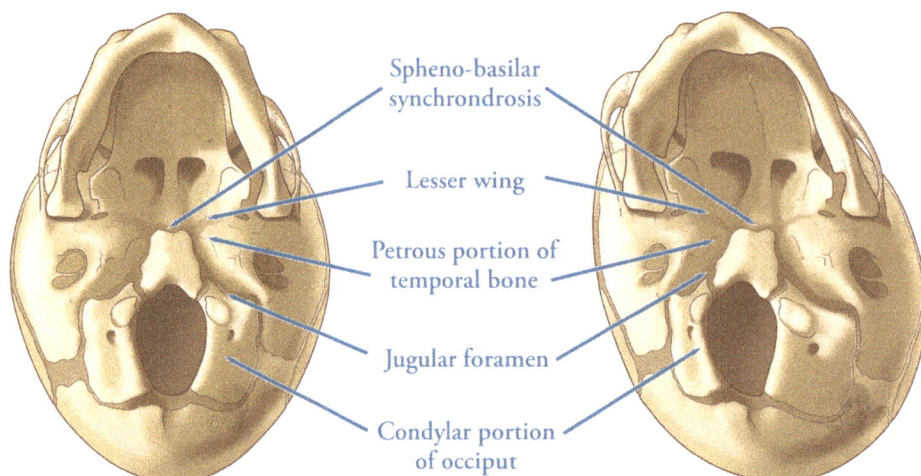

Spheno-basilar synchrondrosis

Lesser wing

Petrous portion of temporal bone

Jugular foramen

Condylar portion of occiput

Figure 5.13 Infant Skull

The atlas and axis vertebrae have several components at the neonate stage, with each component cranial plate being encapsulated by periosteal dura, which is a fascial continuation of the spinal and cranial dura. They provide reinforcement adding enormous strength and flexibility to the structures they support.

The periosteal dura allows the bone to grow to maturity and then becomes the suture between the adjacent cranial bones that make up the cranium. Similarly, the vertebral bones go through the same process, and especially at the atlanto-occipital junction where the weight bearing dynamics required to hold the head above the spinal column and embrace the spinal cord and the brainstem, are enormous.

Neonatally, the cranial bones that require massive strength and versatility are made up of cartilage (later to become bone) and membrane (later to remain as membrane). The major vessels, both blood and nerve carrying vessels, make their passage through cartilage and then are ensured of structural support when the cartilage becomes bone in maturity.

Counterclockwise torque appears to be most common type of cranial torque, and is referred to in a paper by the author, 'Normal Benign Cranial Distortion and Brain Drainage through the Venous Sinus System' (19 May 2017), which looks at: the hydrodynamics caused by blood and CSF flow through the venous sinuses; and the routes taken by the superior sagittal sinus through the right transverse sinus into the right sigmoid sinus exiting the right inferior jugular vein. The blood would appear to flow through this system in a clockwise helical motion to the right brachiocephalic vein. The inferior sagittal sinus drains into the left transverse sinus, left sigmoid sinus and the left inferior jugular vein, in a clockwise helical motion to the left brachiocephalic vein. This clockwise torsional movement of fluid would create a counterclockwise motion of the dural membrane system in the RTM, which is why there is a benign counterclockwise torque in the cranium, that would appear to be predisposed in all of us. These findings are consistent over 13 years of clinical evaluation, with MRIs indicating that the torque is present intraumatised or pathological studies.

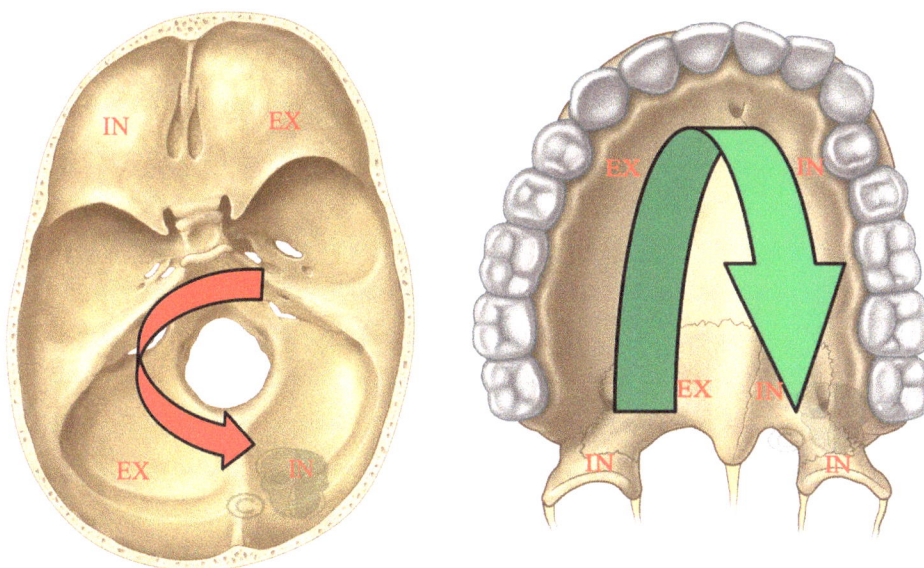

Figure 5.14 (left) Counterclockwise Torque; (right) Clockwise Correction

CHAPTER 6

CRANIAL SCANNING

Many years of clinical practice have allowed the author to develop a scanning method to evaluate more accurately a patient's most immediate needs, thereby attempting to remedy that particular deficit. The process is complete when the clinician explores what physiologically 'feels' at risk. This method utilises 'muscle testing' to evaluate those needs and, in particular, 'therapy localisation' as the pathway to establish accuracy.

Once the testing method is regularly practised and established, there will be a marked change in the areas identified for treatment and where diagnosis leads. For instance, the cranio fascial distortion plays a major role in what you are trying to achieve clinically, and so strict adherence to your clinical protocols is imperative.

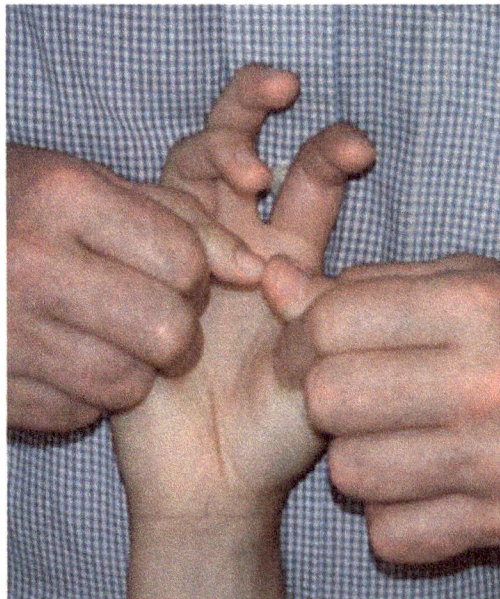

Figure 6.1 Testing Pathway, Opponens Policis and Flexor Pollicis Brevis: Thumb–little finger are the testing components for cranial scanning

TESTING FORMAT

The next stage involves testing the patient's right thumb and little finger held together, with the doctor trying to pull them apart. These two digits are used is because they are rarely not a testable component. For young children of about six (due to compliability) to the most geriatric of patients, shoulder and cervical complications very rarely affect these two digits. For babies and for children up to six years old, the mother can be used as a surrogate. The doctor tests the mother's thumb and little finger (while she is holding her baby) with therapy localising the areas that the doctor needs to test again using the mother's other hand. This has been tried and tested and works very well in practice.

With the thumb and little finger in contact, have the patient keep the head in a forward position, then move the eyes left and test. This movement will usually be strong. Then have the patient move eyes to the right and re-test. Invariably, patient resistance will weaken in this position, the indication being: cranio fascial torsion. As most patients tested have a counterclockwise torque, so moving the eyes left follows the torque and does not compromise the medial rectus muscle – the convergence muscle. When moving the eyes right, this counters the torque and so the medial rectus muscle has to do more work and becomes compromised.

The same can be achieved by taking the doctor's index finger from a midline position over the nose and taking the finger posterior towards the eyes, to demonstrate the patient's ability to perform convergence of the eyes. The right eye will perform without difficulty, but the left eye will not converge. This is due to the cranio fascial torque. These two tests, normally performed upright, may be performed while the patient lies down, as will be demonstrated in due course, and are the simplest and most effective way to test for cranio fascial torque. At the patient's first presentation test all the other parameters to give the doctor a full pre-assessment of the patient's current condition This provides a format to establish the problems that the patient displays on this first visit. This is vital giving the doctor full appreciation of stages in treatment from beginning to end thus allowing the doctor to show the patient what has been achieved at a later date. At this point, as the brain is confused and sends mixed messages to the body when being tested, the clinician will have to translate a plethora of confused findings. If treated without following the testing format, the doctor may apply the wrong treatment protocol. This will inevitably lead to inappropriate outcomes and will further confuse the body, the doctor and certainly the patient. Take control as the doctor and approach diagnosis in a rigorous and disciplined manner.

Cranial Scanning Points

   a. Left and right TMJs
   b. Glabella
   c. Bregma
   d. Lambda
   e. Tentorial notch
   f. Transverse sinus
   g. VVP, sub-occipital cavernous sinus, atlanto-occipital membrane
   h. C1, C2 and C3
   i. Anterior temporalis
   j. Medial temporalis
   k. Posterior temporalis
   l. Left greater wing of the sphenoid
   m. Temporo-sphenoid line
   n. Incisors
   o. Canines
   p. Left SCM and right upper trapezius
   q. Right SCM and left upper trapezius
   r. Upper right quadrant – neurologic tooth
   s. Lower right quadrant – neurologic tooth
   t. Upper left quadrant – neurologic tooth
   u. Lower left quadrant – neurologic tooth
   v. Mid-sternum – biomechanical
   w. Epigastric – electro-magnetic indicator

x. Umbilicus – chemical indicator

y. CN III oculomotor. Eyes left and eyes right – convergence

Document all these findings as these are the pre-examination findings.

LEFT AND RIGHT TMJS

Changes in the TMJs will occur when the mandibular condylar head is found superior and posterior in the TMJ, compressing the retrodiscal tissue. In the initial stages this will register in the mandibular and maxillary branches of the trigeminal nerve and then into the trigeminal ganglion as a joint that is congested and possibly inflamed. The articular disc starts to be stretched and possibly loses its contact over the condylar head, or becomes detached from its origin and/or insertion within the joint space. As time progresses, the articular disc will become detached, either bunching up behind or in front of the condyle, reducing smooth articular motion, resulting in popping or clicking of the condyle within the joint space. Regressive pressure on the retrodiscal tissue causes abnormal percussion on the tympanic membrane, the ossicles and the internal auditory meatus. All of these physical changes will register as a positive indicator on either or both TMJs and should be documented.

GLABELLA

This is the anterior pole, the attachment for the falx cerebri at the crista galli of the ethmoid bone. The glabella lies at the most inferior position of the metopic suture in the neonate and is corrupted by falls onto the frontal area as an infant. Trauma to this area can affect the ethmoid-sphenoid junction, displacing the falx cerebri, affecting the superior and inferior sagittal sinus and disrupt drainage through the arachnoid granulations of CSF; this is an exacerbation of cranio fascial distortion. The nasal and maxillae can also be disturbed and affect the nasal chonchi and frontal sinuses, causing congestion and difficulty in breathing. If the falls include the face, the premaxilla is disturbed and the incisors erupt in an asymmetric fashion causing a switch – 'neurologic chaos' – this phenomenon occurs when the body fails to respond to sensory input and is generally caused by a lack of neurological coordination between the left and right hemispheres where confusion reigns throughout the corpus callosum. This is alleviated through cranio fascial correction.

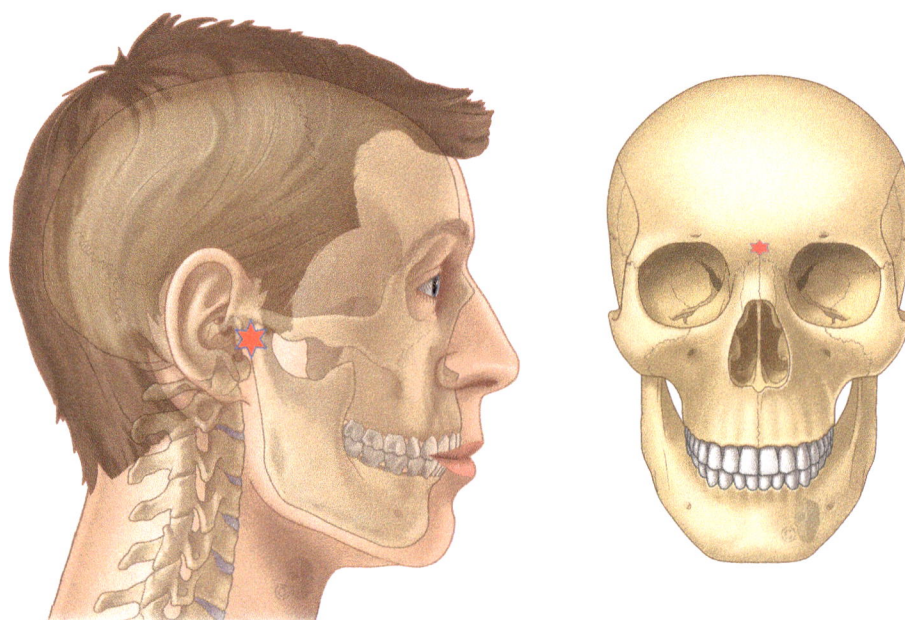

Figure 6.2 (left) Right Temporomandibular Joint; (right) Glabella: Terminal point for superior sagittal sinus

BREGMA AND LAMBDA

The bregma is created by/seated in the anterior fontanelle, and the lambda is created seated in the posterior fontanelle. Both are fascial in nature, being the anastomoses of the periosteum and the endosteum at those fontanelles, and as such become dural attachments for the superior sagittal sinus which, as mentioned, has its origin at the crista galli of the ethmoid bone and anchors at the fascia of the confluence of the sinuses at the internal occipital protuberance. The bregma lies at the confluence of the frontal and both parietal bones, while the lambda lies at the junction of the two parietal bones and the occiput. Cranio fascial torsion becomes evident with any skull trauma (contacts with the frontal, parietal and occiput) in early life and becomes increasingly emphasised with later trauma. Torsion of the falx cerebri manifests at both the bregma and lambda and indicates that those anchor points are under stress, possibly losing their ability to drain CSF and blood efficiently. This is also evident in forceps and ventouse birth processes. Changes to the falx cerebri change the midline of the cerebrum and cerebellum. All the intracranial organs that lie underneath the falx cerebri – the cingulated gyrus, the corpus callosum, the fornix, the caudate nucleus, the hippocampus, the thalamus, the hypothalamus and of course the ventricular system – also become distorted.

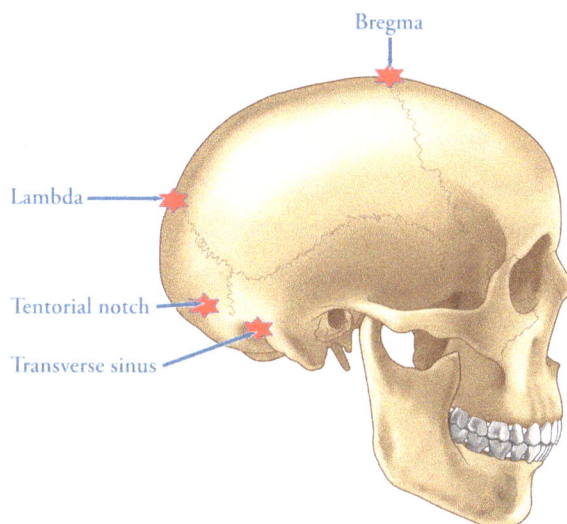

Figure 6.3 Bregma, Lambda, Tentorial Notch, Transverse Sinus

TENTORIAL NOTCH

This point lies at the junction of the transverse sinus, which is encapsulated by the tentorium cerebelli and attaches internally at the squama of the occiput. Externally, the tentorial notch lies off the midline at a level just superior to the external nuchal line on the external squama. The posterior pole represents the anterior anchor point of the tentorium cerebelli at the anterior and posterior clinoid processes of the sphenoid bone. Changes through cranio fascial torque alter the ethmoid-sphenoid junction and disrupt inter-pole activity as well as the vertical and horizontal dynamics of the falx cerebri and the tentorium cerebelli. Drainage of the sinuses is a major concern due to the change in these dynamics. The tentorial groove which controls the brainstem, pons and part of the cerebellum also has a bearing on how those organs function, as the tentorium cerebellum distorts. Drainage through the tentorium cerebelli, which encapsulates the confluence of the sinuses, the superior petrosal sinuses at the petrous portion of the temporal bone, the transverse sinuses, the sigmoid sinuses and the downward drainage of the internal jugular vein, all have to be considered with tentorium cerebelli distortion.

TRANSVERSE SINUS – OPTIONAL

The contact point for the transverse sinus lies lateral to the tentorial notch, and on the same level, just on the occipitomastoid suture. The transverse sinus leaves the confluence of the sinuses and becomes the sigmoid sinus, as it turns caudalward, before becoming the internal jugular vein, and exits through the jugular foramen. It adheres to the squama of the occiput, encapsulated by the tentorium cerebelli, then joins the sigmoid sinus at the junction of the petrous portion of the temporal bone, still encapsulated by the tentorium cerebelli and follows the border of the tentorium cerebelli. Disruption of the tentorium, from changes in the cranio fascial torque, will obstruct and congest the transverse sinus. This is a point of verification as to the status of the transverse sinus.

VERTEBRAL VENOUS PLEXUS, ATLANTO-OCCIPITAL MEMBRANE

This point is on the foramen magnum, just lateral to the midline on the atlanto-occipital membrane which covers the vertebral venous plexus and houses the entry point of the vertebral arteries. The atlanto-occipital membrane attaches to the base of the occiput, covers the VVP, the auxiliary plexus and the vertebral arteries. Changes in the cranio fascial torque, affect the spinal dura, C1, C2 and C3, distorting the atlas and attachments at the foramen magnum, and subsequently the atlanto-occipital membrane, obstructing drainage of the VVP, auxiliary plexus and the arterial flow of the vertebral arteries into the brain.

CERVICAL 1, 2 AND 3 – TRIGEMINAL SPINAL NUCLEUS

Changes in the dental-occlusion affect the trigeminal ganglion – through the maxillary and mandibular branches of the trigeminal – the mesencephalic and pontine nuclei, then the spinal nucleus at the levels of C1, C2 and C3. These changes at the upper cervical level should be monitored closely, as without changing the malocclusion, these vertebrae will come under a compensation, and will always be present. Constant presentation of a repeated subluxation at the atlas should give warning of an ongoing malocclusion.

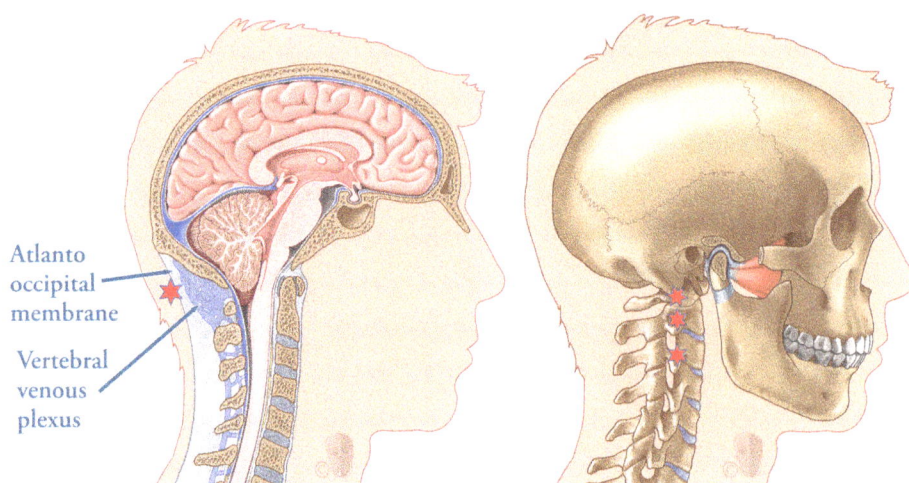

Atlanto occipital membrane

Vertebral venous plexus

Figure 6.4 (left) Vertebral Venous Plexus, Atlanto-Occipital Membrane; (right) Trigeminal Spinal Nucleus: C1, C2 and C3

ANTERIOR TEMPORALIS

If this indicator is present, check to see if the other anterior temporalis is involved. If so, the bilateral indicators suggest the mandible is being pulled forward into an anterior position. If the contralateral posterior temporalis is an indicator, the mandible is being pulled forward on the anterior temporalis indicator side but is pulled posterior on the contralateral posterior indicator side, meaning the mandible is rotating towards the posterior temporalis indicator side.

MEDIAL TEMPORALIS

Positive bilateral indicators on the medial temporalis suggest the mandible is pulled superior, possibly due to a lack of support at the 4s and 5s – bilaterally, placing the condylar heads up and back into the TMJ. If only one medial temporalis is indicated, then the 4s and 5s on that side are intruded and not offering support to the mandible on that side. If the contralateral indicator is absent, the 4s and 5s on that side are giving support to the mandible, so the mandible will present as horizontally skewed, putting pressure into the contralateral TMJ and possibly compressing the retrodiscal tissue.

POSTERIOR TEMPORALIS

Positive bilateral indicators on the posterior temporalis indicate that the mandible is being pulled posterior up into the TMJ. This could mean a total loss of posterior support, and a loss of dentition producing a loss of height in the TMJ. A unilateral posterior temporalis indicator will mean a loss of posterior support (6s, 7s and/or 8s), and the mandible will be protruded, the condyle forced up and back into the TMJ and the retrodiscal tissue will be compromised. Combinations of anterior temporalis indicators can occur and have been discussed.

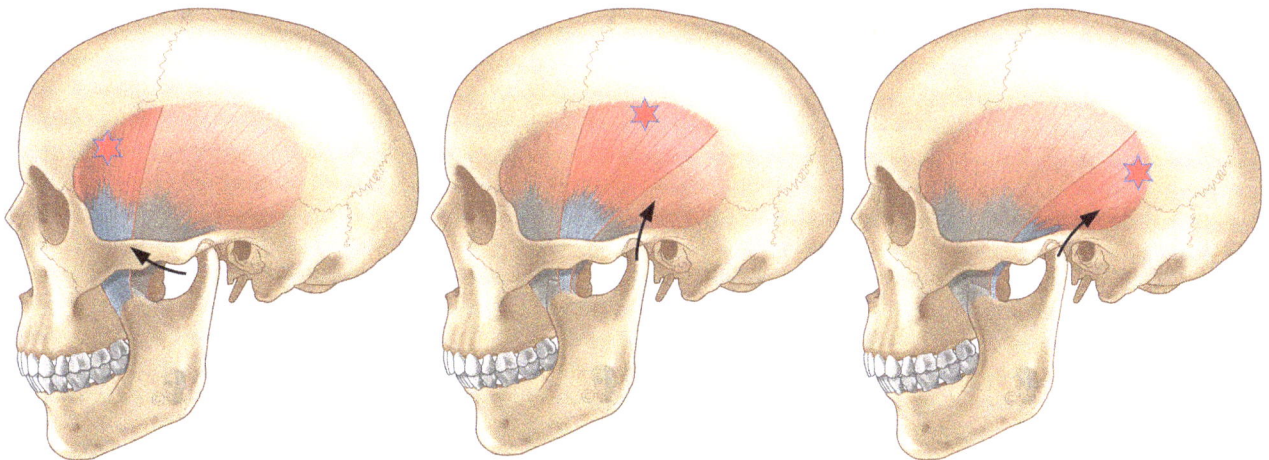

Figure 6.5 (left) Anterior Temporalis; (centre) Medial Temporalis; (right) Posterior Temporalis

LEFT GREATER WING OF THE SPHENOID

A positive indicator at the greater wing of the sphenoid will indicate how the greater wing is positioned. In most cases the greater wing of the sphenoid on the left side will be inferior and posterior, meaning that the superior orbital fissure is compressed, the ocular orbit is posterior and smaller, compressing the eye and all the fascia and membranes surrounding the eye. This will lead to poor drainage of the lacrimal gland and possibly gives rise to pterygiums – triangular patches of hypertrophied bulbar subconjunctival tissue, extending from the medial canthus to the border of the cornea. The pterygoid plates will be pulled posterior and inferior changing the torsion of the medial and lateral pterygoid muscles and changing the relationship of the condyle in the temporomandibular fossa which, by virtue of the left external temporal bone, has pulled the TMJ posterior forcing the mandible into a left deviation. Challenging the position of the greater wing superior and medial will confirm where it needs to be moved.

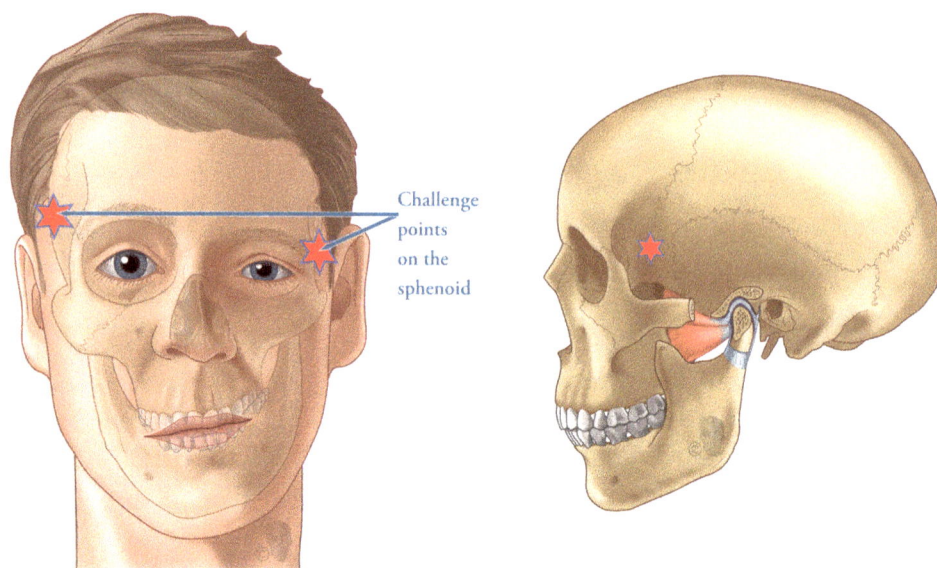

Challenge points on the sphenoid

Figure 6.6. (left) Greater Wing of Sphenoid Contact Points: Challenge points on the greater wing – anterior, posterior, inferior and superior collapsed left sphenoid. Compressed left temporomandibular fossa; (right) Left Greater Wing of the Sphenoid

INCISORS

Positive indicators at either the medial or lateral incisors or both, will indicate incisal interference on either of the teeth that test positive – 1s and 2s. This means the mandible is forward of its juxtaposition, or a loss of posterior teeth, either retruded or loss of dentition. There may be a combination of other indicators, such as the temporalis muscles.

CANINES

Indicators of either canine (3s) will implicate the ipsilateral trapezius muscle or the contralateral SCM of the indicator tooth. Loss of canine guidance means there is no contact for that canine on the one below, so those muscles will react to try and compensate. If both canines lose their guidance, the mandible can go into a crossbite, or slide into incisal interference.

320

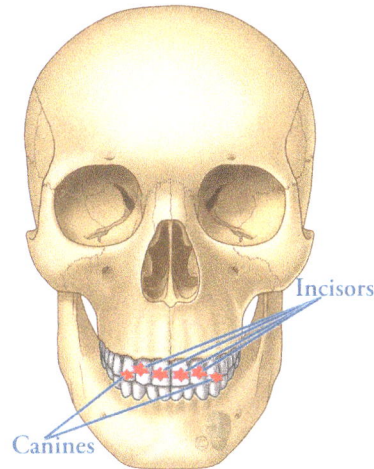

Figure 6.7 Incisors and Canines

LEFT SCM AND RIGHT UPPER TRAPEZIUS

If the right canine is indicated as positive, it will implicate the right upper trapezius and the left SCM. With the patient lying down supine, the doctor will test the right psoas muscle, while the (patient) therapy localises (TLs) the right upper canine, which in this case is positive. The clinician will then test the right upper trapezius muscle by asking the patient to pinch the muscle. A positive on this muscle will indicate a weakness of the upper right trapezius meaning the opposite trapezius will pull the head to the left.

The left SCM is then tested by the patient pinching the belly of the SCM and will be positive meaning the right SCM is strong and pulls the rotated head left. Now, when the patient touches the right upper canine simultaneously with either the right upper trapezius or the left SCM, the test will be negative, indicating the circuit is now closed and confirming the original non-contact on that canine.

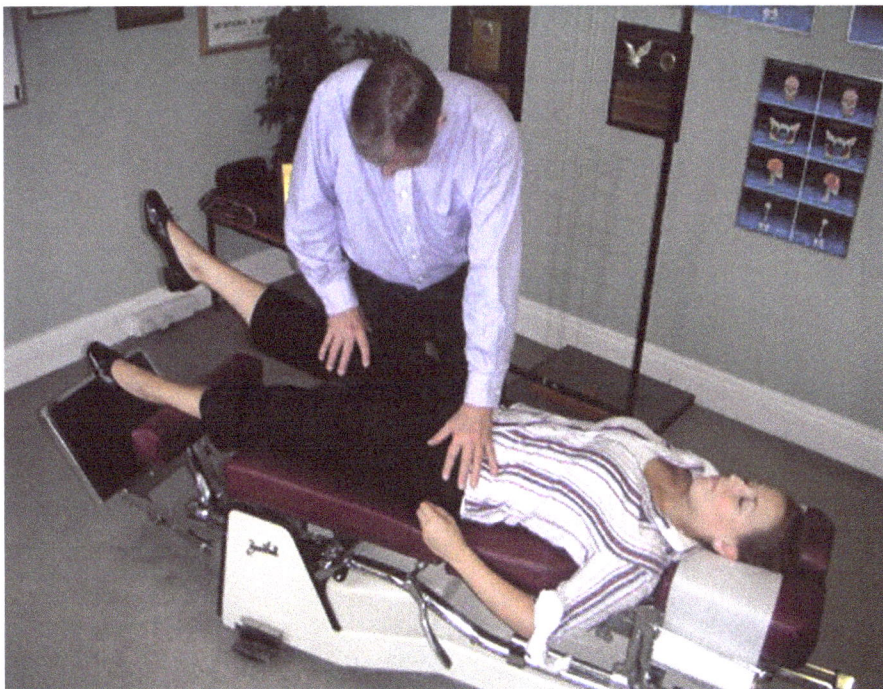

Figure 6.8 Right Psoas Muscle Test

RIGHT SCM AND LEFT UPPER TRAPEZIUS

If the left canine is indicated as positive, it will implicate the left upper trapezius and the right SCM. With the patient lying down supine, the doctor will again test the right psoas muscle, while the patient TLs the left upper canine, in this case being positive. The clinician will then test the left upper trapezius muscle by asking the patient to pinch the muscle. A positive on this muscle will indicate a weakness of the upper left trapezius meaning the opposite trapezius will pull the head to the right.

The right SCM is then tested, by the clinician pinching the belly of the SCM and a positive will mean the left SCM is strong and pulls the rotated head right. Now when the patient touches the left upper canine, simultaneously with either the left upper trapezius, or the right SCM, the test will be negative, indicating the circuit is now closed confirming the original non-contact on that canine.

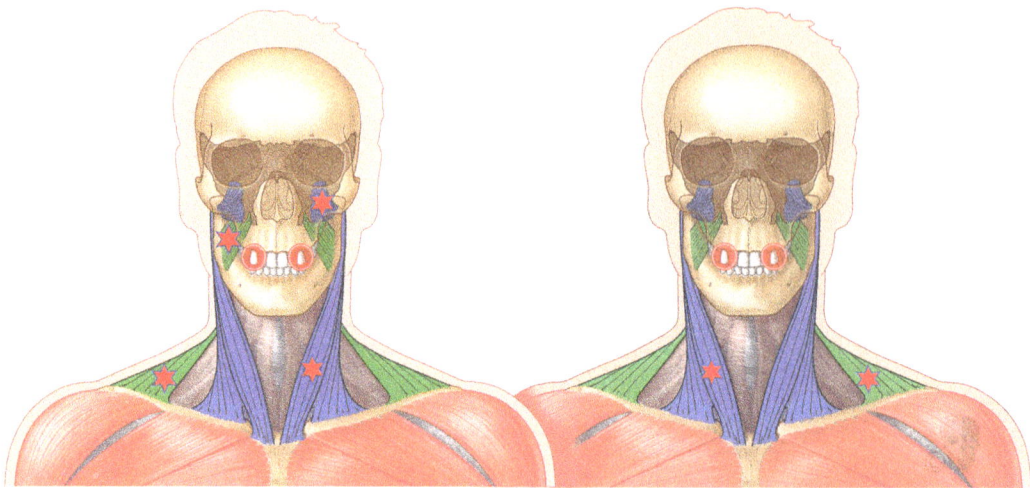

Figure 6.9 (left) Left SCM and Right Upper Trapezius: Right canine control;
(right) Right SCM and Left Upper Trapezius: Left canine control

RIGHT UPPER QUADRANT

The patient's right index finger covers the buccal tooth surfaces and the gums simultaneously on the right upper quadrant, with the jaw in an open position, ensuring that no other contact is made with the face, jaw or any other quadrant, with any of the other fingers. If the indicator is negative, there are no neurologic teeth in that quadrant.

If there is a positive indicator on that quadrant, each tooth is then individually tested from 8, 7, 6, 5, 4, 3, 2 down to 1, to isolate the neurologic tooth. One or possibly more of these teeth may be positive. The patient then holds that tooth between the thumb and index finger, while the doctor tests that tooth in the superior, inferior, clockwise and counterclockwise direction. The direction in which the indicator strengthens is the position in which the correction is made. The doctor then holds the offending tooth in the position that strengthens the indicator, and presses the tooth into that position, and into the alveolus, while the patient goes through three respiratory phases. When that is completed the doctor tests the involved quadrant again, and the individual teeth. This should now be a negative indicator, and that quadrant is clear. If that indicator does not clear, then check to find out if there is another neurologic tooth present in that quadrant. If there is, repeat the same procedure once more. The objective is to clear all the quadrants in this manner.

The neurologic tooth refers to:

- A tooth fracture, either horizontal or in most cases a vertical fracture, indicating dental evaluation and restoration, to clear that tooth
- Or the gumline, indicating bleeding, pus formation, or similar breakdown of the gingiva surrounding that tooth. This again may require dental intervention to clear the problem.

OPGs (orthopantomagraph) of the upper and lower teeth will indicate any changes in the socket, loss of dentition, loss of bone at the tooth root, fractures of the tooth or sites of infection that may have been missed on earlier evaluation.

Occasionally, this form of evaluation on the neurologic tooth uncovers sites of infection and tooth decay that would not necessarily be exposed with ordinary investigations.

RIGHT LOWER, LEFT UPPER AND LEFT LOWER QUADRANTS

Follow the same protocols as outlined above.

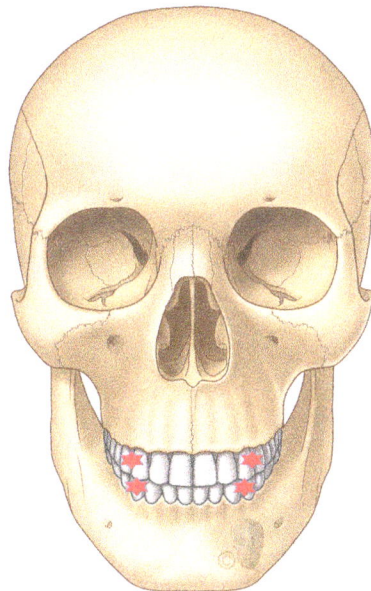

Figure 6.10 Upper and Lower Quadrants

MIDSTERNUM

This is a non-specific indicator showing the presence of a biomechanical disruption. Check plumb line analysis for biomechanical disruption to the pelvis and spine.

EPIGASTRIC

This is an electro-magnetic indicator at the level of the solar plexus – sympathetic overload, indicating stress and possibly adrenal fatigue. Balance autonomic responses to sympathetic and parasympathetics.

UMBILICUS

This is a chemical indicator, suggesting digestive overloads, incompatibility of digestive function, possibly an involvement at the iliocaecal valve. More TL at various abdominal indicators will produce more realistic and accurate data, such as I-C valve, ampulla of Vater, pancreatic duct, pancreatic head, ascending colon, transverse colon, descending colon and sigmoid colon. Check temporo-sphenoidal (TS) line for any visceral involvement. These indicators should also coincide with the occipital line fibres 1, 2 and 3, and areas on the fibres 1 to 7.

Chiropractic manipulative reflex technique (CMRT) from the chiropractic standpoint of normal physiology achieves optimal results when the combined effects of the CNS integrate normally with the autonomic nervous systems (parasympathetic and sympathetic nervous systems), and the peripheral nervous system.

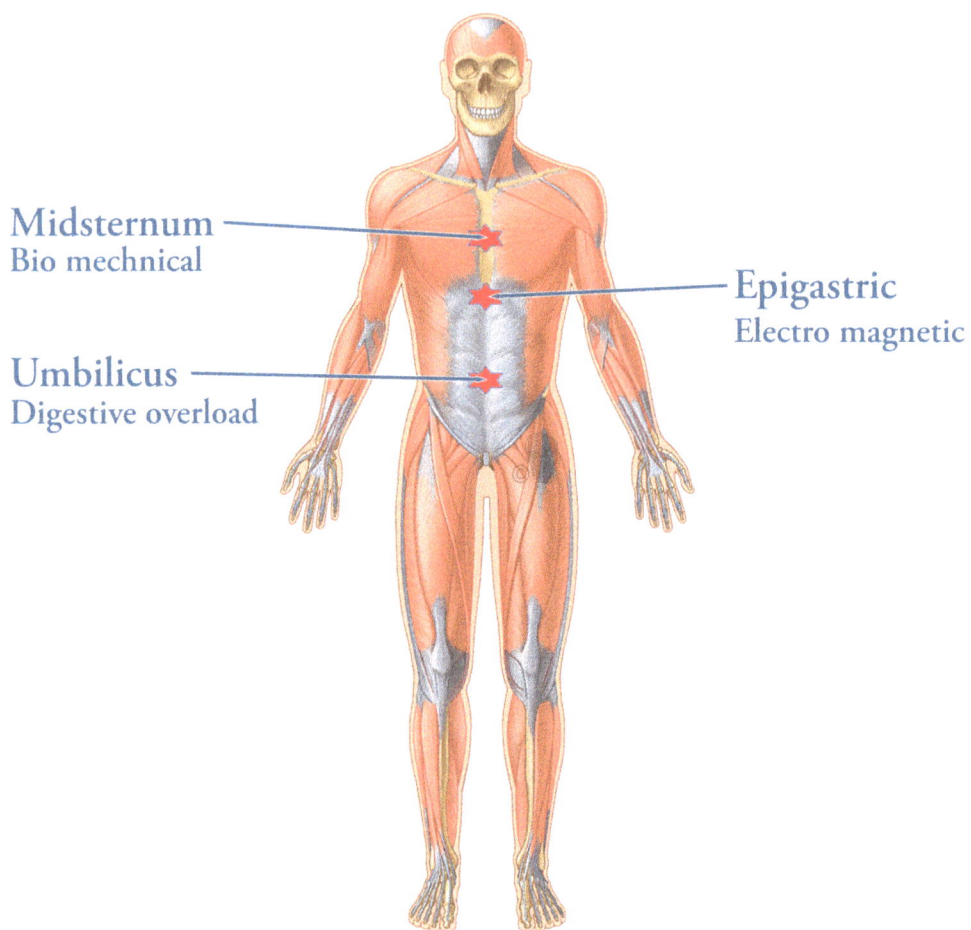

Midsternum
Bio mechnical

Umbilicus
Digestive overload

Epigastric
Electro magnetic

Figure 6.11 Sternum, Epigastric and Umbilicus

TEMPORO-SPHENOIDAL LINE

Each organ or system has a specific occipital area (1 to 7) and a specific line fibre (1, 2 or 3) coupled with specific organ reflex points and vertebral level (i.e. cervical, thoracic, lumbar or sacral), which the clinician must clear in order to reinstate homeostatic function. The temporo-sphenoidal line is found on the border of the greater wing of the sphenoid at the spheno-temporal border, the pterion and the sphenofrontal border. Each indicator represents an organ and vertebral level, which can then be identified more accurately by therapy localising the organ area on the abdomen as indicated.

The expression of normal nervous system integrity is dependent on the stable and balanced biomechanics of the skeletal system, primarily the pelvis, spine, cranium and a normal maxillary mandibular occlusion. Deviations of any of these components will lead to a neurological deficit affecting the brain, spinal cord, cranial nerves and spinal nerves and their ganglia, and will ultimately result in disease or lack of homeostasis.

CMRT (soft tissue orthopaedics) was devised by Dr Major Bertram DeJarnette and embellished by Dr Mel Rees as a visceral technique to complement the structural work as defined in Sacro Occipital Technique. The utilisation of the occipital fibre analysis combined with visceral reflexes earmarks visceral components that are dysfunctional and thereby inhibiting the neurological response to repair and heal.

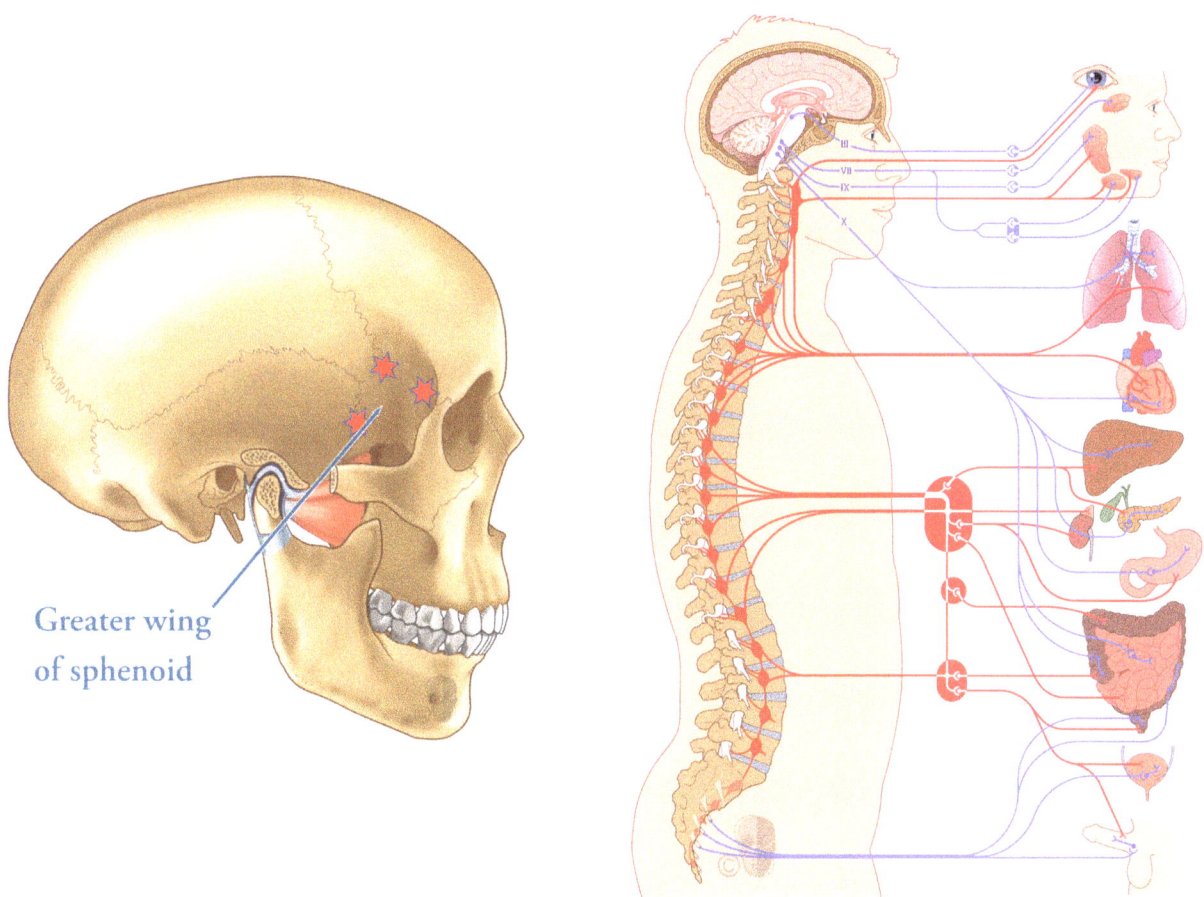

Greater wing of sphenoid

Figure 6.12 Temporo Sphenoidal Line: (left) CMRT levels contact points; (right) Active area indicates organ involvement

CN III – OCULOMOTOR – CONVERGENCE

With the patient in a standing position facing the doctor, the testing thumb-finger indicator is checked and should be negative. Ask the patient to roll the eyes to the left, while keeping the head straight, and check the indicator. This is usually negative. Then ask the patient to roll the eyes to the right, with the head straight, and again check the indicator. If this indicator is positive, the patient has a cranial counterclockwise torque.

Thus with a clockwise torque the eyes rolling left will produce a positive indicator. If there is a counterclockwise torque, the oculomotor nerve – feeding the medial rectus muscle – will have no difficulty in moving to the left as that is the direction of torque, while the eyes rolling right will be pulling against the torque, and will not be able to accommodate that position.

This will also be confirmed by checking the convergence of the eyes. The doctor's index finger moves from a midline towards the eyes; both eyes should converge to the midline. If counterclockwise torque is present, the left eye will NOT converge, weakening the medial rectus muscle, and indicating that cranio fascial counterclockwise torque is present. This is also confirmed by the internal rotation of the feet, when the patient is lying supine, and the feet are internally rotated. The left foot will internally rotate with ease, while the right foot will be restricted.

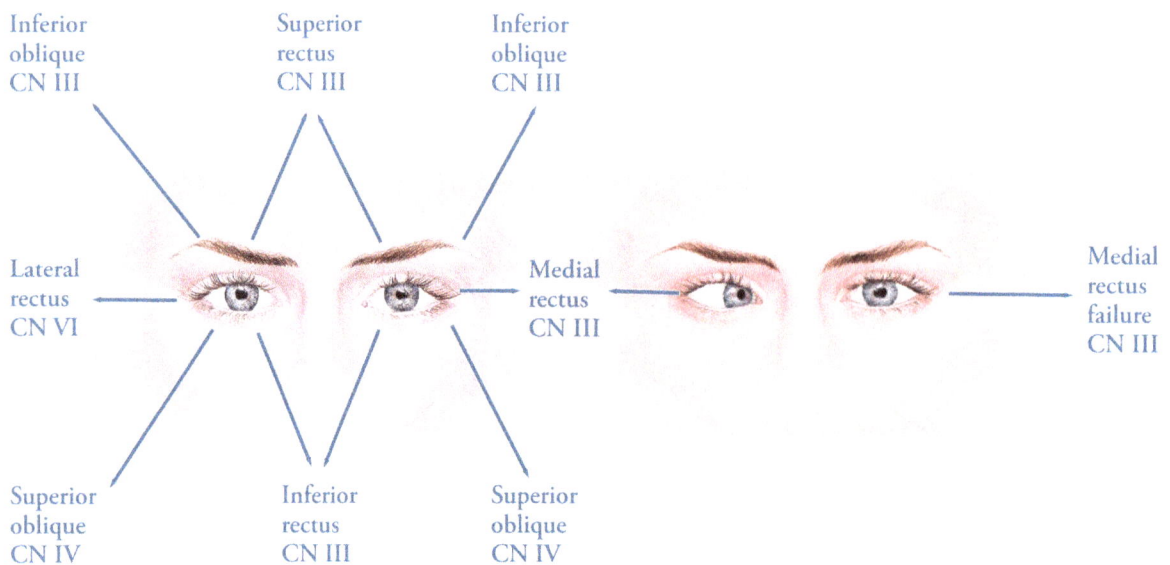

Figure 6.13 Inability for Ocular Convergence

CONCLUSION

This chapter explains the procedure of cranial scanning, the process of applying the scan and the indicators that show the doctor where the problems lie. This is a practical technique requiring regular implementation in order to gain proficiency but vital to the correct diagnosis of underlying problems and future treatment protocols.

This also allows the doctor independence to supervise the diagnosis, treatment and outcome for the patient, without recourse to previous medical assessment or more importantly, anecdotal and subjective input about the condition by the patient himself.

The list of indicators for cranial scanning are:

- Left and right TMJs
- Glabella
- Bregma
- Lambda
- Tentorial notch

- Transverse sinus
- VVP, sub-occipital cavernous sinus, atlanto-occipital membrane
- C1, C2 and C3
- Anterior temporalis
- Medial temporalis
- Posterior temporalis
- Left greater wing of the sphenoid
- Temporo-sphenoid line
- Incisors
- Canines
- Left SCM and right upper trapezius
- Right SCM and left upper trapezius
- Upper right quadrant – neurologic tooth
- Lower right quadrant – neurologic tooth
- Upper left quadrant – neurologic tooth
- Lower left quadrant – neurologic tooth
- Mid-sternum
- Epigastric
- Umbilicus
- CN III oculomotor. Eyes left and eyes right – convergence

CHAPTER 7

VISUAL ANALYSIS OF THE PATIENT

AND TREATMENT PROTOCOL

THE PLUMB LINE

Standing a patient in a plumb line will show how the body reacts to gravity as the patient strays away from the midline.

The smooth and non-smooth coupling should also be noted – pelvic, shoulder and head levels – horizontally as well as rotationally, denoting the presence of bilateral sacroiliac rotation, sacroiliac lesion, or a lumbo-sacral disc lesion.

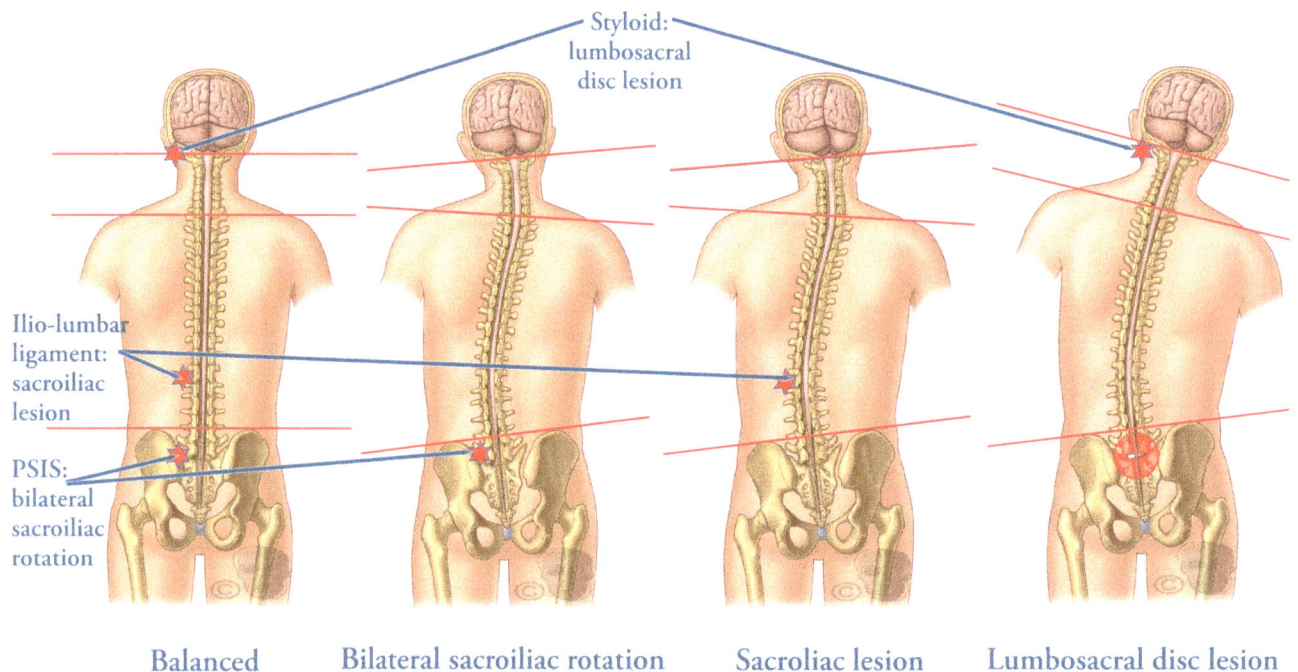

Figure 7.1 The Plumb Line

The lateral or anterior to posterior (A to P) motion of the body to delineate between a bilateral sacroiliac rotation and a sacroiliac lesion, and the non-smooth, static posture of a lumbosacral disc lesion, are specific data that give one an idea of the gravitational pull on the body. The palpable first rib motion of the neck and head in a flexion and extension defines a bilateral sacroiliac rotation (both rib heads will move together, as the two sacroiliac joints are functional and supportive), or a sacroiliac lesion (only one rib head will move, as one sacroiliac joint has become compromised, and will not weight bear as designed, nor function properly, and so slips on the offending side, exposing the non-supportive rib head – the unilateral rib head).

With the patient standing in front of you with both arms outstretched horizontally, press the arms towards the floor and, notwithstanding any upper extremity issues, the arms will weaken. Cotton rolls are placed between the teeth, covering both the left and right occlusal surfaces, and the test is repeated. If the strength returns to the arms in this test mode, a descending major is present, indicating a stomatognathic major, which may involve dentition, jaw to jaw relationship, TMJD or a neuro-muscular involvement.

PLUMB LINE SCANNING

Bilateral sacroiliac rotation – A to P sway, PSIS, bilateral rib heads, smooth coupling

Sacroiliac lesion – Lateral sway, ilio lumbar, unilateral rib head, smooth coupling

Lumbosacral disc lesion – antalgic posture, styloid indicator, non-smooth coupling

FIRST VISIT – REMOVE CRANIO FASCIAL TORQUE ONLY

Once all the pre-tests and checks have been performed, on the first visit the doctor will only remove the cranio fascial torque. Once completed, ask the patient to walk around the room and then post-test all the same parameters. The patient and doctor will be amazed at the changes that have taken place using this apparently innocuous intracranial procedure. Sacroiliac lesions can become bilateral sacroiliac rotations, the entire membrane system will be reinstated, balance as well as leg length can change with the patient aware of immediate improvement. The author cannot overemphasise the importance of following this first procedure as so many chiropractors become confused with mixed treatment categories, switching and ineffective protocols. Cranio fascial torque has been long ignored and should become the first diagnostic protocol when embarking on this kind of treatment.

SECOND VISIT (1 WEEK LATER) – REPEAT PARAMETER CHECKS

The same format is followed. Check all the parameters as on the first visit to see what is happening, what has changed, what is still persistent in the testing. Complete documentation.

Follow the treatment protocol, block the pelvis, following the usual category protocol and finish with the 8-Step cranial drainage protocol and the Howat Sweep.

THIRD VISIT (2 WEEKS LATER) – REPEAT PARAMETER CHECKS

The same format is followed. Check all the parameters as on the first and second visits to see what is happening, what has changed, and what is still persistent in the testing. Complete documentation.

Follow the treatment protocol, block the pelvis following the usual category protocol, introduce the 6-point CMRT visceral clearing (this is important as the body is now going through a detoxifying process and needs to have visceral clearing), and finish with the 8-Step cranial drainage protocol and the Howat Sweep.

FOURTH VISIT (3–4 WEEKS LATER) – REPEAT PARAMETER CHECKS

The same format is followed. Check all the parameters as on the first, second and third visits to see what is happening, what has changed, and what is still persistent in the testing. Complete documentation.

The treatment protocols will now include the blocking, 6-point CMRT, muscle work (psoas, etc.) and lymphatic drainage, then finish up with the 8-Step cranial drainage and the Howat Sweep.

Treatment visits are initially stretched out to give the body time to heal and re-adjust to new parameters that have been initiated by the treatment protocol. Hereafter, keeping patient visits to a monthly or bi-monthly visit regime is a matter of clinical judgement and one's expertise. Remember that cranio fascial torque has been present since birth, possibly exacerbated by skeletal and cranial trauma, followed by dental insults with orthodontics and orthopaedics through puberty, whiplash injuries and emotional and hormonal strain, vaccinations and any other drugs that pass through the blood brain barrier, creating cytotoxic oedema. Cranio fascial torque has been intrinsic to this body over many years, given poor eating habits, lifestyle, psychological trauma and ever-present underlying stress any healing process will last more than a matter of weeks. This is in addition to the trauma disrupting brain drainage, leaving the ventricular system and all the adjacent intracranial organs congested and vulnerable to cytotoxic effects (as well as the ravages of MS, Parkinson's disease, dementia, Alzheimer's disease and stroke). Patients have to be educated in these matters. This type of chiropractic care not only resolves ad hoc problems, but may also be employed prophylacticly using the cranial scanning and treatment protocols outlined above. It is unacceptable for the chiropractor to leave cranio fascial distortions and torque untreated given the inevitable difficulties and potentially life-threatening conditions the patient risks in the future.

CONCLUSION

The plumb line presents the doctor with a very important asset in the consulting room. It represents a clear idea of how the patient presents, and accurate details of the plumb line position vertically should be noted. Horizontal lines representing the levels of the head, shoulders and pelvis should also be noted, referring to smooth and non-smooth coupling.

Smooth coupling refers to a dural torque, or a sacroiliac lesion, whereas a non-smooth coupling indicates a lower lumbar disc lesion.

The treatment protocols described a first visit, what to do and look for, and what treatment to administer on that visit. If cranio fascial torque is evident, it is recommended that only that is taken care of on the first visit. Outlines of how to proceed on following visits is detailed once the cranio fascial torque has been removed.

The doctor will note that the time lapse between visits is extended, in most cases, as the body needs time to re-adjust to the removal of the torque, before changing other indicators too quickly. Clinical assessment is vital, and with more acute patients, time lapses between visits can be reduced.

THE DISLOCATED BRAIN

PART VI

CRANIO BRAIN

DYNAMICS

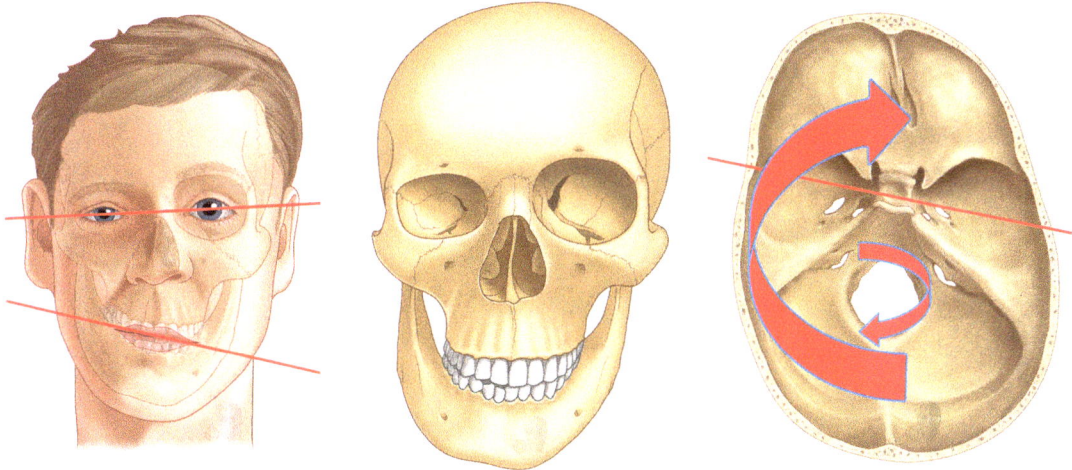

CONTENTS PART VI

ILLUSTRATIONS PART VI

INTRODUCTION TO PART VI

The purpose of this chapter is to examine the internal dynamics of the brain components derived from the neural tube. It will show how the ventricular system – the two laterals, the third and the fourth ventricles – is found to be central to these components and how the action and stability of the dominant system is foremost to the homeostasis of the brain. The choroid plexuses of the four ventricles produce cerebrospinal fluid (CSF), which flows through the interventricular foramen of Monro in the lateral ventricles, into the third ventricle, and then from the aqueduct of Sylvius into the fourth ventricle. From here there are two apertures; the apertures of Luschka and Magendie which take CSF into the cisterns, the cerebellum, and then finally into the central canal of the spinal cord.

Under normal circumstances, in benign asymmetry of the brain, CSF flows in a normal circulatory motion through the dominant system as described above. In the case of brain trauma and upper cervical trauma however, the drainage process eliminating blood and CSF from the brain becomes more tenuous, and a stagnation of fluid occurs. With this slowing effect taking place at the base of the cranium, CSF and blood flow may be reversed by back pressure. These fluids subsequently pool in the dominant system, changing its stable structural format. This alteration in structure has an influence on all the adjacent organs, nuclei and communicating fibres, affecting their ability to perform as they should. The result is a change in neurological function, which in turn creates stasis within the brain and produces a myriad of neurological symptoms and conditions that clinicians encounter regularly. There exists a modern misconception in medical philosophy that physical trauma is the cause of these problems, and that this can be resolved and reversed using a cocktail of chemicals. This is where the narrative needs to change.

CHAPTER 1

CRANIO BRAIN DYNAMICS

In reviewing the literature available, the author has concluded that forces directed to the skull and upper cervical spine – from birth trauma to every other unexpected traumatic incident – has an impact on one's life. With current diagnostic tools such so-called minor traumas to these areas are not able to be measured They do not warrant investigation, nor are they recognised as a threat to homeostasis.

Anyone who has dealt with a fracture to the anatomy, regardless of where it occurs in the body, will be satisfied with the reduction of the fracture, before applying a cast to keep that area immobilised thereby allowing it to mend. After removal of the cast physiotherapy and rehabilitation will encourage, the musculo-skeletal area to return 'to normal'. On closer evaluation and observation, the force applied to a fracture site first goes into a strain, followed by a sprain and finally with more force – a fracture. Unless the strain and sprain above and below the fracture site are reduced by reinstating the bones into their juxtaposition, the joints above and below never return to their full optimum function. The fracture of an ulna or radius will ultimately affect and compromise the carpal tunnel or the elbow joint or both resulting many years later in so-called 'repetitive strain injury'. The 'tennis/golf elbow' and the 'carpal tunnel syndrome' are both well documented problems, which usually lead to surgery. Earlier intervention of strain and sprain reduction would reduce that outcome.

This analogy is applicable to the cranial vault, where forces of a varying dynamic collide with or hit the skull; the strain and sprain at the cranial sutural level goes a long way before that force causes a fracture of the cranial plate. In the meantime, the periosteum and the endosteum of that cranial plate twist with the strain, are exacerbated by the sprain This distorts the external muscle and fascial structures outside the skull, and simultaneously distorts the internal fascia inside the skull. This internal fascia includes the meningeal dura, the dura mater, the pia mater and the arachnoid mater, including the subdural and subarachnoid cavities. This fascial torque also includes the falx cerebri, the tentorium cerebellum, the falx cerebelli and the diaphragma sellae – in effect, the reciprocal tension membranes (RTM), the supportive and balancing membrane system that holds the brain in place. This fascial distortion then goes further into the brain, warping or twisting the fibres and pathways that traverse the brain connecting organs, glands, nuclei and complete systems.

This trauma is not ascribed relevance as it cannot be measured and is therefore ignored. Further traumas of this nature and complexity occur many times throughout one's life, accumulating and subsequently changing the dynamic role that the brain plays. This discussion has so far dealt with the mature cranium and its established cranial sutures. The infant cranium is made up of the anterior and posterior fontanelles and the two posterior-lateral fontanelles, which close a few months after birth, but the former only close between 18 months and two years after birth. At this stage of infant development, the child has frequently fallen whilst learning to walk with the skull subjected to many 'minor' traumas before full closure of the fontanelles. Arguably the infant skull is designed to absorb many of these shocks but the the concern is that the fascial distortions occuring at this age become permanent fixtures in the brain, lay down a template for further intrusive problems. Understandably, medical literature concentrates on life-threatening traumatic brain injuries, which certainly produce a cascade of neurological changes that can last a lifetime. Due to lack of diagnostic ability there is insufficient concern with the myriad minor traumas that occur throughout life and have an accumulative effect on brain physiology. Consider the four-year-old who is placed on the back of a Shetland pony and bounces around without control, falls off then is replaced on the pony, only for the whole process to be repeated. Hitting the ground from that height is dismissed as part of growing up, but the impact, the whiplash, and the torsional and rotational dynamics to the head caused by that fall are considerable in a growing and developing child. The ventricular system, the cingulate gyrus, the corpus callosum, the caudate nucleus, the fornix, the thalamus and the hippocampus, as well as the drainage process of the venous sinus system must all be affected.

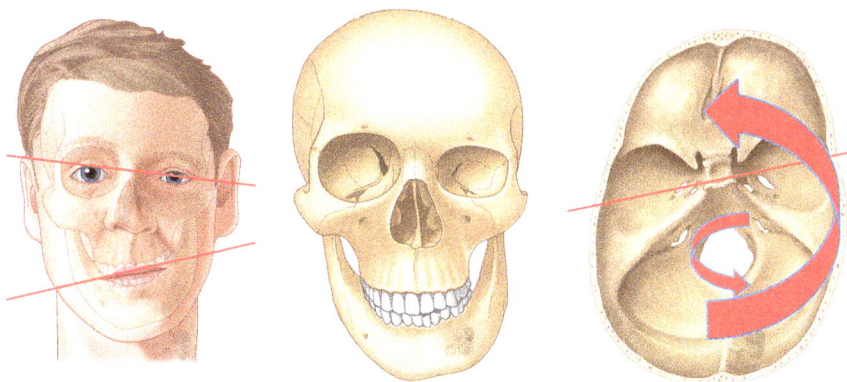

Figure 1.1 Normal Counterclockwise Torque Smooth Coupling: Right sphenoid greater wing, anterior and superior; larger and more prominent right eye; diaschisis increasing torque of the brainstem

Minor traumas – the strains and sprains of the cranial sutures in the cranial vault – that are overlooked due to lack of diagnostics, but when repeated over and over throughout life, are accumulative and physiologically damaging.

In an age where youngsters are introduced to active sports and are involved in the rough and tumble of growing up in our civilised society, these overlooked 'minor traumas' are ignored.

The minor traumas described above alter the integrity of neurological fibres transmitting information from brain to spinal cord and vice versa, via junction boxes such as the thalamus. Association fibres radiate throughout the brain from the thalamus. Commissural fibres link the left and right hemispheres of the brain through the corpus callosum, the fornix and the hippocampus.

The benign asymmetry of the brain allows the functional movement of arterial blood into the brain and venous blood out of the brain. This completes the vascular cycle of replenishing the brain and removing its toxins. This represents balanced haemodynamic function in a counterclockwise movement, due in part to the larger superior sagittal sinus flowing into the larger right transverse and sigmoid sinuses, with the smaller inferior sagittal sinus flowing into the smaller left transverse and sigmoid sinuses, as described earlier.

External traumatic forces or diaschisis into the brain can exacerbate this counterclockwise motion, changing dural membrane tonus. This causes reduction of vascular flow and static fluid retention. On the other hand, a necrotic external traumatic force produces a clockwise torsion against the haemodynamic balance, strangulating the internal cranial organs in close proximity to the tentorial incisura, the falx cerebri, the tentorium cerebellum, the falx cerebelli and the diaphragma sellae. This force is probably more damaging to the neurophysiology of the brain, as the delicate neural fibre system becomes corkscrewed and constricted resulting in gradual necrosis of those invaluable pathways. The pathways involved and the organs they nurture, will ultimately determine the debilitating syndrome that manifests itself.

Interestingly, the commonalities shared by Alzheimer's, Parkinson's disease, multiple sclerosis and dementia and their idiosyncratic symptoms may fall into this category.

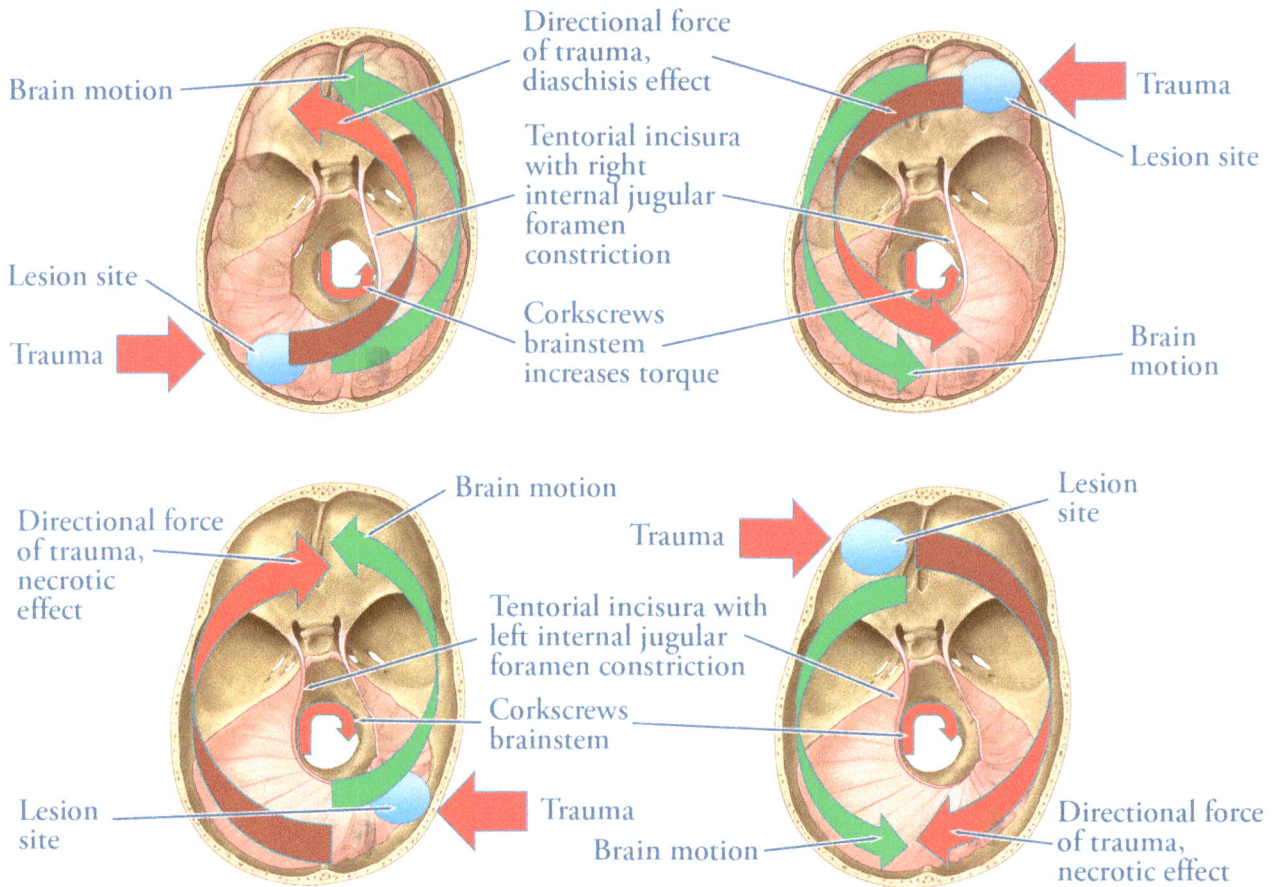

Figure 1.2 (top) Brain Trauma and Diaschisis, Smooth Coupling Force: Counterclockwise torque with counterclockwise torque, increases counterclockwise torque; (bottom) Brain Trauma and Necrosis, Non-Smooth Coupling Force: Clockwise torque against benign counterclockwise torque corkscrews the brainstem and ventricular system

When major pathways weave their way through the brain and are influenced by torsional clockwise or counterclockwise dynamics, the transmission capability of individual fibres must be questioned. They will either stimulate or inhibit the end organ producing symptoms that guide the diagnosis which, to a large degree, becomes superfluous to the end result as these are secondary issues.

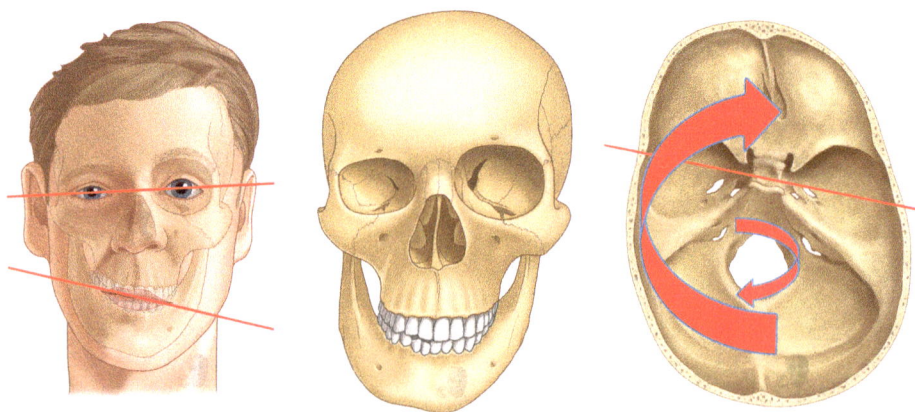

Figure 1.3 Abnormal Counterclockwise Torque Non-Smooth Coupling: Left sphenoid greater wing, anterior and superior; larger and more prominent left eye; necrotic brainstem corkscrew

CHRONIC TRAUMATIC ENCEPHALOPATHY (CTE)

Recent discoveries by neurophysiologists and pathologists show that CTE is a degenerative brain disease increased by repetitive brain trauma evident in contact sports such as rugby, American football and soccer. With CTE, the presence of 'toxic tau protein' is becoming more evident, and although not quantifiable in living humans, it is evident in pathological brain slides taken from the cadavers of people who have been involved in these sports.

The toxic protein, tau, builds up in nerve cells and astrocytes found deep in the sulci of the cerebral cortex and in perivascular sites in the frontal lobe – causing changes in memory, judgement and concentration – and in the medial temporal lobes – affecting behavioural changes in emotion and anger management.

Tau builds up in the brain where traumatic forces are applied, namely in close proximity to the base of the RTM and the influence they have in distorting the brain balance – as at the base of the falx cerebri – separating the cerebral hemispheres, and centrally located above the cingulate gyrus, the supracallosal gyrus, the corpus callosum and the lateral ventricles. Forces of concussion and 'sub-concussion' – a state before fully assertive concussion occurs – are sufficient to constitute the formation of tau.

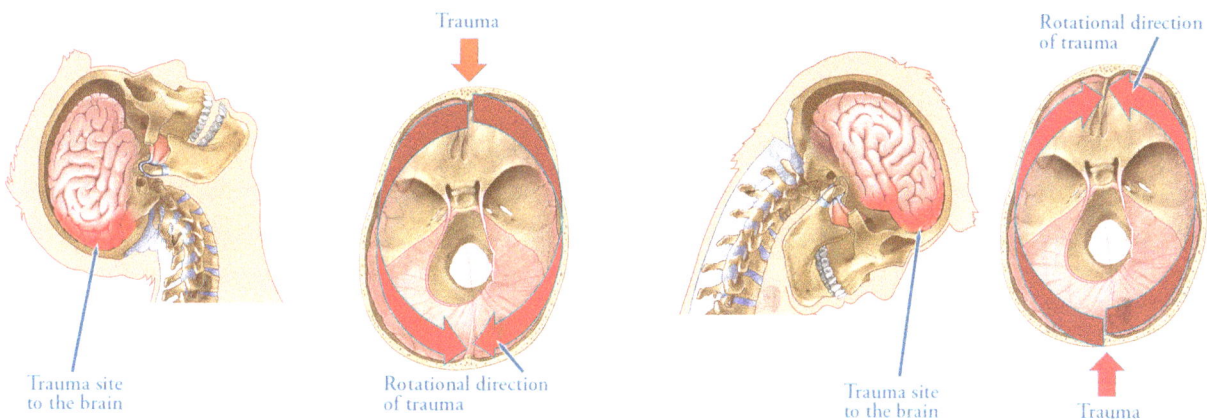

Figure 1.4 Brain Trauma after Whiplash of the Spine: Magnified distortion of tentorial incisura

According to the current research, retirement from contact sport does not diminish spread of the tau protein in the individual, as it continues to disseminate and migrate to the brainstem – disrupting cognition – and altering other areas of the brain.

The CTE process starts with concussion and sub-concussion, followed by more damage by repetitive trauma.

Post-concussion, a manifestation of toxic tau protein in the brain, initiates more insidious spread involving changes in personality, executive decisions and behaviour.

Prolonged manifestation leaves the cerebral cortex with marked shrinkage – damaging areas used for thinking, planning and remembering, as well as the hippocampus crucial to formation of new memories. The size of the ventricles will also show an increase in size.

These traumas are dynamically produced as a result of physical forces, and those forces also have to be addressed physically to reinstate function. The medical world has too often sought to heal physiological damage through chemical intervention when the problems of dynamic trauma are mechanical in essence.

If these conditions linger for thirty or forty years, necrotic brain tissue will be the result.

ASSUMPTION OF A SYMMETRIC BRAIN AND MEMBRANES

The symmetric brain shows the tentorium cerebellum and the attachments to the petrosal ridges laterally on the temporal bones, encapsulating the superior petrosal sinuses bilaterally. The anterior margins of the tentorium cerebellum anchor at the body of the sphenoid at the anterior and posterior clinoid processes. These are also the attachments of the diaphragma sellae, the encapsulating layer around the hypophyseal stalk of the pituitary gland.

The tentorial incisura anchors at the straight sinus and moves anteriorly, separating into two enveloping borders encasing the cerebellum, brain stem and pons to anchor at the clinoid processes on the sphenoid body.

The tentorium cerebellum has its posterior border along the interior border of the occiput at the transverse sulci, encapsulating the transvers sinuses and the sigmoid sinuses bilaterally.

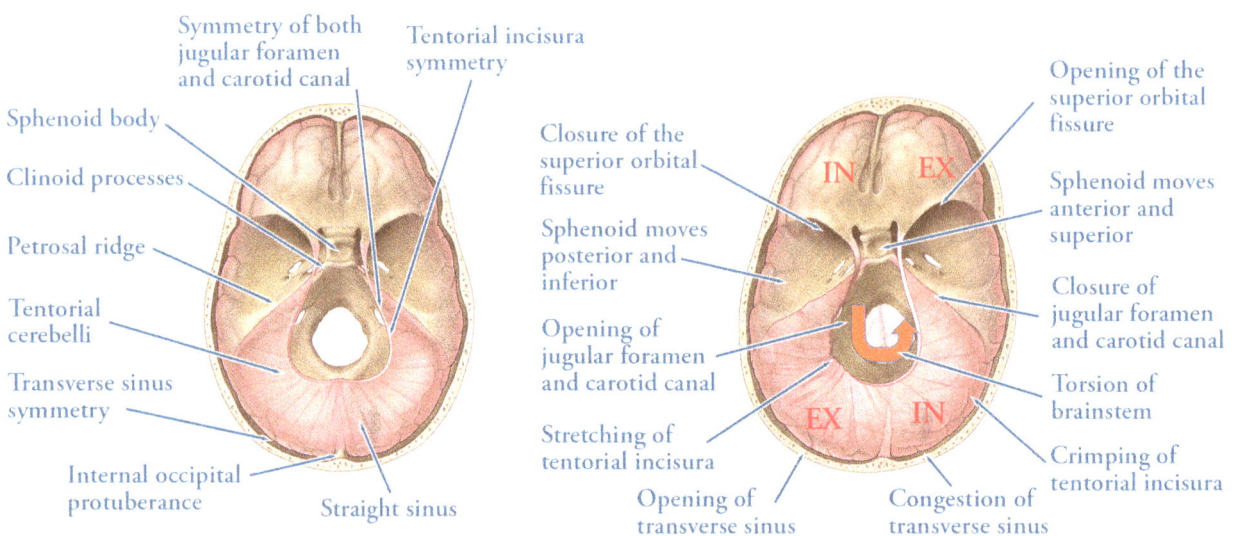

Figure 1.5 (left) Symmetric Brain and Membranes: Tentorial incisura and sphenoid in symmetric brain; (right) Traumatic Counterclockwise Torque of the Brain and Membranes

HAEMODYNAMIC BENIGN ASSYMETRY OF THE BRAIN

The haemodynamic asymmetry of the brain begins in utero, driving a counterclockwise torque of the brain thereby influencing the RTM and ultimately the helical drainage process.

In the cranium, the right frontal bone presents as an external rotation opposite the left external occiput, which is coupled with a left external temporal bone, producing a larger jugular foramen and carotid canal on that left side. The left glenoid fossa is also relatively posterior to the right glenoid fossa, causing the mandible to deviate to the left on opening. The opposing right internal temporal bone creates a smaller jugular foramen and carotid canals, on the right side.

This counterclockwise torsion takes the right sphenoid's greater wing into a superior/anterior position opening the superior orbital fissure, while the left sphenoid greater wing moves posterior/inferior closing the superior orbital fissure. The pterygoid plates on the left are posterior to the right pterygoid plates, which influence the internal (medial) pterygoid and external (lateral) pterygoid muscles and their activity on the condylar and ramus portion of their respective mandibles.

The cranial fascial torsion that results from this early phenomenon means that the brain components become influenced by the torque. The midline position of the two lateral, third and fourth ventricles, warp and twist further with resultant influence on all the adjacent and neighbouring organs. These are primarily the cingulate cortex and the supracallosal gyrus, lying on top of the corpus callosum, the roof of the lateral ventricles. The organ lying under the lateral ventricle is the caudate nucleus, while the lateral borders of the third ventricle provide support for the thalamus and hypothalamus and the fourth ventricle interfaces with the cerebellum.

Consequently, the cerebellum and the prefrontal lobes rely on a spontaneously generated electrical pulse to make sense of both incoming sensory information and to generate appropriate motor responses. Learning and behavioural disabilities, under the term 'developmental dyspraxia' include poor balance, difficulty with both fine and gross motor skills, problems with vision, motor planning and perception, poor body awareness, and difficulty with reading, writing and speech. Poor social skills and emotional/behavioural difficulties, together with the physiological problems detailed above may all be regarded as the legacy of cranio fascial distortion.

APOPTOSIS

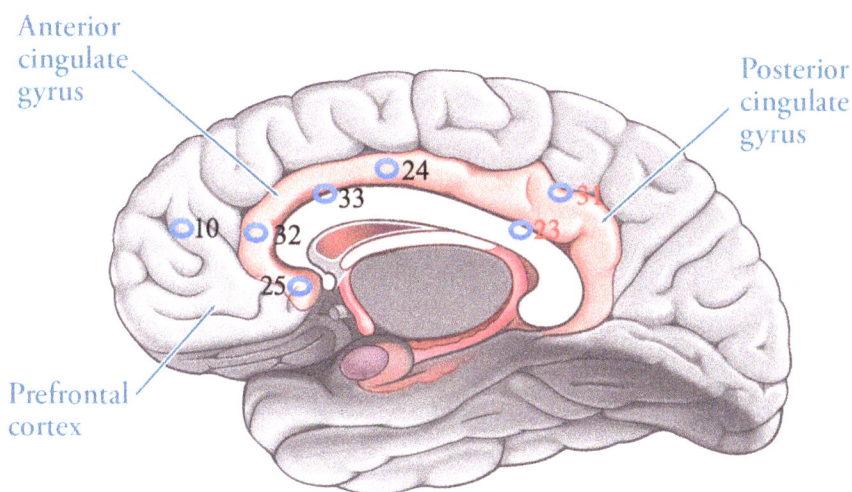

Figure 1.6 Brodmann's Areas: Associated with cingulate gyrus executive function and with prefrontal cortex

Apoptosis is a term coined in 2004 by Robin Pauc to cover the development, migration and synaptogenesis of the second-generation of specialised neurons that start to develop four months after birth in the human brain. The most notable and best researched second-generation cell is the VEN spindle cells.

The anterior cingulate cortex contains a class of spindle-shaped neurons that are found only in humans and the great apes, and thus are a recent evolutionary specialisation probably related to the the function described below. The spindle cells appear to be widely connected with diverse parts of the brain and may have a role in the coordination essential in developing the capacity to focus on difficult problems. Furthermore, they emerge postnatally and their survival may be enhanced or reduced by environmental conditions of enrichment or stress, thus potentially influencing adult competence or dysfunction in emotional self-control and problem-solving capacity.[1]

Studies have shown that dyspraxia manifests as a prominent symptom in association with each of the following primary 'conditions' and that no case of dyslexia, dyspraxia, attention deficit disorder (ADD), attention deficit hyperactivity disorder (ADHD), obsessive compulsive disorder (OCD) or Tourette's

1 The Anterior Cingulate Cortex. The Evolution of an Interface between Emotion and Cognition, John M. Allman,[a] Atiya Hakeem,[a] Joseph M. Erwin,[b] Esther Nimchinsky[c] and Patrick Hof[d]

syndrome was found in isolation. Everything the human brain does requires very precise natural timing/ordering and this unconscious capability is critical to our brain's ability to plan and sequence thoughts and actions and connect them to their consequences. Thus, the sequencing generated in the brainstem and thalamus of the brain is an important foundation of our ability to attend, learn and process information, and physically execute actions.

Taken individually, the right side of the brain deals with one's position in space. It is this side of the brain that shows developmental delay in 98% of children with problems, possibly due to the relatively minor accidental traumas experienced by the immature brain.

Recent research would suggest that more than 30% of children diagnosed as suffering from dyslexia may, in fact, have convergence insufficiency, possibly due to the closure of the left superior orbital fissure, and the effect of compression of the oculomotor nerve on the medial rectus muscle.

Tourette's syndrome, OCD, ADD, ADHD, phobias, anxiety and autism may be symptoms of a right prefrontal cortex that is struggling to develop correctly. Interestingly, the bulk of the second wave of brain cells developing some four months after birth end up in the right prefrontal cortex and in those areas of brain that have been implicated in developmental delay. This is possibly due to fascial torque of the falx cerebri which lies superior to the anterior cingulate gyrus, and separates the gyri through the midline.

ADHD is now considered to be due to sub-optimal function in the anterior cingulate gyrus. In 98% of boys it is the right cerebral hemisphere that is at fault. It is of interest to note that the anterior cingulate gyrus is one of the sites in the human brain where von Economo neurons (VENs) are found and where a great many of these neurons (one of the second wave brain cells) migrate. The symptoms associated with ADD, ADHD, and Tourette's all seem to originate in this area.

Developmental delay, as the name would imply, is a slowing or delay in the maturation of the brain in general but more specifically in the development, migration and synaptogenesis of the second wave of brain cells that includes the VENs.

DIASCHISIS

Diaschisis is defined as a sudden inhibition of function. This is produced by an acute focal disturbance in a portion of the brain at a distance from the original site of injury, but anatomically connected with it through fibre tracts.

Diaschisis can come in many forms and from many focal points of trauma, and although leading to many physiological changes these are ultimately provoked by the focal lesion. In the following examples, trauma to the cerebellum (focal lesion) may lead to physiological changes at the prefrontal lobe. This is where cognitive and emotional changes are identified and could be caused by changes in neural fibre communications, possibly at a time when the frontal lobe is immature and the spindle cell configuration is not established. Conversely, the focal lesion could occur at the prefrontal lobe or the anterior cingulate gyrus with ramifications at the cerebellum, initiating changes in fine motor skills and motor function.

Cranio fascial distortion may also be similarly viewed; in many areas the focal lesion could be caused by changes in the RTM – the falx cerebri, tentorium cerebellum, falx cerebellum and the diaphragma sellae. These RTM, as previously discussed, have roots in all the midline cranial organs, with the central organ – the ventricular system – and all the adjacent supportive organs. Changes in the reciprocal torsion of these strong dural attachments will bring changes to the organs, the neural fibre structures and their communications, and their neuro-vascular drainage processes. All these components are similar in presentation to a Diaschisis Torque.

While the benign asymmetry of the cranium is already established by haemodynamic forces in utero, the pre-cursory fascial torque has ramifications in all directions – anterior, posterior and laterally. Even when additional forces in the guise of minor traumas are applied, the incidence of diaschisis occurs in all aspects. When the traumatic forces are applied in a counterclockwise direction, they exacerbate the fascial torque on the membranes and intensify subsequent neurological complications. This is a 'smooth coupling' and necessitates correction in a 'de-torque' process with a favourable and resolved outcome.

For instance, the sphenoid bone will present as a left greater wing in a posterior and inferior position, and a smaller retracted eye with poor eye convergence, delivered by a closed superior orbital fissure on that side. Conversely, the right greater wing will appear anterior and superior, with a larger and more prominent eye, with good convergence of the right eye, as a result of an opening of the superior orbital fissure. Since the haemodynamic process of counterclockwise development occurs 'in utero', the prime benign template is already established prior to external trauma. The clinician will therefore find most patients to be counterclockwise in presentation.

However, when the traumatic forces are applied in a clockwise direction, the outcome due to the fascial torque on the membranes cause intensified neurological complications that are varied and multiple. This is a non-smooth coupling, presenting a complicated and difficult outcome, and needs to be corrected carefully and in a prescribed order, determined by the indicators as they present.

Remember, these traumatic changes occur through physical dynamics and thus have to be reinstated by similarly physical dynamics. They are primary causes and have to be addressed using the counter-dynamics.

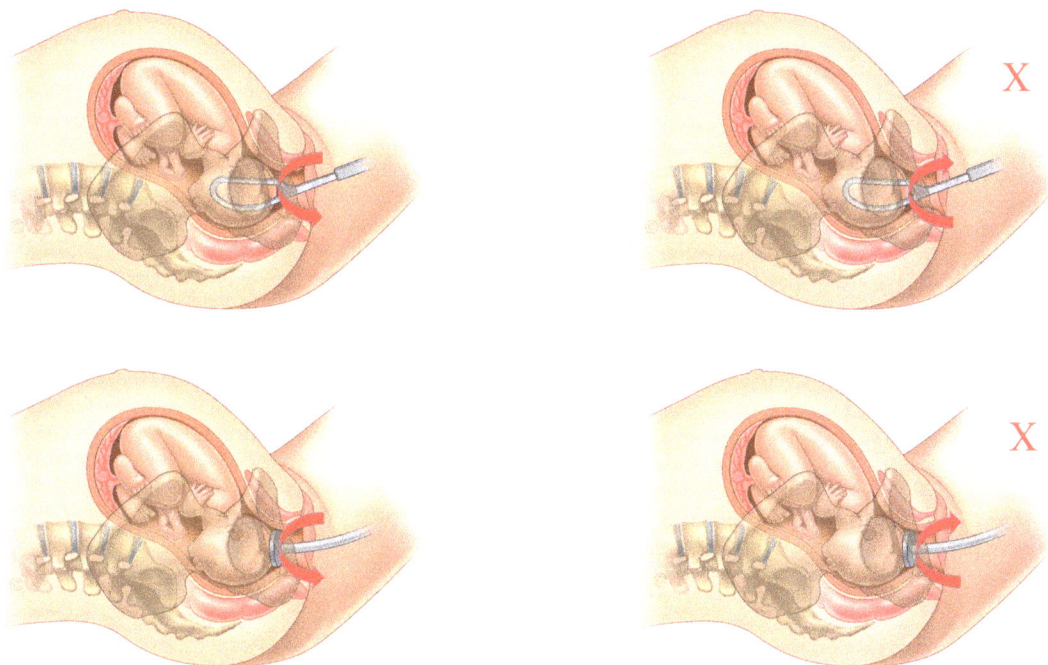

Figure 1.7 Directional Torque: Counterclockwise produces diaschisis at the brainstem, clockwise produces necrosis at the brainstem and should be discouraged – (top row) forceps, also causes contusion at the lateral and anterior fontanelles; (bottom row) ventouse, also produces contusion at the superior sagittal sinus

NECROSIS AND APOPTOSIS

Necrosis is cell death triggered by factors including infection and trauma.

Apoptosis is defined as a form of cell death, generated by normal changes and misalignment in a healthy body.

In the context of these two types of cell death, one should consider the severe changes that occurring when the brainstem becomes severely torqued (eg. the corkscrew or strangulation process possibly induced by ventouse or forceps delivery).

The forces applied to the cranium in a clockwise torque to extract an infant stuck in the birth canal is an example of conflicting dynamics. The resultant forces can simulate a severe strangulation process, where extraction of the infant is successful, but the damage to neural fibres, spinothalamic and corticospinal pathways can be devastating. In the context of diaschisis, this has to be one of the most severe forms of neural damage to cells, resulting in apoptosis and damage repair, but could also involve necrotic outcomes through loss of oxygen and vascular supply. This is necrotic torque.

Therefore, from a dynamic standpoint, extraction from the birth canal by forceps or ventouse, should be applied in a counterclockwise direction, thereby mirroring the counterclockwise direction of the existing membrane This will increase/reinforce the already established torque further stretching the neural membranes and fibres and following the natural fascial torsion.

In contrast, the extraction using clockwise force promotes tearing and disruption resulting in a potential necrotic state with severe neurological complications impending. This type of damage to the brainstem, with resultant influence on the cerebellum and pons, and the circle of Willis could be the underlying aetiology of conditions that will take years to establish, such as Alzheimer's disease, dementia, multiple sclerosis, Parkinson's disease and stroke.

CHAPTER 2

TENTORIAL INCISURA

Probably one of the most important and influential membranes of the cranium is the tentorial incisura. The tentorium cerebellum is the crescent-shaped sceptre of the meningeal dura that horizontally separates the occipital lobes superiorly and the cerebellum inferiorly. Its interior concave border is free and between it and the dorsum sellae of the sphenoid there is a large oval opening called the tentorial incisura which is occupied by the midbrain and the anterior part of the superior vermis of the cerebellum. At the petrosphenoid articulation and beneath the cavernous sinuses is a recess that is created by an anterio-lateral evagination of the lower section of the tentorial membrane called the trigeminal cave. It forms a dural pocket that enfolds with the roots and sensory ganglion of the trigeminal nerve.

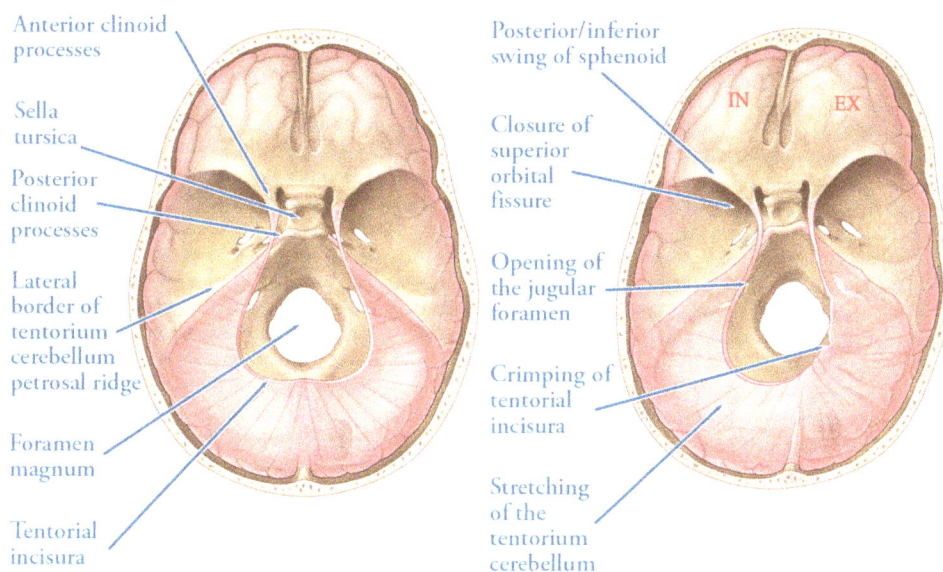

Figure 2.1 (left) Effects of the Tentorial Incisura; (right) Torsion of the Tentorial Incisura

The vertical torsion displayed by the falx cerebelli affects the cerebellar hemispheres, and cerebellar dysfunction is characterised by awkwardness in intentional movements:

- Ataxia – awkwardness in gait and posture
- Asthenia – muscles tire more easily
- Tremors – emphasised jerky movement
- Nystagmus – oscillating movement of the eye, tremors
- Basal ganglion disorders – are Parkinson's chorea (rigid tremor)
- Athetosis – a succession of slow writhing movements
- Hemiballismus – jumping about on one side of the body.

Changes at the pons and the brainstem are brought about by restriction of the dural membrane at the foramen magnum and the endosteal dural membranes and, of course, CSF changes at the cisterna basalis, magnus and pontis that provide the brainstem with a waterbed. Changes in the status of the tentorial incisura will cause irregular balance to these cisterna as well as the pons and brainstem.

CRANIAL FLOOR VENOUS SINUSES

The anterior inferior drainage of the brain occurs at the cavernous and intercavernous sinuses that drain through the basilar plexus and the superior and inferior petrosal sinuses into that transverse sinus and the sigmoid sinus, respectively.

The anterior superior drainage of the brain occurs via the superior and inferior sagittal sinuses that drain into the confluence of the sinuses and then through the transverse sinus, the sigmoid sinus and into the internal jugular vein. Around the foramen magnum the vertebral venous sinuses collect blood from the basilar plexus, the occipital vein and the sub-occipital cavernous sinus.

With cranio fascial distortion the left external temporal gives a far greater drainage potential than the right internal temporal, so the left transverse sinus and the sigmoid sinus leading into the internal jugular vein carry a greater volume of ischaemic blood than their counterpart on the right. This potential is created by the open jugular foramen on the left following the external temporal and occipital bones, while the jugular foramen on the right is more constricted following the internal temporal and internal occiput. The depression of the greater wing of the sphenoid also allows more drainage potential than the elevated greater wing on the right, which affects the left cavernous sinus, removing more ischaemic blood from that area than on the right side.

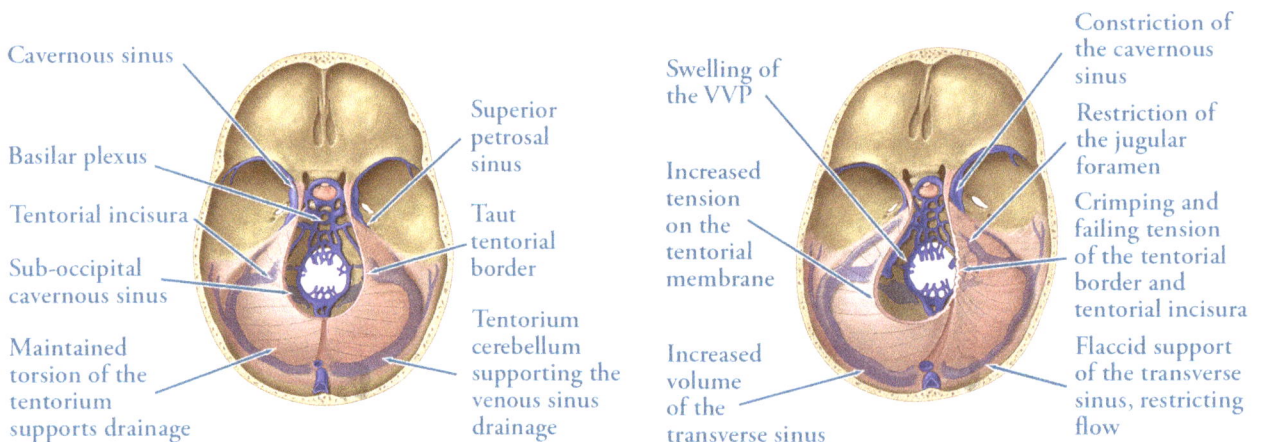

Figure 2.2 (left) Venous Sinus Drainage: Supported by the tentorium cerebellum; (right) Torsion of the Tentorial Incisura: Drainage reduction

TENTORIAL VENOUS DRAINAGE

The tentorium cerebellum encapsulates both the transverse and sigmoid sinuses along the internal occipital boundaries and the petrous portion of the temporal bone, which is where the tentorium is anchored. As the cranio fascial distortion comes into effect, the left temporal and occipital bones move into external rotation and the bilateral taut tentorium is now subjected to a torsional twist giving a far greater surface area on the left, opening the transverse and sigmoid sinuses. This allows for a greater volume of blood than its counterpart on the right that now becomes more flaccid and crimped distorting the transverse and sigmoid sinuses as the right temporal and occipital bones go into internal rotation, thus reducing venous flow.

OPTIC CHIASMA AND OPTIC TRACT

Cranial nerve two, the optic nerve, takes information from both retinae and transfers that information through the optic chiasma to the occipital lobe where the visual centres are maintained. The optic chiasma takes information from each eye, both central and peripheral, medially and laterally, combining one half of each nerve's axons entering the opposite tract, making it a partial decussation at the chiasma. This system allows for parts of both eyes that attend to both visual fields, left and right, to be processed in the brain. The information transfers to right brain and vice versa.

From the retina, the optic nerve fibres traverse the optic chiasma, and move into the lateral geniculate nucleus/body that is a relay centre in the thalamus for the visual pathway. From here it becomes the primary visual cortex in the occipital lobe. The lateral geniculate nucleus lies adjacent to the medial geniculate nucleus (the acoustic nerve nucleus is part of the auditory thalamus and represents the thalamic relay between the inferior colliculus and the auditory cortex) and both are attached to the pulvinar.

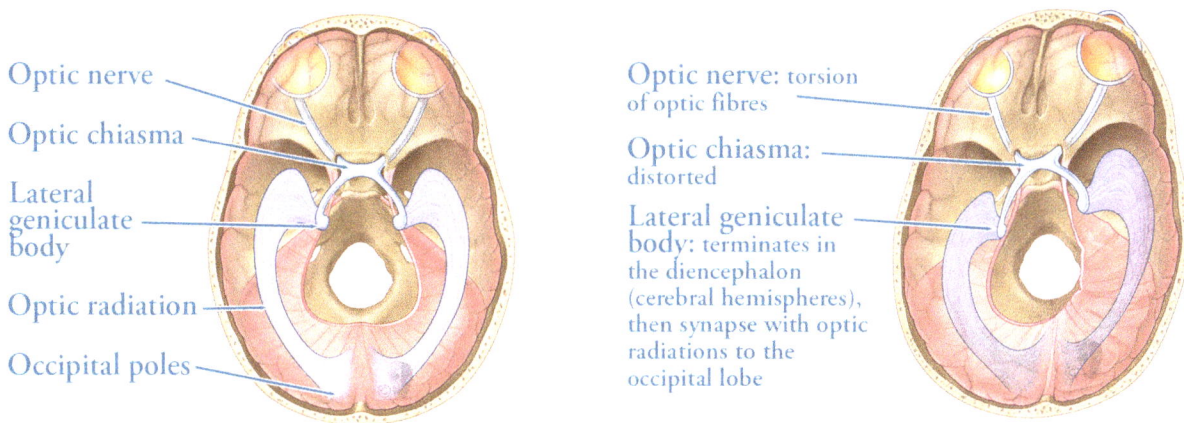

Optic nerve

Optic chiasma

Lateral geniculate body

Optic radiation

Occipital poles

Optic nerve: torsion of optic fibres

Optic chiasma: distorted

Lateral geniculate body: terminates in the diencephalon (cerebral hemispheres), then synapse with optic radiations to the occipital lobe

Figure 2.3 Sight Nerve Pathways: entire system consists of nerve fibres; (right) Torsion of the Tentorial Incisura: Distorts and stretches system of nerve fibres

PITUITARY

The pituitary is a small endocrine gland that is an extension of the hypothalamus at the base of the brain and is found in the sella tursica of the body of the sphenoid bone. The diaphragma sellae is a horizontal layer of dura that is an extension of the tentorium cerebellum and secures the hypophyseal stalk of the pituitary in the sella tursica, between the anterior and posterior clinoid processes of the sphenoid bone. The pituitary is made up of two lobes – the anterior and the posterior lobe. When cranio fascial distortion occurs, the tentorial incisura and diaphragma sellae become distorted twisting the hypophyseal stalk – the infundibulum – reducing the blood flow and affecting the parvocellular neuro-secretory system.

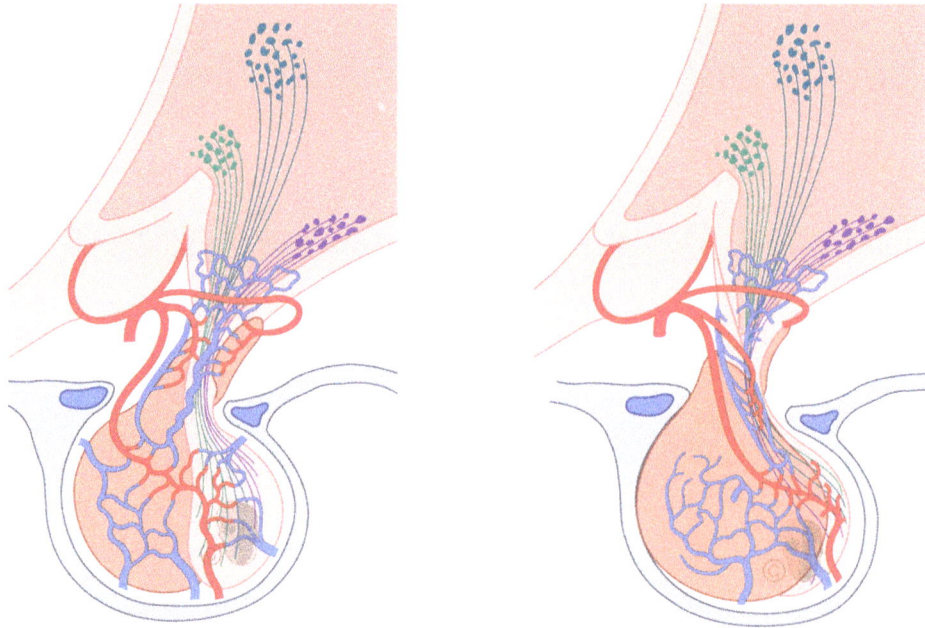

Figure 2.4 Pituitary: (left) Textbook symmetry; (right) Strangling of the hypophyseal stalk

CORPUS CALLOSUM

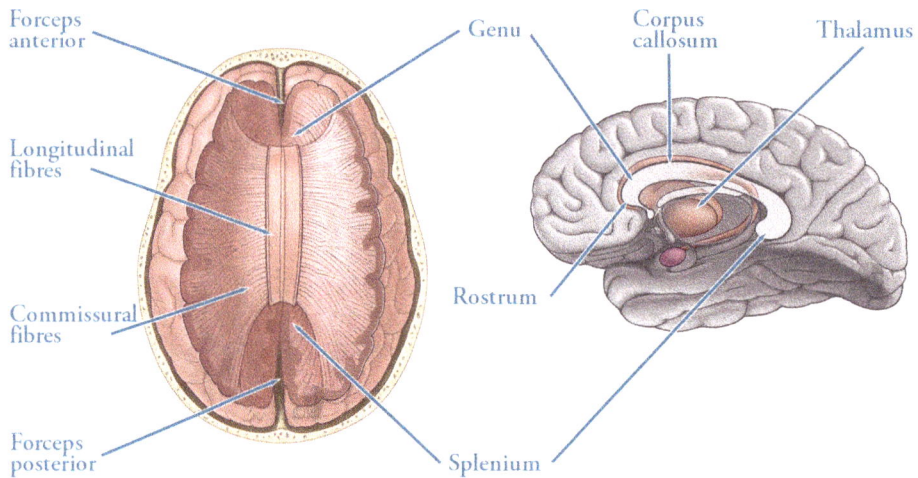

Figure 2.5 Corpus Callosum: Related to coordination and complex problem solving

The corpus callosum is a wide flat bundle of neural fibres beneath the cortex. It connects left and right cerebral hemispheres and facilitates interhemispheric communication. It is the largest white matter structure in the brain. The posterior part of the corpus callosum is called the splenium, the anterior part is called the genu, and the part in between is called the body. The part between the body and the splenium is the lamina terminalis, which represents the cephalic end of the early neural tube and extends from the roof plate of the diencephalon to the optic chiasma. There are three different types of fibre:

Commissural fibres

These fibres pass from one hemisphere to the other. The largest group of these fibres integrates and facilitates the information being passed from one cerebral hemisphere to the other and provides the most important integrative pathways to the brain.

Association fibres

These fibres connect areas of the cerebral cortex within the same hemisphere. They are white matter fibres that run from between the front and the back of the brain.

Projection fibres

These fibres connect the cerebrum and other parts of the brain and/or spinal cord. They are white fibres deep within the subconscious core that project up into the conscious cortical areas – where our subconscious emotions enter our consciousness.

This fibrous network is jeopardised by tentorial incisura torsion.

HYPOTHALAMUS

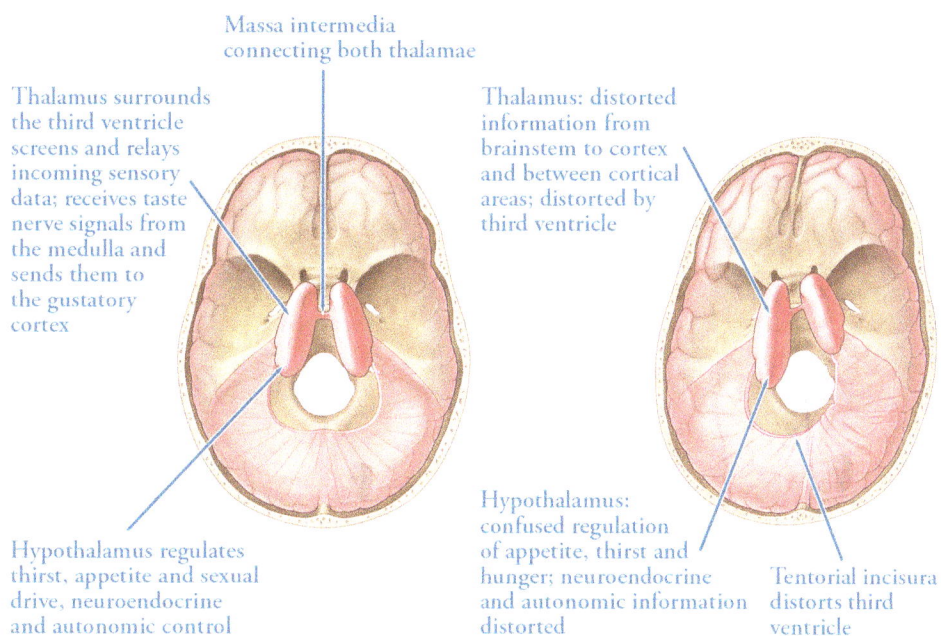

Massa intermedia connecting both thalamae

Thalamus surrounds the third ventricle screens and relays incoming sensory data; receives taste nerve signals from the medulla and sends them to the gustatory cortex

Thalamus: distorted information from brainstem to cortex and between cortical areas; distorted by third ventricle

Hypothalamus regulates thirst, appetite and sexual drive, neuroendocrine and autonomic control

Hypothalamus: confused regulation of appetite, thirst and hunger; neuroendocrine and autonomic information distorted

Tentorial incisura distorts third ventricle

Figure 2.6 Thalamus and Hypothalamus; (right) Torsion of the Tentorial Incisura

The hypothalamus is the section of the brain responsible for the production of many of the body's essential hormones and chemical substances that help control different cells and organs. Physiological functions such as temperature regulation, thirst, hunger, sleep, sex drive, mood, blood pressure, respiration, intestinal peristalsis and the release of other hormones within the body are controlled by the hormones from the hypothalamus. It has master control of body metabolism because it is in charge not only of the autonomic nervous system, but also of the nearby pituitary gland.

The hypothalamus has central control over visceral autonomic functions, regulating thirst, appetite and sexual drive through neuroendocrine and autonomic control. The thalamus screens and relays incoming sensory data, receiving taste nerve signals from the medulla and sends them to the gustatory cortex. The hypothalamus and the thalamus are adjacent organs to the third ventricle, and tentorial incisura distortion will torsion the ventricular system, compromising the connecting fibre conduction of neural information.

Torsion of the thalamus by the tentorial incisura disrupts information from the brainstem to the cerebral cortical areas, so while the hypothalamus propagates confused regulation controls of appetite, thirst and hunger, the neuroendocrine system and the autonomics produce distorted information.

THE LIMBIC SYSTEM

The limbic system is the centre of our subconscious emotional processing and comprises the cingulate gyrus, lying just above the corpus callosum, the orbitofrontal and subcallosal gyri of the basal frontal lobes as well as the dentate and hippocampal gyri, and the parahippocampal, entorhinal and perirhinal cortices of the medial temporal lobes. The falx cerebri comes off the straight sinus, houses the superior and inferior sagittal sinuses, and attaches to the crista galli of the ethmoid bone anteriorly, and divides the cingulate gyrus, the supracallosal gyrus and the corpus callosum. When the tentorial incisura torsions, it pulls the falx cerebri with it distorting the midline organs and systems.

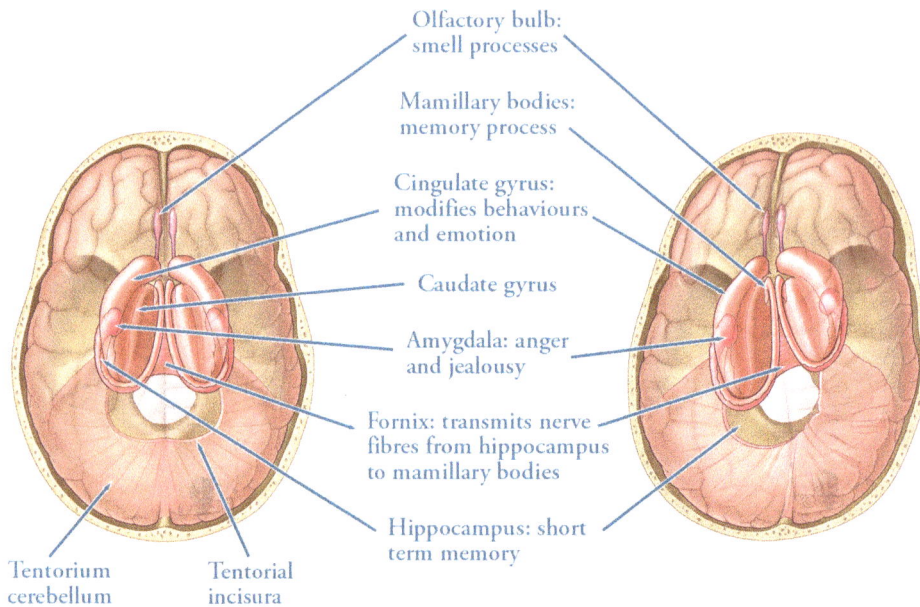

Olfactory bulb: smell processes

Mamillary bodies: memory process

Cingulate gyrus: modifies behaviours and emotion

Caudate gyrus

Amygdala: anger and jealousy

Fornix: transmits nerve fibres from hippocampus to mamillary bodies

Hippocampus: short term memory

Tentorium cerebellum

Tentorial incisura

Figure 2.7 Limbic System; (right) Torsion of the Tentorial Incisura: Effects on all of the limbic system

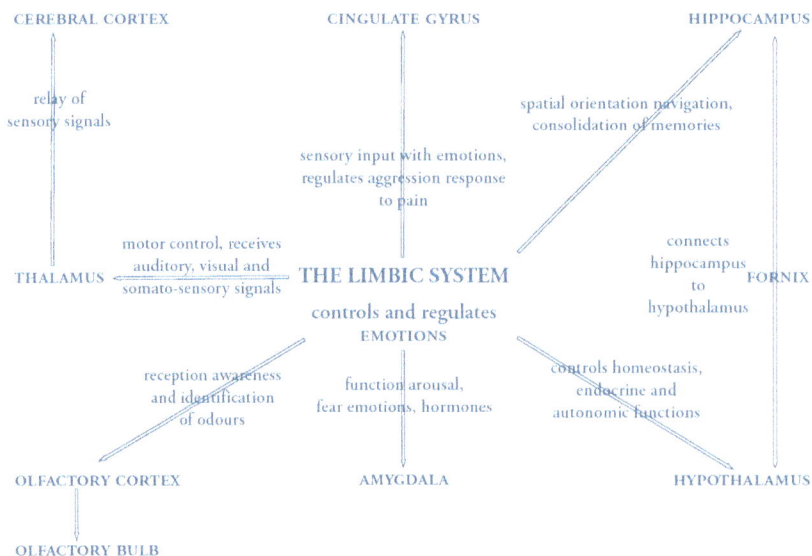

CEREBRAL CORTEX

relay of sensory signals

CINGULATE GYRUS

sensory input with emotions, regulates aggression response to pain

HIPPOCAMPUS

spatial orientation navigation, consolidation of memories

THALAMUS

motor control, receives auditory, visual and somato-sensory signals

THE LIMBIC SYSTEM

controls and regulates EMOTIONS

connects hippocampus to hypothalamus

FORNIX

reception awareness and identification of odours

function arousal, fear emotions, hormones

controls homeostasis, endocrine and autonomic functions

OLFACTORY CORTEX

AMYGDALA

HYPOTHALAMUS

OLFACTORY BULB

Figure 2.8 Limbic System

352

MIDBRAIN-PONS-MEDULLA

The tentorial incisura has almost a direct linkage to this part of the brain, housing the spinal cord at the brainstem, immediately inferior to the pons, the peduncles and the colliculi. This level of the brain also provides the nuclei for the trigeminal and vagus nerves, the two fundamental controlling mixed nerve complexes of the body, as well as the oculomotor nerve controlling ocular convergence.

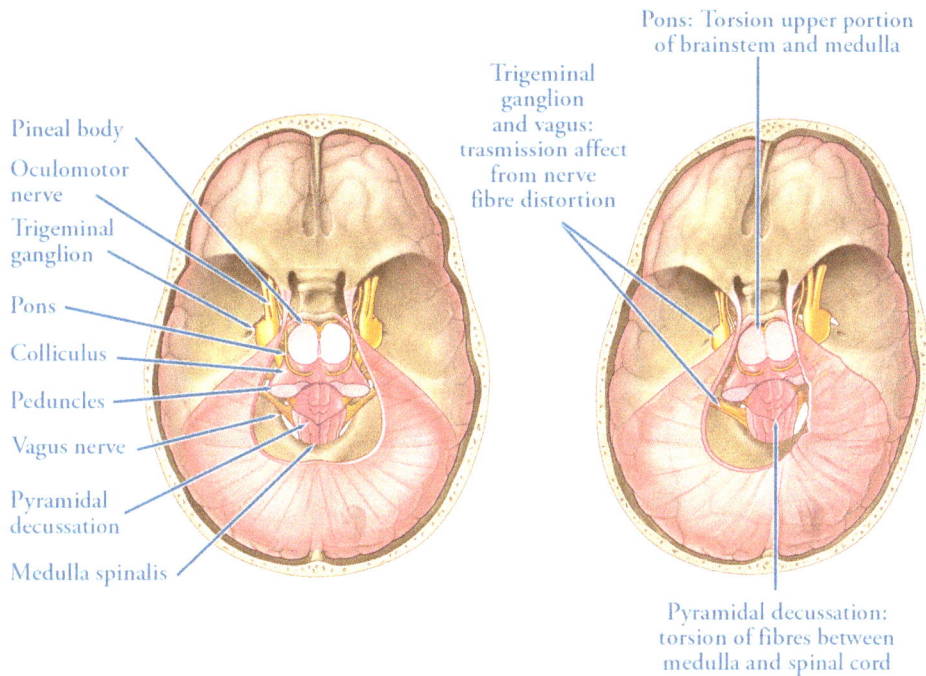

Figure 2.9 Cranial Nerves and Midbrain; (right) Torsion of the Tentorial Incisura: misplaces brainstem, pons and medulla

BRAIN COMPONENTS

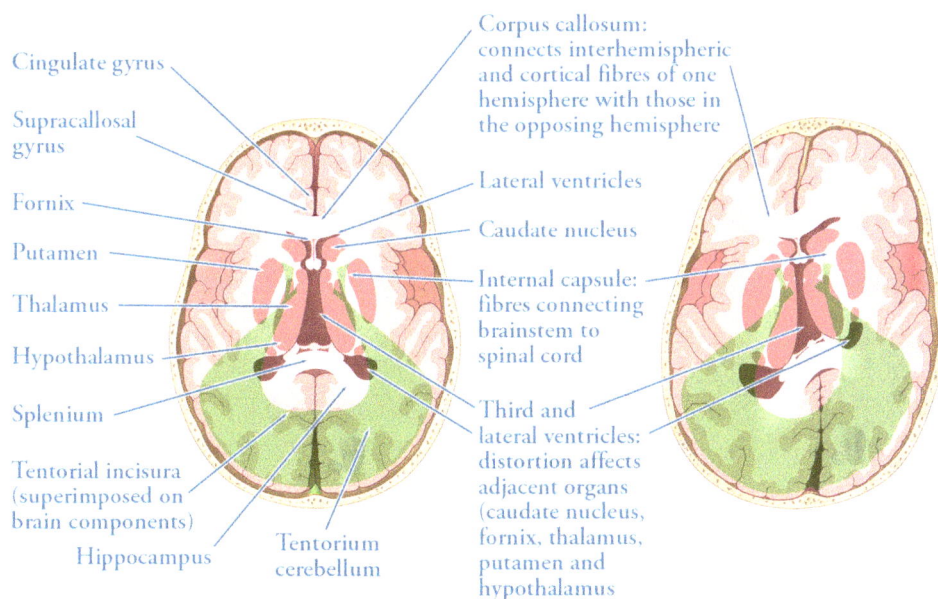

Figure 2.10 Superior View of Brain Components; (right) Torsion of the Tentorial Incisura: distorts projection, association and radiation fibres

CONCLUSION

The strategic positioning of the tentorial incisura shows the massive influence it has on the central brain organs surrounding the ventricular system which, as the origin of CSF embryologically, has been placed at the centre of the midbrain.

Cranio fascial changes to the dynamics of the tentorial incisura position serve as a constant torque on all the central organs that come under its influence from birth.

CTE exacerbates that torque and changes the fundamental bio-chemistry of the nerve cell, perivascular spaces, astrocytes and the deep sulci sites of the cerebral cortex.

This chapter demonstrates the devastating effects occuring when the tentorial incisura becomes torqued. The complications to nerve fibres, communicating neurological pathways and brain systems cannot be underestimated and may in fact, form the basis for many neurodegenerative conditions that appear later in life.

CHAPTER 3

FUNCTIONAL AREAS OF THE CEREBRAL CORTEX

FUNCTIONAL AREAS OF THE CEREBRAL CORTEX

The primary somatosensory cortex and the primary motor cortex are separated by the central sulcus or Rolandic sulcus, which divides the frontal and parietal lobes. The face, hands, arms and trunk are on the lateral convexities, while the legs and feet are in the interhemispheric fissure.

Cortical association fibres convey information to Wernicke's area in the dominant (usually left) hemisphere via the medial geniculate body in the thalamus. Lesions in Wernicke's area cause deficits in language comprehension (receptive or sensory aphasia), or Wernicke's aphasia as a result of acoustic interpretation.

Broca's area is located in the left frontal lobe adjacent to the areas of the primary motor cortex involving the lips, tongue, face and larynx. Lesions in Broca's areas cause deficits in speech production.

The optic chiasma relays nerve fibres through the lateral geniculate body of the thalamus, then radiation fibres transmit into the primary visual cortex. These fibres involved in the motor transmission can be affected by cranio fascial torsion and affect the medial rectus muscle and reduce convergence.

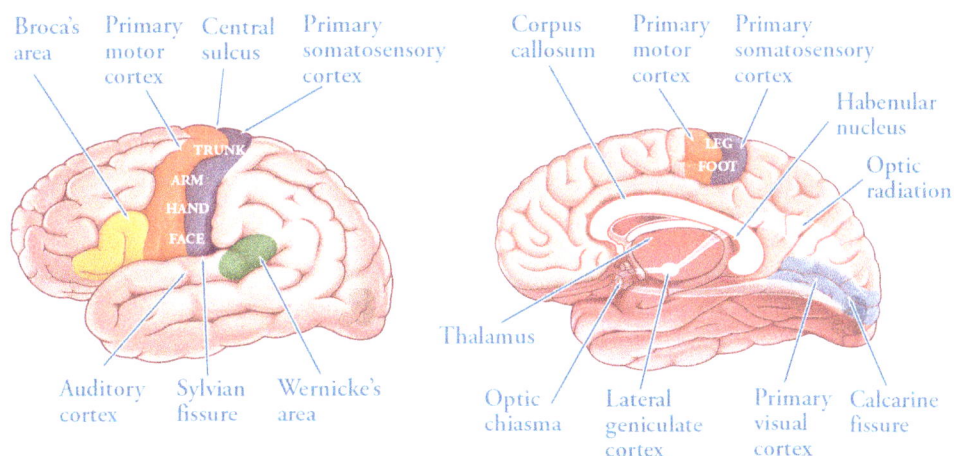

Figure 3.1 Functional Areas of the Cerebral Cortex: (left) Lateral view of the left hemisphere; (right) medial view of the right hemisphere showing the visual components

TRANSVERSE PLANE OF NORMAL MIDBRAIN

This transverse plane of the midbrain shows the intricate positioning and important relationship of the intracranial structures.

White matter is made up of three different types of fibres: commissural, association and projection fibres. The commissural fibres run from the right to the left side and from the left to the right side connecting the two cerebral hemispheres. Below the longitudinal sulcus lies the band of fibres that make up the corpus callosum. These interhemispheric fibres that cross the corpus callosum connect a cortical column of one hemisphere with cortical columns in exactly the same area in the opposite hemisphere.

Each hemisphere has a specialised capability to interpret and process specific types of information. On many occasions information processed in both hemispheres must be integrated to provide a higher level of function in order to achieve maximum results. This might involve logical capabilities and analysis (derived from the left hemisphere) coupled with spatial layout and aesthetic arrangement (derived from the right hemisphere), as required by an engineering or architectural type problem. To achieve this, both hemispheres must coordinate and integrate their activities, a function dependent on the exact precision of nerve conduction and transmission through the fibres crossing the corpus callosum – one of the most important integrative pathways in the brain.

The base of the corpus callosum provides the roof the lateral ventricles. The two lateral ventricles are coupled with the third ventricle by the interventricular foramen of Monro. Separating the anterior horns of the lateral ventricles is the septum pellucidum: a thin, triangular, vertical membrane, which runs as a sheet from the corpus callosum down to the fornix.

The fornix, part of the limbic system, is a C-shaped bundle of afferent fibres taking information from structures in the diencephalon and basal forebrain to the hippocampus, and is closely correlated to recall memory, rather than recognition memory. The C-shape of the fornix mimics the C-shape of the corpus callosum where the two anterior columns of the fornix curve inferiorly, anterior to the interventricular foramen of Monro, posterior to the anterior commissure, through the grey matter in the lateral walls of the third ventricle to join the mammillary bodies at the base of the brain.

The posterior columns of the fornix curve posteriorly together where they are intimately connected to the under surface of the corpus callosum, before diverging from each other to curve around the posterior aspect of the thalamus and pass inferiorly and anteriorly into the temporal horn of the lateral ventricle. From here the columns move along the concavity of the hippocampus, the fimbria of the hippocampus and into the parahippocampal gyrus. These fibres of the pre-commissural fornix arch down in front of the interventricular foramen of Monro, in the lateral wall of the third ventricle where it ends in the mammillary bodies.

The third C-shaped organ that mimics the corpus callosum and the fornix is the basal ganglia. The basal ganglia are a collection of grey matter nuclei located deep within the white matter of the cerebral hemispheres. The main component of the basal ganglia is the caudate nucleus – a paired organ – which underpins the lateral and inferior walls of the lateral ventricles. The head, body and tail of the caudate terminates in the amygdala, which lies just anterior to the tip of the caudate tail in the temporal lobe. These parts of the basal ganglia follow the under surface of the lateral ventricles on both sides of the midline, lying above the lentiform nucleus – consisting of the putamen and the globus pallidus. The caudate nucleus and the lentiform nucleus are separated by projection fibres of the internal capsule. The thalamus lies underneath the caudate body and acts as the lateral wall of the lateral ventricles.

TRANSVERSE PLANE OF TORQUED MIDBRAIN

Cranial torque ultimately changes the midline position of all the cranial organs, but more specifically changes the ability of the brain to drain venous blood through the transverse and sigmoid sinuses and the internal jugular vein. This back up of venous blood means the ventricular system becomes engorged and changes the two lateral, third and fourth ventricular boundaries which then impinge on the organs that lie in close contact. Here we look at changes to the commissural fibres of the corpus callosum and their inability to process information accurately from either side of the cerebral hemispheres. Similarly affected are the fornix and its commissural fibres, the caudate nucleus and the combined nuclei, the septum pellucidum, the thalamus and its ability to act as the junction box between the cortex and the medulla and pons, as well as all cortico-spinal and spinal thalamic tracts. Association, projection and commissural fibres will all be corrupted by these changes.

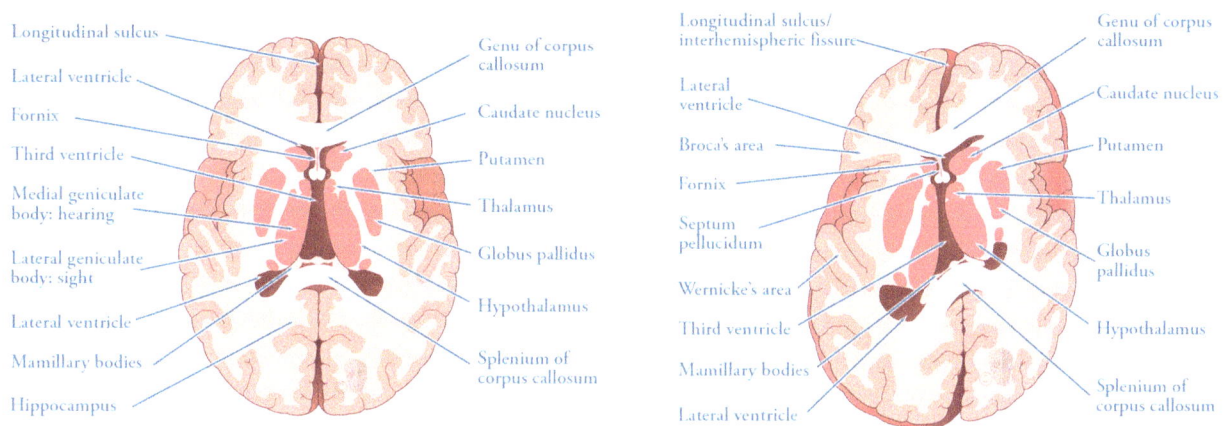

Figure 3.2 Transverse View of Midbrain: (right) normal; (left) torqued

CORONAL VIEW OF THE TEXTBOOK NORMAL DIENCEPHALON

The midline organs shown in this view include the cingulated cortex, the corpus callosum, the fornix body, the two lateral ventricles, the third ventricle and the fourth ventricle.

Separating the anterior horns of the lateral ventricles is the septum pellucidum; a thin, triangular, vertical membrane, which runs as a sheet from the corpus callosum down to the fornix.

Underpinning the lateral ventricles are the caudate nucleus, separated from the lentiform nucleus (the putamen and the globus pallidus) by the projection fibres of the internal capsule, terminating in the anterior commissure under which lie the hippocampus and the pineal bodies. The thalamus and the hypothalamus lie against the lateral walls of the third ventricle.

CORONAL VIEW OF TORQUED DIENCEPHALON

The influence of benign asymmetrical cranial torsion changes the midline dramatically. All the cranial organs on both sides of the midline have a commissural fibre connection with their opposite half. The RTM will change the symmetric position of the organs, but more importantly their commissural contact across the midline becomes corrupted and changes efficient neurological transmission. The central cranial components, the midbrain, the pons and the medulla come under the influence of the tentorial incisura (tentorial notch), the junction of the falx cerebri at the straight sinus, where the tentorium forms a 'tent-like' opening, to allow the passage of the central components.

The torque on the tentorial incisura affects the midbrain, pons and the medulla oblongata as it prepares to move through the foramen magnum. This influences the cranial nerve nuclei, the projection fibres that pass from thalamus to spinal cord and vice versa, and the corona radiata fibres that serve the cortico-thalamic tracts.

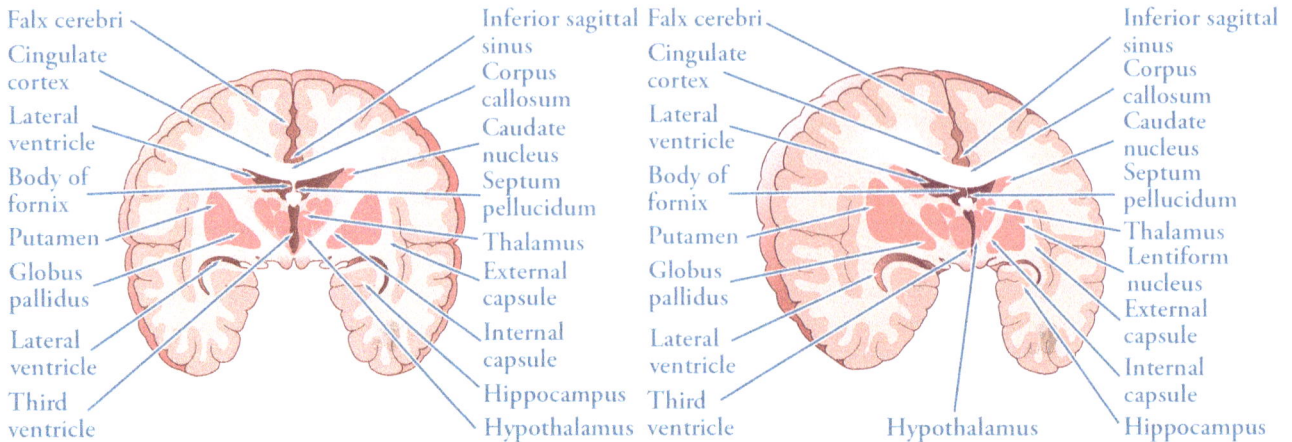

Left diagram labels: Falx cerebri, Cingulate cortex, Lateral ventricle, Body of fornix, Putamen, Globus pallidus, Lateral ventricle, Third ventricle, Inferior sagittal sinus, Corpus callosum, Caudate nucleus, Septum pellucidum, Thalamus, External capsule, Internal capsule, Hippocampus, Hypothalamus

Right diagram labels: Falx cerebri, Cingulate cortex, Lateral ventricle, Body of fornix, Putamen, Globus pallidus, Lateral ventricle, Third ventricle, Hypothalamus, Inferior sagittal sinus, Corpus callosum, Caudate nucleus, Septum pellucidum, Thalamus, Lentiform nucleus, External capsule, Internal capsule, Hippocampus

Figure 3.3 Coronal View of the Diencephalon: (left) normal; (right) torque, central core distorted

ANATOMY OF THE CRANIAL FORAMINA

The dura mater that surrounds the brain is frequently described as consisting of two layers – an external or endosteal layer, and an internal or meningeal layer. Because these two layers are indistinguishable, except in a few cases, it is more practicable to describe the dura as one layer – the endocranium.

The dura is particularly adherent at the base – the foramen magnum and the upper three cervical vertebrae, the sutures and the foramina, where it becomes continuous with the pericranium.

The four RTM – the falx cerebri, the falx cerebelli, the tentorium cerebellum and the diaphragma sellae – are continuous swathes of dura that anchor the brain in position and provide a vascular drainage system at the outer border of these membranes.

The falx cerebri is sickle-shaped and occupies the longitudinal fissure between the cerebral hemispheres, and is anchored anteriorly at the crista galli of the ethmoid bone. At its superior and inferior borders it encloses the superior sagittal and inferior sagittal sinuses.

The tentorium cerebellum anchors at the anterior and posterior clinoid processes of the body of the sphenoid bone, separating the cerebral hemispheres from the cerebellum (also separating the two occipital lobes) and encases the superior and inferior petrosal sinuses laterally at the petrous portion of the temporal bones. It also continues to attach at the occiput where it encases the two transverse and sigmoid sinuses before entering the internal jugular veins at the jugular foramen. The tentorial notch (tentorial incisura) contains the midbrain, part of the cerebellum and the subarachnoid space. Changes in cranio fascial support will affect the position of these cranial components.

The falx cerebelli is also sickle-shaped and lies as a continuation of the falx cerebri, separated at the straight sinus, also adherent to the occiput encapsulating the occipital sinus.

The diaphragma sellae is a horizontal piece of dura that covers the sella turcica, surrounds the hypophyseal stalk and encases the pituitary.

The dura of these RTM and the endosteal dura of the cranial openings and apertures are flexible, can become distorted and therefore play a crucial role in all the nerves, arteries, veins and cranial structures that traverse these areas and affect the transmission of fluid and nerve fibres transmitting through them.

When studying the arrow-shaped petrous portion of the temporal bone, as it attaches between the basilar part of the occiput – where it forms the jugular foramen – and the body of the sphenoid, this junction comprises one of the most congested areas of the cranium, involving the dural attachments, the endosteum and the periosteum.

In the neonate cranium, the sutures of the three parts of the temporal bone – the squama (membrane), the tympanic ring and the petrous portion (both cartilage) – begin life as three separate bones encapsulated by dura in the form of periosteum and endosteum.

The occiput consists of four components; the basilar portion (cartilage), the two condylar areas (cartilage) and the occipital squama (cartilage from the foramen magnum to the transverse sinus attachment, and then membrane from the superior part of the transverse sinus attachment to the lambda). These four components start life as individual bones encapsulated by dura in the form of periosteum and endosteum.

The sphenoid bone consists of three components: the body and the lesser wings (cartilage), and the pterygoid plates and greater wings (membrane). These three bones start life as individual components encapsulated by dura in the form of periosteum and endosteum.

As growth and development takes place and the individual components merge into three cranial bones (the temporal, the occiput and the sphenoid) The dura, the periosteum and endosteum merge into a matrix of fascia, both internally and externally of the cranium, and so become influenced by any fascial distortion that is present. When the right temporal bone becomes internally rotated, it narrows the jugular foramen, the internal auditory meatus of the temporal bone and enlarges the superior orbital fissure of the sphenoid, the greater wing of the sphenoid is then elevated and the hypoglossal canal at the occiput becomes narrowed. At the same time the left temporal bone becomes externally rotated, it opens the jugular foramen, the internal auditory meatus of the temporal bone and narrows the superior orbital fissure of the sphenoid. The greater wing of the sphenoid is then depressed and the hypoglossal canal at the occiput becomes open. The basilar part of the occiput fuses with the sphenoid body at the sphenobasilar synchondrosis at the age of twenty-five and becomes a continuous bone.

The tentorial notch (incisura) is pulled towards the left external temporal bone, pulling with it the midbrain (part of the cerebellum and the subarachnoid space) away from the midline thus distorting the radiation fibres of the spinal thalamic tract and the midbrain nuclei.

SAGITTAL VIEW OF THE BRAIN – PROJECTION FIBRES

Projection Fibres and Radiation Fibres

These fibres connect the cerebral cortex with the lower part of the brain or brainstem and the spinal cord, in both directions.

The corticopetal (afferent) fibres include:

• Geniculocalcarine radiation from the lateral geniculate body to the calcarine cortex
• Auditory radiation from the medial geniculate body to the auditory cortex
• Thalamic radiations from the thalamic nuclei to specific cerebrocortical areas.

The corticofugal (efferent) fibres proceed from the cerebral cortex to the thalamus, brainstem or spinal cord.

Internal Capsule

Most of the nerve fibres interconnecting the cerebral cortex with centres in the brainstem, the spinal cord and the thalamus, pass through the interval between the thalamus and caudate nucleus medially and lentiform nucleus laterally. This region at the upper end of the brainstem, forms a compact band and is called the internal capsule. Above, the internal capsule is continuous with corona radiata and below, with the crus cerebri of midbrain.

As seen on the horizontal section, the internal capsule consists of:

• Anterior limb, which lies between the caudate nucleus medially and the anterior part of the lentiform nucleus laterally

• Posterior limb, which lies between the thalamus medially and the posterior part of the lentiform nucleus laterally

• Genu, where both limbs meet.

In addition, some fibres of the internal capsule lie behind the posterior end of the lentiform nucleus constituting its retrolentiform part whereas other fibres, which pass below the lentiform nucleus (not medial to it), constitute the sublentiform part.

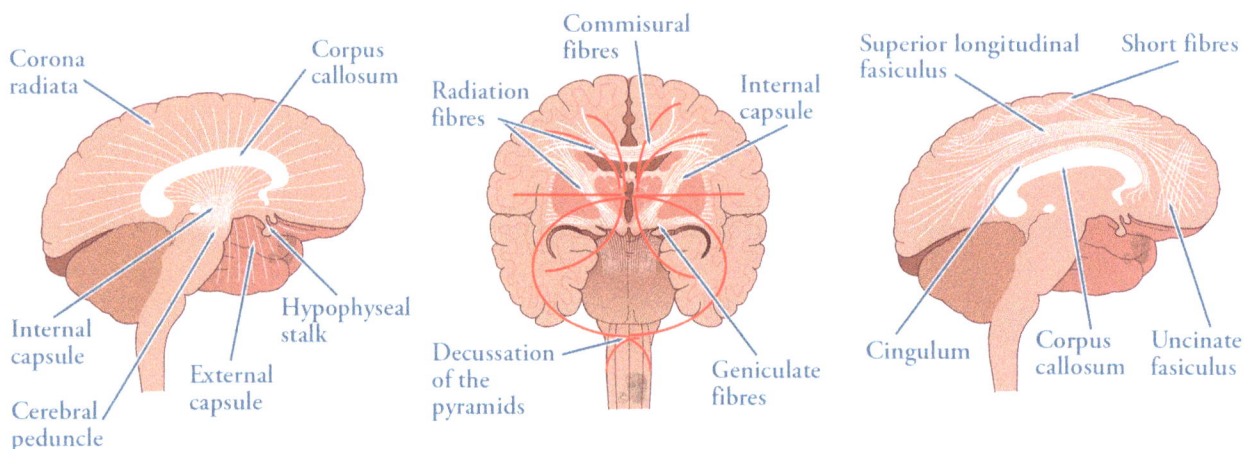

Figure 3.4 (left) Sagittal View of the Brain: Projection fibres; (centre) Radiation Fibre Formation: Reticular formation fibres transmit from thalamus to cortex; (right) Sagittal View of the Brain: Association fibres

SAGITTAL VIEW OF THE BRAIN – ASSOCIATION FIBRES

Association Fibres

These fibres connect the various cortical regions of a cerebral hemisphere; they permit the cortex to function as a coordinated whole.

Short association fibres

Short association fibres, or U fibres, connect adjacent gyri.

Types:

• Intracortical fibres – located in the deeper portions of the white matter
• Subcortical fibres – located just beneath the cortex.

Long association fibres

Long association fibres connect more widely separated areas.

Types:

- Uncinate fasciculus connects the inferior frontal lobe gyri with the anterior temporal lobe
- Cingulum, a white band within the cingulate gyrus, connects the frontal and parietal lobe with the parahippocampal gyrus
- Arcuate fasciculus sweeps around the insula and connects the superior and middle frontal convolutions (containing the speech motor area) with the temporal lobe (containing the speech comprehension area)
- Superior longitudinal fasciculus connects portions of the frontal lobe with occipital and temporal areas
- Inferior longitudinal fasciculus connects the temporal and occipital lobes
- Occipitofrontal fasciculus extends backwards from the frontal lobe, radiating into the temporal and occipital lobes.

Coronal View of Diencephalon – Commissural Fibres

The commissural fibres interconnect the corresponding regions of the two cerebral hemispheres. They are as follows:

- Corpus callosum
- Anterior commissure
- Posterior commissure
- Fornix
- Habenular commissure.

Corpus callosum

The corpus callosum comprises the largest bundle of fibres; most of these arise from parts of the neocortex of one cerebral hemisphere and terminate in the corresponding parts of the opposite cerebral hemisphere. It lies at the bottom of the longitudinal fissure. It is divided into:

- Rostrum – a thin lamina of nerve fibres that connects the genu to the upper end of the lamina terminalis
- Genu – the curved anterior end
- Body or trunk – which arches posteriorly and ends as the thickened enlargement called the splenium.

Traced laterally, the fibres of the genu curve forward into the frontal lobes and form the forceps minor. The fibres of the body extend laterally as the radiation of the corpus callosum. The fibres from the splenium run backwards into the occipital lobe and form the forceps major.

Anterior commissure

The anterior commissure is situated in the anterior wall of the third ventricle at the upper end of the lamina terminalis. The fibres passing through the commissure interconnect the olfactory bulbs of the two cerebral hemispheres. Other fibres interconnect the parahippocampal gyri and other parts of the temporal lobe.

Posterior commissure

It lies in the inferior lamina of the stalk of the pineal gland immediately above the opening of the cerebral aqueduct into the third ventricle.

Fornix

This is a prominent bundle of fibres seen on the medial aspect of the cerebral hemisphere. It is made up of fibres arising from the hippocampus. The body of the fornix is suspended from the corpus callosum by the septum pellucidum. The nerve fibres arise from the alveus, a thin layer of white matter covering the surface of the hippocampus and then converge to form the fimbria. The fimbriae form the posterior column or crus of the fornix arching below the corpus callosum. The two crura then come together in the midline to form the body of the fornix. The two crura are interconnected by fibres passing from one to the other – hippocampal commissure or commissure of the fornix which actually joins the two hippocampi. The anterior end of the body of fornix also divides into anterior columns or pillars. Each anterior column of the fornix turns downwards just in front of the interventricular foramen and passes through the hypothalamus to reach the mamillary body.

Habenular commissure

This is a small bundle of nerve fibres that cross the midline in the superior stalk of the pineal gland. The commissure is associated with the habenular nucleus. The habenula originally denoted the stalk of the pineal gland (pineal habenula; pedunculus of pineal body), but gradually came to refer to a neighbouring group of nerve cells with which the pineal gland was believed to be associated, the habenular nucleus.

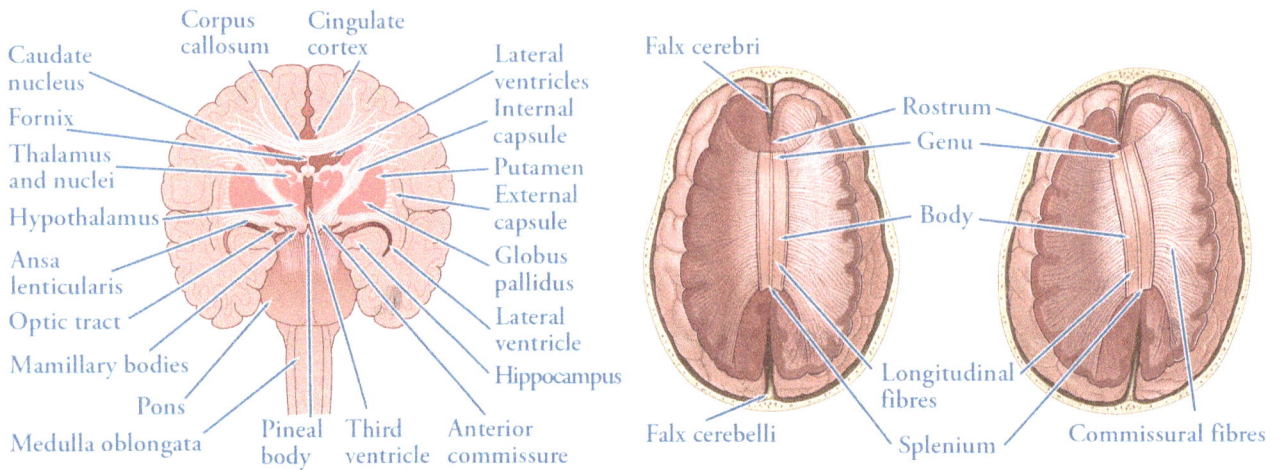

Figure 3.5 (left) Coronal View of the Diencephalon; (right) Corpus Callosum: Torsion of the falx cerebri on right

CONCLUSION

The dura is particularly adherent at the base – the foramen magnum and the upper three cervical vertebrae, the sutures and the foramina where it becomes continuous with the pericranium.

The four RTM – the falx cerebri, the falx cerebelli, the tentorium cerebellum and the diaphragma sellae – are continuous swathes of dura that anchor the brain in position. The tentorial notch (tentorial incisura) contains the midbrain, part of the cerebellum and the subarachnoid space.

In the neonate cranium, the sutures of the three parts of the temporal bone – the squama (membrane), the tympanic ring and the petrous portion (both cartilage) – begin life as three separate bones encapsulated by dura in the form of periosteum and endosteum.

The occiput consists of four components; the basilar portion (cartilage), the two condylar areas (cartilage) and the occipital squama (cartilage from the foramen magnum to the transverse sinus attachment, and then membrane from the superior part of the transverse sinus attachment to the lambda).

The sphenoid bone consists of three components; the body and the lesser wings (cartilage), and the pterygoid plates and greater wings (membrane).

This chapter illustrates the various companion organs adjacent to the central ventricular system and examines how the cranio fascial torsion affects the distortion of the midline organs and the impact of those organs from resultant swelling and disfiguration of the dominant system.

Central to the ventricles are the supportive organs that are primarily responsible for the neurological pathways set up by the central nervous system to connect the cerebral cortex with the spinal cord, through the junction box, the thalamus. Note how the thalamus and the hypothalamus, support the lateral walls of the third ventricle. The fornix and the caudate nucleus (both of which are C-shaped) support the floor of the lateral ventricles, while the limbic system, also C-shaped, along with the hippocampus, are supported by the fornix.

The corpus callosum, also a C-shaped organ, lies over the lateral ventricles and forms the roof of the lateral ventricles. Lying on top of the corpus callosum, is the cingulate gyrus, another C-shaped organ which forms the midline attachment to the inferior sagittal sinus at the base of the falx cerebri.

All these aforementioned organs encapsulate the thalamus and hypothalamus, which consist of many nuclei that are central to cortex/cord communications, as well as between each other. Memory recall, emotions, temperature control, CSF production, pH control and so on are all controlled through these central organs.

Cranial fascial distortion of the tentorial incisura/notch – the horizontal component – and the falx cerebri – the vertical component – changes the juxtaposition of all these organs and the commissural, projection and radiation fibres thereby stretching, compressing and compromising their innate ability to communicate neurologically with one another.

CHAPTER 4

EMBRYOLOGICAL NEUROANATOMY OF THE BRAIN

EMBRYOLOGICAL NEUROANATOMY OF THE BRAIN

The far-reaching effects of cranio fascial dynamics (CFD) are often misunderstood and are overlooked in our understanding of the brain and its many physiological or pathophysiological functions. It is therefore vital to appreciate the fundamental cranial development: how on the 16th day of foetal development the first indentation to occur is the primitive streak (neural groove) primed to grow into the future brain and spinal cord. From here onwards as the embryo becomes a foetus and the brain components evolve, all the neural parts and organs are developed within this first compartment.

The central nervous system appears at the beginning of week 3 as a slipper-shaped plate of thickened ectoderm (the neural plate) and is located in the mid dorsal region in front of the primitive streak. Its lateral edges soon become elevated to form the neural folds. With further development, the neural folds become more elevated, approach each other in the midline, and finally fuse, thus forming the neural tube. This fusion begins in the cervical region and proceeds in a somewhat irregular fashion in the cephalic and caudal directions. The cephalic end shows three dilations, the primary brain vesicles:

a. The prosencephalon or forebrain
b. The mesencephalon or membrane
c. The rhombencephalon or hindbrain.

Simultaneously it forms two flexures; the cervical flexure at the junction of the hindbrain, and the spinal cord and the cephalic flexure, located in the midbrain region.

By week five, the three primary brain vesicles become enlarged to form the five secondary brain vesicles.

a. The prosencephalon consists of two parts:

- Telencephalon or end brain – formed by a mid-portion and two lateral outer pockets – the primitive cerebral hemispheres, and the lateral ventricles
- Diencephalon, characterised by the outgrowth of the optic vesicle, forms the interventricular foraman of Monro

b. The mesencephalon is separated from the rhombencephalon by a deep furrow – the rhombencephalon isthmus – and forms the third ventricle

c. The rhombencephalon consists of two parts:

- Metencephalon – later to become the pons and cerebellum, and the aqueduct of Sylvius
- Myelencephalon– the fourth ventricle.

These two flexures are separated by the pontine flexure.

The lumen of the spinal cord, the central canal, is continuous with that of the brain vesicles.

The cavity of the rhombencephalon becomes the fourth ventricle.

The cavity of the mesencephalon becomes the third ventricle.

The cavity of the cerebral hemispheres becomes the lateral ventricles.

The lumen of the mesencephalon joins the third and fourth ventricles and is known as the aqueduct of Sylvius, while the lateral ventricles communicate with the third ventricle through the interventricular foramen of Monro.

The Spinal cord

During the neural groove stage, and immediately after the closure of the tube a collection layer of neuroepithelial tissue evolves, becoming primitive nerve cells or neuroblasts, and form an inner layer known as the mantle layer which later forms the grey matter of the spinal cord. The outermost layer of the spinal cord becomes known as the marginal layer and as a result of myelination of these nerve fibres becomes the white matter of the spinal cord.

The continuous thickening of the ventral mantle layer produces the basal plates containing the ventral motor horn cells forming the motor areas of the spinal cord, while the dorsal thickening produces the alar plates that form the sensory areas. The dorsal and ventral midline portions of the neural tube are known as the roof and floor plates and serve as a pathway for nerve fibres crossing from one side to the other.

In the third month of development the spinal cord extends the entire length of the embryo and the spinal nerves pass through the intervertebral foramen at their level of origin. In the adult the spinal cord terminates at the level of L2, forming the filum terminale, which anchors the spinal cord at the level of the second sacral body, while the extension of the spinal cord continues in the form of a horse's tail – the cauda equina.

The Brain

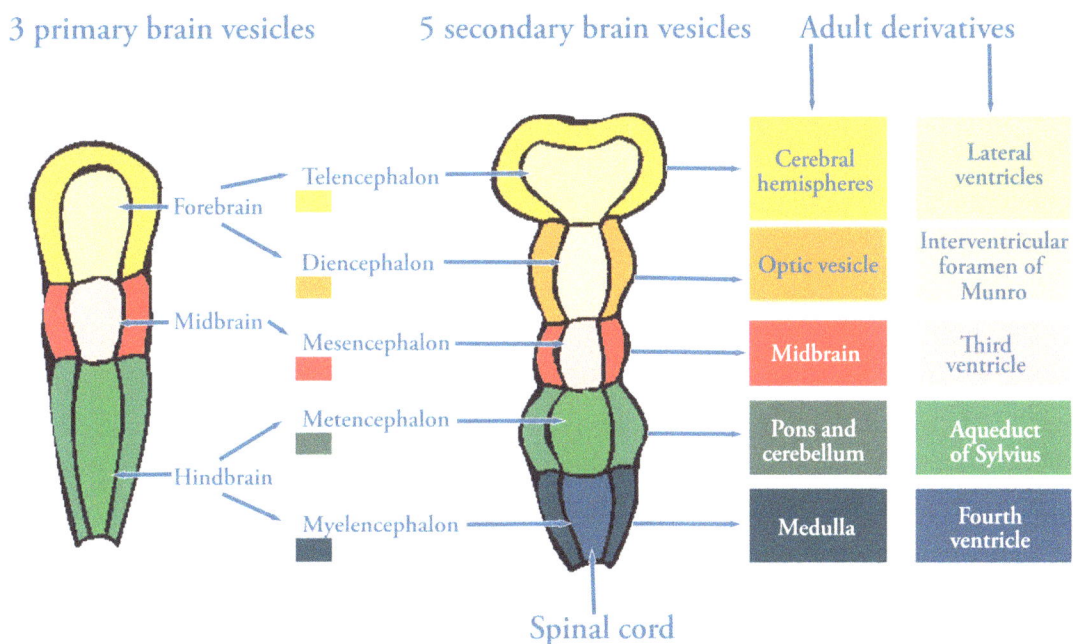

Figure 4.1 Vesicles of the Brain at Five Weeks: The ventricular system becomes the central core support of the brain

Distinct basal and alar plates representing the motor and sensory areas are found respectively on either side of the midline in the brain vesicles, while the sulcus limitans forms the dividing line between motor and sensory areas and is present in the rhombencephalon and the mesencephalon.

The rhombencephalon

The rhombencephalon consists of the myelencephalon, the most caudal of the brain vesicles, and the metencephalon that extends from the pontine flexure to the rhombencephalic isthmus.

The myelencephalon

This brain vessel gives rise to the medulla oblongata. The basal plate similar to that of the spinal cord contains the motor nuclei. These motor nuclei are divided into three groups:

a. A medial somatic efferent group – contains the motor neurons which form the cephalic continuation of the anterior horn cells to become the somatic efferent motor column and represents the neurons of the hypoglossal nerve supplying the musculature of the tongue. In the metencephalon and the mesencephalon the column represents the neurons of the abducens, trochlear and oculomotor nerves supplying eye musculature.
b. An intermediate special visceral efferent group – extends into the metencephalon forming the special visceral efferent motor column and supplies motor neurons into the striated muscles of the branchial arches, while in the myelencephalon the column is presented by the neurons of the accessory, the vagus and glossopharyngeal nerves.
c. A lateral general visceral efferent group – contains the motor neurons which supply the involuntary musculature of the respiratory tract, intestinal tract and the heart.

The alar plate contains three groups of sensory relay nuclei. The most lateral of the ear and the surface of the head by way of the vestibulocochlear and trigeminal nerves. The intermediate or special visceral afferent group receives impulses from the taste buds of the tongue and from the palate, oropharynx and epiglottis. The medial, or general visceral afferent groups, receive interoceptive information from the gastrointestinal tract and the heart.

The roof plate of the myelencephalon consists of a single layer of ependymal cells covered by the vascular mesenchyme – the pia mater. These two combined are known as the tela choroidea, which become invaginated tufts underlying the ventricular cavity to form the choroid plexus that produces CSF for the central nervous system.

The metencephalon

This too is characterised by basal (motor) and alar (sensory) plates, but two new components are formed:

a. The cerebellum which acts as a coordination centre for posture and movement
b. The pons which serves as a nerve pathway between the spinal cord and the cerebral and cerebellar cortices.

Each basal plate of the metencephalon contains three groups of motor neurons:

a. The medial somatic efferent group which gives rise to the nucleus of the abducens nerve
b. A special visceral efferent group containing the nuclei of the trigeminal and facial nerves and which also innervates the musculature of the first and second branchial arches
c. The general visceral efferent group which supplies the submandibular and sublingual glands.

The alar plates of the metencephalon contain three groups of sensory nuclei:

a. A lateral somatic afferent group which contains neurons of the trigeminal nerve and the vestibulocochlear complex
b. A special visceral afferent group
c. The general visceral afferent group.

The mesencephalon

The mesencephalon consists of a basal plate containing two groups of motor nuclei:

a. A medial somatic different group represented by the oculomotor and trochlear nerves, which innervate eye musculature

b. A small general visual efferent group represented by the nucleus of Edinger-Westphal which innervates the sphincter papillary muscle.

The marginal layer of each basal plate forms the crus cerebri that serves as a pathway for the nerve fibres descending from the cerebral cortex to the lower centres of the pons and spinal cord.

The alar plates of the mesencephalon divide into the anterior (superior) colliculus which function as correlation and reflex centres for the visual impulses, and the posterior (inferior) colliculus which serve as a synaptic relay station for the auditory reflexes.

The diencephalon

The roof plate of the diencephalon consists of a single layer of epidermal cells covered by vascular mesenchymal, and gives rise to the choroid plexus of the third ventricle. The most caudal part of the roof plate develops into the pineal body or epiphysis that serves as a channel through which light and darkness effect endocrinal and behavioural rhythms.

The alar plates form the lateral walls of the diencephalon forming a groove; the hypothalamic sulcus that divides the plate into a dorsal and ventral region, giving rise to the thalamus and the hypothalamus. The hypothalamus serves as a regulation centre for visceral functions such as sleep, digestion, body temperature and emotional behaviour. The mammillary body forms a distinct protuberance on the ventral surface of the hypothalamus on each side of the midline and becomes part of the fornix. Special note should be made of the anatomical characteristics that are developed at this embryological stage, namely the lateral walls of the third ventricle lined by the thalamus and the hypothalamus.

The telencephalon

The development of this secondary brain vesicle produces the cerebral hemispheres and several sub-cortical structures, including the hippocampus and the basal ganglia.

The Basal Ganglia

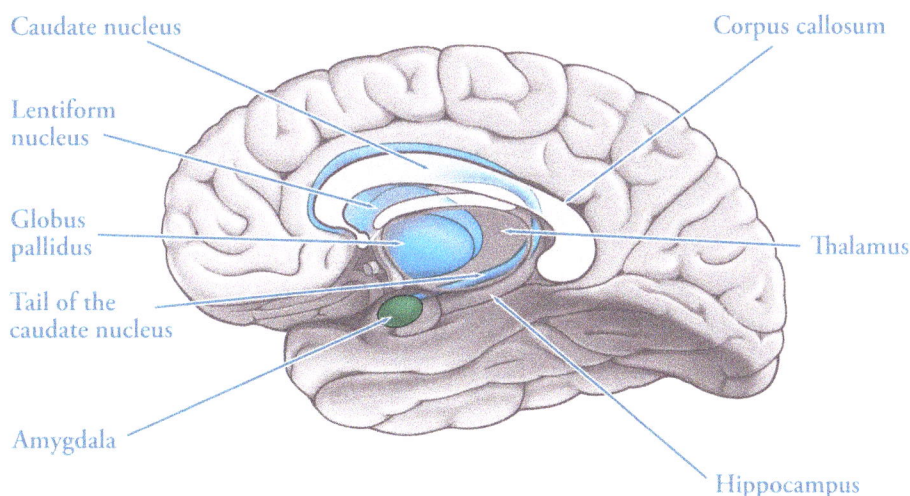

Figure 4.2 Basal Ganglia

Derived from the neural tube in week 3 of embryological development, the basal ganglia nuclei are interconnected with the cerebral cortex, the thalamus and the brainstem and are associated with a variety of functions including control of voluntary motor movements (particularly to control and regulate activities of the motor and premotor cortical areas so that voluntary movements can be performed smoothly), procedural learning, routine behaviours or habits such as bruxism, eye movements, cognition and emotion.

The basal ganglia are a group of paired deep brain nuclei that play a crucial role in the integration and organisation of coordinated motor activity. Along with the cerebellum, the basal ganglia act to turn the desired conscious activity into reality. These are one of the largest groups of brain nuclei consisting of the corpus striatum, which is itself divided into the caudate nucleus, the tailed nucleus and the lentiform nucleus.

The lentiform nucleus is divided into an outer part, the putamen, and an inner part, the globus pallidus. It encloses the more medial thalamus and lies above the subthalamic nucleus and substantia nigra of the midbrain. The dentate nucleus is separated from the lentiform nucleus by a band of white fibres called the internal capsule. The C-shaped caudate nucleus overlays the lentiform nucleus (putamen and globus pallidus) and the thalamus, and is divided into the head, the body and the tail. The tail nucleus terminates in the amygdala (part of the limbic brain nuclei). The caudate nucleus provides the floor of the lateral ventricles. The substantia nigra produces the neurotransmitter dopamine, while the subthalamic nucleus produces the neurotransmitter glutamate.

Embryologically the telencephalon produces the caudate nucleus and the putamen. The subthalamic nuclei are derived from the diencephalon, while the substantia nigra are derived from the mesencephalon.

Abnormal functions of the basal ganglia

The importance of these subcortical nuclei for normal brain function and behaviour is emphasised by the numerous and diverse neurological conditions associated with basal ganglia dysfunction, which include: disorders of behaviour control, such as Tourette's syndrome, hemiballismus, obsessive compulsive disorder, dystonia and addiction; and movement disorders, the most notable of which is Parkinson's disease, which involves the degeneration of the dopamine-producing cells in the substantia nigra pars compacta; and Huntington's disease which primarily involves damage to the striatum.

The basal ganglia, because of its extensive anatomy, becomes subjected to cranio fascial torsion, and transmission of processed neurological information will be reduced and retarded.

HAMBURGER BRAIN – SIX LEVELS

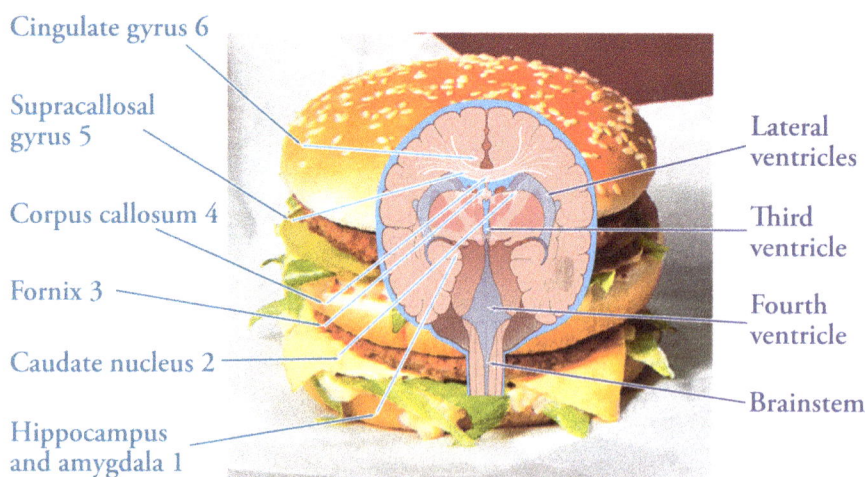

Figure 4.3 The Hamburger Brain: Six levels of crescent-shaped organs that make up the brain; the ventricular system is the central organ that provides the lift shaft and connects all the levels

The analogy of a six-layered hamburger to depict the brain shows how the six crescent-shaped systems are so integrated, with the 'lift-shaft' going through the middle representing the ventricular system – the two laterals, the third and fourth ventricles. Embryologically the neural tube is central to the brain formation as it becomes the ventricular system, surrounded eventually by the other central brain organ systems, namely, the:

- Cingulate gyrus
- Supracallosal gyrus
- Corpus callosum
- Fornix
- Caudate nucleus
- Hippocampus
- Amygdala.

More specifically this model shows the influence the dominant system has on the central brain organs in maintaining their neurological networks, nerve fibres and organ systems.

The Hippocampus and Amygdala

The hippocampus is part of the limbic system and is involved in the consolidation of information for the short-term to long-term memory and in spatial memory that enables navigation. Extensive evidence supports the view that the hippocampal formation, hippocampus and the dentate charges are indeed essential for processing information in short-term memory, particularly the consolidation of memory traces for transfer to long-term memory.

The hippocampus in each temporal lobe has an arm; the fornix that arches up to lie just below the corpus callosum before diving deep into the brain ending at the mammillary bodies. They protrude from the bottom of the brain and suggest that the left hippocampus is involved in symbolic digital processing and auditory short-term memory, while the right hippocampus is largely involved with visuospatial processing and visual short-term memory. The fornix is the major output path over the hippocampus to the mammillary bodies and via radiations from the fornix to many areas of the limbic system and the cerebral cortex.

Abnormal function of the hippocampus

In Alzheimer's disease, the hippocampus is one of the first regions of the brain to suffer damage; memory loss and disorientation are included among the early symptoms. Damage to the hippocampus can also result from oxygen starvation (hypoxia), encephalitis or medial temporal lobe epilepsy. People with extensive bilateral hippocampal damage may experience anterograde amnesia – the inability to form and retain new memories.

The hippocampus in schizophrenic patients has been found to be smaller in size when compared with controls of the same age group, and similarly the caudate and putamen have been found to be smaller in volume in the longitudinal study of schizophrenic patients, while the volume of grey matter is smaller, the size of the lateral and third ventricles is larger in schizophrenic patients. This could possibly be attributed to ventricular engorgement, expanding the size of the ventricles, through loss of CSF drainage through the venous sinus system, causing displacement of adjacent midline organs such as the caudate nucleus, the thalamus, the fornix, the hippocampus, the corpus callosum and ultimately the cingulated cortex.

The Amygdala

The amygdalae are considered part of the limbic system and are shown to perform a primary role in the processing of memory decision-making and emotional reactions. They are two almond-shaped groups of nuclei located deep and medially within the temporal lobes of the brain. The right amygdala is concerned with negative emotions, especially fear and sadness, while the left amygdala is able to induce either pleasant (happiness) or unpleasant (anxiety, sadness and fear) emotions. Although the right and left portions of the amygdala have independent memory systems, they are able to combine their functions to store, encode and interpret emotions – the right amygdala particularly has a role in association of time and places with emotional properties. The amygdalae are primarily responsible for our deepest emotions of fear, rage, pain and pleasure and our reactions to punishment, as well as behaviours relating to species survival, sexual arousal and the desire to nurture the young and helpless.

Abnormal function of the amygdala

Brain damage to the amygdala plays a role in trustworthiness, and damage tends to confuse trust and betrayal, thus patients 'place trust' in those having done them wrong. Overall, the amygdaloid function has a great deal to do with the process of learning. If excitement is encoded around it, learning can become a joy. A fearful encoding can produce the opposite result.

The overall functioning capability of the amygdala, and its integral association with the limbic system, means that its overall efficiency is retarded by cranio facial torsion.

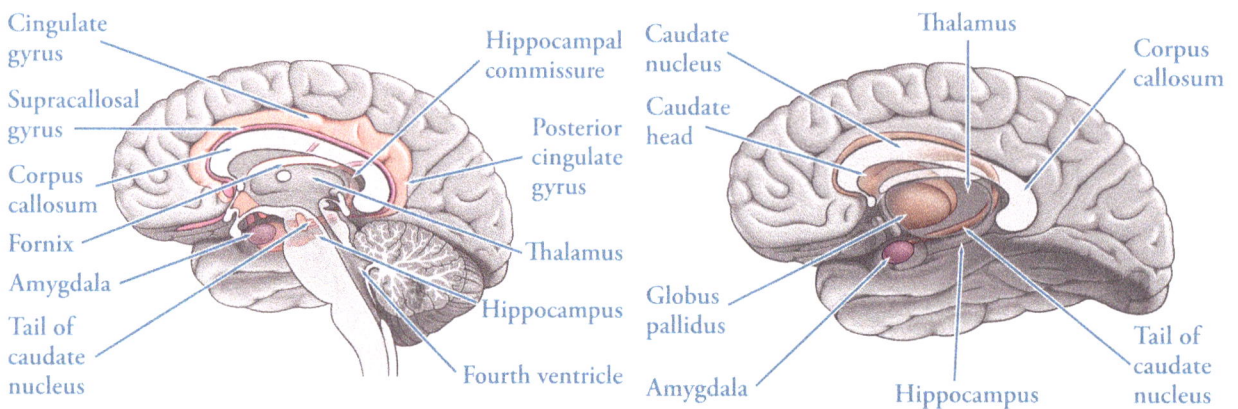

Cingulate gyrus
Supracallosal gyrus
Corpus callosum
Fornix
Amygdala
Tail of caudate nucleus
Hippocampal commissure
Posterior cingulate gyrus
Thalamus
Hippocampus
Fourth ventricle
Caudate nucleus
Caudate head
Globus pallidus
Amygdala
Thalamus
Corpus callosum
Hippocampus
Tail of caudate nucleus

Figure 4.4 (left) 1st Floor, Hippocampus and Amygdala: The C-shaped hippocampus and amygdala and their connections to the cingulate gyrus; (right) 2nd Floor, Caudate Nucleus: Storing and processing memories using past experiences to influence future actions and decisions

The Caudate Nucleus

The caudate nuclei are located near the centre of the brain, one in each hemisphere, and resemble a C-shaped structure with a wider head at the front tapering to a body and a tail. The head and body of the caudate nucleus form part of the floor of the anterior horn of the lateral ventricle, while the tail curves back, forming the roof of the inferior horn of the lateral ventricle. The caudate nucleus is highly innervated by dopamine neurons that originate from the substantia nigra, located in the midbrain, containing cell projections to the caudate and putamen and utilise the neurotransmitter dopamine.

The caudate nucleus and the putamen send their axonal signals back to the globus pallidus, the output component of the basal ganglia. The globus pallidus, in turn, forwards the signals to the ventral anterior nucleus of the thalamus. The thalamus then relays the signals to the motor and premotor cortex of the cerebrum, where the motor cortex provides the executive commands for movement while the premotor cortex provides the programmes to write and store in memory when they need to be retrieved. The C-shaped structure of the caudate nucleus resembles the C-shaped structure of the fornix, both straddling the central organ of the brain, the thalamus.

Abnormal function of the caudate nucleus

The C-shaped caudate nucleus and fornix change their juxtaposition, as influenced by the distortion of the thalamus and the thalamic nuclei with cranio fascial distortion.

In Alzheimer's disease, a 2013 study has suggested a link between Alzheimer's patients and the caudate nucleus. MRI images were used to establish the volume of the caudate nucleus in patients with Alzheimer's and normal volunteers. The study found a significant reduction in the caudate nucleus volume in Alzheimer's patients.

Parkinson's disease depletes dopaminergic neurons in the nigrostriatal tract, a dopamine pathway that is connected to the head of the caudate. The substantia nigra sends messages to the caudate nucleus and the putamen of the basal ganglia, which also receives additional input from the entire neocortex including association and primary sensory areas.

ADHD draws a relationship between caudate asymmetry and symptoms related to ADHD.

Schizophrenia – Smaller absolute and relative volumes of white matter in the caudate nucleus have been linked to patients diagnosed with schizophrenia.

OCD patients have increased grey matter volume in the bilateral lenticular nuclei, extending to the caudate nucleus with decreasing grey matter volume in the bilateral dorsal medial frontal/anterior cingulated gyri. The findings of these patients contrast with those suffering from other anxiety disorders who showed evidence of decreased (rather than increased) grey matter volume in the bilateral lenticular/caudate nuclei, as well as decreased grey matter volume in the bilateral dorsal medial frontal/anterior cingulated gyri.

This could be attributed to ventricular engorgement expanding the size of the ventricles, through loss of CSF drainage through the venous sinus system. Such engorgement leads to displacement of adjacent midline organs such as the caudate nucleus, the thalamus, the fornix, the hippocampus, the corpus callosum and ultimately the cingulate cortex. This displacement and distortion alters neurological pathways, association and radiation fibres, and over a period of time affects their physiological function.

The Fornix

The fornix is the major output pathway of the hippocampus transmitting information held in short-term memory to other areas of the limbic system and cortical association areas for further processing or to be laid down as a long-term memory.

The fornix is a C-shaped bundle of nerve fibres in the brain that acts as the major output tract of the hippocampus and is a part of the limbic system. These fibres begin in the hippocampus on each side of the brain, embedded in the temporal lobes, as a separate left and right side, forming the crura of the fornix which come together in the midline of the brain at the hippocampal commissure (commissure of the fornix), forming the body of the fornix. In between the two lateral bodies of the fornix lies the terminal lamina, which creates the commissure plate, a structure that gives rise to supporting the corpus callosum, the septum pellucidum (separating the two lateral ventricles) and the body of the fornix. The fornix then travels anteriorly and divides again at the anterior commissure, into two columns – as the front anterior pillars.

These fibres of the precommissural fornix arch down in front of the interventricular foramen of Monro in the lateral wall of the third ventricle where they end in the mammillary bodies.

The posterior fibres then split into two posterior crura from the post commissural fornix on each side and continue to curve around the posterior end of the thalamus into the temporal horn of the lateral ventricle. Like the corpus callosum, the fornix has commissural fibres (the hippocampal commissure) that allow the left hippocampus and the right hippocampus to communicate with each other and thus to coordinate their activities.

Abnormal function of the fornix

The function of the fornix has been found to correlate most closely with recall memory rather than with recognition memory. This means that damage to the fornix can cause difficulty in recalling long-term information such as details of past events, but has little effect on the ability to recognise. The fornix is also a communicating organ relaying information from the left side of the brain to the right side of the brain and vice versa, and through a series of commissural fibres – like the corpus callosum which it supports – also communicating from the left side of the brain to the right side of the brain and vice versa.

The commissural membranes and the information they convey will come under duress as a result of fascial torsion changing their juxtaposition. This may be aggravated by the torsion of the tentorium cerebellum (as the sphenoid twists to accommodate the torsion of the skull) the change in the vomer dynamics and the asymmetric pull on the pterygoid plates by the lateral and medial pterygoid muscles, through a long standing and repeated malocclusion.

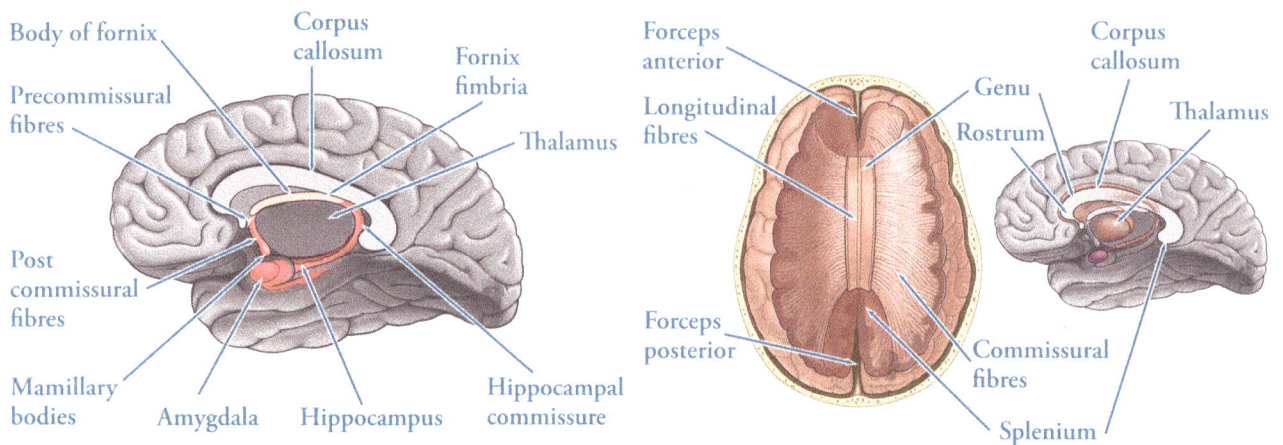

Figure 4.5 (left) 3rd Floor, Fornix: Supports the corpus callosum and the hippocampus; (right) 4th Floor, Corpus Callosum: Related to coordination and complex problem solving

The Corpus Callosum

This C-shaped organ contains the largest fibre bundle in the brain made up of commissural fibres that communicate between the brain hemispheres.

The anterior–posterior dimension of the corpus callosum is made up of the following regions where the genu connects the frontal lobes of the brain, the body connects the temporal lobes of the brain and the splenium connect the occipital lobes of the brain. The commissural fibres transfer motor, sensory and cognitive information between the brain hemispheres. Anatomically the corpus callosum is located underneath the cerebrum at the midline of the brain, and occupies the interhemispheric fissure, the deep furrow that separates the brain hemispheres.

Abnormal function of the corpus callosum

Developmental disorders of the corpus callosum can cause social and mental behavioural issues and delays in attaining developmental milestones in young children (walking, talking and reading), as well as clumsiness and poor motor coordination, particularly in skills requiring coordination of left and right hands and feet. A typical sensitivity to specific sensory input (for example, food textures or certain types of touch) often results in low pain threshold. Typically, the following symptoms may be attributed to corpus callosum disorders: quirky personality traits, poor parenting, ADHD, autism spectrum disorders, non-verbal learning disability, specific learning disabilities or psychiatric disorders.

As the corpus callosum is a midline organ it becomes subjected to cranio fascial torsion and therefore loses its dynamic symmetry. The commissural fibres deviate from their juxtaposition, becoming stretched or compressed, and in essence become poor transmitters of nerve function, disrupting the overall processing capability of the corpus callosum.

The Supracallosal Gyrus or the Indusium Griseum

The indusium griseum is a thin layer of grey matter embedded in the medial and lateral longitudinal striae of the corpus callosum. It is an extension of the hippocampus which follows the splenium and then curves around the genu and rostrum of the corpus callosum, ending in the subcallosal gyrus or the precommissural septum, on the inferior aspect of the corpus callosum.

The indusium griseum is made up of radial fibres that connect between the transverse fibres of the corpus callosum transmitting between the left and right side of the brain, and the longitudinal fibres of the cingulate gyrus that follow the brain and transmit from anterior to posterior, and vice versa – the afferent and efferent tracts from the hippocampus. These fibres are also connected to the fornix fimbria, the mamillary bodies, habenular commissure, the hippocampus commissures and the subcallosal gyrus. The supracallosal gyrus (indusium griseum) and the subcallosal gyrus encapsulate the corpus callosum and would appear to act as an interface between the cingulate gyrus and the corpus callosum. The subcallosal gyrus connects anteriorly with the olfactory trigone and is limited anteriorly by the anterior parolfactory gyrus.

Abnormal function of the supracallosal gyrus

There is nothing in the research literature that alludes to significant changes to the indusium griseum, apart from the fact that Alzheimer's disease has been investigated, but with no real significance. However, the indusium griseum (with radial fibres) would appear to act as a transmitting mechanism between the corpus callosum (with lateral commissural fibres) and the cingulate gyrus (with longitudinal commissural fibres). Note that the floor of the corpus callosum is provided by the lateral ventricles, and the caudate nucleus provides the lateral walls of the lateral ventricles. This suggests that disruption to vascular flow must compromise the dominant system by engorgement of the fourth, third and the lateral ventricles sufficient to change its shape. Similarly, as the torque of the tentorial incisura changes midline organ position, the corpus callosum commissural activity must be modified.

The Supracallosal is also influenced superiorly by the falx cerebri that encapsulates the inferior sagittal sinus at the superior cingulate gyrus midline and will change its position when the falx cerebri is torqued – part of the RTM distortion. This change will therefore affect the indusium griseum radial communication fibres, and as such will change the commissural activity of the cingulate gyrus and all the other commissural connections and their interrelationships, including the hippocampus.

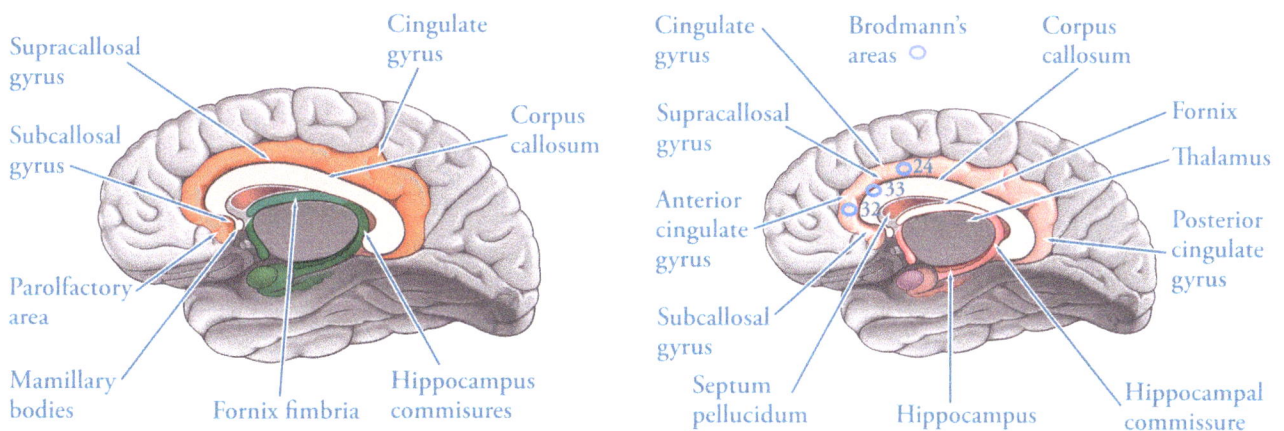

Figure 4.6 (left) 5th Floor, Supracallosal Gyrus: Made up of radial fibres of the corpus callosum, left and right side of brain, and longitudinal fibres of the cingulate gyrus to hippocampus, memory recall; (right) 6th Floor, Cingulate Gyrus: Involved in survival behaviour

The Cingulate Gyrus

The cingulate gyrus is situated in the medial aspect of the cerebral cortex lying immediately above the corpus callosum and is considered to be part of the limbic system involved with emotion formation and processing, learning and memory, and plays a role in executive function and respiratory control.

The anterior cingulate cortex corresponds to Brodman's areas 24, 32 and 33, and is continued anteriorly to the subgenual area 25 – located below the genu of the corpus callosum. The anterior cingulate cortex primarily receives its afferent axons from the trilaminar and midline thalamic nuclei.

The posterior cingulate cortex corresponds to Brodman's area 23 and 31.

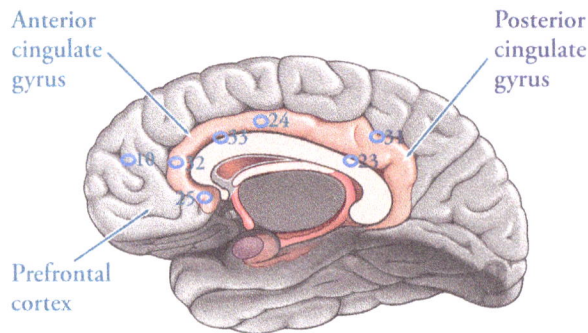

Figure 4.7 Brodmann's Areas: Associated with cingulate gyrus executive function, associated with prefrontal cortex

Abnormal function of the cingulate cortex

Studies have shown that the smaller the size of the anterior cingulate gyrus, the lower the level of social functioning and the higher the psychopathological level in schizophrenic patients. The anterior cingulate gyrus was found to be bilaterally smaller in patients with schizophrenia.

The volume of grey matter in the anterior cingulate gyrus was found to be lower in schizophrenic patients.

As the cingulate cortex is a midline cranial organ lying beneath the cerebral cortex and above the corpus callosum, cranio fascial torsion will affect the relay of information from the anterior singular gyrus through the body into the posterior cingulated gyrus.

The Limbic System

The limbic system is a set of brain structures located on both side of the thalamus immediately beneath the cerebrum and is generated embryologically from structures of the telencephalon, the diencephalon and the mesencephalon. It contains the areas that give birth to our emotions, lays down and retrieves memories and focusses on our survival. The fight/flight response originates here but is expressed in the body by the hypothalamus.

Anatomically, the limbic system is the cortical rim surrounding the diencephalon at the head of the brainstem. The cortical components are known as the limbic lobe and comprise the cingulated gyrus lying just above the corpus callosum, the orbitofrontal and subcallosal gyri of the basal frontal lobes, as well as the dentate and hippocampal gyri and the parahippocampal, entorhinal and perirhinal cortices of the medial temporal lobes.

In addition to the cortical limbic lobe, the limbic system also includes subcortical areas, the mammillary bodies of the hypothalamus, the amygdala bodies of the basal ganglia, the anterior thalamic nuclei of the thalamus and the septal nuclei of the basal forebrain.

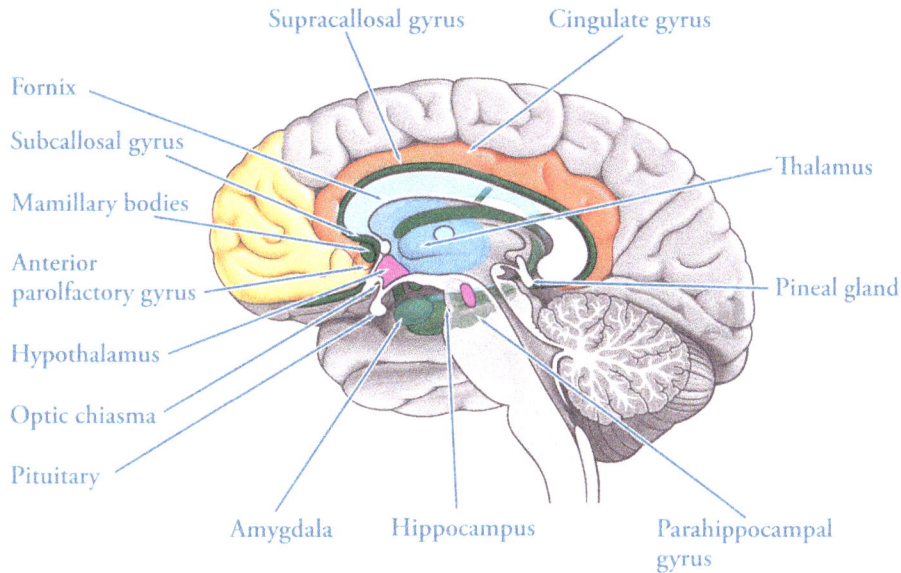

Figure 4.8 The Limbic System: Gathers sensory information, controls memory, emotions and arousal

The cingulate gyrus is a band of tissue lying around the corpus callosum that functions as the major relay centre for the limbic system. Many of the messages coming from the subcortical limbic nuclei are relayed through the cingulate gyrus on the way to the cortex. Likewise, cortical messages to the subconscious limbic system are delivered by the cingulate gyrus. The cingulate gyrus may be regarded as one of the major interfaces between the conscious and the subconscious. The anterior cingulate gyrus appears to be the site where our emotions, feelings, attention and working memory flow together. Also located within the anterior cingulate gyrus is a centre that suppresses our feelings of anger and rage. Destruction of this centre automatically engages the rage centres in the central and hypothalamic nuclei leading to subjects becoming vicious and subject to fits of uncontrolled rage.

The hippocampal formation, which comprises the dentate and hippocampal gyri together, is a central processing unit for memory and ongoing awareness of events. Information held in the hippocampus will be made available to the surrounding parahippocampal, perirhinal and entorhinal cortices, which appraise information against the matrix of previous experiences, sight, sound, smell, touch and taste. Via its interconnections with all of the association areas of the cortex, amygdala and temporal lobe, emotional associations are made. Reactions to this information in any of the senses are registered by the entorhinal cortex and sent back to the hippocampus formation for further consideration. Concurrently, the same information is being processed by the amygdala – the seat of subconscious emotions. Output from the subconscious emotional centres to the hypothalamus and prefrontal cortex generates our feelings and conscious awareness of the experience. In a way, the subcortical brain nuclei assign emotional content to the information, which is then experienced as a specific feeling in the body.

The mammillary bodies play an important role in the storage of conscious memory. They are a major relay station for output of short-term memory centres in the hippocampus to the anterior thalamus and anterior cingulate gyrus which, in turn, have rich connections to the association memory area of the cortex. The mammillary bodies also receive input from the taste areas of the brain and control our behaviours relating to eating.

Other areas involved in the limbic system include the olfactory bulbs, hippocampus, hypothalamus, amygdala, anterior thalamic nuclei, the fornix, columns of the fornix, mammillary body, septum pellucidum, habenular commissure, cingulate gyrus, parahippocampal gyrus, limbic cortex and midbrain limbic areas.

The limbic system supports a variety of functions including emotion, behaviour, motivation, long-term memory and olfaction, and parts of the brain that regulate visceral and autonomic process.

The following structures are considered part of the limbic system.

- Cortical Areas:
  - Limbic lobe
  - Orbitofrontal cortex – decision states and operation making
  - Piriform cortex – the olfactory system
  - Entorhinal cortex – memory and associative components
  - Hippocampus – consolidation of new memories
  - Fornix – connecting hippocampus with other brain structures

- Subcortical Areas:
  - Septal nuclei – pleasure zones
  - Amygdala – emotional process
  - Nucleus accumbens – reward, pleasure and addiction

- Diencephalic Structures:
  - Hypothalamus – centre for the limbic system, connected with the frontal lobes, septal nuclei and the brainstem reticular formation via the medial forebrain bundle, the hippocampus via the amygdala and with the thalamus via the mammillothalamic fasciculus regulates a number of autonomic processes
  - Mammillary bodies – part of the hypothalamus that receives signals from the hippocampus via the fornix and projects them to the thalamus
  - Anterior nuclei of the thalamus – receives input from the mammillary bodies involving memory processing.

Abnormal function of the limbic system

Some of the disorders associated with the limbic system are epilepsy and schizophrenia. Is also by the widespread connections of the limbic system to the hypothalamus, basal ganglia, and thalamus and cerebral cortex, that emotions have such profound effects on the viscera or gut functions (ulcers); muscle tone and posture (tired neck and hunched shoulders); sensory states (aversion to noxious sights, sound, smells and taste); and overall sensory states that define our mood. Because of the size of the limbic system and all the various cranial components that make up this system, central cranial torsion affects the frontal, parietal and temporal lobes, where most of these cranial components are embedded, and have fibrous insertions. Thus the entire limbic system becomes subjected to cranio fascial disturbance. The cranio fascial torsion therefore corrupts the limbic system's ability to function normally.

The Reticular Formation

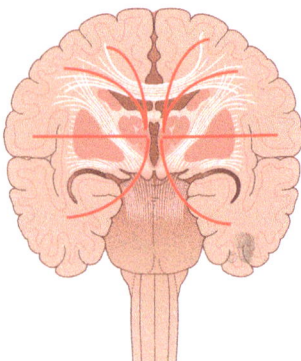

The reticular formation is a set of interconnected nuclei that are located throughout the brainstem which play a crucial role in maintaining behavioural arousal and consciousness. The medial and lateral reticular formation are two columns of neuronal nuclei with ill-defined boundaries that send projections through the medulla and into the mesencephalon (midbrain). The nuclei can be differentiated by function, cell type and projections of efferent or afferent nerves.

Figure 4.9 Reticular Formation: Fibres transmit from thalamus to cortex

376

Somatic motor control – these tracts function in maintaining tone balance and posture especially during body movements. The reticular formation also relays visual and aural signals to the cerebellum so that they can integrate stimuli into motor coordination.

Cardiovascular control – reticular formation includes the cardiac and vasomotor centres of the medulla oblongata.

Pain modulation – signals from the lower body reach the cerebral cortex.

Sleep and consciousness – projections to the thalamus and cerebral cortex allow control over the sensory signals from the cerebrum and from our conscious attention, alertness and sleep.

Habituation – modulate activity of the cerebral cortex as part of the reticular activating system – the brain learns to ignore repetitive meaningless stimuli while remaining sensitive to others.

Dural torque from the attachments at C3, C2 and C1 through the foramen magnum, influences the pons, the brainstem and the mesencephalon twisting the membrane system and has an adverse effect on the projection fibres of the reticular formation, potentially modifying these neurological pathways.

Abnormal function of the reticular formation

Mass lesions in the brainstem can cause severe alterations in the level of consciousness because of their effect on the reticular formation. Lesions in the reticular formation have been found in the brains of people who have post-polio syndrome, and in some imaging studies have shown abnormality in the area in people with chronic fatigue syndrome indicating a high likelihood that damage to the reticular formation is responsible for the fatigue associated with these syndromes. Again cranio fascial torsion plays a major role in allowing the reticular formation to function at its optimal level, applying torsion on the projection and radiating fibres that transmit information from the pons to the cerebral cortex.

The Septum Pellucidum

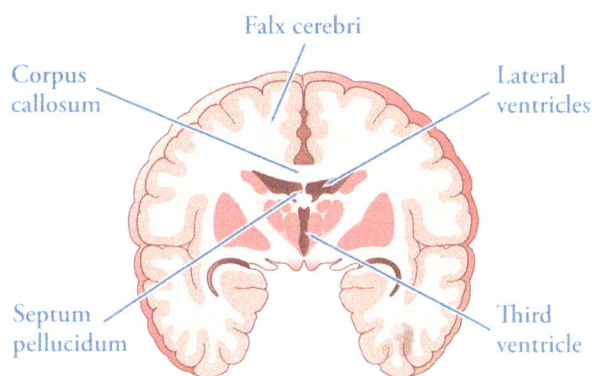

Figure 4.10 Septum Pellucidum: Lateral ventricles separated by the septum pellucidum

The septum pellucidum is located in the midline of the brain between the cerebral hemispheres and is attached superiorly to the corpus callosum and inferiorly to the anterior part of the fornix. On either side of the septum are the two lateral ventricles. It also lies underneath the other vertical brain separator and supporter, the falx cerebri, and so becomes the second vertical vector to be challenged by a clockwise/counterclockwise torque when the long axis of the skull is changed.

Abnormal function of the septum pellucidum

The third vertical vector included in this discourse is the vomer, supporting the ethmoid and the sphenoid body superiorly, while anchored below on the maxillae and the palatines of the palate. All these vertical membranes come under powerful dynamic forces when their juxtaposition is challenged by torsion through the midline of the skull, the brain and the occlusion. Also to be noted is the volume of CSF in the lateral ventricles, and how that volume changes with the advent of cranio fascial torsion. The interventricular foramen of Monroe, being a central vessel between the two lateral ventricles also torques and when restricted, retards the flow of CSF into and out of the lateral ventricles. Lower down in the same central position lies the aqueduct of Sylvius feeding CSF into the third ventricle. This volume change will also have repercussions on the septum pellucidum, and higher up on the corpus callosum forming the roof of the lateral ventricles.

Intracranial pressure

Intracranial pressure (ICP) is the pressure inside the skull on brain tissue exerted by CSF and is normally 7-15 mmHg. The components inside the cranium consist of blood-CSF and brain tissue and are responsible for volume equilibration, such that any increase in volume of one of the cranial constituents must compensate by a decrease in volume of another. One of the most damaging aspects of brain trauma and other similar conditions is an elevated intracranial pressure. An increase in pressure, most commonly due to head injury leading to intracranial haematoma with cerebral oedema, can crush brain tissue, shift brain structures, contribute to hydrocephalus, cause brain herniation and restrict blood supply to the brain. It is also a cause of reflex bradycardia. Small increases in the volume of vascular irrigation of the brain do not lead to an immediate increase in intracranial pressure. CSF may be displaced into the spinal canal; similarly the falx cerebri has the slight ability to stretch between the hemispheres and the tentorium cerebellum to stretch between the hemispheres and cerebellum.

However, once the ICP has reached about 25 mmHg, small increases in brain volume can lead to marked elevations in ICP; this is due to failure of intracranial compliance. It is the author's view that this slow increase in ICP created by retention of CSF over many years has the effect of changing the brain tissue, rearranging its juxtaposition and decreasing the size of various nuclei as a result of increased volume and pressure, particularly in the third and lateral ventricles.

Traumatic brain injury is a devastating problem with both high subsequent morbidity and high mortality. Injury to the brain occurs both at the time of initial trauma (primary injury) and subsequently due to the ongoing cerebral ischaemia (secondary injury). Cerebral oedema, CSF hypertension, circulatory hypotension, and hypoxic conditions are well recognised causes of the secondary injury, and the raised intracranial pressure is seen frequently after the original severe diffuse brain injury leads to cerebral ischaemia by compromising cerebral perfusion.

Cerebral perfusion pressure (CPP) is the pressure of blood flowing to the brain and is normally fairly consistent due to the autoregulation. If the level of ICP is increased it can cause ischaemia by decreasing the CPP. The body's response to a fall in CPP is to raise the systemic blood pressure and dilate cerebral blood vessels. This results in increased cerebral blood volume that increases ICP lowering CPP further and causing a vicious cycle. This results in widespread reduction in cerebral flow and perfusion, eventually leading to ischaemia and brain infarction. Increased blood pressure can also make intracranial haemorrhages bleed faster and also increases the ICP.

Severely raised ICP, if caused by a unilateral space-occupying lesion (e.g. haematoma) can result in midline shift, and are dangerous sequela in which the brain moves towards one side as the result of massive swelling in the cerebral hemisphere. A midline shift can compress the ventricles and lead to hydrocephalus. Increased ICP, combined with a space occupying process, can cause brainstem herniation (tonsillar ectopia) where the brainstem is forced through the foramen magnum.

Causes of increased intracranial pressure

The following are the causes of ICP and the mechanisms that influence that increase:

a. Space invading lesions such as brain tumours, infarction with oedema, contusions, subdural or epidural haematomas or abscesses, can lead to deformity and misplacement of adjacent brain tissue.

b. Generalised brain swelling as in ischaemic-anoxic states which tend to decrease the cerebral perfusion pressure with minimal tissue shifts.

c. An increase in venous pressure as a result of venous sinus thrombosis, heart failure or obstruction of the auxiliary plexus, the vertebral venous plexus and the jugular veins.

d. Obstruction of flow such as hydrocephalus, or subarachnoid space at the base of the brain, blockage in the ventricles (tonsillar ectopia – Arnold-Chiari malformation), extensive meningeal disease or obstruction in cerebral convexities and superior sagittal sinus (decreased absorption).

e. An increase in CSF production can occur in meningitis, subarachnoid haemorrhage, or choroid plexus tumour.

f. Craniosynostosis – abnormal skull formation as a result of birth trauma.

g. Torsion of the dural membrane system is involved in all of the aforementioned cases. Trauma suffered by the cranium combined with a whiplash type trauma to the cervical spine (atlanto-occipital membrane and the dural membrane attachments) will exacerbate congestion of CSF flow. It will especially affect drainage through the vertebral venous plexus and inferior jugular veins, creating a back pressure of CSF from the internal jugular vein, the sigmoid sinus, and the transverse sinus to the confluences of the sinuses. This build up of pressure also affects the inferior and superior sagittal sinuses, the diploic veins and the cavernous sinuses, ultimately affecting the drainage of the dominant system. As there are no valves involved in the venous sinus system and CSF flows backwards and forwards on a pressure gradient, the ultimate obstruction is an engorgement of CSF from the fourth ventricle through the aqueduct of Sylvius, the third ventricle, the interventricular foramen of Monro and the two lateral ventricles.

THE BLOOD–BRAIN BARRIER (BBB)

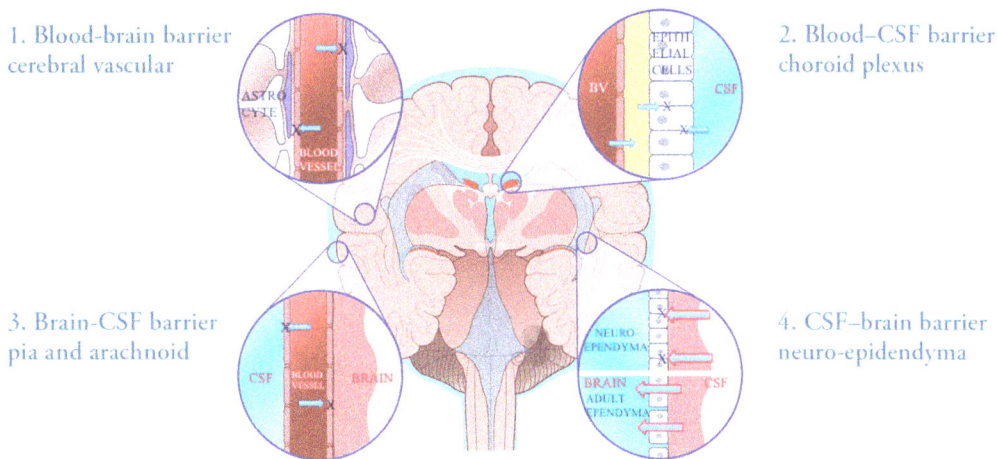

1. Blood-brain barrier cerebral vascular

2. Blood–CSF barrier choroid plexus

3. Brain-CSF barrier pia and arachnoid

4. CSF–brain barrier neuro-epidendyma

Figure 4.11 The Blood-Brain Barrier

The blood–brain barrier (BBB) is a dynamic interface that separates the brain circuitry system and protects the central nervous system from potentially harmful chemicals, while regulating transport of essential molecules and maintaining a stable environment.

The BBB is formed by highly specialised endothelial cells that line the brain capillaries and block transducer signals from the vascular system and from the brain. It allows passage of water, some gases, and lipid soluble molecules by passive diffusion, as well as the selective transport of molecules such as glucose and amino acids that are crucial to neural function.

However, unlike other blood vessels in the body, the endothelial cells in the brain are tightly woven together, creating a nearly impermeable boundary between the brain and bloodstream. The structure and function of the BBB is dependent upon the complex interplay between the different cell types such as the endothelial cells, astrocytes and pericytes, and the extracellular matrix of the brain and blood flow in the capillaries.

Tight junctions between the cerebral endothelial cells form a diffusion barrier, which selectively excludes most blood-borne substances from entering the brain. Astrocyte end-feet tightly sheath the vessel wall and appear to be critical for the function and maintenance of the 'tight junction barrier'.

Dysfunction of the BBB, for example, the impairment of the tight junction seal, complicates a number of neurological diseases including stroke and non-inflammatory disorders. Increased BBB permeability in hypoxia-ischaemia, ischaemia and inflammatory mechanisms, involving the BBB in septic encephalopathy, HIV-induced dementia, multiple sclerosis and Alzheimer's disease. The BBB is distinct from the quite similar blood-CSF barrier, which is a function of the choroidal cells in the choroid plexus, and from the blood retinal barrier that can be considered a part of the whole realm of such barriers.

Four types of barrier have been defined:

a. The blood–brain barrier – involves cerebral vascular capillaries and brain endothelial cells connected by tight junctions
b. The blood–CSF barrier – involves the choroid plexus epithelium of the third ventricle and the two lateral ventricles
c. The brain–CSF barrier – in the meninges of the brain between the pia mater and the epithelium of the arachnoid mater
d. The CSF–brain barrier – on the marginal borders of the ventricles through the neural ependymal layer into brain tissue.

Several areas of the human brain are not in the BBB and include the roof of the third and fourth ventricles, capillaries in the pineal gland on the roof of the diencephalon and the pineal gland (a small independent gland located near the centre of the brain between the two halves of the thalamus). The pineal gland produces melatonin, a serotonin derived hormone, which modulates sleep patterns in both the circadian and seasonal cycles.

CRANIO FASCIAL DISTORTION

The existence of the blood–brain barrier and the importance of the brain requiring a strict regime of selected and specific nutrition to perform and survive should be a question that concerns every clinician working in this very complex area. The primary question that arises from the aforementioned discussion, is, 'How do we preserve this most vital organ and its systems to the optimum?'

The first concern seems to manifest 'in utero' as teratogenic complications such as the maternal use of alcohol, smoking and recreational drugs which have provided scientists with an abundant amount of information over the years.

The second concern is the universal approach of the pharmaceutical industry driven by a commercial push for profit. Governments need these corporates to conduct vital research and development but sometimes research is not taken to its conclusion, or results are supressed (tobacco and thalidomide being prime examples).

Vaccines are generally seen as beneficial. Their use in infants however, and their ability to cross the blood–brain barrier at an age when the brain immaturity has not been consolidated deserves more investigation. Increased incidence of children with 'behavioural' issues and delayed development remains a concern.

Similarly, there is a growing realisation that anti-bacterial agents have reached their peak in effectiveness giving rise to the digestive anomalies. Younger generations are suffering with the effective loss of gut bacteria resulting in poor nutrition harvesting for the brain.

Senior citizens are also facing a tsunami of cardiovascular and cholesterol controlling drugs, that are questionable in the benefits they claim to resolve.

The other major issue already mentioned is the inadequacy of conventional medicine to measure or explain, unless very obvious, the advent of trauma and its damaging effect on the central nervous system and brain integrity. Symptomatic syndromes and diagnoses that cover a plethora of neurological changes are only addressed by pharmaceutical remedies which fail to improve the outcomes for these patients. The iatrogenic effect of these protocols is already changing the autoimmune systems of millions of people, who just do not 'cope'.

When CFD change through trauma and membrane distortion takes place, neurological systems fail and if not corrected, change life patterns forever. The mere change of the RTM affects the central organ of the brain – the two lateral, third and fourth ventricles. When torsion is applied to the ventricular system, changes occur in CSF production and circulation, and in adjacent cranial organs such as the thalamus and hypothalamus, affecting neural transmission 'junction boxes' throughout the brain and spinal cord. Because of their interdependence, systems such as the cingulate gyrus, the supracallosal gyrus, the corpus callosum, the caudate nucleus, the fornix, the basal ganglia and the limbic system fail. Retrieval and processing ability slow down and a myriad of changes occur, creating the 'syndrome' diagnosis.

The blood–brain barrier with its tightly woven barrier of endothelial cells, the cerebral vascular capillaries, the choroid plexus epithelial cells, the pia mater, the epithelium of the arachnoid mater and the marginal borders of the ventricles through the neuro ependymal layer into brain tissue, are all implicated by a cranio fascial assault. This ultimately loosens the barrier and makes it more susceptible to agents trying to cross it. The literature suggests that once this barrier has been breached, the susceptibility for more traffic is increased.

Once the blood–brain barrier has been traversed, the brain becomes vulnerable to an assortment of infiltrating chemicals, causing cytotoxic oedema located in the brain substance. They also interact with each other so that toxicity increases, destroying the myelin sheath and creating a necrotic environment and brain damage. Its occurrence and location determines the disruption in neurological function and so produces more symptomatic diversity, encouraging further pharmaceutical intervention and 'brain chaos'. This has become a pharmaceutical nightmare and without a change in approach, the young with their vaccinations and the elderly with their toxic cocktails, are both going to require sustained care. CFD is about changing this serious scenario and realising that early intervention can change these brain-membrane dynamics.

The BBB acts very effectively to protect the brain from most pathogens. Examples of pathogens that can traverse the BBB and the diseases they cause include, toxoplasmosis gondii, which causes toxoplasmosis, spirochetes like borrelia that causes Lyme disease, group B streptococci that causes meningitis in newborns, and Treponema pallidum that causes syphilis.

Meningitis

When the meninges are inflamed, the blood–brain barrier may be disrupted. This disruption may increase the penetration of various substances including either toxins or antibiotics into the brain. Antibiotics used to treat meningitis may aggravate the inflammatory response of the central system by releasing neurotoxins from the cell walls of bacteria – like lipo-polysaccharides.

Epilepsy

Epilepsy is a common neurological disease characterised by recurrent and sometimes untreatable seizures. Several clinical and experimental data have implicated the failure of the blood–brain barrier function in triggering chronic or acute seizures.

Multiple Sclerosis

Multiple Sclerosis (MS) is considered to be an autoimmune neurodegenerative disorder in which the immune system attacks the myelin that protects and electrically insulates the neurons of the central and peripheral nervous systems. Normally, a person's nervous system would be inaccessible to the white blood cells due to the blood–brain barrier. However, MRIs have shown that when a person is undergoing an MS 'attack', the blood–brain barrier has broken down in a section of the brain or spinal cord, allowing white blood cells called the 'T' lymphocytes to crossover and attack the myelin. It is sometimes been suggested that, rather than being a disease of the immune system, MS is a disease of the blood–brain barrier. Weakening of the blood–brain barrier may be a result of a disturbance in endothelial cells on the inside of the blood vessel due to which the production of protein P-glycoprotein is not working well. It is believed that oxidative stress plays an important role in the breakdown of the barrier. Antioxidants such as lipoic acid may be able to stabilise a weakening of the blood–brain barrier.

Alzheimer's Disease

There is evidence to suggest that disruption of the blood–brain barrier in Alzheimer's disease patients allows blood plasma containing amyloid beta to enter the brain where the amyloid beta adheres preferentially to the surface of astrocytes. Eventually the astrocytes are overwhelmed, die, rupture and disintegrate, leaving behind the soluble amyloid beta 42 plaque. Thus Alzheimer's disease may be caused or likely aggravated by a breakdown in the blood–brain barrier.

Cerebral Oedema

Cerebral oedema is the accumulation of excess water in the extracellular space of the brain, which can result when hypoxia causes the blood–brain barrier to open.

Systemic Inflammation

Inflammation in the body may lead to effects on the brain via the blood–brain barrier. During systemic inflammation, whether in the form of infection or sterile inflammation, the BBB may undergo changes that may be disruptive or nondisruptive. These changes may also induce auxiliary disease of the brain, for example, in multiple sclerosis and Alzheimer's disease, and may be part of the reason why patients with these conditions deteriorated during the infection. Patients with neurological disease may influence the BBB and may be abnormally sensitive to the effect of systemic inflammation.

CONCLUSION

The developing brain has three main divisions:

- Forebrain or prosencephalon
- Midbrain or metencephalon
- Hindbrain or rhombencephalon.

The forebrain or prosencephalon is the largest part of the nervous system in humans and is subdivided into telencephalon and the diencephalon.

The telencephalon is made up of:

- Cerebral hemispheres

- Cerebral cortex
- Subcortical white matter
- Basal ganglia
- Basal forebrain nuclei.

The diencephalon halon is made up of:

- Thalamus
- Hypothalamus
- Epithalamus.

The mesencephalon is a relatively short and narrow region connecting the forebrain and hindbrain and consists of:

- Cerebral peduncles
- Midbrain tectum
- Midbrain tegmentum.

The rhombencephalon consists of the:

- Metencephalon – pons and cerebellum
- Myelencephalon – medulla.

The midbrain, pons and medulla together form a connection between the forebrain and the spinal cord.

A summary of the growth and development of the various vesicles is:

Week 3 – The neural tube

- Neural plate
- Neural grove
- Neural tube
- The brain

Week 4 – Primary vesicle

- Prosencephalon
- Mesencephalon
- Rhombencephalon

Week 5 – Secondary vesicles

- Telencephalon
- Diencephalon
- Mesencephalon
- Metencephalon
- Myelencephalon
- Adult Status – adult structure.

Telencephalon – rhinencephalon, amygdala, hippocampus, cerebrum, basal ganglia, lateral ventricle.

Diencephalon – epithalamus, thalamus, subthalamus, pineal, retina, interventricular foramen of Monro.

Mesencephalon – tectum, cerebral peduncle, pretectum, third ventricle, brainstem, midbrain.

Metencephalon – brainstem pons, cerebellum, aqueduct of Sylvius.

Myelencephalon – brainstem medulla, medulla oblongata, fourth ventricle.

Brain Organs and their Abnormal Functions and Effects

- Basal ganglia – problems controlling speech, movement and posture
- Hippocampus – influences memories and ability to form new memories
- Amygdala – poor decision making and impaired emotional memories
- Fornix – difficulty recalling long-term information and details of past events
- Caudate nucleus – cognitive impairment, depression and movement issues
- Cingulate gyrus – person struggles to associate certain actions with emotions such as fear and sadness
- Limbic system – poor performance in relationships; low self-esteem
- Cortical areas – cortical strokes can result in neglect, aphasia and hemianopia
- Reticular formation – results in prolonged sleep or inactivity; loss of neurotransmitter – norepinephron
- Septum pellucidum – learning difficulties, behavioural changes, seizures and visual changes
- Intracranial pressure – intracranial hypertension; headaches
- Blood–brain barrier – tight endothelial cells are loosened and harmful substances may cross through the barrier.

THE DISLOCATED BRAIN

PART VII

PHYSIOLOGY OF THE HOWAT 8-STEP PROTOCOL

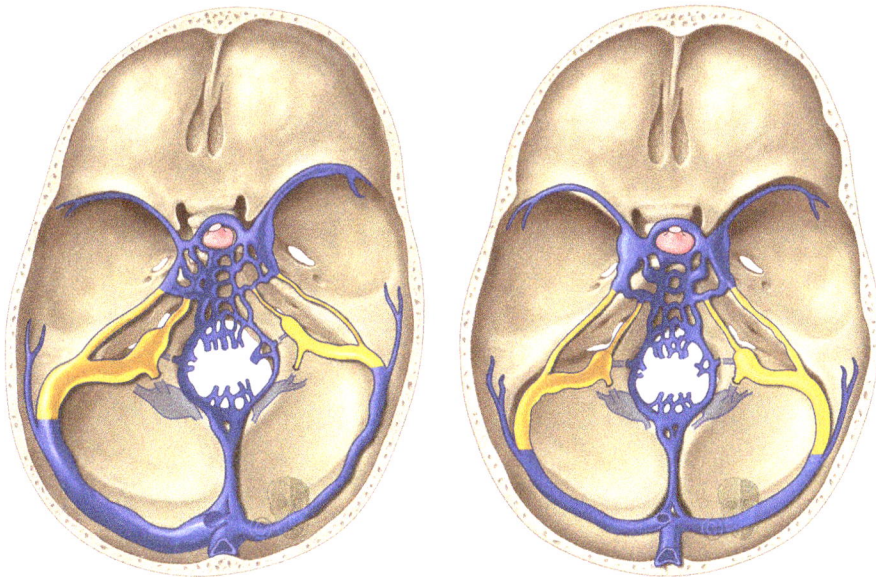

CONTENTS PART VII

ILLUSTRATIONS PART VII

PHYSIOLOGY OF THE HOWAT 8-STEP PROTOCOL

OF CRANIO FASCIAL DYNAMICS© (HPCFD)

As a conclusion to this book, it is pertinent to show that cranio fascial dynamics (CFD) has an alternative protocol to addressing the problems and consequences of TBI no matter what shape or size it comes in.

In the first place, having covered all the possible aetiologies of this huge subject, it is important to realise that TBIs of whatever size have an impact on all our lives.

The severely traumatised have a life to live with the terrible outcomes of the trauma that are sometimes evident, but for the most part are obscured and hidden for many years, then a gradual deterioration and realisation that things are not the 'same'.

The others – the innocent bystanders – live with the gradual changes in mood, behaviour, personality and the physical deviations that their nearest and dearest now portray and become the carers as well as the spouse, parent or child in a life-long incarceration that has no let-up.

To bring together the ventricular system (the controller of cerebrospinal fluid – CSF) and the cerebral perfusion aspect of brain function or dysfunction as the case maybe, the author has tried to show the complications of TBIs and how he thinks that a dialogue and narrative needs to take place with all parties concerned in an attempt to change ideas and practices to bring a better outcome to humanity.

In his opinion, there needs to be an understanding of what a physical trauma looks like and there needs to be a physical resolution to change the status quo, before all the other modalities come into play.

Chapter 3 describes the HPCFD in an attempt to take the 'traumatic CFD' situation into a functional 'benign' resolution to help the body heal. Anyone working in this field knows full well that the practitioner, of whatever discipline, relies on the inherent recuperative powers of the body to heal that body to the best of its optimum ability. The understanding of removing neurological interference means the outcome can never be vouched for, as everyone is 'wired' similarly, but differently. By removing neurological interferences, the body has the format and the competence to make the required changes to enable that system to 'heal'. One can never predict the outcome.

Elastoplast and mercurochrome have never healed a cut – just kept the wound clean. The 'healing' body potential brings both parts of the cut skin together to create new cells and tissue, and a scar. We do not possess that capability in our arsenal.

CHAPTER 1

THE VENTRICULAR SYSTEM

The ventricular system consists of four ventricles, the two lateral ventricles, the third and the fourth ventricle. CSF is generated in the choroid plexuses of each ventricle, by cuboid epithelial cells, which remove plasma from the blood and form the CSF where the consistency and exact chemical composition of the fluid can be controlled.

The volume of the CSF remains a constant within the ventricles.

Drainage of the ventricles flows through the interventricular foramen of Monro, from the lateral ventricles to the third ventricle and then through the aqueduct of Sylvius to the fourth ventricle. The CSF then flows through the two lateral apertures of Lushka and the medial aperture of Madgendie into the subarachnoid cisterns of the brain, bathing the brain between the pia mater and the arachnoid mater. Small projections of arachnoid mater project into the dura mater to form the arachnoid granulations, where it is drains into the superior sagittal sinus of the venous sinuses and finally into the internal jugular vein. The fourth aperture to drain CSF from the fourth ventricle is the central canal which drains into the spinal canal of the spinal cord.

FUNCTIONS OF CSF

- Protection of brain tissue from neural damage in cranial injuries
- The buoyancy of the brain is created by the CSF in the ventricles and the subarachnoid space. The low specific gravity in CSF keeps the brain which usually weighs about 1,400 grams buoyant and reduces its weight to 25 grams. This buoyancy allows the brain to exist in neutral buoyancy, allowing it to maintain its density without being impaired by its own weight and prevents the brain from compressing the cisterns and the vertebral venous plexus at the base of the cranium. CSF also acts as a diffusion medium for the transport of neurotransmitters and neuroendocrine substances
- Production of CSF remains a constant at 500 mls/day and while the subarachnoid space around the spinal cord and the brain contain only 135 to 150 mls, the remainder is drained into the superior sagittal sinus through the arachnoid granulations, creating a rate of turn over for CSF of about 3.7 times a day. This continuous flow of CSF allows a dilution of the of larger, lipid-insoluble molecules penetrating the brain and CSF.

CHANGES IN THE STATUS OF THE VENTRICULAR SYSTEM

When an injury or illness alters the circulation of CSF, one or more of the ventricles becomes enlarged as CSF accumulates. In an adult, the skull is rigid and cannot expand, so the pressure in the brain may increase profoundly.

Normal pressure hydrocephalus (NPH) results from the gradual blockage of the CSF-draining pathways in the brain. The ventricles enlarge to handle the increased volume of CSF, thus compressing the brain from within and eventually damaging or destroying the brain tissue. NPH owes its name to the fact that the ventricles inside the brain become enlarged with little or no increase in pressure.

NPH can occur as the result of head injury. Unfortunately, the cause of the majority of NPH cases is unknown, making it difficult to diagnose and understand. Compounding this difficulty is the fact that some of the symptoms of NPH are similar to the effects of the aging process, as well as diseases such as Alzheimer's and Parkinson's, and a small percentage suffer with dementia. The brain may shrink in older patients or those with Alzheimer's disease, and CSF volume increases to fill the extra space. In these instances, the ventricles are enlarged, but the pressure usually is normal.

Trauma to the Ventricular System – Hydrocephalus

- Trauma to the brain can result in blood clots within the ventricles preventing CSF flow out of the cranial space is the main cause of acute hydrocephalus
- Similarly, inflammation-mediated adhesions, which obstruct the reuptake of CSF, are the main causes of chronic hydrocephalus
- In traumatic brain injury (TBI) patients, both mechanisms can lead to the development of post-traumatic hydrocephalus (PTH)
- The long-term effects of TBIs can result in the atrophy of the cerebral cortex, thalamus, hypothalamus, temporal lobes and brain stem, resulting in ventricular enlargement, as well as tau protein deposits found in the sulci and perivascular spaces of the cerebral cortex
- Post-traumatic ventriculomegaly is a frequent and early finding in patients with moderate (mTBI) or severe TBI
- Compromised ventricular function can result in higher volumes of CSF within the ventricles, giving rise to intracranial pressure – internal ventricular ICP and a decrease in cerebral perfusion
- Conversely, intracranial pressure, can be reduced by the ventricles displacing CSF through the central canal – external ventricular ICP. This reduction of intracranial pressure will lead to an increase of cerebral perfusion.

Concussion and Cerebral Perfusion

Concussion is the prelude to changing the brain status in many dimensions. These are factors to be aware of when applying the Howat 8-Step Protocol. The fact is that 70% of mTBI result in changes to 'cerebral perfusion'.(Perfusion is the passage of fluid through the circulatory system or lymphatic system to an organ or a tissue, usually referring to the delivery of blood to a capillary bed in tissue)

The cranium contains CSF, blood and brain tissue. When the cranium becomes traumatised, the CSF and blood retain their separate volumes and cannot be compressed. The brain tissue swells from the trauma, resulting in its compression, caused by intracranial pressure (ICP) thereby effecting the permeability of the tissue and reduces the cerebral blood flow (CBF) and cerebral perfusion pressure (CPP).

Intra-cranial pressure
• Bruised brain swelling in confined cranium
• CSF and Blood cannot compress - Therefore compression of brain tissue
• Cerebral perfusion pressure- poor permeability – ischemia
• Autoregulation increases heart rate Increases cerebral perfusion - stroke

Decrease in brain drainage
• Venous sinus congestion
• Atlanto-occipital membrane distortion
• Internal jugular vein constriction

Brain core distortion
• Ventricular system stagnation
• Spinal canal constriction
• Brain blood flow autoregulation is abolished in traumatic brain injury
• Autoregulation controlled by cardiovascular nucleus tractus solitarii with parasympathetic preganglionic neurons in the pons

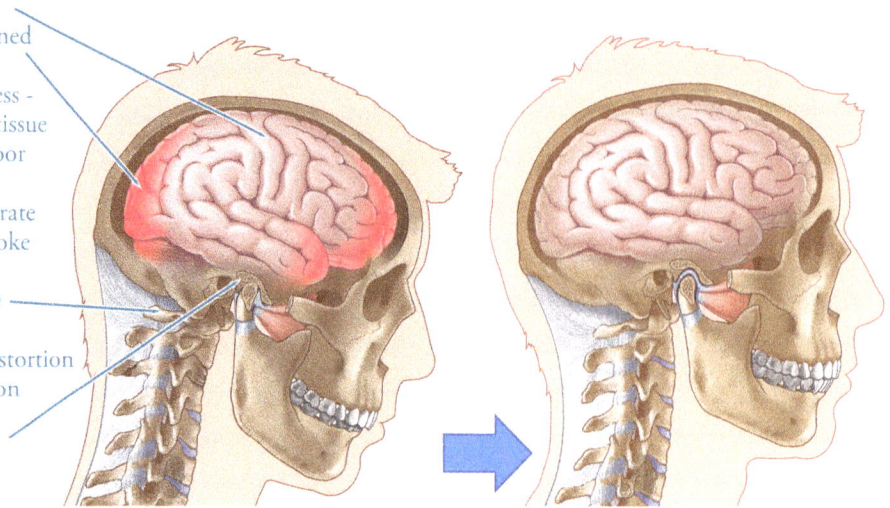

Figure 1.1 Loss of Cerebral Perfusion

Were this to continue, ischemia would result and tissue damage would follow suite. To reverse this process autoregulation kicks in, increasing the heart rate and vasodilation of the cerebral blood vessels, thereby increasing cerebral blood flow and cerebral perfusion. The outcome of this process means that with a further increase in ICP, increased heart rate, increased CBF increases the onset of a stroke or a cerebral bleed.

The cardio-accelerator centres (the sympathetic component of the cardiovascular centre in the medulla oblongata):

• Stimulate cardiac function by regulating heart rate and stroke volume via sympathetic stimulation from the cardiac accelerator nerve
• Autoregulation then tries to reverse the process, decreasing heart rate and CBF
• This becomes a 'vicious cycle', fluctuations of increase and decrease, but ultimately leads to ischemia and brain infarction, or a 'stroke'.

The cardio-inhibitor centres (parasympathetic component of the cardiovascular centre in the medulla oblongata):

• Slow cardiac function by decreasing heart rate and stroke volume via parasympathetic stimulation from the vagus nerve
• Autoregulation is controlled by the cardiovascular nucleus tractus solitarii with parasympathetic preganglionic neurons in the pons.
• The vasomotor centres, found in the medulla oblongata, control vessel tone or contraction of the smooth muscle in the tunica media. Changes in diameter affect peripheral resistance, pressure and flow, which affect cardiac output. The majority of these neurons act via the release of the neurotransmitter norepinephrine from sympathetic neurons.

Brain core distortion
• Ventricular system stagnation
• Spinal canal constriction
• Brain blood flow autoregulation is abolished in traumatic brain injury
• Autoregulation controlled by cardiovascular nucleus tractus solitarii with parasympathetic preganglionic neurons in the pons

Neurological regulation of blood pressure and flow depends on the cardiovascular centres located in the medulla oblongata. This cluster of neurons responds to changes in blood pressure as well as blood concentrations of oxygen, carbon dioxide and hydrogen ions. The cardiovascular centre contains three distinct paired components

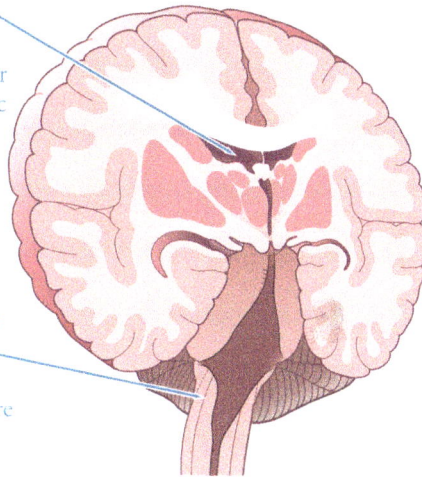

Figure 1.2 Resultant TBI causes brain core distortion

Within this physiological oscillation several developments take place:

a. The trauma force will whiplash the upper cervical spine and the brain stem, constricting the atlanto-occipital membrane, restricting arterial inflow of the vertebral arteries and constricting the outflow of the vertebral venous plexus – stagnation of the internal vascular dynamics.

b. The cranium membranes will torque, further reducing the venous outflow from the cavernous sinuses, the transverse and sigmoid sinuses and the internal jugular vein – torque of the tentorium cerebelli and tentorial incisura.

c. Intracranial pressure results compressing the brain tissue and its permeability, reducing CBF and CPP, while the brain swells from the trauma.

d. The internal brain core organs, primarily the ventricular system, torques and changes its boundaries, effecting the cerebellum, pons, cerebral and cerebellar peduncles around the fourth ventricle, the thalamus and the hypothalamus around the third ventricle. Ventricular stagnation leads to central canal constriction and loss of drainage into the spinal canal.

e. Neurological pathways become distorted, twist and occlude, changing nerve transmission and communications, altering the brain's ability to retrieve, process and disseminate information.

f. Brain chaos results and if not reversed, lays the path open to neurological syndromes and cardiovascular diseases later in life, with the prospect of an accumulation of further traumas superimposed on the original insult.

The mTBI effect has many direct and indirect consequences to brain and neurological function. The early consequences of the initial insult change the volumes of the internal cranial dynamics within the confined restraints of the cranium itself.

This insult not only changes the biomechanics of the cervico-cranial junction and the spinal column, but more importantly the neurological components of the spinal cord, the medulla oblongata, the pons, the cerebral and cerebellar peduncles and the midbrain.

This physical upset has huge ramifications on the outcome of brain irrigation, in the first instance, in a diminishment of brain drainage, resulting from brain swelling, oedema and a change in the reciprocal tension membranes (RTM) status. The RTM are responsible for the encapsulated vessels of the venous sinus system and are ultimately in control of brain drainage. Linked to this is the ventricular system, which may lose its bouncy potential and sink into the cisterns around the base of the brain, compressing the internal vertebral venous plexus. This is not usually a situation that is considered in mTBIs.

The blood and CSF are a constant in volume capacity and do not change. However, the change in brain dimensions is the critical variable that alters autoregulation and cerebral perfusion beyond the proportions that the cranium can cope with. In the precursor to brain function – before the insult – normal homeostatic brain irrigation effectively maintains the normal blood flow, arterial inflow and venous outflow. While the arterial inflow reduces, through the vertebral arteries pathways through the atlanto-occipital membrane, that membrane distortion also restricts the venous outflow through the internal and external vertebral venous plexus.

• The **cardio-accelerator centres** stimulate cardiac function by regulating heart rate and stroke volume via **sympathetic stimulation from the cardiac accelerator nerve**

• The **cardio-inhibitor centres** slow cardiac function by decreasing heart rate and stroke volume via **parasympathetic stimulation from the vagus nerve**

• The **vasomotor centres** control vessel tone or contraction of the smooth muscle in the tunica media. Changes in diameter affect peripheral resistance, pressure, and flow, which affect cardiac output. The majority of these neurons act via the **release of the neurotransmitter norepinephrine from sympathetic neurons**

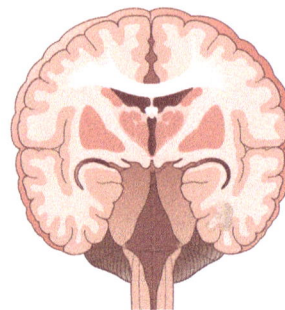

Textbook symmetry

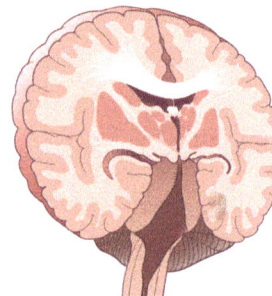

Traumatic CFD

Figure 1.3 Cardio-accelerator and Inhibitor

The sequencing of reinstating the traumatic CFD is important as there are two basic problems that need to be restored, namely, the drainage and the fascial torque.

One also has to establish where the major problem, or the primary, exists and then produces secondary and tertiary consequences. Without establishing the primary, one is dealing with compensation and adaptation, and not addressing a faulty premise.

CHAPTER 2

FASCIAL TORQUE AND BRAIN DRAINAGE

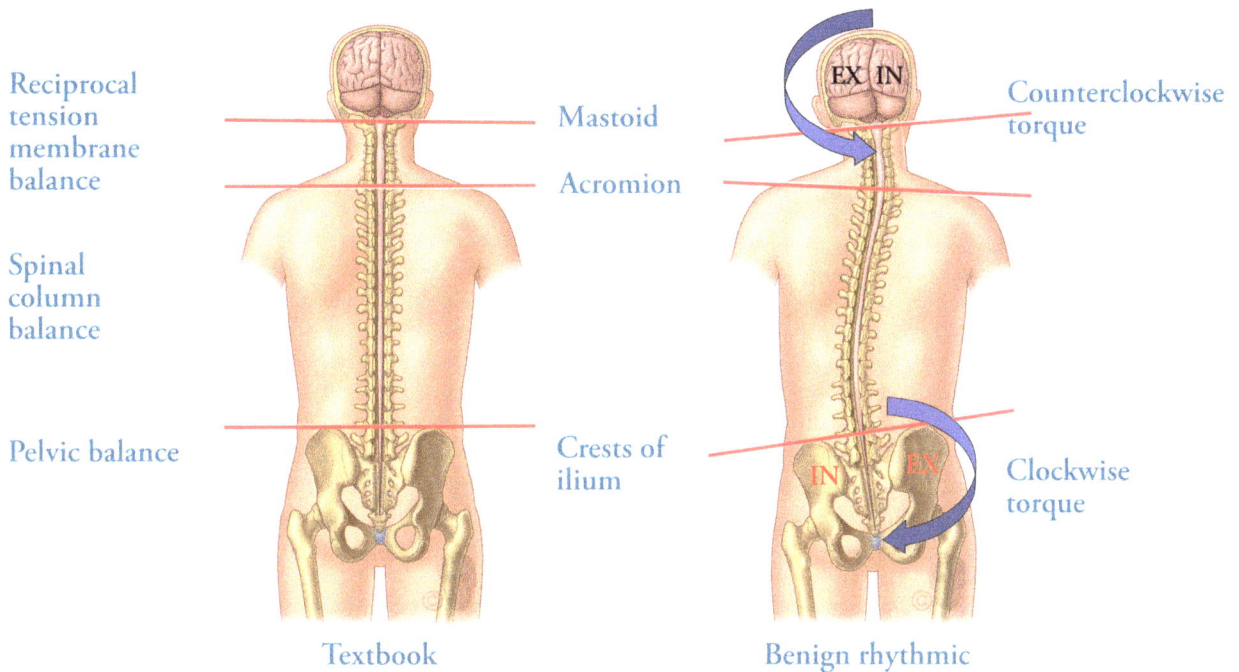

Reciprocal tension membrane balance

Spinal column balance

Pelvic balance

Mastoid

Acromion

Crests of ilium

Textbook

EX IN

IN EX

Counterclockwise torque

Clockwise torque

Benign rhythmic

Figure 2.1 Fascial Torque and Brain Drainage

The final objective is to have benign rhythmic and diaphragmatic respiration in both fascial torque and drainage perspectives, where no clinical deviants are present. The process illustrated in this chapter shows the various components of the brain reversing a traumatic CFD to a benign CFD, moving from a clinical positive to a non-clinical negative. Utilising the protocols of the HPCFD to reduce the trauma and their indicators to a haemodynamic benign motion is the precursor to changing and returning the dynamics towards homeostasis.

MUSCLE SYSTEMS

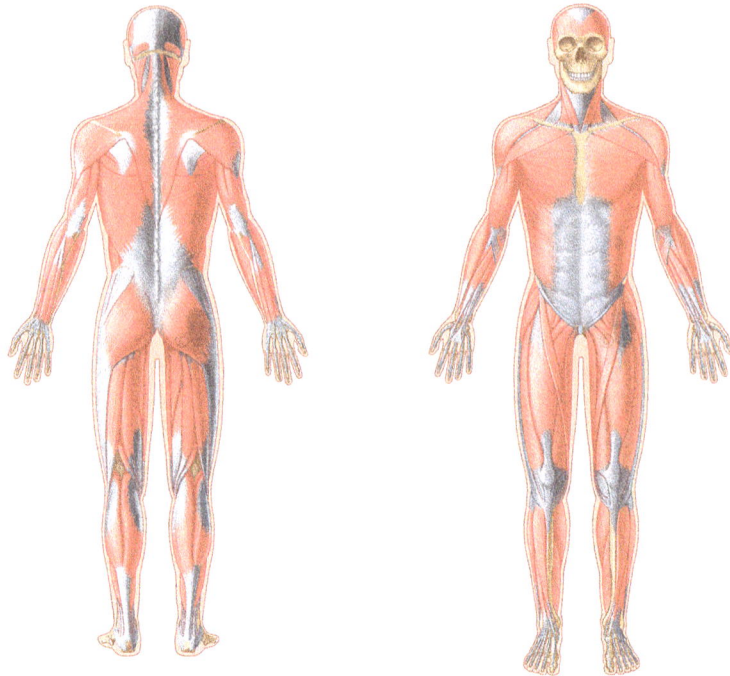

Figure 2.2 Textbook Symmetric Body Musculature

The muscle systems involved are defined by the bio-mechanical needs that they service. The bio-mechanical diversification can be driven by compensation and adaptation from the primary, or may themselves have been the result of direct trauma.

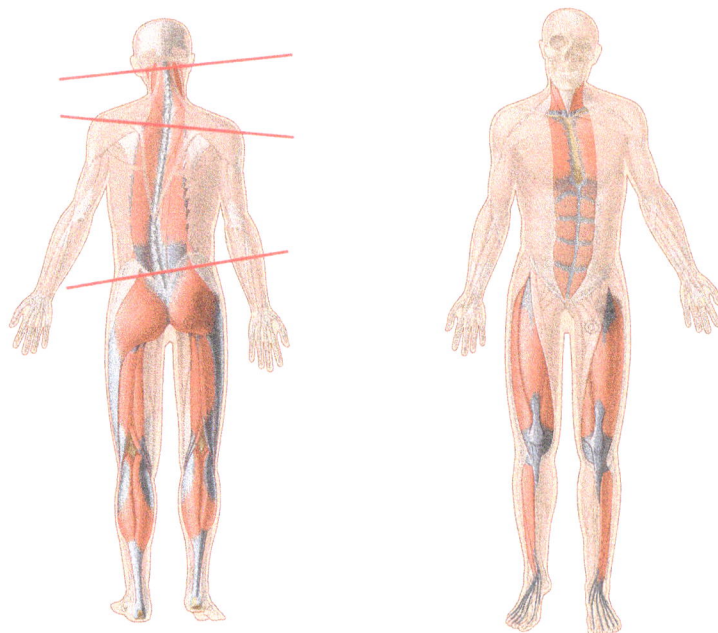

Figure 2.3 Central Core Muscle Groups in Benign Rhythmic Respiration

These muscle groups are central core muscles that link the sacrum to the superior nuchal line of the occiput and establish the 'sacro-occipital pump', primarily driving the spinal canal of the fourth ventricle in circulating CSF. Opposite the superior nuchal line attachment of the erector spinae muscles, lies the transverse groove on the interior wall of the occiput where the tentorium cerebelli (encapsulating the transverse and sigmoid sinuses) attaches – the horizontal reciprocal tension membrane. The reciprocal rhythmic motion of these two muscle groups (erector spinae and tentorium cerebelli) is a major factor in balance, equilibrium and drainage.

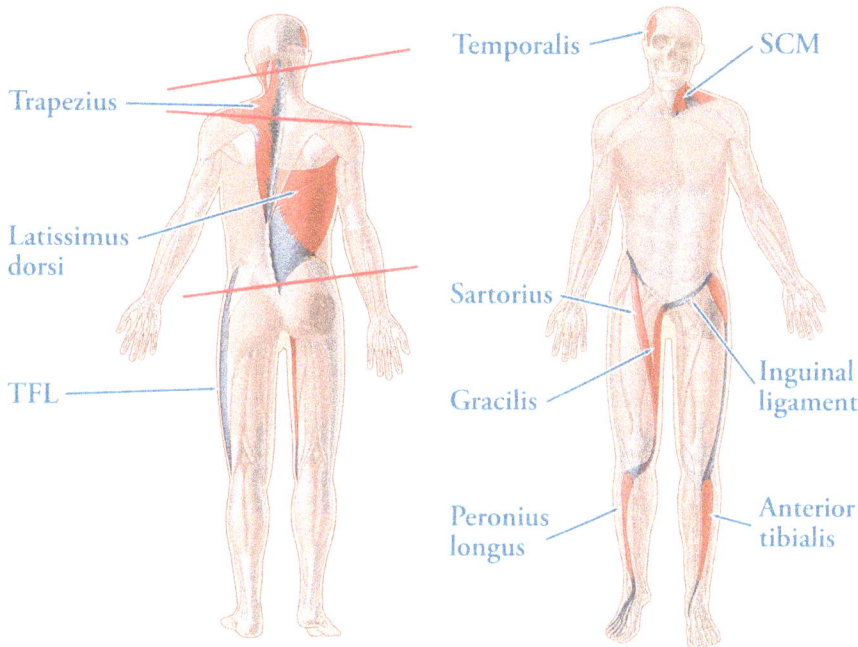

Figure 2.4 Lateral Muscle Groups in Traumatic CFD

The traumatic CFD now recruits the lateral muscle groups, incapacitating the lateral components of the body and cranium, more by compensation from the primary than direct trauma, creating imbalance, loss of equilibrium and corrupt drainage.

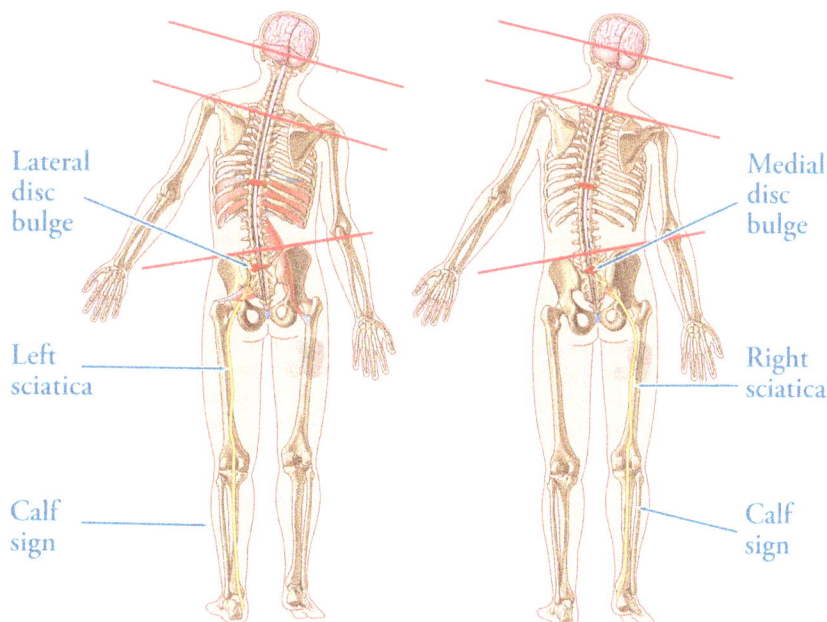

Figure 2.5 Muscle Groups in Lumbosacral Disc Lesion: Psoas and piriformis muscles

A failure of traumatic CFD to accommodate, moves to a stage of physical breakdown in the biomechanical structures, bringing the body to a standstill. Lumbar 5 reciprocates with the atlas (C1), severely disrupting the atlanto-occipital membrane, the arterial inflow (vertebral arteries) and the venous outflow (vertebral venous plexus), and negates the fourth ventricle and spinal canal drainage of CSF.

A clinical assessment of all these complexities has to be undertaken first, to ensure that the 'sacro-occipital pump mechanism' is able to work at the optimum level to achieve maximum irrigation potential before the cranium is released. However, the primary is almost always found to be a descending major, which then compensates and adapts into the ascending components. It is therefore essential to establish where the primary cause is located, before embarking on a treatment protocol.

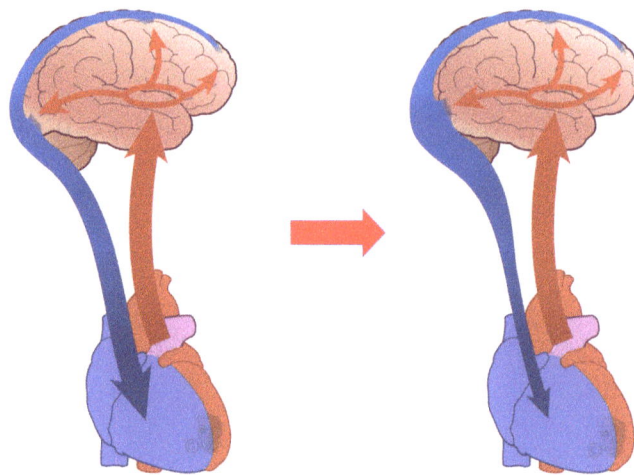

Figure 2.6 Whiplash Reduces Brain Drainage

The insult of mild traumatic brain injury damages the function of the cervico-cranial junction from an osseous standpoint, inhibiting the brain drainage as already discussed. More importantly, it changes the internal central core components of the brain – a neurological outcome. The spinal cord, the medulla oblongata, the pons, the cerebral and cerebellar peduncles, along with the fourth ventricle and the midbrain, thalamus and hypothalamus, and the third ventricle, become torqued and displaced by the traumatic force. The central brain core structures are intimately integrated with the frontal, parietal, temporal and occipital lobes, and their neural pathways are all implicated.

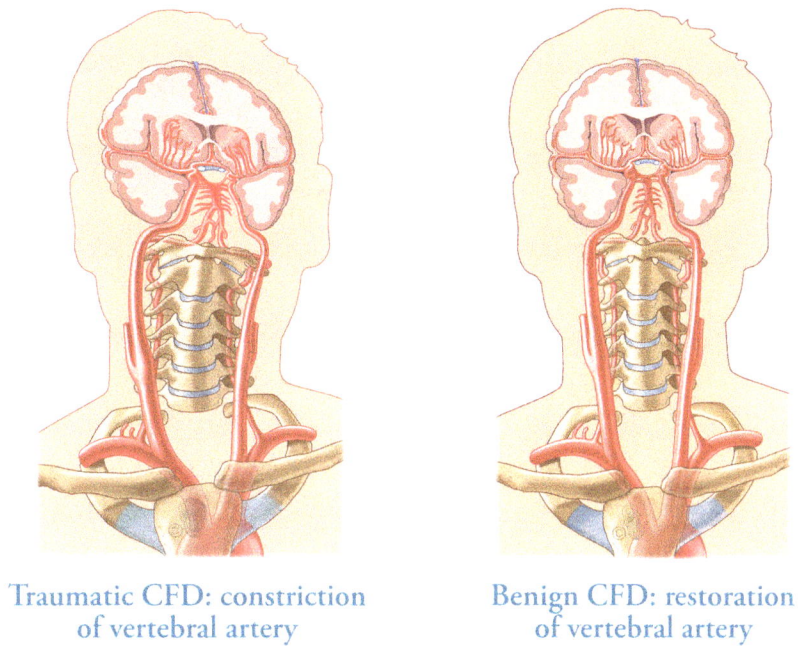

Traumatic CFD: constriction
of vertebral artery

Benign CFD: restoration
of vertebral artery

Figure 2.7 Circulation of the Vertebral Artery: Activate the cervical spine to release the veterbral artery

Arterial inflow is essential to maintain the posterior branches of the circle of Willis. The two vertebral arteries form the basilar artery going into the foramen magnum to feed the pontine arteries, before joining the posterior circulatory branch of the circle of Willis.

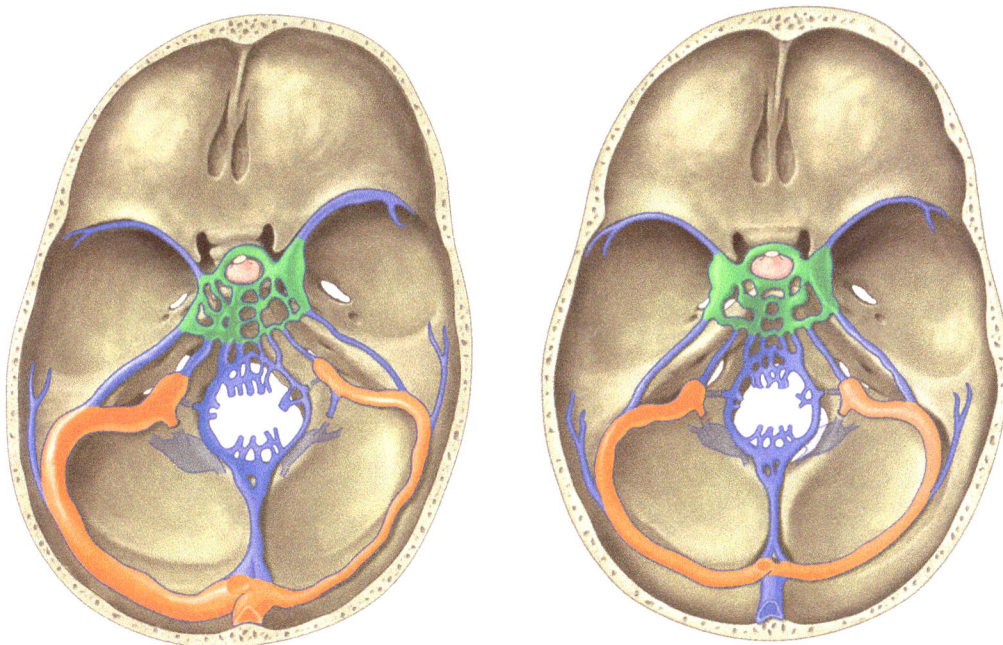

Figure 2.8 Establishing Drainage of the Vertebral Venous Plexus

Reinstating the drainage of the vertebral venous plexus is vital to brain drainage, which is adversely affected by the whiplash effect of the cervico-cranial junction. The constriction or occlusion of the spinal canal into the spinal cord must also be considered, as well as the spinal nucleus of the trigeminal nerve.

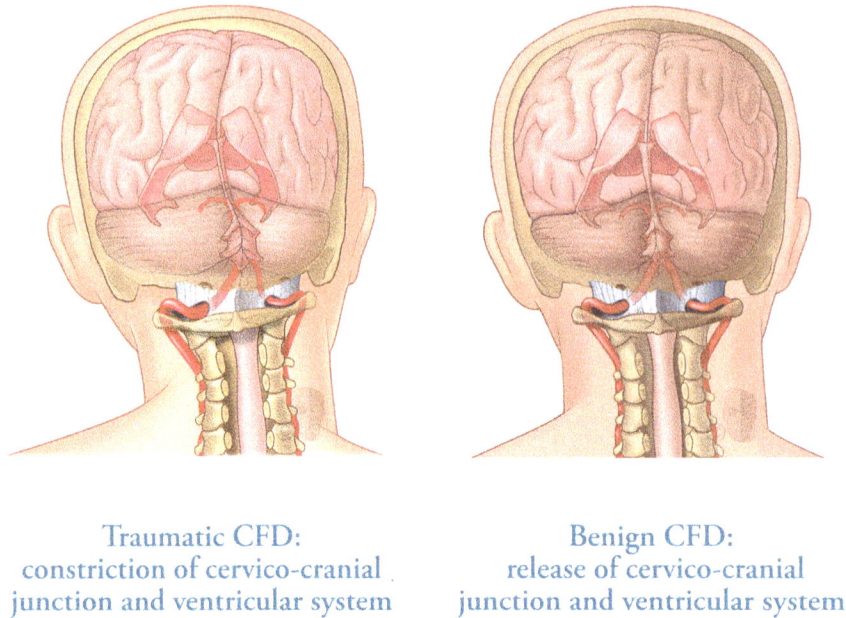

Traumatic CFD:
constriction of cervico-cranial
junction and ventricular system

Benign CFD:
release of cervico-cranial
junction and ventricular system

Figure 2.9 Balance of the Atlanto-Occipital Membrane and Atlas

This encapsulating membrane, attached to the ring of the atlas below and the foramen magnum above, is responsible for both arterial inflow and venous outflow, as well as neurological complications to the medulla oblongata (respiratory and cardiac centres) and the spinal cord.

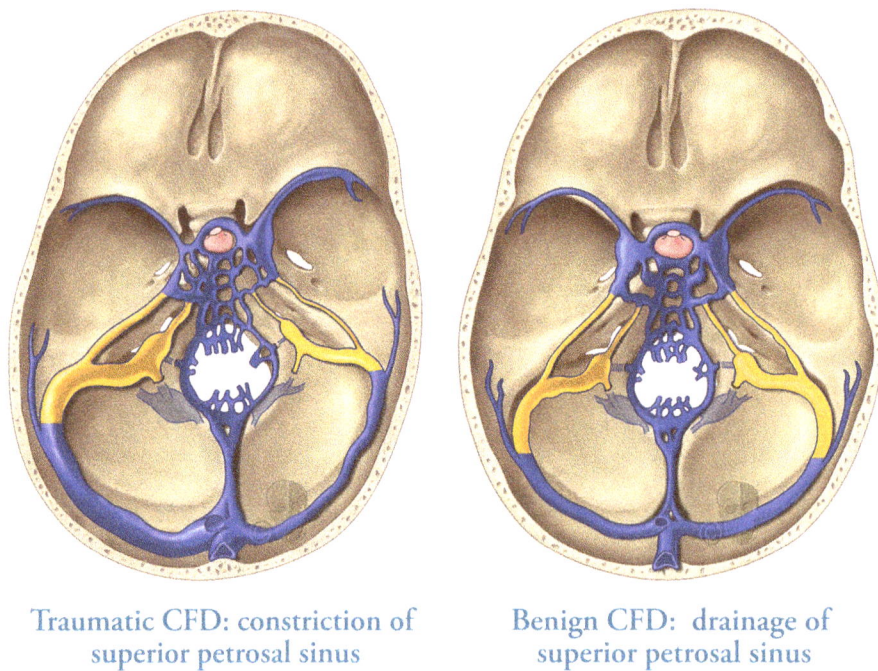

Traumatic CFD: constriction of
superior petrosal sinus

Benign CFD: drainage of
superior petrosal sinus

Figure 2.10 Temporal Bone – Superior Petrosal Sinus

The petrous ridge of the temporal bone anchors the tentorium cerebelli, while encapsulating the superior petrosal sinus, one of the main drainage sinuses for the cavernous and intercavernous sinuses, leading into the jugular bulb of the sigmoid sinus before exiting through the internal jugular vein at the jugular foramen.

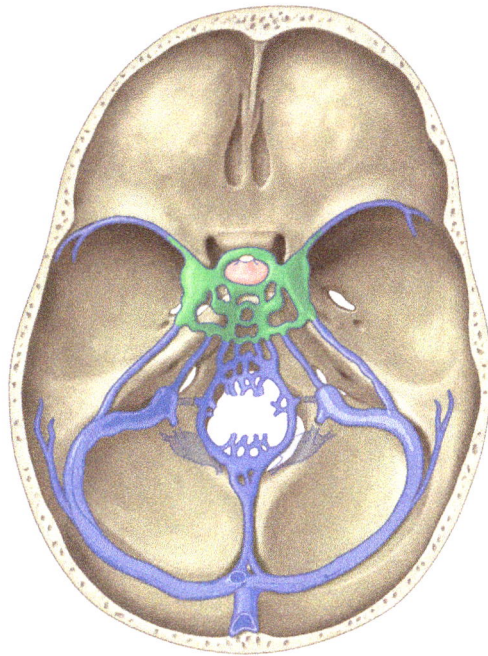

Figure 2.11 Drainage of the Cavernous Sinus

The cavernous and intercavernous sinuses surround the body of the sphenoid, principally the sella turcica, and represent the dural venous sinuses in the inferior part of the brain. The veins of the face and ocular orbit drain into the cavernous sinus through the superior ophthalmic vein.

The cavernous and intercavernous sinuses drain into the basilar plexus and the vertebral venous plexus at the anterior foramen magnum, then laterally through the inferior and superior petrosal sinuses of the temporal bone, before exiting through the sigmoid sinuses into the internal jugular vein.

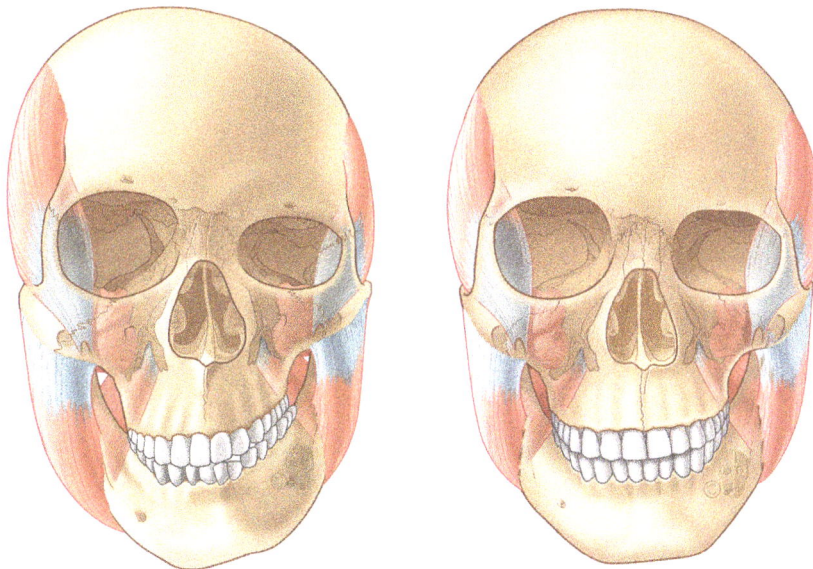

Traumatic CFD: crossbite
and TMJ dysfunction

Benign CFD: restored TMJ
and balanced cranium

Figure 2.12 Decompression of the Temporomandibular Joint

Traumatic CFD cause the left temporal bone to move into external rotation, moving the mandibular fossa relatively more posterior than the right temporomandibular joint (TMJ). This means that as the mandible translates it deviates to the left on opening before coming back into the midline. On closure the mandible will move towards the left and close, creating a crossbite malocclusion and activating the trigeminal ganglion as a result. In turn, this activates the mesencephalic nucleus, the pontine nucleus and the spinal nucleus, changing the atlas and the atlanto-occipital membrane. This mandibular deviation also impacts on the medial and lateral pterygoid muscles, deviating the pterygoid plates and the sphenoid.

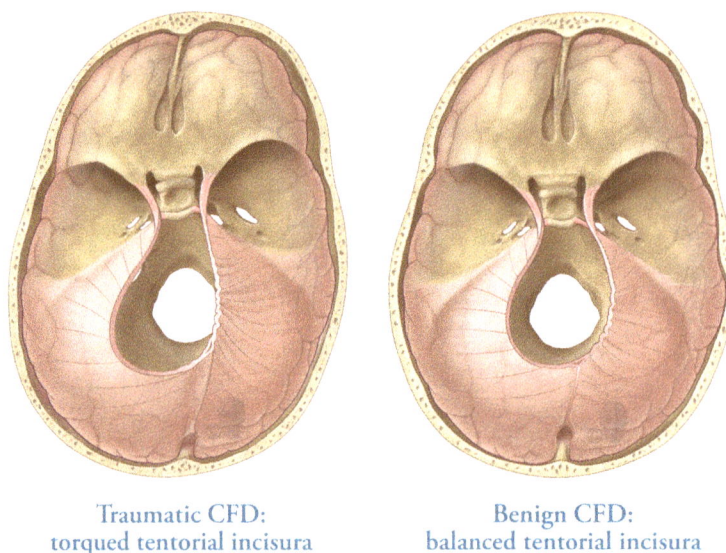

Traumatic CFD:
torqued tentorial incisura

Benign CFD:
balanced tentorial incisura

Figure 2.13 Tentorial Incisura and Tentorium Cerebelli

The tentorial incisura, as has been mentioned, possibly has more influence on the central brain components than any other dural membrane. With traumatic CFD the tentorial incisura is pulled anteriorly on the right internal rotated temporal bone, following the counterclockwise motion of the brain, but on the left, the pull posterior and lateral is significant to move the tentorial incisura across the path of the central core brain components, distorting these components and the ventricular system. The lateral anchor points of the tentorium cerebelli at the petrous portion of the temporal bone, also crimp the superior petrosal sinus on the right, inhibiting drainage.

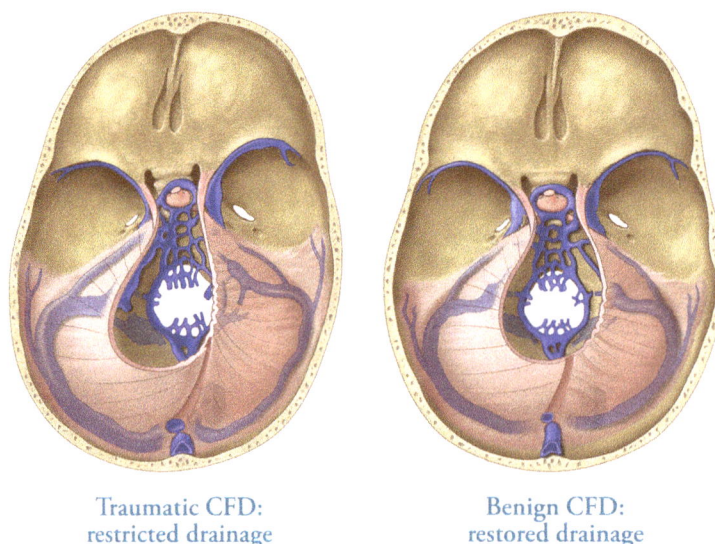

Traumatic CFD:
restricted drainage

Benign CFD:
restored drainage

Figure 2.14 Tentorial Incisura and Tentorium Cerebellum Drainage

The encapsulation of the right transverse and sigmoid sinuses by the tentorium cerebelli, also becomes crimped by the internally rotated temporal/occipital bones at the right transverse groove of the occiput, reducing brain drainage in the right internal jugular vein. On the left external temporal/occipital bones the pull laterally of the tentorium cerebelli opens the transverse and sigmoid sinuses, but as these vessels are smaller on the left than their counterparts on the right, there becomes a venous congestion bottleneck, which reduces brain drainage.

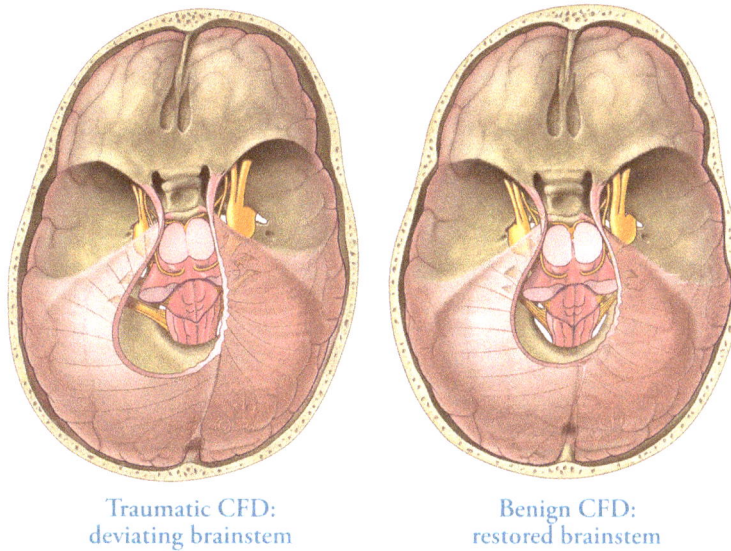

Traumatic CFD:
deviating brainstem

Benign CFD:
restored brainstem

Figure 2.15 Tentorial Incisura and Tentorium Cerebellum: Brainstem

The tentorial incisura pulls the central core brain components to the left, away from the midline, thereby distorting and torquing those components. These are the medulla oblongata, the pons, the cerebral and cerebellar peduncles and the midbrain. These are all neural pathways, along with the thalamus and the hypothalamus – the junction boxes, receiving and disseminating neurological communications. The breakdown in these nerve conduits being able to perform must be seriously in question.

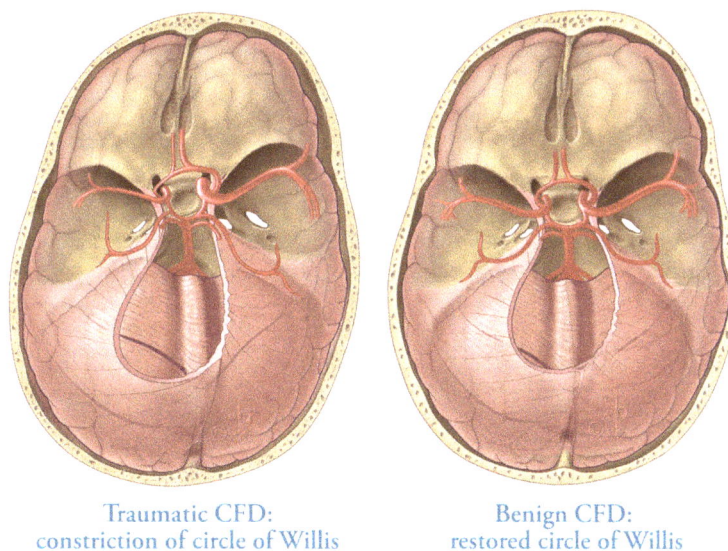

Traumatic CFD:
constriction of circle of Willis

Benign CFD:
restored circle of Willis

Figure 2.16 Tentorial Incisura and Tentorium Cerebellum: Circle of Willis

405

The anterior space of the tentorial incisura controls the circle of Willis, particularly the anterior cerebral artery and the middle cerebral artery, both fed by the internal carotid artery and posterior communicating artery. The distortion therefore of the tentorial incisura must come into serious consideration, as the incidence of aneurisms in this area is extremely high. About 60% of saccular aneurisms occur in the circle of Willis. The posterior space of the tentorial incisura controls the great vein of Galen and the straight sinus, draining into the confluence of the sinuses.

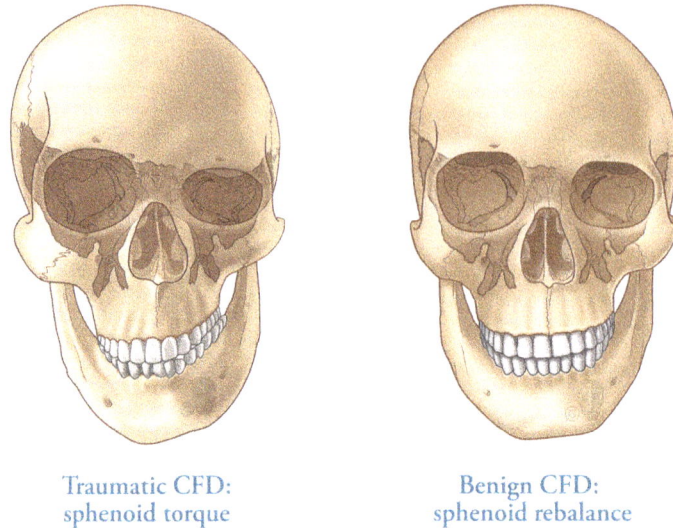

Traumatic CFD:
sphenoid torque

Benign CFD:
sphenoid rebalance

Figure 2.17 Sphenoid and Cranial Torque

Traumatic CFD is a gross counterclockwise motion of the skull, inflicting changes in all the internal structures. One of the steps in the Howat 8-Step Protocol is to de-torque the cranial membrane system, and try to return the membrane influence to that of a benign CFD. The cranial membranes come under scrutiny over all the aspects discussed above, all of which affect the homeostatic balance of the brain.

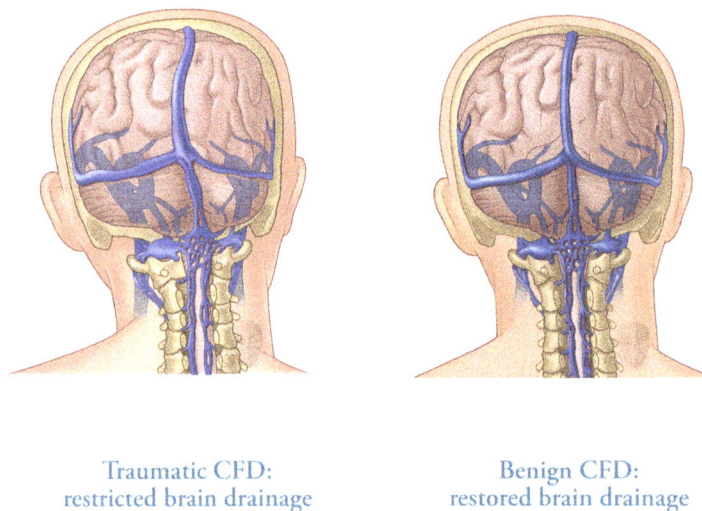

Traumatic CFD:
restricted brain drainage

Benign CFD:
restored brain drainage

Figure 2.18 Confluence of the Sinuses and Venous Sinus Drainage

Traumatic CFD is the main reason that brain drainage is restricted and reduced. The brain irrigation system works when the volume of blood into the brain equals the volume of blood leaving the brain. When that changes through traumatic CFD, the cerebral perfusion is reduced, autoregulation diminishes and stagnation occurs, with the cytotoxic waste being retained. The process in the Howat 8-Step Protocol is to remove obstructions from the occluded vessels such that the floodplain may indeed flood and improve the drainage potential.

The confluence of the sinuses is one of the exit points where venous blood can be retained, along with the transverse and sigmoid sinuses and the internal jugular vein.

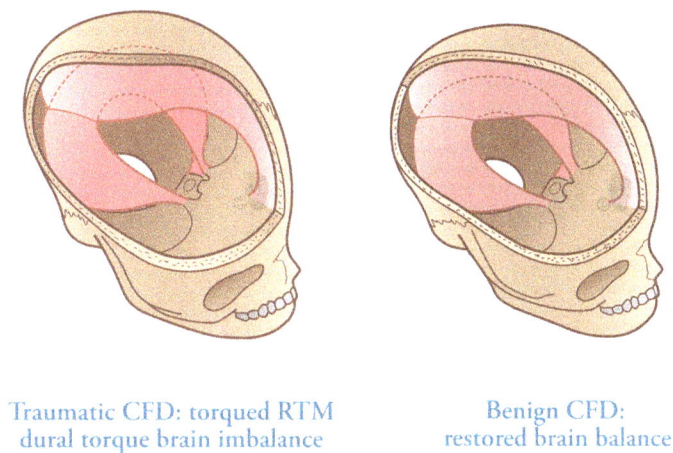

Traumatic CFD: torqued RTM
dural torque brain imbalance

Benign CFD:
restored brain balance

Figure 2.19 Benign Cranio Fascial Dynamics

The RTM are responsible for all of the brain drainage, through the venous sinus system vessels, all of which are encapsulated within the dural membrane system. To de-torque the cranial membranes increases the potential for the venous sinus system to drain and create irrigation for the brain.

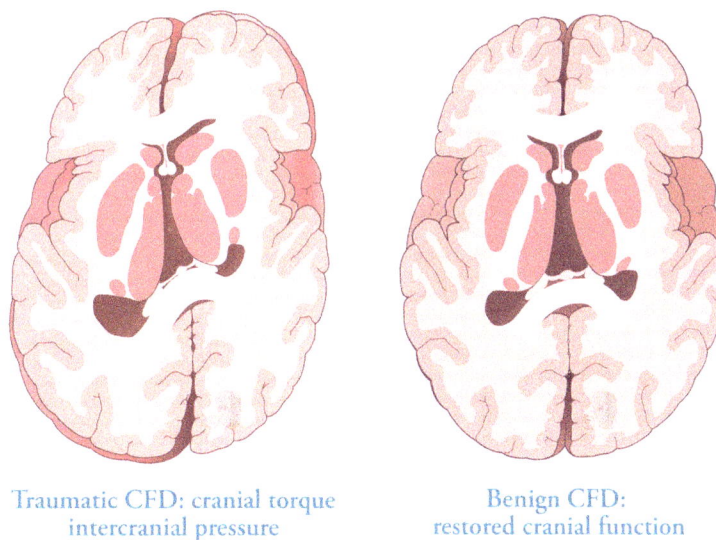

Traumatic CFD: cranial torque
intercranial pressure

Benign CFD:
restored cranial function

Figure 2.20 Cranial Torque and Intracranial Pressure

By reducing the volume of retained venous sinus blood, the intracranial pressure is reduced, cerebral perfusion and autoregulation are increased. These factors are the concern of the neurology world. If brain drainage is not accomplished, these factors remain unchanged and the process of regaining vital neurological pathways goes unchallenged. Instead, the brain is infused with various drugs that increase the cytotoxic waste within the blood–brain barrier, and a stagnation over many years produces the fatal neurological syndromes that result.

Major neurological pathways join the cortex to the thalamus and to the cerebellum. The ventricular system surrounded by the brainstem anteriorly and the cerebellum, fornix, caudate nucleus, hippocampus and amygdala, posteriorly. The cerebral peduncles are the anterior part of the midbrain that connects the remainder of the brainstem to the thalami.

They are paired and run to and from the cerebrum assisting in refining motor movements, learning of new motor skills and converting proprioceptive information into balance and posture maintenance. The cerebellar peduncles consist of three pairs, the superior cerebellar peduncles join the cerebellum to the midbrain, the middle cerebellar peduncles join the cerebellum to the pons and the inferior cerebellar peduncles join the medulla oblongata to the cerebellum. These major pathways are all affected by torque of the brainstem and changes to the ventricular system by cranio fascial distortion.

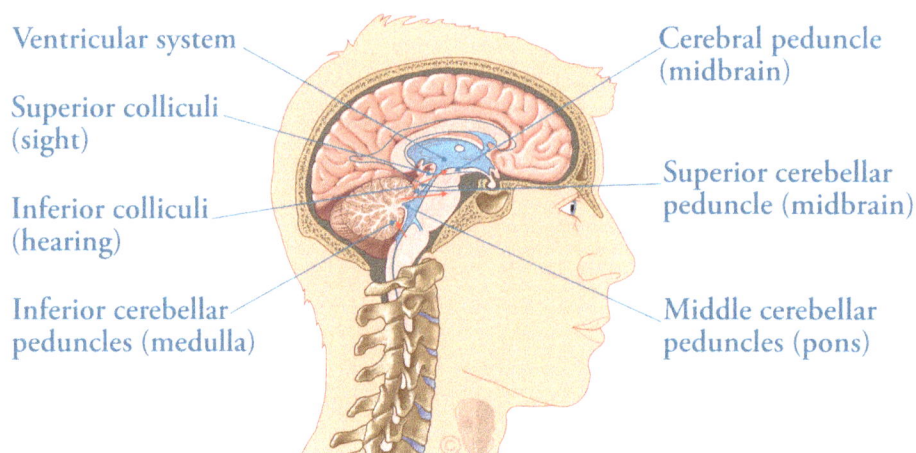

Figure 2.21 Major Neurological Pathways from Cortex –Thalamus –Cerebellum: Central brain core components surround the ventricular system

CONCLUSION

The Howat 8-Step Protocol has been developed to counter the effects of TBI, by reversing the traumatic CFD that occurs with this type of injury. The knock-on effects of a TBI are multifactorial and invade all the various components of a healthy brain, so to reinstate these various components, an unwinding procedure takes place. The body's innate intelligence survives by not having interferences, and so the disentangling process allows the impediments to re-establish a 'near normal' situation to develop, along with the healing progression. This may not happen immediately, but with time restoration will be achieved in a more homeostatic environment.

Traumatic brain injury applies to every living being on this earth, and may possibly be the initiator of many conditions that are never investigated in this manner. Our sophisticated first-world countries need to talk about this and rethink how to change minds and protocols that are being passed on from generation to generation, with the same narrative.

CHAPTER 3

THE NEUROPHYSIOLOGY OF THE HPCFD

The Howat 8-Step Protocol of Cranio Fascial Dynamics (HPCFD) is a procedure designed to address the complexities of traumatic brain injuries. It deals with the intricacies of the brain's irrigation system, whereby the volume of the arterial blood into the brain must equal the volume of venous blood out of the brain, in order to create homeostasis.

The dural meningeal membranes (collectively referred to as the reciprocal tension membranes (RTM) – falx cerebelli, falx cerebri, tentorium cerebelli and diaphragma sellae) support, separate and balance the brain.

The brainstem (medulla oblongata, pons and midbrain), a continuation of the spinal cord, is the core communication centre of the brain. The thalamus and hypothalamus act as 'junction boxes', transmitting neurological information from the cerebral cortex to the spinal cord and vice versa and from the cerebral cortex to the cerebellum and spinal cord and vice versa.

Trauma is any sort of artificial interference to the normal birth process. Whiplash trauma of any description and at any age has the propensity to change the dynamics of the central core brainstem and the balance of the RTM and can ultimately change the ability for the brain to drain. The accumulation and superimposition of trauma throughout life will result in irrevocable damage to brain function and change these dynamics. Over time, if nothing is done to change the status quo and to reverse these traumas, severe life-changing syndromes – which are identified clinically on a daily basis – may be the result.

THE PHYSICAL DYNAMICS OF THE HPCFD

The two factors of drainage and membrane torque are the essence of the 8-Step Protocol. The first four steps are designed to enhance venous drainage in a methodical manner, by clearing the 'floodplain' first and then moving further in towards the slopes and finally to the head of the 'river'. In anatomical terms, the internal jugular vein is cleared first, then the sigmoid sinus (and its tributaries, the superior petrosal sinus and jugular bulb), then the transverse sinus, the confluence of the sinuses, followed by the superior sagittal sinus, the inferior sagittal sinus and the cavernous sinus.

The last four steps involve the de-torqueing process, starting with the temporal bones, repositioning the tentorial incisura, the sphenoid bone and finally the RTM.

This whole process, from one to eight steps, involves more than the physical dynamics of venous drainage and de-torqueing the RTM.

THE NEUROLOGICAL DYNAMICS OF THE HPCFD

The fact that the process involves sensory and motor branches of all the cranial nerves which feed back to the brainstem where their individual nuclei are sourced, makes the HPCFD a neurological process in its aetiology.

Sensory nerves feed into sensory receptors – dendrites of sensory neurons specialised in receiving special kinds of stimuli conduct sensory information to the central nervous system, where the information is processed. These are synonymous with afferent nerves.

Motor nerves conduct signals from the CNS to their target muscles and glands. These are synonymous with efferent nerves.

Mixed nerves contain both afferent and efferent axons, and thus conduct both incoming sensory information and outgoing muscle commands in the same nerve bundle.

Special visceral motor neurons, known as branchial motor neurons, are involved in facial expression, mastication, phonation and swallowing and are associated with the cranial motor nerves:

- oculomotor nerve CN III (M)
- trochlear nerve CN IV (M)
- abducens nerve CN VI (M)
- hypoglossal nerve CN XII (M).

In the stomatognathic system, mechanoreceptors innervate a wide range of oral tissue, including:

- periodontal ligament
- perioral skin, lips and mucosa
- gingiva
- palate
- tongue
- jaw muscles
- temporomandibular joint.

The four mixed cranial nerves involved in the stomatognathic system involve:

- trigeminal CN V (M&S)
- facial CN VII (M&S)
- glossopharyngeal CN IX (M&S)
- vagus CN X (M&S).

The cranial nerves have their nuclei in the brainstem:

- midbrain
  - oculomotor CN III (M)
  - trochlear CN IV (M)
- pons
  - trigeminal CN V (M&S)
  - abducens CN VI (M)
  - facial CN VII (M&S)
  - vestibulocochlear CN VIII (S)
- medulla oblongata
  - glossopharyngeal CN IX (M&S)

- vagus CN X (M&S)
- spinal accessory CN XI (M)
- hypoglossal CN XII (M).

SENSORY NERVES

The amount of sensory innervation found in the stomatognathic system and incorporated in the HPCFD, relates back to the brainstem and fires those sensory receptors in the brainstem to activate the sensory nerves they feed. The result of this 'new' stimulation from the HPCFD process is to bring the muscles and mucosa they stimulate back into a homeostatic environment.

This also involves an arousal of sensations throughout the body, which may have been retarded by trauma, and will include exteroception – stimulus outside the body – and interoception – stimulus within the body.

Primary stimuli or senses include sight, hearing, smell, touch and taste, all conveyed by four essential sensory faculties:

- chemoreceptors – respond to chemical stimulus
- photoreceptors – respond to light
- thermoreceptors – respond to fluctuations in temperature.
- mechanoreceptors – respond to mechanical stimulus, such as pressure, touch, vibration and cutaneous tension.

There are four types of mechanoreceptors that are specialised to provide information to the CNS:

- Pacinian corpuscles
- Merkel's disks
- Ruffini's corpuscles
- Meissner's corpuscles.

Additional senses include the stimuli that are also changed and interfered with in fascial distortion (traumatic CFD) and include:

- nociception – pain from tissue damage
- equilibrioception – balance involving movement, direction and acceleration/retardation to maintain postural balance and equilibrium
- proprioception – awareness of where the body and limbs are in space
- chronoception – perception of a sense of time.

From the spinal cord, the ascending or afferent nerve pathways include:

- dorsal column medial lemniscus system
  - gracile fasciculus/medial part of the dorsal column – lower body to cortex
  - cuneate fasciculus/lateral part of the dorsal column – upper body to cortex
- anterolateral system (conscious)
  - lateral spinothalamic tract –pain and thermal stimuli
  - anterior spinothalamic tract –pressure and crude touch
  - dorsal spinothalamic tract – vibration and proprioception
- spinocerebellar tracts (unconscious)
  - posterior spinocerebellar tract – proprioception in joints and muscles

- anterior spinocerebellar tract – proprioception in joints and muscles
- spinotectal tract – midbrain – tactile, pain and thermal stimuli
- spinoreticular tract – reticular formation
- spino-olivary tract – information to cerebellum.

MOTOR NERVES

A motor neuron, or efferent neuron, is a neuron whose cell body is located in the motor cortex of the frontal lobe, brainstem (medulla oblongata, the pons and the midbrain) or the spinal cord, and whose axon (fibre) projects to the spinal cord or outside of the spinal cord, to directly or indirectly control effector organs, mainly muscles and glands. There are two types of motor neuron: upper motor neurons and lower motor neurons.

The upper motor neuron is the motor system that is confined to the CNS and is responsible for the initiation of voluntary movement, the maintenance of muscle tone for support of the body against gravity, and the regulation of posture to provide a stable background upon which to initiate voluntary movement.

Upper motor neurons originate in the motor cortex located in the precentral gyrus of the frontal lobe, and terminate within the medulla oblongata or the spinal cord. The axons of these cells descend from the cortex to form the corticospinal tract. Upper motor neurons in the cerebral cortex reside in several adjacent and highly interconnected areas in the frontal lobe, which together mediate the planning and initiation of complex temporal sequences of voluntary movements.

The upper motor neurons synapse in the spinal cord with anterior horn cells of lower motor neurons, usually via interneurons. Anterior horn cells are the cell bodies of the lower motor neurons and are located in the grey matter of the spinal cord. Damage to upper motor neurons can result in spasticity and exaggerated reflexes.

An upper motor neuron descends in the spinal cord to the level of the appropriate spinal nerve root and synapses with a lower motor neuron, each of whose axons innervate a fibre of skeletal muscle.

The lower motor neuron is responsible for transmitting the signal from the upper motor neuron to the effector muscle to perform a movement. Any lesion that damages or destroys the upper motor neuron and its influence over the lower motor neuron is termed an upper motor neuron lesion. Such a lesion is damaging to the cortex, internal capsule, brain stem or spinal cord above the area of the lower motor neuron. A lower motor neuron lesion is a lesion which affects nerve fibres travelling from the anterior horn of the spinal cord to the associated muscle(s).

When differentiating between upper and lower motor neuron disease, remember that upper motor neurons are responsible for motor movement, whereas lower motor neurons prevent excessive muscle movement. Upper motor disorders usually cause spasticity; lower motor disorders usually cause flaccidity.

The upper motor neuron syndrome refers to a combination of resulting symptoms, such as muscle weakness, decreased muscle control, easy fatigability, altered muscle tone and exaggerated deep tendon reflexes (also known as spasticity), all of which can occur after a brain or spinal cord injury.

Axons from upper motor neurons synapse on to interneurons in the spinal cord and occasionally directly on to lower motor neurons. The axons from the lower motor neurons are fibres that carry signals from the spinal cord to the effectors. These motor descending efferent tracts include:

- pyramidal tracts
  - lateral corticospinal tracts – skilled motor activities
  - anterior corticospinal tracts – skilled motor activities
  - corticobulbar tracts –brainstem – to nuclei of CN V, VII, XI and XII

- extrapyramidal tracts
  - rubrospinal tracts (inhibitory) – promote flexor and inhibits extensor muscles
  - vestibulospinal tracts – support balance and posture
  - tectospinal tracts (excitatory) – facilitate postural movements from visual stimuli
  - reticulospinal tracts –regulate voluntary movements and reflexes
  - olivospinal tract – information from cerebellum.

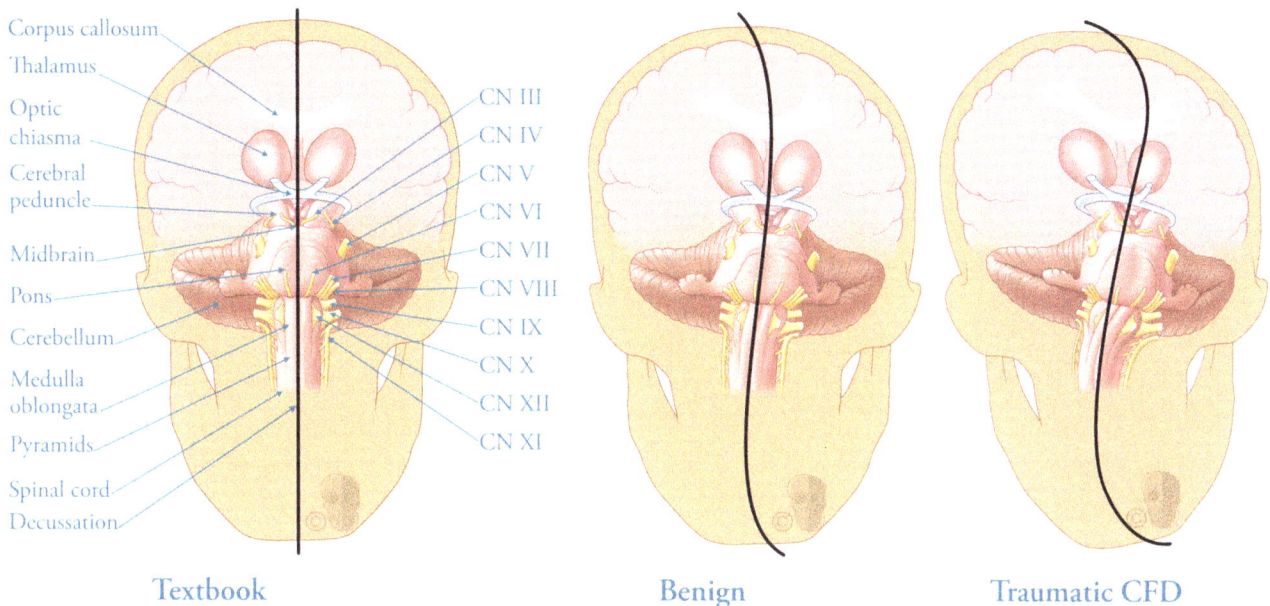

Corpus callosum
Thalamus
Optic chiasma
Cerebral peduncle
Midbrain
Pons
Cerebellum
Medulla oblongata
Pyramids
Spinal cord
Decussation

CN III
CN IV
CN V
CN VI
CN VII
CN VIII
CN IX
CN X
CN XII
CN XI

Textbook   Benign   Traumatic CFD

Figure 3.1 Brainstem – Midbrain, Pons and Medulla Oblongata: The brainstem is the pathway to all the ascending and descending spinal tracts

THE NEUROPHYSIOLOGY OF THE HPCFD©

Found within the HPCFD's neurophysiology is the breakdown of all the neurological stimuli – motor, sensory and mixed – as discussed above (see Table 3.1).

While the 8-Step Protocol is divided into two groups of four steps – with the first four dedicated to brain drainage and the second four to de-torqueing the cranium – the actual format of each step is involved in stimulating the stomatognathic system in its entirety. The tactile activity of having a finger inside the intra-oral cavity with the many contacts on various components within that cavity (including mucosa, muscles, osseous structures, periosteum and dural membranes) and their insertion points, creates stimulus along the various nerves to motor and sensory nuclei in the brainstem. Quite apart from the cranial nerves involved in the process, the meningeal dura and the periosteal dura are directly and indirectly stimulated by following the protocol.

The physical drainage of the brain through the venous sinus system, relies on those venous sinus vessels being cleared and opened by removing the physical torque initiated by traumatic CFD and by attempting to reinstate the brainstem in its juxtaposition. Opening the internal jugular veins, the basilar plexus, the vertebral venous plexus, the confluence of the sinuses, the transverse sinuses, the sigmoid sinuses and the internal jugular veins, allows the venous blood to drain through the foramen magnum and the jugular foramen, allowing the irrigation status of the brain to be re-established and to achieve vascular homeostasis (i.e. equal volumes of arterial blood in and equal volumes of venous blood out).

The action of the physical drainage also stimulates the cranial nerves, their motor and sensory components, the meningeal and endosteal dura and the cranial bones. This includes their muscle activity, the vascular vessels involved, the fascia and, primarily, the nuclei situated in the brainstem. All this stimulus ultimately retreats to the medulla oblongata, the pons and the midbrain, the source of the major nuclei, where the reaction to the stimulus activates the homeostasis required by the brain to function at its optimum level. Despite past trauma that has torqued the brain (particularly the brainstem), resulting in disturbed neurological dysfunction, the provocation and motivation by the inherent recuperative powers in the body to re-establish the neurological pathways come to the fore. This occurs through the cranial nerve nuclei at the medulla oblongata, the pons and the midbrain. The most important of the nuclei are the trigeminal (the pons) and the vagus (the medulla oblongata), where the vast majority of the activity in the 8-Step Protocol culminates.

The devastating effect of the central core brain component twisting that occurs in traumatic CFD creates numerous undiagnosed and devastating toxic neurological sequelae. The fact that the brainstem can be influenced by the position of the tentorial incisura after trauma raises the question of where the influence is greater in the brainstem and to what degree its components are directly traumatised. This could be: in the midbrain, thereby implicating the cranial nerve nuclei of the oculomotor and the trochlear nerves; in the pons, implicating the trigeminal, abducens, facial and cochlear nerves; or in the medulla oblongata, implicating the glossopharyngeal, vagus, spinal accessory and hypoglossal nerves.

This poses the question, do these origins of the cranial nerves in their respective positions within the brainstem have a direct impact on the neurological outcome of the serious syndromes that appear 30 years later? Does this influence on the pons, for instance, have a direct implication for trigeminal nerve activity in the head? Or maybe in the medulla oblongata, where the implication is vagus nerve interruption to the balance of the body's neurological function? These are serious consequences when bringing the cerebral and cerebellar peduncles into the equation.

The application of the HPCFD through the nuclei of the brainstem maximises the neurological potential of the neurophysiology of the brain. This process takes all of three minutes.

During the restorative protocols, the patient is constantly inhaling and exhaling, in conjunction with the feet flexing and extending, thereby continually stimulating the sacro-occipital pump, activating the ventricular system and moving CSF.

The phrenic nerve at C4 controls the diaphragm, which is constantly moving the ilia into external and internal rotation, again in conjunction with the sacro-occipital pump.

The flexion and extension of the occiput activates the nuchal ligament externally at the nuchal line on the external occipital protuberance and the internal occipital protuberance internally. This latter action flexes the falx cerebelli and the falx cerebri, activating the superior and inferior sagittal sinuses and consequently the anterior and inferior superior drainage of the brain. This flexion and extension of the internal occipital protuberance activates the straight sinus, the common border with the falx cerebelli, the falx cerebri and the tentorium cerebelli. This action activates the transverse and sigmoid sinuses, draining into the internal jugular vein and ultimately the brain, through the jugular foramen.

The activation of the falx cerebri and the tentorium cerebelli, brings the ethmoid and sphenoid into a flexion and extension phase as the anterior and posterior poles. This last activity is brought about by the vomer, with its attachments superior/anterior on the ethmoid, superior/posterior on the sphenoid, the inferior/anterior on the maxillae and inferior/posterior at the palatines.

While this linear diaphragmatic pulse continues through the management of these protocols at the rate of 18 to 20 pulses a minute (total about 60 cycles), the cardiovascular pulse is superimposed at the rate of 68 to 72 pulses a minute (total about 210 pulses).

This combined activity brings about linear respiration at the sacro-occipital pump and the RTM, the irrigation system is fully triggered, the cardiovascular pulse is creating a counterclockwise motion through the drainage of the internal jugular veins. Both pulses create a homeostatic environment.

In addition, the intra-oral activity is stimulating the:

- meningeal dura – innervated by the ipsilateral trigeminal ganglion (pons) and endosteal dura; covered by nociceptive nerve endings – trigeminal ganglion (pons)
- mucosa – innervated by the trigeminal nerve (pons), palatine and maxillary bones and the palate; innervated by the trigeminal and the maxillary branch of the trigeminal (pons)
- masticatory muscles – innervated by the facial nerve and mandibular branch of the trigeminal (pons)
- pterygoid plates and pterygoid muscles – innervated by the mandibular branch of the trigeminal nerve (pons)
- tentorial incisura – innervated by the ophthalmic branch of the trigeminal nerve (pons)
- tongue – stimulated by the hypoglossal nerve (medulla oblongata)
- temporo mandibular joint – innervated by the mandibular branch of the trigeminal nerve, facial nerve and spinal trigeminal nucleus (all pons)
- temporomandibular ligament – trigeminal ganglion (pons)
- stylomandibular ligament – trigeminal ganglion (pons)
- sphenomandibular ligament – trigeminal ganglion (pons)
- larynx – vagus nerve (medulla oblongata)
- pharynx – vagus nerve (medulla oblongata)
- throat – glossopharyngeal nerve and vagus nerve (both medulla oblongata)
- upper trapezius muscle – spinal accessory nerve (medulla oblongata)
- SCM – spinal accessory nerve (medulla oblongata)
- splenius muscle – suboccipital nerve, C I
- suboccipitalis muscle – suboccipital nerve, C I
- semispinalis – suboccipital nerve, C I
- erector spinae muscles – posterior branch of spinal nerves, C I to L5
- latissimus dorsi muscles – thoracodorsal, C6 to C8.

This comprehensive list of the intra-oral components, their activity through diaphragmatic and cardiovascular pulses, the stimulus through motor and sensory nerves, the de-torqueing effect on the cranium changing the meningeal and periosteal dura, the change in muscle tonus and the activation of the ten major nuclei at the brainstem, all combine in a very short time to recalibrate and reset those components to their pre-trauma juxtapositions. The author assumes, through his experience, that these pre-trauma juxtapositions facilitate the healing capabilities of the body to reinstate a homeostatic environment and to allow the body to cope and live within its own physiological adaptive range. This assumption is based on clinical observation and the absence of symptoms after protocols have been implemented.

Techniques for measuring pre- and post-clinical data have been tried with various instruments (see Part IV, Chapter 8). All clinical data elicit changes before and after treatment and new instrumentation is being looked at to find a more suitable and consistent method of measurement. Remarkable changes have been shown with thermal imaging, but these results are more visual than analytical. In time, the sophistication of measuring these changes will be available digitally, so patience must prevail.

CONCLUSION

The HPCFD is used to treat all the brain components and membranes, muscles of the cranium, the vascular components, the sensory and motor nerves culminating at the brainstem where the cranial nuclei invest.

This also includes the cerebral and cerebellar peduncles and the cerebellum, as well as the ascending and descending spinal tracts that either traverse the brainstem, have their sensory termination in the brainstem or their motor origins above or in the brainstem – when that is traumatised, the neurological implications can be complex. While the protocols are being initiated, the patient is breathing and activating the sacro-occipital pump circulating CSF and activating the spinal dura and all 31 pairs of spinal nerve roots – the autonomic nervous system. The eight steps form a neurological sequence of events, which is why the HPCFD must be a mandatory first step in all cranial and chiropractic techniques, as a precursor to removing the 'basic and primary neurological interference' – a fact that practitioners would be encouraged to utilise.

The HPCFD must be the pre-emptive treatment of choice for removal of brain interference, only then should other techniques be implemented if there is to be a realistic prospect of a truly positive outcome for the patient (see Table 3.1, which depicts the full flow chart for HPCFD and all the neurological consequences of intra-oral corrections).

Table 3.1 The neurophysiology of the Howat 8-Step Protocol of Cranio Fascial Dynamics© in TBI

PROTOCOL STEPS	AREAS INVOLVED IN THE PROTOCOL		ACTION
DRAINAGE **STEP 1**	Preparing for venous drainage through foramen magnum into the cervical spine CSF from 4th ventricle into the spinal canal of the spinal cord	Cervical spine Stretching the spinal cord and the brainstem –medulla oblongata, pons and midbrain *Foramen magnum*	Mobilising cervical spine Flotation of the brain's ventricular system reduces the weight of the brain by 25 g
STEP 2	Atlanto-occipital membrane junction Vertebral arteries to basilar artery Anterior and posterior spinal arteries Dural veins and the vertebral venous plexus	Upper cervical spine Stretching the spinal cord and the brainstem –medulla oblongata, pons and midbrain *Foramen magnum* Spheno-basilar synchrondrosis	Drainage of VVP Internal jugular vein Anterior and posterior spinal arteries Dural veins
STEP 3	Petrous ridge – temporal bone Basilar part of occiput Body of sphenoid	Temporal rotation Lateral tentorium cerebelli Cranial apertures *Jugular foramen, foramen ovale, foramen rotundum, foramen lacerum*	Drainage of cavernous and intercavernous sinuses – basilar plexus and superior petrosal and inferior petrosal veins into sigmoid sinus and then into the internal jugular vein
STEP 4	Drainage of cavernous and intercavernous sinuses Drainage of basilar plexus Drainage of superior petrosal sinus Drainage of internal jugular vein	Central inferior drainage Anterior superior drainage Superior sagittal sinus Anterior inferior drainage Inferior sagittal sinus Cranial apeture *Cavernous sinus contents*	Drainage of cavernous and intercavernous sinuses – sphenoid bone Confluence of the sinuses – occiput Transverse and sigmoid sinuses – occiput Internal jugular vein – jugular foramen Ultimately the superior and inferior sagittal sinuses
DE-TORQUE **STEP 5**	Decompression of temporo mandibular joint centralising tentorial incisura	Temporo-mandibular joint Cranial apertures *Jugular foramen, petrous ridge, sphenoid body diaphragma sellae, foramen lacerum, foramen ovale, foramen rotundum*	Sphenoid body Sphenoid – superior orbital fissure TMJ – mandibular fossa – retro-discal tissue and the articular disc Temporal – temporalis muscle Parietal – temporalis muscle Muscles of mastication Release the trigeminal ganglion
STEP 6	Jugular foramen open Temporal Occiput Sphenoid	Cranial apertures *Jugular foramen, carotid canal, foramen lacerum, foramen ovale, foramen rotundum*	CN IX, CN X and CN XI and internal jugular vein Tentorial incisura Posterior attachments of tentorium cerebelli Brainstem – medulla, pons and midbrain Sphenoid – mastoid and vestibular mechanism
STEP 7	Sphenoid – long axis – greater wings Fronto-maxillae – ethmoid – sphenoid Tentorium cerebelli – falx cerebri and falx cerebelli Diaphragma sellae	Sphenoid – central bone of the cranium Cranial apertures *Superior orbital fissure, jugular foramen, foramen lacerum, foramen ovale, foramen rotundum*	Superior orbital fissure Anterior and posterior pivots – RTM Palatine and maxillae Straight sinus and interior occipital protuberance Body of sphenoid – anterior and posterior clinoid processes
STEP 8	**Howat Sweep – Neurological Rebalancing** This is a compilation of neurological pathways and conduits re-established by the combined actions of all eight steps coming together at the source of the cranial nuclei: medulla oblongata, the pons and midbrain. These pathways include: Superior colliculi – lateral geniculate body Inferior colliculi – medial geniculate body Both parts of the tectum: paired cerebral peduncles – anterior and laterally Three pairs of cerebellar peduncles: Superior – cerebellum to midbrain Middle – cerebellum to pons Inferior – medulla oblongata to cerebellum	Brainstem and midbrain Medulla oblongata Pons Midbrain Cranial apertures *Superior orbital fissure, jugular foramen, foramen lacerum, foramen ovale, foramen rotundum, foramen magnum, foramen spinosum, cavernous sinus*	**Internal influence** Medial and lateral pterygoid muscles Palatines – inferior surface Maxillae – inferior surface Sphenoid – de-torque Tentorium cerebelli – posterior anchor Tentorium cerebelli – lateral anchor Tentorial incisura – reposition Straight sinus – reposition Falx cerebelli – reposition **External influence** Foramen magnum Atlanto-occipital membrane Cervical spine Multifides muscles – hypertonic Erector spinae

CRANIAL BONES	NEUROLOGY	MUSCLES INVOLVED IN ACTION	BRAINSTEM NUCLEI
Occiput Atlas C1, C2 and C3	Trigeminal spinal nucleus located in the upper cervical spine at C1, C2 and C3 Ventricular system	General musculature Erector spinae (Steps 1 & 2) Nuchal ligament (Steps 1 & 2) Upper trapezius (Steps 1 & 2) Sternocleidomastoid (Steps 1 & 2) Digastricus (anterior and posterior belly)	Pons – after the mesencephalic Pontine and spinal nucleus Midbrain, pons and medulla oblongata
Occiput Atlas Axis	Spinal cord and brain stem Medulla oblongata Pons and the midbrain	Submandibular Omohyoideus – stylohyoideus Carotid triangle and submandibular triangle	Brainstem – medulla oblongata Pons and midbrain
Temporal – petrous ridge Occiput – basilar part Sphenoid – body	Houses internal auditory meatus Acoustic: cochlear – special afferent Vestibular – special afferent CN VIII – vestibulocochlear/acoustic nerve	Submental triangle Occipital triangle Deep cervical flexors Scalene muscles	vestibulocochlear CN VIII go to pons
Nuchal line of occiput Palate – maxillae and palatine Occipito-mastoid suture	Ophthalmic Nerve (CN V.1) is joined by filaments from the cavernous plexus – sympathetic and then communicates with oculomotor (CN III), trochlear (CN IV) and abducens nerves (CN VI) and recurrent filament that passes between the layers of the tentorium	Upper trapezius Temporalis SCM Tentorium cerebelli	CN VI go to pons CN III go to midbrain CN IV go to midbrain CN VI go to pons
Mandible – ramus Temporal TMJ Sphenoid – greater – wings Sphenoid body Parietal	Medial pterygoid (M) – CN V.3 Tensor tympani veli palatini (S) – CN V.3 Tensor tympani (S) – CN V.3 Meningeal branch (S) – CN V.3 Masseteric nerve (M) – CN V.3 Deep temporal nerves – anterior and posterior (M) – CN V.3 Buccal nerve (S) – CN V.3 Lateral pterygoid (M) nerve – CN V.3 Auriculo nerve (S) CN X medulla Lingual nerve (S) – CN V.3 Inferior alveolar nerve (S) and (M) – CN V.3 Mental nerve (S) – CN V.3 Mylohyoid nerve (S) – CN V.3 and CN VII Digastric (M) – anterior CN V.3 and posterior CN VII Deep temporalis nerve (M) – CN V.3 Temporalis nerve (M) – CN V.3	**Specific musculature** Temporalis (M) – CN V.3 Masseter (M) – CN V.3 Buccinator (M) – CN V.3 Internal pterygoid – CN V.3 External pterygoid (M) – CN V.3	All CN V.3 go to pons CN X go to medulla oblongata
Pterygoid plate – sphenoid – bone Mastoid process Temporal – bone Sphenoid Ethmoid and sphenoid Occiput Temporal	Closure of jugular foramen Distortion of the brainstem Medulla oblongata – CN IX, CN X, CN XI and CN XII Pons – CN V, CN VI, CN VII and CN VIII Midbrain – CN III and CN IV Open passage for CN III, CN IV, CN V and CN VI Relocation of RTM Activation of the vomer Drainage of superior and inferior sagittal sinuses Reduce mandibular deviation	Glossopharyngeal CN IX – medulla Vagus CN X – medulla oblongata Spinal accessory – CN XI – medulla SCM and temporalis Internal pterygoid External pterygoid Muscles attached to the cranium Cervical muscles attached to cranium	Glossopharyngeal CN IX – medulla oblongata Vagus CN X – medulla oblongata Spinal accessory – CN XI – medulla oblongata Hypoglossal CN XII – medulla oblongata Oculomotor – CN III – midbrain Trigeminal CN V – pons Vagus nerve – CN X – medulla oblongata Multifidus – posterior ramus spinal nerves
Sphenoid Palatine Maxilla Vomer Occiput Temporal Left temporal external EOP – occiput Occipital sinus sulci	Sphenopalatine ganglion provides passage Greater palatine nerve (S) – hard palate Lesser palatine nerve (S) – soft palate Nasopalatine (S) mouth, soft palate tonsils Uvula	Oculomotor activates medial rectus muscle homologous with multifidus muscles of the spine. When oculomotor fails (superior orbital fissure) hypotonicity occurs in the multifidus innervated by the medial branch nerve of the level ramus of the spinal nerve at each level. Both these muscles are lateral and respond similarly. When the eye moves right, the multifidus contracts and moves the spine right. Both are ipsilateral muscles. The contralateral side causes side bending and rotation – enhancing fascial torque on that side. Hence external rotation of the right ilium and short right leg	CN V.3 mandibular branch – trigeminal – pons CN V.2 maxillary nerve from mouth through foramen rotundum to pons CN IX – glossopharyngeal (S) post third of the stylopharyngeus (M) CN IX – medulla oblongata Parotid gland (S) CN IX – tractus solitarius Medulla oblongata Carotid sinus (M) – CN IX – nucleus ambiguus Tympanic membrane (S) CN V.3 – pons Auricular Branch (S) CN X medulla oblongata and facial nerve CN V11 – pons

BIBLIOGRAPHY

Allman JM, Hakeem A, Erwin JM, Nimchinsky E, Hof P (2001). The anterior cingulate cortex. The evolution of an interface between emotion and cognition. *Ann N Y Acad Sci* May;935:107-17. PMID: 11411161.

Alzheimer's Association, Brain Tour Cortex Hippocampus Ventricles: http://alz.org/alzheimers_disease_4719.asp

Awasthi S, Hallene KL, Fazio V, Singhal SS, Cucullo L, Awasthi YC, Dini G, Janigro D (2005). RLIP76, a non-ABC transporter, and drug resistance in epilepsy. *BMC Neuroscience* 6:61. doi:10.1186/1471-2202-6-61. PMC 1249579. PMID 16188027

Beam TR, Allen JC (1977). Blood, brain, and cerebrospinal fluid concentrations of several antibiotics in rabbits with intact and inflamed meninges. *Antimicrobial Agents and Chemotherapy* 12(6):710–6. doi:10.1128/AAC.12.6.710. PMC 430009. PMID 931369.

Boyer P, Phillips JL, Rousseau FL, Ilivitsky S (2007). Hippocampal abnormalities and memory deficits: new evidence of a strong pathophysiological link in schizophrenia. *Brain Research Reviews* 54(1):92–112. doi:10.1016/j.brainresrev.2006.12.008. PMID 17306884.

Costain G, Ho A, Crawley AP, Mikulis DJ, Brzustowicz LM, Chow EWC, Bassett AS (2010). Reduced gray matter in the anterior cingulate gyrus in familial schizophrenia: A preliminary report. *Schizophrenia Research* 122(1–3):81–84. doi:10.1016/j.schres.2010.06.014.PMC 3129334. PMID 20638248.

Davie CA (2008). A review of Parkinson's disease. *Br. Med. Bull.*, 86(1), 109–27. PMID 18398010. doi: PMID 18398010.

de la Monte SM, Wands JR (2005). Review of insulin and insulin-like growth factor expression, signaling, and malfunction in the central nervous system: relevance to Alzheimer's disease *J Alzheimer's Dis* 7:45-61. PMID: 15750214 doi: 10.3233/jad-2005-7106.

de la Monte SM, Wands JR (2008). Alzheimer's disease is type 3 diabetes – evidence reviewed. *J Diabetes Sci Technol* 2:1101–13. PMID 19885299. PMCID PMC2769828 doi: 10.1177/193229680800200619

Dickson D, Weller RO (2011). *Neurodegeneration: The molecular pathology of dementia and movement disorders* (2nd ed.). John Wiley & Sons.

Fujiwara H, Hirao K, Namiki C, Yamada M, Shimizu M, Fukuyama H, Hayashi T, Murai T (2007). Anterior cingulate pathology and social cognition in schizophrenia: A study of gray matter, white matter and sulcal morphometry. *NeuroImage* 36(4):1236–1245. doi:10.1016/j.neuroimage.2007.03.068. PMID 17524666.

Fusar-Poli P, Smieskova R, Kempton MJ, Ho BC, Andreasen NC, Borgwardt S (2013). Progressive brain changes in schizophrenia related to antipsychotic treatment? A meta-analysis of longitudinal MRI studies. *Neuroscience & Biobehavioral Reviews* 37:1680–1691. doi:10.1016/j.neubiorev.2013.06.001. PMC 3964856. PMID 23769814.

Ghajar J (2000). Traumatic brain injury. *Lancet* 356 (9233):923–9. doi:10.1016/S0140-6736(00)02689-1. PMID 11036909.

Glorieux FH, Pettifor JM, Juppner H (2003) *Pediatric bone : Biology & Diseases*. San Diego: Academic Press.

Gray's Anatomy, 'The Confluence of the Sinuses Gross', 28th ed. Lea & Fabiger.

Hansen ES, Hasselblach S, Law I, Bolwig TG (2002). The caudate nucleus in obsessive-compulsive disorder. Reduced metabolism following treatment with paroxetine: a PET study. *International Journal of Neuropsychopharmacology* 5(1):1–10. doi:10.1017/S1461145701002681. PMID 12057027.

Harrison PJ (2004). The hippocampus in schizophrenia: a review of the neuropathological evidence and its pathophysiological implications. *Psychopharmacology* 174(1):151–62. doi:10.1007/s00213-003-1761-y. PMID 15205886.

Haznedar MM, Buchsbaum MS, Hazlett EA, Shihabuddin L, New A, Siever LJ (2004). Cingulate gyrus volume and metabolism in the schizophrenia spectrum. *Schizophrenia Research* 71 (2–3):249–262. doi:10.1016/j.schres.2004.02.025. PMID 15474896.

Hendrie CA, Pickles AR (2009). Depression as an evolutionary adaptation: Implications for the development of preclinical models. *Medical Hypotheses* 72, 342–347. PMID 19153014. doi:10.1016/j.mehy.2008.09.053.

Hendrie CA, Pickles AR (2010). Depression as an evolutionary adaptation: Anatomical organisation around the third ventricle. *Medical Hypotheses* 74, 735–740. PMID 19931308. doi:10.1016/j.mehy.2009.10.026.

Ho BC, Andreasen NC, Ziebell S, Pierson R, Magnotta V (2011). Long-term Antipsychotic Treatment and Brain Volumes. Arch. Gen. *Psychiatry* 68:128–37. doi:10.1001/archgenpsychiatry.2010.199. PMC 3476840. PMID 21300943.

Husseini KM, Quiroz JA, Sporn J, Payne JL, Denicoff K, Gray NA, Zarate Jr. CA, Charney DS (2003). Enhancing neuronal plasticity and cellular resilience to develop novel, improved therapeutics for difficult-to-treat depression. *Biological Psychiatry* 53:707–742. doi:10.1016/s0006-3223(03)00117-3.

Jiji S, Karavallil A, Smitha AK, Gupta VP, Ramapurath SJ (2013). Segmentation and volumetric analysis of the caudate nucleus in Alzheimer's disease. *European Journal of Radiology* 82(9):1525–1530. doi:10.1016/j.ejrad.2013.03.012. PMID 23664648. doi:10.1016/j.ejrad.2013.03.012.

Kempton MJ, Geddes JR, Ettinger U et al. (2008). Meta-analysis, Database, and Meta-regression of 98 Structural Imaging Studies in Bipolar Disorder. *Archives of General Psychiatry* 65:1017–1032. doi: 10.1001/archpsyc.65.9.1017.

Kempton MJ, Salvador Z, Munafò MR, Geddes JR, Simmons A, Frangou S, Williams SC (2011). Structural Neuroimaging Studies in Major Depressive Disorder: Meta-analysis and Comparison With Bipolar Disorder. *Arch Gen Psychiatry* 68(7): 675–90. doi:10.1001/archgenpsychiatry.2011.60. PMID 21727252.

Kolb B, Whishaw IQ (2001). *An Introduction to Brain and Behavior*. 4th ed. New York: Worth Publishers.

Led AB, May WB (1977). Arthritic Symptoms Related to Position and Function of the Mandible. *Basal Facts* 2:66.

Löscher W, Potschka H (2005). Drug resistance in brain diseases and the role of drug efflux transporters. *Nature Reviews Neuroscience* 6(8):591–602. doi:10.1038/nrn1728. PMID 16025095.

Miller AH, Maletic V, Raison C L (2009). Inflammation and its discontents: the role of cytokines in the pathophysiology of major depression. *Biological Psychiatry* 65 (9): 732–741. PMC 2680424. PMID 19150053. doi:10.1016/j.biopsych.2008.11.029.

Minikel E (2013) Cell Biology 11: Apoptosis & Necrosis. *Bios-e-16*. Notes from lecture 11 of Harvard Extension's Cell Biology Course. https://www.cureffi.org/2013/04/28/cell-biology-11-apoptosis-necrosis/

Mosby's Medical Dictionary, 9th edition. © 2009, Elsevier.

Mortazavi M M, Adeeb N, Griessenauer C J, Sheikh H, Shahidi S, Tubbs RI, Tubbs RS (2013). The ventricular system of the brain: a comprehensive review of its history, anatomy, histology, embryology, and surgical considerations. *Child's Nervous System* 30(1):19–35. doi:10.1007/s00381-013-2321-3. ISSN 0256-7040.

MRI database at www.bipolardatabase.org and at www.depressiondatabase.org

Nagele RG (2006). Alzheimer's disease: new mechanisms for an old problem. *UMDNJ Research* 7(2). Archived from the original on 2011-09-17. Retrieved 2011-07-22.

National Institute of Neurological Disorders and Stroke, Dementia with Lewy Bodies Information Page. https://www.ninds.nih.gov/Disorders/All-Disorders/Dementia-Lewy-Bodies-Information-Page.

Nestor S, Rupsingh R, Borrie M, Smith M, Accomazzi V, Wells J, Fogarty J, Bartha R. (2008). Ventricular enlargement as a possible measure of Alzheimer's disease progression validated using the Alzheimer's disease neuroimaging initiative database. *Brain* 131(9):2443–2454. doi:10.1093/brain/awn146.

Nizet V, Kim KS, Stins M, Jonas M, Chi EY, Nguyen D, Rubens CE (1997). Invasion of brain microvascular endothelial cells by group B streptococci. *Infection and Immunity* 65(12): 5074–5081. PMC 175731. PMID 9393798.

Raison CL, Capuron L, Miller AH (2006). Cytokines sing the blues: inflammation and the pathogenesis of depression. *Trends in Immunology* 27 (1): 24–31. PMC 3392963. PMID 16316783. doi:10.1016/j.it.2005.11.006.

Raza, MW, Shad A, Pedler SJ, Karamat KA (2005). Penetration and activity of antibiotics in brain abscess. *Journal of the College of Physicians and Surgeons Pakistan* 15(3):165–7. PMID 15808097.

Schrimsher GW, Billingsley RL, Jackson EF, Moore BD III (2002). Caudate nucleus volume asymmetry predicts attention-deficit hyperactivity disorder (ADHD) symptomatology in children. *Journal of Child Neurology* 17(12):877–884. doi:10.1177/08830738020170122001.

Sheline Y (2003). Neuroimaging studies of mood disorder effects on the brain. *Biological Psychiatry* 54, 338–352. PMID 12893109. doi:10.1016/s0006-3223(03)00347-0.

Steiner LA, Andrews PJ (2006). Monitoring the injured brain: ICP and CBF. *British Journal of Anaesthesia* 97(1):26–38. doi:10.1093/bja/ael110 PMID 16698860.

Takase K, Tamagaki C, Okugawa G, Nobuhara K, Minami T, Sugimoto T, Sawada S, Kinoshita T (2004). Reduced white matter volume of the caudate nucleus in patients with schizophrenia. *Neuropsychobiology* 50(4):296–300. doi:10.1159/000080956.

Tortora GJ, Funke BR, Case CL (2010). *Microbiology: An Introduction*. San Francisco: Benjamin Cummings.

Upledger JE, Vredevoogd JD. (1983). *Craniosacral Therapy*. Eastland Press.

Van Sorge NM (2012). Defense at the border: the blood–brain barrier versus bacterial foreigners. *Future Microbiol* (3):383–394. doi:10.2217/fmb.12.1.# PMC 3589978. PMID 22393891.

Varatharaj A, Galea I (2016). The blood–brain barrier in systemic inflammation. *Brain, Behavior, and Immunity* 60:1-12. doi:10.1016/j.bbi.2016.03.010. PMID 26995317.

Waubant, E (2006). Biomarkers indicative of blood–brain barrier disruption in multiple sclerosis. *Disease Markers* 22(4):235–44. doi:10.1155/2006/709869. PMC 3850823. PMID 17124345.

Wikipedia.org My thanks to Wikipedia.org for supplying and confirming some of the material and references for this book. Wikipedia continues to be a constant source of vital and relevant material to the healing arts professions, without whose supportive information, one would be sorely stretched.

Wright IC, Rabe-Hesketh S, Woodruff PW, David AS, Murray RM, Bullmore ET (2000). Meta-analysis of regional brain volumes in schizophrenia. *Am J Psychiatry* 157(1): 16–25. doi:10.1176/ajp.157.1.16. PMID 10618008

Zipser BD, Johanson CE, Gonzalez L, Berzin TM, Tavares R, Hulette CM, Vitek MP, Hovanesian V, Stopa EG (2007). Microvascular injury and blood–brain barrier leakage in Alzheimer's disease. *Neurobiology of Aging* 28(7):977–86. doi:10.1016/j.neurobiolaging.2006.05.016. PMID 16782234.

Zysk G (2001). Pneumolysin is the main inducer of cytotoxicity to brain microvascular endothelial cells caused by streptococcus pneumoniae. *Infection and Immunity* 69(2):845–852. doi:10.1128/IAI.69.2.845-852.2001. PMC 97961. PMID 11159977.

ABOUT THE AUTHOR

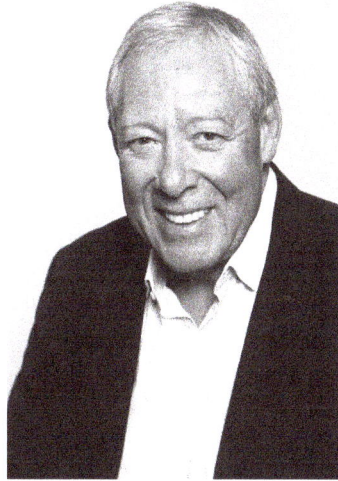

Born to parents of a Scottish lineage, Jonathan Howat's father David arrived in Rhodesia with his family in 1911. His mother, Elspeth, arrived in South Africa with her family in the 1820s. She was a classics teacher. Jonathan was born in 1947 in Salisbury, Southern Rhodesia. His father spent five years in the Western Desert during the Second World War as Adjutant of 237 Rhodesia Squadron. He returned to Southern Rhodesia to practise chiropractic.

Jonathan's primary education was at Milton Junior School in Bulawayo. His secondary education took place at Falcon College, a boarding school in an abandoned gold mine near Essexvale, in the Matabeleland bush.

His chiropractic career started in 1970 after he graduated from the Palmer College of Chiropractic Medicine. Jonathan returned to Rhodesia to join his father, who had graduated in 1938 from what was then the Palmer School of Chiropractic. He spent a very happy 15 years under David's guidance and tutelage. Jonathan aquired skills using the Gonstead technique and HIO (hole-in-one, upper cervical specific, created by Dr BJ Palmer in the 1930s) and soon built a busy practice, seeing several hundred patients a week.

The Rhodesian Terrorist War started in 1974 and, like all Rhodesian men, Jonathan was conscripted into the Rhodesian Army. He served as a paratrooper medic with the Selous Scouts until the war ended with Zimbabwean Independence in 1980. Matabeleland then became the focus of Mugabe's Korean-trained 5th Brigade who terrorised and killed over 50,000 Matabele. With his wonderful wife, Arline, and his three children, Josh, Kate and Juliet, Jonathan decided to leave their homeland and parents to emigrate to the United Kingdom in 1984 to start a new life. They arrived at Heathrow in London with several suitcases and £70.

While still in Bulawayo, Jonathan had been investigating other forms of chiropractic treatment and one day his father passed him a letter inviting him to a SOT (sacro-occipital technique) seminar with David Denton, in Bexhill, in England. Jonathan flew the next day to London and participated in what was to be a life changer.

Dr Major Bertram DeJarnette was the founder and developer of SOT, which introduced Jonathan to a chiropractic method of assessing symptoms and problems before correcting them. DeJarnette's engineering insight into the biology of the body was original and groundbreaking, and his logical appreciation of how to address these complexities resulted in SOT. Jonathan returned home and turned his practice around 180 degrees. He spent every night for the next year going through Gray's *Anatomy* and Guyton's *Physiology* until he had completely mastered SOT.

After the move to the UK, Jonathan became involved in teaching SOT, along with Drs Nelson and Cameron DeCamp, and having taken all the relevant exams and received his Diplomate in Craniopathy in 1985, Jonathan formed SOTO Europe, a sister organisation to SORSI (USA), PAAC (Japan), SOTO Australia/Asia. SOTO Europe now teaches over 400 chiropractors.

Jonathan wrote his first book, *The Anatomy and Physiology of Sacro Occipital Technique*, in 1999, accompanied by charts, brochures and videos. He continued to teach this magnificent work around the world – Japan, Australia, USA, South Africa, South America and Europe.

His Oxford Chiropractic Clinic in Headington, Oxford, became a showcase for SOT. Over the next 28 years, young men and women who practised with Jonathan went on to teach and lecture in SOTO Europe, in France, Italy, Holland, Germany, Scandinavia and the UK. They are still a constant force within SOT and he is eternally grateful for their continued support. Their enthusiasm and dedication are what made SOTO Europe such a powerful chiropractic platform.

Jonathan had spent 15 years with the Rhodesian Chiropractic Association in many capacities and ultimately became its President for several years, and after its transition to the Zimbabwe Chiropractic Association. After arriving in the UK he spent several years working with The British Chiropractic Association in different capacities and was finally invited to the Executive Board. After the foundation of SOTO Europe, he became its President for several years, then chaired the Education Committee, writing and developing the education programme with numerous and dedicated members of that committee. He was also on the Executive Board of SORSI (USA) in the late 1980s and early 1990s, culminating in the formation of SOTO International, when he was installed as its first president. This is an international group of SOT chiropractors bringing SOT to a formal understanding of how it should be taught, with the same curriculum and examinations across the globe. Fortunately, this ethos has been maintained.

In 2004, he received a revelation by The Lord in a dream, showing an internal view of a distorted mouth and its correction, giving him an immediate insight into how the cranium and brain really worked, with the sphenoid being the central bone of the skull and the key to the cranium and all the cranial fascia that controlled the internal brain components.

For too long, he felt, science had based its learning of the body segmentally, rather than systemically, leaving the student with no way of understanding the intricacies of brain physiology. He decided to take this concept forward and called it 'Cranial Fascial Dynamics (CFD)' and spent many years developing the hypothesis and model into an entirely different application of understanding how the brain develops from the embryological principles and reversing the fascial distortions that occur through trauma.

Jonathan wrote *Chiropractic – Cranial Fascial Dynamics* in 2010, which outlined the importance of the ventricular system and the central core components that surround it. The Howat Protocols of Cranial Fascial Dynamics were formed in 2019 to teach practitioners how to recognise and identify the fascial torque component, how to reduce it as much as possible, and how to allow the body's inherent recuperative powers to re-establish normal physiological function, within its own capability. Naturally, time is a major factor and an absolute reversal of major syndromes – such as Parkinson's, Alzheimer's, dementia and multiple sclerosis – after years of fundamental nerve tissue damage may not be feasible. Nevertheless, addressing the seat of original trauma is always beneficial to the recipient. This reversal is the ethos of CFD and the results have all been documented in this work over the last 17 years, culminating in the Howat Protocols of Cranio Fascial Dynamics.

During his 50 years in chiropractic, Jonathan has been blessed by and recognised for his work in the profession in many ways, for which he is eternally grateful, but a lifetime's work is not complete without the amazing support and dedication he has had from his family – Arline, his rock, and Josh, Kate and Juliet. The wealth of knowledge, ingenuity and passion they have collectively given to Jonathan in his quest to accomplish CFD in its totality, has been remarkable and without their love, loyalty and enthusiasm his achievements would have never happened.

Index

temporomandibular joint dysfunction (TMJD) 49, 51, 156, 233, 284, 292, 294, 297, 300, 329

tic douloureux 51, 98, 233, 295

tremors 37, 264, 347

trigeminal neuralgia 51, 98, 233

Cranial bones

ethmoid 25–26, 41, 50, 55–60, 64, 68–69, 73, 90, 95, 99, 103, 127, 132–133, 137, 141, 152, 160, 179–180, 218, 220–221, 223, 228, 229, 232, 289, 295, 316–317, 352, 358, 377. *See also* Crista galli

frontal bone 24–25, 46, 76, 80, 87, 90–91, 93, 125–127, 137, 149, 153, 210, 231, 236, 286–287, 342

mandible 16, 24, 45–47, 49–50, 62, 65, 71, 73, 75–77, 81, 87, 89–90, 96–98, 103, 119, 121, 129–131, 136, 153, 158, 158–159, 176, 178, 181, 200, 207, 221, 229, 243, 284–285, 287, 289–292, 295–301, 303–311, 319–320, 342, 404

mandibular ramus 73, 178

maxillae 16, 45, 56–57, 59–60, 65, 71–73, 76–77, 81, 83–85, 87, 89–91, 94–96, 101–103, 127, 129, 132–133, 136, 157–158, 171, 178, 180, 220–221, 232, 285, 287, 289, 295, 298, 300, 305, 310, 311, 316, 377

nasal bones 87, 112, 130

occipital–condyles 24, 46, 49, 51, 62, 68, 75, 77, 87, 90, 98, 119, 156, 176, 232–233, 288, 290, 295–296, 301, 305–307, 316, 319, 320

occipital–external occipital protuberance 44, 52–53, 116, 151, 177, 179

occipital–internal occipital protuberance 25, 26, 41, 52, 54–56, 68, 116–118, 123, 152, 179, 203, 218, 223, 295, 317

occiput–nuchal line 52, 54, 176–177, 179–180, 317

occiput–superior nuchal line 116–118, 151, 178, 399

palatines 57, 59–60, 91, 133, 180–181, 220–221, 232, 289, 377

parietal 112, 125, 137

parietal–anterior fontanelle–bregma 41, 45–46, 125, 317. *See* Bregma

parietal–posterior fontanelle–lambda 23, 41, 125, 317, 338. *See* Lambda

sphenoid

    anterior and posterior clinoid processes 26, 28, 41, 47, 49, 59–60, 68, 90, 120, 122, 160, 179, 205, 218, 223, 240, 242, 245, 317, 342, 349, 358

    greater wings 25, 49, 53, 96, 103, 120–121, 125, 137, 171, 181, 219, 242, 292, 359, 362

    lesser wings 47–50, 53–54, 62, 120–121, 137, 171, 294, 359, 362

    pterygoid plates 49–50, 53, 57, 62, 75, 78, 87, 89–91, 95–96, 103, 121, 136, 156, 171, 180–181, 220–221, 232, 237, 245, 292, 320, 342, 359, 362, 372, 404

    sella turcica 28, 41, 46–47, 49, 57, 68, 95, 110, 120, 122–123, 160, 170, 204–205, 218, 227, 242, 245, 358, 403

    sphenoid body 25, 47–48, 54, 59–60, 68, 118, 122, 133, 180, 204–205, 218, 220–221, 223, 233, 237, 240, 243–244, 295, 342, 359, 377

temporal 24–26, 38–40, 46–47, 49–51, 53, 56, 64–66, 69, 72, 76, 80, 83, 87, 90, 95, 97, 100, 103, 114–115, 118–120, 123, 138, 151, 159, 166–167, 171–172, 177–178, 200, 204–205, 218–219, 223, 231–232, 237, 241, 243–244, 292, 295, 305, 312, 317–318, 320, 342, 348, 359, 362, 402–404

temporal–glenoid/mandibular fossa 24, 46, 49, 51, 75, 77, 89, 96, 103, 118–119, 121, 156, 158, 232, 233, 237, 241, 243, 290, 296–298, 301, 305–306, 308, 342, 404

temporal–mastoid portion 50, 54, 89, 98, 100, 172, 178–179, 210

temporal–petrous portion 25–26, 38–40, 49–50, 54, 56, 72, 90, 95, 103, 114, 118–120, 123, 137, 151, 159, 172, 178–179, 200, 204–205, 218–219, 223, 240–241, 245, 295, 312, 317–318, 348, 358–359, 362, 404

temporal squama 50, 89, 119

temporal–styloid process 65

vomer 56–57, 59–60, 73, 95, 103, 132–133, 136, 160, 180–181, 220–221, 289, 295, 372, 377

zygomatic/malar 45, 65, 119, 127–129, 159, 210

Cranial nerves (CN). *See* Central nervous system

Cranial sutures

coronal 45, 125

frontozygomatic 45

lambdoid suture 115, 125

maxillo-frontal 45

metopic suture 91, 127, 149, 316

squamosal suture 125

temporozygomatic 45

Cranial torque 94, 102, 149, 273, 312–313

clockwise–necrotic 166, 172, 180, 326, 346

Foramen magnum. *See* **Apertures**

temporalis 80, 98, 125, 158, 176, 178–179, 289, 303–305, 320

upper trapezius 64, 98, 158, 177–178, 308–309, 315, 321

www.ingramcontent.com/pod-product-compliance
Lightning Source LLC
Chambersburg PA
CBHW050521230326
R18018400001BA/R180184PG41597CBX00001BA/1